Converting peak flow values between Wright and EU scales

Find old peak flow reading on bottom of graph and read off value for a new EU scale meter on the vertical axis.

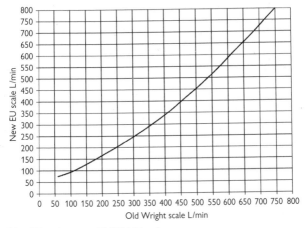

New EU scale versus Old Wright scale.

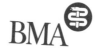

OXFORD MEDICAL PUBLICATIONS

Oxford Handbook of
Occupational Health

Published and forthcoming Oxford Handbooks

Oxford Handbook of
Occupational Health

Second Edition

Edited by

Dr Julia Smedley

Consultant Occupational Physician,
Lead consultant Occupational Health,
University Hospital Southampton
NHS Foundation Trust, and
Honorary Senior Lecturer,
University of Southampton, UK

Dr Finlay Dick

Senior Occupational Physician,
Capita Health and Wellbeing,
Aberdeen, and Honorary
Senior Lecturer in Occupational
Medicine, University of
Aberdeen, UK

Dr Steven Sadhra

Senior Lecturer and Director
of Education for Occupational
Health, Institute of Occupational
and Environmental Medicine,
College of Medical and
Dental Sciences, University of
Birmingham, UK

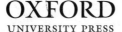

OXFORD
UNIVERSITY PRESS

OXFORD
UNIVERSITY PRESS

Great Clarendon Street, Oxford, OX2 6DP,
United Kingdom

Oxford University Press is a department of the University of Oxford.
It furthers the University's objective of excellence in research, scholarship,
and education by publishing worldwide. Oxford is a registered trade mark of
Oxford University Press in the UK and in certain other countries

First edition published 2007
Second edition published 2013

Impression: 1

British Library Cataloguing in Publication Data
Data available

ISBN 978–0–19–965162–7

Printed in China by
C&C Offset Printing Co. Ltd.

Preface

This second edition of the former newcomer to the handbook series covers the broad field of occupational health (OH) and wellbeing. It is aimed primarily at occupational health professionals from all disciplines, including general practitioners (GPs) who practise OH on a sessional basis and a new breed of non-medical case managers who advise on occupational rehabilitation. The book will also be useful for trainees in occupational medicine who are preparing for professional examinations.

We have retained the basic structure and features of the first edition which received good feedback from readers. Six main areas (occupational hazards, occupational diseases, OH practice, specialist disciplines, practical procedures, and emergencies) are covered in twelve sections. The new edition still provides a 'quick look-up' tool (particularly for specific hazards and diseases), and gives a structured overview of some important operational issues such as service provision and the legal framework. The specialist chapters (occupational hygiene, toxicology, epidemiology, environmental medicine, and safety science) aim to give an overall approach to problem-solving, helping to identify the need for (and interpretation of) specialist advice. The inevitable overlap between topics has been minimized by cross-referencing other pages in the handbook, but we have deliberately retained limited duplication where this avoids excessive 'flitting' between pages.

The new material for the second edition reflects developments in the field of OH and the increasing web-based information store. The principal changes are:

- The updating and signposting of evidence-based and other important guidance where applicable for each topic, including more web references than the previous edition
- A new emphasis on wellbeing to reflect the changing role of OH practitioners in optimizing health at work, and minimizing the negative impact of work loss on health
- New pages on managing chronic pain, psychological therapies, managing psychiatric emergencies, REACH legislation, obesity, policy writing, voice disorders, and evidence-based guidelines in OH.

We hope that the second edition will be as successful as the first, and look forward to hearing your feedback via the OUP website (⅏ http://www.oup.com/uk/medicine/handbooks). We are particularly interested in views on the overall emphasis and level of detail of pages, and any topics that we have omitted.

JS
FD
SS

January 2012

Acknowledgements

We would like to give special thanks to those who supported us during the revision of this handbook.

JS is indebted to her tolerant and supportive family, Andrew, Ben, and Alex. FD thanks his family, Smita, Ananya, Cara, and Rohan for their encouragement and support. SS thanks his family, in particular his parents Tarsem Singh and Gurdev Kaur for their encouragement and for the work ethic they instilled in him.

We also thank Michael Hawkes from OUP who helped to keep us on track.

Contributors
The following colleagues kindly gave up their time to update topics, or to contribute the initial drafts for new topics or chapters.

Professor Jon Ayres, Dr David Brown, Dr John Cherrie, Professor David Coggon, Dr Hilary Cross, Dr Steve Deacon, Dr Mike Doig, Dr Clive Harker, Dr Kit Harling, Dr Max Henderson, Professor Craig Jackson, Dr Bob Jefferson, Professor Susan Klein, Professor Diana Kloss, Professor Ewan Macdonald, Dr Ira Madan, Dr Stuart Mitchell, Professor Keith Palmer, Dr Cathy Price, Dr Paul Sclare, Dr Alan Smith, Dr Jon Spiro, Dr Andrew Wheatley, and Dr Nerys Williams.

Expert advisers
We are particularly grateful to Dr Fortune Ncube who gave extremely helpful comments on fitness for exposure prone procedures.

Foreword

The plain clear message at the centre of this authoritative text is that occupational medicine is preventive medicine practised in the workplace—safeguarding and promoting health and wellbeing among the workforce. Occupational health is now seen as a major aspect of public health. Specialist services have a responsibility both to respond effectively to unforeseen threats to individual and population health arising in the context of working life, and wherever possible to act to prevent work-related ill-health.

Whilst the Handbook is a detailed and comprehensive text for specialists in occupational health it also meets important needs of a much wider readership. The tenets of occupational health are increasingly observed by other health professionals, and by farseeing employers, largely because of evidence that being in work is generally good for health and wellbeing and worklessness is harmful, and also because not being wholly fit is still compatible with work of the right kind.

The Handbook reinforces the view that safeguarding health at work, preventing loss of occupation as a result of ill health, and supporting prompt treatment and rehabilitation to enable people to return to work following absence through illness or injury, are not for occupational health services alone. They are joint enterprises requiring collaboration between employers and occupational health services, the services set up under health and safety legislation, and the NHS.

Issues arising in the practice of occupational health are not limited to specialists in this discipline. They are also the concerns of other people whose advice and actions can influence the balance of understanding between employer and employee, especially when the employee is a patient under the care of other health professionals.

The Handbook is a source of guidance on the occupational significance of many health conditions. This information serves to strengthen clinical management, relieving uncertainty about the implications of illness for working life, and enabling sound advice on the steps to be taken for the best outcome. The Handbook contains information that should be readily accessible to any professional in primary and secondary health care.

At a time marked by an inescapable awareness of serious inequalities in health and life chances, and a climate of economic stringency, we have become familiar with the costs, burdens, and social consequences of impaired health among working age people.

There is widening recognition of the interplay of health with work and of work and the conditions of work with health, and of the many factors that influence health, health beliefs, and behaviour. Often they are deeply embedded in the history and culture of societies. Some can be changed for the better and that is what the practice of a more fully engaged occupation health discipline aims to do. Such engagement requires further changes in culture and in practice, and in the education and training of professionals in health care, and in business and management, necessary to bring about those changes. The Handbook provides a vade mecum in this task.

Professor Dame Carol Black
National Director for Health and Work

June 2012

Contents

List of contributors

Professor Jon Ayres
Professor of Environmental and
Respiratory Medicine, Institute of
Occupational and Environmental
Medicine, University of
Birmingham, UK

Dr David Brown
Consultant Occupational
Physician, EDF-Energy Nuclear
Generation, Gloucester, UK

Dr John Cherrie
Research Director, Institute of
Occupational Medicine,
Edinburgh, UK

Professor David Coggon
Professor of Occupational and
Environmental Medicine, MRC
Lifecourse Epidemiology Unit,
University of Southampton,
Southampton, UK

Dr Hilary Cross
Honorary Senior Lecturer
in Occupational Toxicology,
Institute of Occupational and
Environmental Medicine, College
of Medical and Dental Sciences,
University of Birmingham, UK

Dr Steve Deacon
Consultant Occupational
Physician, Avondale Medical
Consultancy Ltd, Waltham on the
Wolds, Leicestershire, UK

Dr Finlay Dick
Senior Occupational Physician,
Capita Health and Wellbeing,
Aberdeen, and Honorary
Senior Lecturer in Occupational
Medicine, University of
Aberdeen, UK

Dr Mike Doig
Regional Medical Manager,
Chevron Corporation,
London, UK

Dr Clive Harker
Consultant Occupational Physician,
Occmed Ltd, Carlisle, UK

Dr Kit Harling
Retired Consultant Occupational
Physician, Devon, UK

Dr Max Henderson
Consultant Psychiatrist, Institute
of Psychiatry, Kings and The
Maudsley, Senior Lecturer in
Epidemiological & Occupational
Psychiatry, Kings College London,
Institute of Psychiatry, Weston
Education Centre, London, UK

Professor Craig Jackson
Professor of Occupational Health
Psychology/Head of Psychology,
Birmingham City University,
Birmingham, UK

Dr Bob Jefferson
Consultant in Environmental
Medicine & Deputy Director,
Medical Toxicology Centre,
Newcastle University, UK

Professor Susan Klein
Director, Aberdeen Centre for
Trauma Research, Institute for
Health & Welfare Research,
Robert Gordon University,
Aberdeen, UK

Professor D Kloss MBE
Hon. FFOM, Barrister and Chair,
Council for Work and Health,
Manchester, UK

Professor Ewan Macdonald
Head of Healthy Working Lives
Research Group, University of
Glasgow, UK

Dr Ira Madan
Consultant and Honorary
Senior Lecturer in Occupational
Medicine, Guy's and St Thomas's
NHS (Foundation) Trust,
London, UK

Dr Stuart Mitchell
Head of Aeromedical Centre
and Occupational Health Safety
Regulation Group, UK Civil
Aviation Authority, Gatwick
Airport, UK

Professor Keith Palmer
Professor of Occupational
Medicine & Honorary Consultant
Occupational Physician, MRC
Lifecourse Epidemiology Unit,
University of Southampton, UK

Dr Cathy Price
Consultant in Chronic Pain
Management, University Hospital
Southampton NHS Foundation
Trust, Southampton, UK

Dr Steven Sadhra
Senior Lecturer and Director
of Education for Occupational
Health, Institute of Occupational
and Environmental Medicine,
College of Medical and
Dental Sciences, University of
Birmingham, UK

Dr Paul Sclare
Consultant in Adult Psychiatry,
NHS Grampian, Cornhill Hospital,
Aberdeen, UK

Dr Julia Smedley
Consultant Occupational
Physician, Lead consultant
Occupational Health, University
Hospital Southampton NHS
Foundation Trust, and Honorary
Senior Lecturer, University of
Southampton, UK

Dr Alan Smith
Lighting Consultant, Honorary
Research Fellow, Institute of
Occupational and Environmental
Medicine, College of Medical and
Dental Sciences, University of
Birmingham, UK

Dr Jon Spiro
Independent Specialist in
Occupational Medicine, UK

Dr Andrew Wheatley
Honorary Senior Research Fellow,
Institute of Occupational and
Environmental Medicine,
College of Medical and
Dental Sciences,
University of Birmingham, UK

Dr Nerys Williams
Independent Consultant
Occupational Physician and
NHS Non Executive Director, UK

Symbols and abbreviations

↑	Increased
↓	Decreased
►	Important
⚠	Warning
●	Controversial
📖	Book reference
℘	Web reference
♂	Male
♀	Female
A(8)	8-h energy equivalent acceleration (of vibration)
AAS	atomic absorption spectroscopy
ABS	acrylonitrile-butadiene-styrene plastic
AC	air conduction (of sound in hearing)
ACD	allergic contact dermatitis
ACDP	Advisory Committee on Dangerous Pathogens
ACE-R	Addenbrooke's Cognitive Examination—Revised
ACGIH®	American Conference of Governmental Industrial Hygienists
AChE	acetyl cholinesterase
ACOP	Approved Code of Practice
ACTS	Advisory Committee on Toxic Substances
AD	Alzheimer's disease
ADS	approved dosimetry service
AED	automated external defibrillator
AER	auditory evoked response
ahw	frequency-weighted measurement (of hand-transmitted vibration)
AIDS	acquired immunodeficiency syndrome
ALARP	as low as reasonably practicable
ALA-D	δ-aminolaevulinic acid dehydratase
AlkPhos	alkaline phosphatase
ALL	acute lymphoblastic leukaemia
ALT	alanine aminotransferase

AMED	HSE approved medical examiner of divers
AML	acute myeloid leukaemia
ANOVA	analysis of variance
ANR	active noise reduction (in hearing protectors)
AP	anteroposterior (usually of a chest X-ray)
APrV	assigned protection value (of respiratory protective equipment)
APF	assigned protection factor
APV	assumed protection values (of hearing protectors)
ARDS	adult respiratory distress syndrome
ARF	acute renal failure
ART	assessment of repetitive tasks tool
ART	anti-retroviral therapy
ASH	Action on Smoking and Health (UK charity)
ASHRAE	American Society of Heating, Refrigerating and Air-conditioning Engineers Scale
AST	aspartate aminotransferase
ATM	automated teller machine
AtW	Access to Work scheme
AUDIT	Alcohol Use Disorders Identification Test
B_{12}	vitamin B_{12}
BA	breathing apparatus
BAT	biological tolerance values (Germany)
BATNEEC	best available techniques not entailing excessive cost
BBV	blood-borne viruses
BC	bone conduction of sound in hearing
BCG	Bacillus Calmette–Guérin—a tuberculosis vaccine
BCME	bis-chloromethyl ether
BDI-II	Beck Depression Inventory
BEIs®	Biological Exposure Indices (USA)
BeLPT	blood beryllium lymphocyte proliferation test
BEM	biological effect monitoring
BM	biological monitoring
BMA	British Medical Association
BMGV	Biological Monitoring Guidance Value (UK)
BMI	body mass index (kg/m^2)
BOHRF	British Occupational Health Research Foundation
BOHS	British Occupational Hygiene Society

bp	boiling point
Bq	becquerel (rate of transformations in radioactive material)
BS	British Standard
BSE	bovine spongiform encephalopathy
BSIF	British Safety Industry Federation
BTPS	body temperature and pressure standard
CAA	Civil Aviation Authority (UK)
CABG	coronary artery bypass graft
CAPS	Clinician-Administered Assessment Scale for PTSD
CAR	Control of Asbestos at Work Regulations 2006
CAS	Chemical Abstracts Service registry number
Carc	carcinogen
CBD	chronic beryllium disease
CBI	Confederation of British Industry
CBRN	chemical, biological, radiological, and nuclear
CBT	cognitive behavioural therapy
CCHF	Crimean/Congo haemorrhagic fever
CD	compact disk
Cd	candela
CDC	Centers for Disease Control and Prevention (USA)
CDSC	Communicable Disease Surveillance Centre
CDT	carbohydrate deficient transferrin
CE	Conformité Européene
CEN	European Committee for Standardization
CET	corrected effective temperature
CFS	chronic fatigue syndrome
CHIP	Chemical (Hazards Information and Packaging for Supply) Regulations
CIBSE	Chartered Institution of Building Service Engineers
CIDR	Coal Mines (Control of Inhalable Dust) Regulations 2007
CISD	critical incident stress debriefing
CJD	Creutzfeldt–Jakob disease
CLAW	Control of Lead at Work Regulations
clo	clothing insulation (unit of measurement)
CLP	Classification, Labelling and Packaging of Substances and Mixtures
CML	chronic myeloid leukaemia
CMV	cytomegalovirus

CNAWRs	Control of Noise at Work Regulations 2005
CNS	central nervous system
COMAH	Control of Major Accident Hazards Regulations
COPD	chronic obstructive pulmonary disease
COSHH	Control of Substances Hazardous to Health Regulations
CoV	coronavirus (see SARS)
CPT	cold provocation test (see HAVS)
CPU	central processing unit
CSA	chemical safety assessment (REACH)
CSM	Committee on Safety of Medicines
CSR	Chemical Safety Report
CT	computed tomography
CTS	carpal tunnel syndrome
CVA	cerebrovascular accident
CVAAS	cold vapour atomic absorption spectroscopy
CWP	coal worker's pneumoconiosis
CXR	chest X-ray
DB	dry-bulb temperature
dB	decibel
DBCP	dibromochloropropane
D&C	dilatation and curettage—a gynaecological procedure
DDA	Disability Discrimination Act
DEEE	Diesel engine exhaust emissions
DEFRA	Department for Environment, Food, and Rural Affairs
DFG	Deutsche Forschungsgemeinschaft (Germany): the German Research Foundation
DH	Department of Health (England)
DIY	do it yourself
dL	decilitre
DNA	deoxyribonucleic acid
DNEL	derived no-effect level (REACH)
DOB	date of birth
DPH	local Director of Public Health—UK
DPT	diptheria, pertussis, tetanus immunization
DSE	display screen equipment
DSEAR	Dangerous Substances and Explosive Atmospheres Regulations
DSM IV	Diagnostic and Statistical Manual of Mental Disorders, 4th edition

DTS	Davidson Trauma Scale
DU	downstream user (REACH)
DVLA	Driver and Vehicle Licensing Agency
DVT	deep venous thrombosis
DWP	Department for Work and Pensions
E	illuminance
EA	Environment Agency
EAA	extrinsic allergic alveolitis
EAGA	Expert Advisory Group on AIDS (UK)
EAP	Employee Assistance Programme
EASA	European Aviation Safety Agency
EAV	exposure action value
EC	elemental carbon
ECG	electrocardiogram
ECHA	Central European Chemical Agency
ECL	exposure control limits (of respirable dust)
EDTA	ethylene diamine tetra-acetic acid
EEF	UK manufacturers' organization
EFQM	European Foundation for Quality Management
EHO	environmental health officer
EH40	list of workplace exposure limits for use with COSHH
EIA	environmental impact assessment
EINECS	European Inventory of Existing Commercial Chemical Substances
EIR	Environmental Information Regulations
ELF	extremely low-frequency fields
ELINCS	European List of Notified Chemical Substances
ELV	exposure limit value
EMA	employment medical adviser
EMDR	eye movement desensitization and reprocessing
EMF	electromagnetic fields
EMG	electromyography
EmT	employment tribunal
ENT	ear, nose, and throat
ENWHP	European Network for Workplace Health Promotion
EPA	Environmental Protection Agency
EPP	exposure prone procedure (of healthcare)
ERPC	evacuation of retained products of conception

ESA	Employment and Support Allowance (UK disability benefit)
ESR	erythrocyte sedimentation rate
ET	effective temperature
ETS	environmental tobacco smoke
EU	European Union
EWI	Expert Witness Institute (UK)
EWTD	European Working Time Directive
FCA	flux cored arc (welding)
FEP	free erythrocyte protoporphyrin
FEV1	forced expiratory volume in 1 second
FFP	ferrous foundry particulate
FFP3	filtering face-piece respirator conforming to EN149:2001 FFP3
FHP	farmer's hypersensitivity pneumonitis
FII	fabricated or induced illness—previously Munchausen's syndrome and Munchausen's syndrome by proxy
FOD	Field Operations Directorate of HSE
FOH	Faculty of Occupational Hygiene
FOM	Faculty of Occupational Medicine
FRP	fibre-reinforced plastic
FSBP	finger systolic blood pressure test
FVC	forced vital capacity
G6PD	glucose-6-phosphate dehydrogenase
GC	gas chromatography
GC-FID	gas chromatography–flame ionization detection
GC-MS	gas chromatography–mass spectroscopy
G-CSF	granulocyte-colony stimulating factor
GDG	Guideline Development Groups
GET	graded exercise therapy
GGT	gamma glutamyl transferase
GI	gastrointestinal
GM	genetic modification
GM	geometric mean
GMC	General Medical Council—UK regulatory body for doctors
GM-CSF	granulocyte-macrophage colony-stimulating factor
GMO	genetically-modified organisms
GMM	genetically-modified micro-organisms

GP	general practitioner
GRADE	Grading of Recommendations Assessment, Development and Evaluation
GSD	geometric standard deviation
GT	globe thermometer temperature
GTC	generalized tonic–clonic convulsions
Gy	gray: unit of absorbed radiation
HAART	highly active anti-retroviral therapy
HACCP	Hazard Analysis and Critical Control Points—of food safety
HADS	Hospital Anxiety and Depression Scale
HAVS	hand–arm vibration syndrome
HBIG	hepatitis B specific immunoglobulin
HBV	hepatitis B virus
HCN	hydrogen cyanide
HCV	hepatitis C virus
HCW	health care worker
HDI	1,6-hexamethylenediisocynate
HDV	hepatitis D virus
HELA	Health and Safety Executive/Local Authority Enforcement Liaison Committee
HEPA	high-efficiency particulate absorption (filters)
HG	hazard group (microbial pathogens)
HGV	heavy goods vehicle
HHG	health hazard group (of substances—based on risk phrases)
HIA	health impact assessment
HIDL	high-intensity discharge lamp
HIV	human immunodeficiency virus
HP	hearing protectors
HML	high, medium, and low frequencies
HP	hypersensitivity pneumonitis
HPA	Health Protection Agency
HPLC	high-performance liquid chromatography
HPS	Health Protection Scotland
HR	human resources (personnel)
HRT	hormone replacement therapy
HSAC	HSE Health Services Advisory Committee
HSC	Health and Safety Commission

HSE	Health and Safety Executive
HSW	Health and Safety at Work etc. Act
HVLV	high-velocity low-volume extraction system
HWDU	Health and Work Development Unit
HWI	Healthy Workplace Initiative
Hz	Hertz
IAPT	Improving access to psychological therapies—a UK National Health Service programme
IARC	International Agency for Research on Cancer
ICAO	International Civil Aviation Organization
ICD-10	International Classification of Diseases, 10th edition
IrCD	irritant contact dermatitis
ICNIRP	International Commission on Non-ionizing Radiation Protection
ICO	Information Commissioner's Office
ICOH	International Commission on Occupational Health
ICP	inductively coupled plasma spectrometry
ICP-AES	inductively coupled plasma atomic emission spectrometry
ICRP	International Commission on Radiation Protection
IEGMP	independent expert group on mobile phones
IES-R	Impact of Event Scale—Revised
IgE	immunoglobulin E
IHD	ischaemic heart disease
IHR	ill-health retirement
IIAC	Industrial Injuries Advisory Council
IIDB	Industrial Injuries Disablement Benefit
ILEA	International League Against Epilepsy
ILI	influenza-like illness
ILO	International Labour Organization
ILS	immediate life support
IM	intramuscular
IOM	Institute of Occupational Medicine (Edinburgh)
IOSH	Institution of Occupational Safety and Health
IPC	Integrated Pollution Control
IPL	intense pulsed light
IR	infrared radiation
IREQ	minimum clothing insulation required in cold environments
IRR	Ionizing Radiation Regulations

ISO	International Standard Organization
IT	information technology
IV	intravenous
IVP	intravenous pyelogram
IVS	identified validated sample (of healthcare workers)
J	joule
KCN	potassium cyanide
L	luminance
L'_A	noise level at the ear
L_{Aeq}	continuous equivalent A-weighted sound pressure level
L_{Cpeak}	peak sound pressure level (pascals)
$L_{EP,d}$	daily personal noise exposure level (Db(A))
LA	A-weighted sound pressure levels
LBP	low back pain
LC	C-weighted sound pressure levels
LD_{50}	lethal dose in 50% of experimental animals
LEV	local exhaust ventilation
LFT	liver function test
LGV	large goods vehicle
LOAEL	lowest observable adverse effect level
LOD	limit of detection
LOLER	Lifting Operations and Lifting Equipment Regulations
LRU	Leptospira Reference Unit
LSA	low specific activity scale
Lx	Lux—a measure of light
MAC	manual handling assessment chart
MAK	maximum allowable concentration of a substance (Germany)
MAPP	major accident prevention policy
MASTA	Medical Advisory Service for Travellers Abroad
MbOCA	dichloro-4,4-methylene dianiline
MCA	Maritime and Coastguard Agency
MDA	4,4-diaminodiphenylmethane
MDHS	methods for the determination of hazardous substances
MDI	methylenebis (phenyl isocyanate)
MDR-TB	multidrug-resistant tuberculosis
ME	myalgic encephalomyelitis
MEDIF	medical information form (fitness to fly)

MEK	methyl ethyl ketone
MHOR	Manual Handling Operations Regulations
MHRA	Medicines and Healthcare Products Regulatory Agency
MHSWR	Management of Health and Safety at Work Regulations
MI	myocardial infarction
M/I	manufacturers and importers
MIG	metal inert gas (welding)
MMA	manual metal arc (welding)
MMMF	machine-made mineral fibre
MMR	measles, mumps, rubella vaccine
MMSE	Mini Mental State Examination
MOD	Ministry of Defence (UK)
MOSS	Musculoskeletal Occupational Surveillance Scheme
MP	Member of Parliament
mp	melting point
MPE	maximum permissible exposure value (of lasers)
MPTP	1-methyl-4-phenyl-1,2,3,6-tetrahydropyridine
MRI	magnetic resonance imaging
MRO	Medical Review Officer (of drug test results)
MRSA	multiresistant Staphylococcus aureus
MS	member states of EU
MSD	musculoskeletal disorder
MSDS	Manufacturer's Safety Data Sheet
MSLA	minimum school-leaving age
mSv	millisieverts
MUC	maximum use concentration (of respirators)
Muta.	mutagen
MWF	metal-working fluid
NaCN	sodium cyanide
NCGC	National Clinical Guideline Centre (UK)
NEBOSH	National Examination Board in Occupational Safety and Health
NEQAS	UK National External Quality Assessment Service
NHS	National Health Service (UK)
NI	National Insurance (UK)
NIBSC	National Institute for Biological Standards and Controls
NICE	National Institute for Health and Clinical Excellence (UK)
NIHL	noise-induced hearing loss

NIOSH	National Institute for Occupational Safety and Health (USA)
nm	nanometre
NMC	Nursing and Midwifery Council
NOx	oxides of nitrogen
NOAEL	no observable adverse effect level
NPIS	National Poisons Information Service
NRL	natural rubber latex
NRPB	National Radiological Protection Board
NRT	nicotine replacement therapy
NRTIs	nucleoside analogue reverse transcriptase inhibitors
NSI	needle stick injury
NTE	neuropathy target esterase
OA	occupational asthma
OA	osteoarthritis
OASYS	computer based analytical tool of serial measurements of peak expiratory flow
OC	organochlorine
OCD	obsessive compulsive disorder
OCP	oral contraceptive pill
OD	occupational dermatitis
ODTS	organic dust toxic syndrome
OEL	occupational exposure limit
OH	occupational health
OHA	occupational health adviser—an occupational health nurse
OHN	occupational health nurse
OHP	occupational health physician
OHS	occupational health service
ONS	Office for National Statistics (UK)
OP	organophosphate
OPCS	Office of Population Censuses and Surveys
OPIDN	organophosphate-induced delayed neuropathy
OPRA	Occupational Physicians Reporting Activity
OSHA	Occupational Safety and Health Administration (USA)
OSSA	Occupational Surveillance Scheme for Audiological Physicians
OSHCR	Occupational Safety and Health Consultants Register
Pa	pascal (SI unit of pressure)
PAP	3-(N-phenylamino)-1,2-propanediol

PAHs	polycylic aromatic hydrocarbons
PBG	porphobilinogen
PBT	persistent bioaccumulative and toxic (REACH)
PC	personal computer
PCBs	polychlorinated biphenyls
PCDF	polychlorinated dibenzofuran
PCR	polymerase chain reaction
PCV	passenger-carrying vehicle
PD	Parkinson's disease
PDA	personal digital assistant—a palmtop computer
pdf	portable document format
PEF	peak expiratory flow
PEP	post-exposure prophylaxis for blood-borne virus exposures
PGD	patient group direction (for vaccine administration)
PHLS	Public Health Laboratory Service (UK)
PHQ9	Patient Health Questionnaire
PI	protease inhibitor
PM2.5	particulate matter <2.5µm in diameter
PM10	particulate matter <10µm in diameter
PMF	progressive massive fibrosis
PMV	predicted mean vote
PPC	pollution prevention and control
PPD	predicted percentage of persons dissatisfied with the thermal environment
PPE	personal protective equipment
ppm	parts per million
PTFE	polytetrafluoroethylene
PTO	power take-off
PTSD	post-traumatic stress disorder
PULHHEEMS	UK military grading scheme: Physique, Upper and Lower limbs, Hearing, Eyesight, Mental function, Stability
PUWER	Provision and Use of Work Equipment Regulations
Pv	velocity pressure (of ventilation systems)
PVA	polyvinyl alcohol
PVC	polyvinyl chloride
QEC	Quick Exposure Check tool
RAST	radio-allergosorbent test

RBP	retinol binding protein
RCN	Royal College of Nursing
RCT	randomized controlled trial
REACH	Registration, Evaluation, Authorization and Restriction of Chemicals
Repr	reproductive toxin
RF	radiofrequency radiation
RIDDOR	Reporting of Injuries, Diseases, and Dangerous Occurrence Regulations
RMM	risk management measures (REACH)
RMO	Review Medical Officer (of drug screen results)
RMP	registered medical practitioner
rms	root mean square
RNA	ribonucleic acid
RO	Responsible Officer (for revalidation of UK doctors)
RPA	radiation protection adviser
RPE	respiratory protective equipment
RPS	radiation protection supervisor
RR	relative risk
RULA	Rapid Upper Limb Assessment tool
SaO_2	oxygen saturation (%)
SARS	severe acute respiratory syndrome
SARs	structure–activity relationships (of toxicology)
SBS	sick building syndrome
SCL	skin contamination layer
SD	standard deviation
SEA	strategic environmental assessment
Sen	sensitizer (term used in HSE publication EH40)
SEPA	Scottish Environmental Protection Agency
SEQOHS	Safe effective quality occupational health service—UK occupational health accreditation scheme
SI	Le Système International d'Unités—the metric system of measurements
SIDAW	Surveillance of Infectious Diseases at Work
SIEF	substance information exchange forum (REACH)
SIGN	Scottish Intercollegiate Guideline Network
Sk	substance can be absorbed through the skin (term used in HSE publication EH40)
SLM	Sound level meter

SMEs	small- and medium-sized enterprises
SMR	standardized mortality ratio
SN	sensorineural—of hand arm vibration syndrome grading
SNR	single rating number (of hearing protection)
SOM	Society of Occupational Medicine
SOP	standard operating procedure
SOSMI	Surveillance of Occupational Stress and Mental Illness
SPRU	Special Pathogens Reference Unit
SSP	statutory sick pay
SSRI	selective serotonin-reuptake inhibitor
STEL	short-term exposure limit
STOT/SE	specific target organ toxicity—single exposure
STOT/RE	specific target organ toxicity—repeated exposure
Sv	Sievert
SVHC	substance of very high concern (REACH)
SWASH	Survey of Workplace Absence Sickness and (Ill) Health -UK
SWI	Self-reported Work-related Illness survey
SWORD	Surveillance of Work-related and Occupational Respiratory Disease
TB	tuberculosis
TDI	toluene-2,4-diisocyanate
TENS	transcutaneous electrical nerve stimulation
THOR	The Health and Occupation Reporting network
TIA	transient ischaemic attack
TIG	tetanus immunoglobulin
TIG	tungsten inert gas (welding)
TLD	thermoluminescent dosemeter
TLV®	threshold limit values
TNT	trinitrotoluene
TOCP	tri-orthocresylphosphate
TOP	termination of pregnancy
TPT	thermal (temperature) perception threshold
Travax	travel health information website—run by Health Protection Scotland
TSE	transmissible spongiform encephalopathy
TST	tuberculin skin test
TTS	temporary threshold shift (of hearing thresholds)
TURP	trans-urethral resection of prostate

TWA	time-weighted average
Twc	Wind Chill Index
UKAP	UK Advisory Panel for health care workers infected with blood-borne viruses
UKAS	UK Accreditation Service
ULD	upper limb disorder
UV	ultraviolet light
UVA	ultraviolet light A
UVB	ultraviolet light B
UVC	ultraviolet light C
vCJD	Variant Creutzfeldt–Jakob disease
VCM	vinyl chloride monomer
VDU	visual display unit
VHF	viral haemorrhagic fever
VO2max	maximal oxygen consumption
VOCs	volatile organic compounds
vPvB	very persistent and very bioaccumulative (REACH)
VPT	vibrotactile perception threshold
VWF	vibration white finger—the vascular component of hand arm vibration syndrome
WB	wet bulb temperature
WBGT	wet bulb globe temperature
WBV	whole-body vibration
WCA	Work Capability Assessment—of entitlement to Employment and Support Allowance in UK
WEL	workplace exposure limit
WHASS	Workplace Health and Safety Survey
WHO	World Health Organization
WRULD	work-related upper limb disorder
XRD	X-ray diffraction
XRF	X-ray fluorescence spectroscopy
ZPP	zinc protoporphyrin

Section 1

Occupational hazards

Physical hazards

Noise1: Legal requirements and risk assessment

Definitions
- *Peak sound pressure level* (L_{Cpeak}): maximum value of the C-weighting sound pressure in pascals (Pa) to which a person is exposed during the working day
- *Daily personal exposure level* ($L_{EP,d}$): daily equivalent A-weighted sound level, expressed in dB (A).
- L_{Aeq}: continuous equivalent A-weighted sound pressure level.
- *dB (A) and dB (C) weighting*: the human ear is more sensitive to certain frequencies than to others. Allowance for this can be made in the electronic circuitry of the sound meter. Certain frequencies can be suppressed and others boosted. This technique is called weighting. The most commonly used weighting is the A weighting because it mimics the response of the human ear. The C weighting should be applied when measuring the peak sound pressure level.

Control of noise at work regulations and exposure limits
The legal requirements are covered in the Control of Noise at Work Regulations 2005 (CNAWRs; see Box 1.1). The exposure action values (EAVs) are the noise exposure levels at which certain actions are required. These actions relate to need for risk assessment, controlling exposure, health surveillance, and the provision of information and training. The exposure limit values (ELVs) are the levels of noise above which employees may not be exposed. The EAVs and ELVs are listed in Table 1.1.

Box 1.1 The general duties under CNAWRs
- A formal risk assessment at or above the lower EAV
- If exposure cannot be reduced by other means, and is likely to above the upper EAV, then ear protection must be provided by the employer and used by employees
- Health surveillance is required if the risk assessment indicates that there is a risk to health from noise (those regularly exposed above the upper EAV) without taking account of noise reduction from use of hearing protectors
- Information, instruction, and training must be provided for those exposed at or the lower EAV.

Table 1.1 Noise exposure limits and action values

Exposure limit type	Daily or weekly personal noise exposure dB (A)	Peak sound pressure dB (C)
Lower EAV	80	135
Upper EAV	85	137
ELV	87	140

Risk assessment and management

Risk assessment
- Systematically identify all noise sources
- Identify individuals exposed to noise
- For those exposed to noise determine daily exposure pattern and exposure duration
- Identify measure used to reduce exposure including protection afforded by ear defenders
- Estimate likely exposure (daily and peak) to noise and compare with limit and action values.

Risk management
- Eliminate/reduce noise exposure where practical
- Provide health surveillance (audiometry) for those at risk
- Give employees information and training on safe work practices and hearing protection
- Maintain noise control equipment and hearing protection
- Record findings and action plan
- Review the following; actual work practices, exposure assessments, health surveillance data, finding from workplace inspections, individual complaints related to noise exposure and new ways to reduce risk.

Noise 2: Instrumentation and determination of $L_{EP,d}$

Instrument types

Sound level meter (SLM)

- Hand held portable instruments with data integrating facility
- Quality (Instrument class) governed by European Standards BS EN 61672–1:2003
- Use windshield to protect microphone against air movement and dirt
- Indicates the following; L_{eq} over the measurement period; L_{Cpeak} and the frequency content of noise (octave band analysis).

Dosimeter (personal sound level meter)

- Easily carried around by operator (Fig. 1.1). Should be placed at least 15cm from the head (avoid reflected sound) and on the side of head where noise levels are higher
- In addition to data from SLM, dosimeters can indicate $L_{EP,d}$ or noise dose expressed as a percentage e.g. 200% dose
- May have data logging facility, enabling the visualization, storage and retrieval of record showing change in sound level with time (work tasks) and data storage.

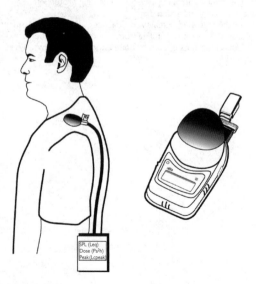

SPL (Leq)
Dose (Pa²h)
Peak (Lcpeak)

Fig. 1.1 Personal noise dosimeters.

Calibrators
- Must provide tight fit around microphone
- Use to check the SLM before and after making measurements
- SLM and calibration should be checked by manufacture at least annually.

Methods for determining L$_{EP,d}$

Personal dosimeter
- Use when the person is highly mobile (e.g. maintenance workers) or where exposure fluctuates greatly
- Place microphone on operators shoulder and on the side of the head where the noise levels are higher and monitor for the duration of shift.

Monitoring tasks/job
- Break the working day in to a number of discrete tasks/jobs and measure representative noise level for each task (L$_{Aeq}$)
- Record time spent conducting each task
- The L$_{Aeq}$ for each task is combined with duration to determine L$_{EP,d}$ using either the ready reckoner or the electronic spreadsheet available on the HSE website (http://www.hse.gov.uk/noise).

Relevant legislation
- The Control of Noise at Work Regulations 2005 (HSE Books)
- Supply of Machinery (Safety) Regulations 1992 (as amended in 1994)
- Provision and Use of Work Equipment Regulations 1998 (amended 1999).

Further information
Health and Safety Executive (1995). *Sound Solutions HSG 138*. HSE Books, Sudbury.

Vibration 1: Whole-body vibration

Common sources

Exposure to whole-body vibration (WBV) arises in workers who drive or ride-on vehicles. Many different vehicle types can give rise to exposure. In the UK, the most common sources are cars, vans, fork-lift trucks, lorries, tractors, buses, loaders, trains, dumpers, and excavators. Other exposures arise from trains, armoured vehicles, off-road vehicles and helicopters.

Occupations and industries

The commonest occupations with exposure are:
• Farm workers
• Drivers of road goods vehicles
• Lift truck drivers.

The commonest industries are:
• Agriculture
• Construction
• Land transport.

Main factors affecting exposure

• Intrinsic vibration of the vehicle (wear and tear, design)
• Seating and vehicle suspension
• Road surface
• Road speed.

Potential health effects

The best recognized effects are on the lumbar spine—non-specific low-back pain (LBP), sciatica, lumbar disc degeneration. A systematic review by NIOSH (1997)[1] described evidence on the association with LBP as 'strong' (15 of 19 studies positive), but there is less certainty about the dose-response relationship.

Other suggested effects include: neck pain and cervical disc degeneration; autonomic disturbance; and disorders of balance and digestion. The evidence for these is much weaker. Motion sickness is well recognized, however.

Risk assessment and monitoring

The Health and Safety Executive (HSE) provides an exposure calculator to facilitate the summation of partial doses from several vehicles (ℜ http://www.hse.gov.uk/vibration/wbv/wbv.xls).

---

1 NIOSH (1997). Musculoskeletal disorders and workplace factors. A critical review of epidemio-logic evidence for work-related musculoskeletal disorders of the neck, upper–extremity and low back, Publication no. 97–141. NIOSH, Cinncinati.

Exposure limits

Two exposure limits are specified in UK and European legislation:

- *An EAV A(8) of 0.5m/s²:* this is the daily amount above which employers must act to control exposure
- *ELV A(8) of 1.15m/s²:* this is the maximum amount an employee may be exposed to on any given day. (HSE advises that the ELV should not be considered a target; rather, the aim should be to reduce exposure as low as reasonably possible.)

Prevention and control

HSE advises that drivers should:

- Adjust their seating
- Avoid rough, poor or uneven surfaces
- Adjust the vehicle speed to suit road conditions.

It also advises on several other measures, including:

- Maintenance of vehicle suspension
- Maintenance of site roadways
- Better choice of seating
- Rest breaks
- Safer systems of work
- Simple health monitoring.

Relevant legislation

Control of Vibration at Work Regulations 2005.

Further information and guidance

HSE web links. Available at: ℘ http://www.hse.gov.uk/vibration/wbv/index.htm
Vibration calculator. Available at: ℘ http://www.hse.gov.uk/vibration/wbv/calculator.htm

Vibration 2: Hand-transmitted vibration

Common sources

Exposure arises from many sources, including concrete breakers, chainsaws, hand-held grinders, metal polishers, power hammers and chisels, needle scalers, scabblers, powered sanders, hammer drills, and even powered lawnmowers and motorcycle handlebars.

Occupations and industries

Occupations where exposure is common include:
- Construction workers
- Metal-working and maintenance fitters
- Welders
- Foresters, shipbuilders
- Foundry workers
- Road workers.

The main industries are construction and heavy engineering. An estimated 1.2 million men in Britain have weekly exposures that may justify health surveillance.

Main factors affecting exposure

- *Tools:* intrinsic properties of the tool (e.g. size, weight, frequency characteristics, balance between reciprocating forces), age of tools, and their maintenance.
- Material being worked
- Type of action at the work interface (e.g. cutting, drilling, grinding)
- Operator technique (e.g. type and force of grip, orientation of the hand-arm).

Potential health effects

- Best-recognized are 2° Raynaud's phenomenon (vibration-induced white finger), sensorineural impairment in the digits and carpal tunnel syndrome
- Other effects to the hand and arm are described (see p. 300, Hand-arm vibration syndrome)
- Workers who use noisy vibratory tools commonly suffer from noise-induced hearing loss, as well as local hand-arm symptoms.

Risk assessment and monitoring

Vibration magnitude is measured in terms of acceleration, averaged (by the root–mean square (rms) method). Frequency-weighted measurements (a_{hw}) are made in three axes relative to the tool handle, using mounted accelerometers, and values (in m/s² rms) are determined for each axis and summated. The procedure is defined in ISO 5349, 1986 (see also ISO 8041 and BS 7482).

Injury is assumed to relate to the total energy entering the hand, so the dose can be re-expressed in terms of the equivalent acceleration imparting the same energy over an 8-h period:

$$A(8) = a_{hw} \sqrt{(t/T(8))} \, \text{m/s}^2$$

where A(8) = the 8-h energy equivalent acceleration, a_{hw} = rms acceleration magnitude after frequency-weighting, t = duration of exposure in a day, and T_8 = 8h (in the same units as t).

Partial doses from >1 tool can be summed to an equivalent daily dose. In practice this requires an inventory of sources, data on vibration magnitude from equipment handbooks or suppliers' information sheets, and an estimate of hand-tool contact times

- HSE provides an exposure ready-reckoner, to estimate A(8) from exposure time and vibration magnitude,[2] and an exposure calculator to facilitate the summation of doses from several tools.[3]

Exposure limits

Two exposure limits are specified in UK and European legislation:
- *EAV A(8) of 2.5m/s²*: the daily amount above which employers must act to control exposure. Health surveillance is required for workers who are regularly exposed above the EAV.
- *ELV A(8) of 5m/s²*: the maximum amount an employee may be exposed to on any given day.

Prevention and control

A number of steps can mitigate the risk in exposed populations. These may be broadly summarized as:
- Avoidance (e.g. doing the job another way)
- Substitution (of tool or material worked)
- Interruption of the pathway (by isolation or vibration-damping)
- Safer systems of work.

Some options include:
- Routine replacement of worn out tool parts
- Proper selection of tools for the task
- The redesign of tools to avoid the need to grip high vibration parts, or to reduce grip force
- Rest breaks to limit exposure times.

Another common approach involves screening for early health effects and limiting further exposure in those with hand-arm vibration syndrome.

Relevant legislation

Control of Vibration at Work Regulations 2005.

Further information and guidance

HSE web links: 🕮 http://www.hse.gov.uk/vibration/hav/index.htm

1 http://www.hse.gov.uk/pubns/indg175.pdf
2 http://www.hse.gov.uk/vibration/hav/readyreckoner.htm
3 http://www.hse.gov.uk/vibration/hav/calculator.htm

Light and lighting 1: effects and illuminance levels

Terms, definitions, and units

- *Luminous intensity* is the term applied to the luminous flux emitted per solid angle and is measured in candela (Cd). The candela is one of the seven basic SI units.
- *Illuminance* (symbol E) is the term given to the amount of light falling on a surface divided by the area over which it is falling and is measured in lux (derivation: lumens/square metre).
- *Luminance* (symbol L) is the flow of light in a given direction from a surface element, measured in Cd/m^2.

Lighting and health

In striving for optimum lighting conditions it is essential to consider the intensity and colour spectrum of the light sources used. Incorrect selection may lead to adverse health and/or psychological effects. The selection of the appropriate illuminance for given visual tasks is vitally important.

- Too much illuminance can lead to the onset of glare
- Too little illuminance can put a strain on the eyes. In some cases the latter causes the individual to adopt uncomfortable working postures which may lead to musculoskeletal problems.

Poor lighting increases risk of fatigue and accidents reduces productivity and increases workers dissatisfaction, which may contribute to worker absenteeism.

Specific health risks

These include, but are not limited to:

- *Infrared and ultraviolet (UV) radiation:* tungsten halogen (desk top lamps) and other high powered lamps e.g. those used in broadcasting studios may emit high levels of UV radiation and cause harm to skin and eyes. These lamps should be fitted with a safety shield or UV filter. For lasers see 📖 p. 26, Non-ionizing radiation 2. Lasers.
- *Blue light hazard (photo retinitis):* this is photochemical damage from exposure to medium to intense strength visible radiation for more than 10s. Blue light hazard is defined as the potential for a photochemical-induced retinal injury from radiation between 400 and 500nm. The damage is irreversible and can lead to blindness. Blue light hazard is particularly important when considering aphakic individuals.
- *Photokeratitis*—a tender eye condition typically following exposure of insufficiently protected eyes to the ultraviolet rays emitted by either natural or artificial sources e.g. welder's arc or some artificial light sources.

Unwanted effects created by lamps and lighting

- *Glare* occurs when one part of the visual field is much brighter than others. There are two major types of glare:
  - *disability glare* where the individual is disabled from carrying out a given visual task

- *discomfort glare* where the individual is not disabled from carrying out a given visual task, but where he/she will experience discomfort, which may be delayed in manifestation.
- *Veiling reflections* is the term applied to the scenario where typically out of focus reflections of light sources are viewed on specular surfaces (typically display screen equipment). This throws a veil of light over the screen making reading of text either difficult or impossible. Veiling reflections is a form of disability glare
- *Flicker* is effectively light modulations at frequencies detectable by the human visual system. This can lead to both discomfort and fatigue and may provoke seizures in photosensitive individuals if the flicker frequency is typical 5–30Hz
- *Stroboscopic effects on rotating machines:* this is the scenario where rotating elements of machinery appear to be stationary or moving in a different manner (possibly in the reverse direction). It is caused by a combination of the rate of oscillations in light output illuminating the rotating element and the rate at which the human visual system can detect movement.

Recommended illuminance values

- The Illuminance requirements of a task depend on performance factors such as level of detail, speed, and accuracy. The Chartered Institute of Building Service Engineers (CIBSE) provides a comprehensive schedule of recommended illuminance values for different workplaces.[1]
- Examples of recommended average illuminance values for work requiring:
  - limited perception of detail (e.g. factories assembling large components, kitchen)—300 lux to 500 lux
  - perception of detail (e.g. offices, metalworking plant)—500 to 750 lux
  - fine detail (e.g. electronic plants)—1000 to 1500 lux.
- Guidance on minimum acceptable levels of lighting is given in the HSE publication *Lighting at work*.[2]

1 CIBSE (2009). http://www.cibse.org/
2 HSE (2002). *Lighting at work*. HSE, Sudbury. Available at: ✆ http://www.hse.gov.uk/pubns/books/ hsg38.htm

Light and lighting 2: Assessment and surveys

Assessing lighting in the workplace

Workplace lighting should meet the following criteria:

- Provides suitable and sufficient illuminance on the work piece
- Provides suitable and sufficient discrimination on the surface colours of objects in the working area
- Prevents the onset of glare (e.g. disability glare)
- Avoids flicker and/or stroboscopic effects
- Avoids the effects of veiling reflections
- Provides sufficient contrast between work piece and background
- Prevents excessive variation in illuminance and luminance within the vicinity of the working areas. Optimally, the ratio of luminance values (task: near surround: far surround) should be 10:3:1.
- Takes into account the requirements of workers with disabilities
- Is located so that access to luminaires (formerly light fittings) and other lighting equipment does not pose a risk to maintenance personnel
- Incorporates appropriate emergency lighting.

Lighting surveys

- It is desirable to have scale drawings of the interior to be surveyed. Alternatively draw a sketch plan of room showing position of work surfaces, windows and luminaires.
- *Record:*
  - visual tasks carried out
  - whether luminaires and windows are clean
  - any luminaires which are damaged or missing
  - whether luminaires or windows cause discomfort or disability glare
  - any flicker from discharge lamps
- Photographs showing areas of particular contention can be extremely useful
- The principle measurements of interest when undertaking a lighting survey are illuminance and luminance. Measuring equipment has to be colour corrected (to compensate for spectral variation) and cosine corrected
- Take illuminance reading at all work stations on every work surface
- During measurements normal workplace lighting should be switched on and natural lighting should be excluded, where possible
- Measurements should be taken 0.80m above floor level.
- The minimum number of measurements can be derived by calculating the room index k

  $$k = L \times W / Hm \times (L + W)$$

where L is the room length, W is the room width, Hm is the height of lamps above working surface. For values of k < 1, 1–2, 2–3, and >3, the minimum number of measurements are 9, 16, 25, and 36, respectively

- Average illuminance is calculated by adding all measurements and dividing by the number of measurements and compared with the CIBSE guidance values
- Comprehensive details of required illuminance values in given locations are provided in CIBSE Code for Lighting.

Further information

BS EN 12464–1 (2011). Light and lighting—lighting of work places. Part 1: indoor work places. Available at: http://shop.bsigroup.com/

BS EN 12464–2 (2007). Light and lighting—lighting of work places. Part 1: outdoor work places. Available at: http://shop.bsigroup.com/

BS 5266–1 (2005). Emergency lighting regulations. Available at: http://shop.bsigroup.com/

CIBSE (2009). *Code for Lighting*. CISE. London. Available at: http://www.cibse.org/

Health and Safety (Display Screen Equipment) Regulations (1992). Available at: http://www.hse.gov.uk/pubns/priced/l26.pdf

HSE (2002). *Lighting at work*, HSG38. HSE Books, Sudbury. Available at: http://www.hse.gov.uk/pubns/books/hsg38.htm

Smith NA (2000). *Lighting for Health and Safety*. Butterworth-Heinemann, Oxford.

Ionizing radiation 1: Types, units, and effects

Routes and sources of exposure
- The hazard from ionizing radiation can arise from:
  - the uniform irradiation of the whole body or part of the body (external radiation)
  - irradiation due to inhaled or absorbed radioactive material, which may concentrate in organs and tissues (internal radiation).
- Natural (background) radiation arises from several sources, including radiation from materials in the earth's crust (e.g. radon in granite strata), cosmic radiation, food, radioactive aerosols, and gases in the atmosphere. The largest dose of radiation, approximately 85% of the total, received by a person living in the UK is due to natural background radiation. Typically, this can amount to 2.2mSv per year (see 📖 p. 16, Units of ionizing radiation).

Sources of ionizing radiation
- *Sealed*: contained or shielded, and present only an external radiation hazard
- *Unsealed*: can be released into the atmosphere because they:
  - are powders, liquids or gases;
  - can contaminate surfaces and be taken into the body by ingestion, inhalation or via the skin, thereby giving rise to an internal radiation hazard, which can be present for variable periods of time.

Types of ionizing radiation
- *Alpha particles:* these are positively charged particles consisting of two protons and two neutrons (the same as a helium atom nucleus) with relatively little energy (they cannot pass through a sheet of paper or intact skin), but capable of causing significant damage to tissue over a short range.
- *Beta particles:* these are electrons and are also charged (negatively). They are much lighter than alpha particles and can pass through paper and skin, although they can be stopped by materials such as glass or thin layers of metal.
- *Neutrons:* these are uncharged particles with intermediate mass and variable energy.
- *Gamma and X-rays:* these are uncharged and without mass. They therefore cause less damage to tissue, but can pass through many materials, although are attenuated by thick layers of lead or concrete.

Units of ionizing radiation
Activity
This indicates the rate of transformations in radioactive material. The unit is the becquerel (Bq).

1 Bq = 1 transformation/s

Absorbed dose

This is the measure of energy deposition in any irradiated material by all types of ionizing radiation, and is expressed as the energy absorbed per unit mass of material. The unit of absorbed dose is the gray (Gy):

$$1\,Gy = 1\,J/kg \text{ of energy deposition.}$$

Dose equivalent

In biological systems, the same absorbed dose of different types of radiation produces different degrees of biological damage. To take account of this, the absorbed dose of each type of radiation is multiplied by a Q (or weighting) factor, which reflects the relative ability of the particular type of radiation to cause damage. The unit of dose equivalent is the sievert (Sv), which is related to the gray as follows:

$$\text{dose equivalent (Sv)} = \text{absorbed dose (Gy)} \times Q.$$

(Occupational doses of radiation are quoted in millisieverts (mSv) in view of the levels of radiation received.)

For beta particles, gamma and X-rays, $Q = 1$. For α particles, $Q = 20$. For neutrons, on average, $Q = 10$.

Effective dose

Similarly, the risk to various tissues varies from one tissue to another; it is not the same for any given equivalent dose. There is thus a weighting factor for each tissue, when multiplied by the equivalent dose, the sum of all such calculations for the various tissues is referred to as the effective dose and is a single measure of the risk of detriment to health.

Health effects

- Damage to tissue sustained by an irradiated individual is termed *'somatic' effects*. These can be acute or delayed. That passed on to descendants is the hereditary effect.
- *Stochastic effects* are those for which risk (the probability of the effect) increases progressively with dose received, but there is no detectable threshold (e.g. induction of carcinogenesis). The risk of developing cancer for radiation workers is calculated as 4% per Sv.
- *Deterministic effects* are those for which the severity of the effect increases progressively with dose and will not occur until a certain threshold of dose has been received (e.g. radiation burn).

Ionizing radiation 2: Principles of radiation protection

Justification
The use of sources of ionizing radiation or radioactive materials must be justified in terms of risk and benefit.

Optimization
Work with sources of ionizing radiation must be such as to reduce risks to levels that are as low as reasonably achievable (in practice, 'achievable' becomes 'practicable').

Dose limits
- Dose limits are recommended by the International Commission on Radiation Protection (ICRP), with the aim of preventing non-stochastic (deterministic) effects and limiting stochastic effects.
- Current dose limits for UK workers and the public are published in the Ionizing Radiations Regulations 1999 and are shown in Table 1.2.

Table 1.2 UK annual dose limits (mSv)

	Annual dose limits		
	Whole body	Skin	Lens of the eye
Radiation workers (classified)	20	500	150
Trainee (under 18)	6	150	50
Radiation workers (non classified)	6	50	15
Others, including members of the public	1	50	15

The dose limit to the abdomen of a woman of reproductive capacity is 13mSv in any consecutive 13-wk period. The dose limit to the fetus once pregnancy has been declared is 1mSv during the period of the pregnancy. From HMSO (1999). *Ionizing Radiations Regulations*. HMSO, London. Available at: ✍ http://www.hse.gov.uk/pubns/books/l121.htm

Ionizing radiation 3: Instrumentation and measurement

Environmental radiation detectors

A wide range of instruments are available. Instruments are based on several types of detectors (gas ionization, solid state detectors, change in chemical systems, and neutron activation) and are used to quantify incident radiation as a count or dose rate. Such detectors include:

- *Installed (fixed) monitors:* used to monitor personal contamination, general radiation, and air contamination level in the working environment
- *Portable (battery operated) monitors:* used to measure levels during specific operations and for contamination surveys.

Devices for personal monitoring

Film badges

- Film is developed and analysed for external radiation dose, in proportion to darkening of the film
- Various filters inside the badge differentiate types of radiation and energies
- Developed film can be stored to provide a permanent record, which can be read again at a later date
- They are no longer widely used as they are less practical and more expensive than TLDs.

Thermoluminescent dosemeters (TLDs)

- Can measure over a wide range for both whole body and extremity (finger) monitoring
- Popular dosemeter for personal monitoring, as they are small and analysis can be performed quickly and automatically
- Not as sensitive to the effects of heat and humidity as film badges
- They are more sensitive to low doses than film badges
- Dose information is destroyed at readout, unlike film badges.

Direct reading instruments

- Use for direct measurement of X-rays or gamma rays
- Self-indicating pocket dosemeters (similar in size to a fountain pen or a radio-pager) are useful for measuring doses in situations where the dose rate is high, allowing a continuous watch to be kept on the rate of accumulation of dose
- Must be calibrated with known dose levels
- Can lose sensitivity with leakage, and tend to be insensitive to low levels of radiation.

Unsealed radiation sources

- *Surface contamination:* monitoring in the work area and on the worker's skin, and clothing is detected by portable and fixed monitors, including before workers leave a controlled area
- *Airborne sampling:* as with dusts, certain types of radioactive material can be sampled on filter paper using a high volume sampler. Particulate or gaseous activity is then measured by scanning the filter for radioactivity using a counter. Radioactive gases can also be collected using a sampling bag or chamber
- *Biological monitoring:* total internal dose is determined in special cases by measuring urine or stool samples. Biological effect monitoring can be done by examining lymphocyte chromosomes from a blood sample.

Ionizing radiation 4: Exposure control

General requirements

- Demarcating specific areas and classification of personnel based on their radiation exposure. For those workers designated 'classified', personal dosimetry and health surveillance are required under the Ionizing Radiations Regulations 1999. Such workers are classified on the basis of a requirement to work in areas where they may receive at least 30% of the legal, or a lower locally imposed, maximum total dose
- Appointing a radiation protection adviser (RPA) and radiation protection supervisors (RPS)
- Arrangement for waste disposal, monitoring exposure, and training on safe work practices and precautions.

Control of external exposure

Exposure to external ionizing radiation can be reduced by time, distance, and shielding.
- *Time:* reduce exposure time to a minimum
- *Distance:* arrange work so that the distance from source to worker is as great as possible. The intensity of point source radiation decreases with increasing distance, obeying the inverse square law
- *Shielding of the worker from radiation:* advice can be obtained from manufacturers or the RPA on the type and thickness of shielding necessary. This is particularly indicated for penetrating radiation, such as gamma and X-rays.

Control of internal exposure

This can be reduced by:
- Containing the source, e.g. in a glove box
- Good housekeeping and personal hygiene
- Uses of personal and respiratory protective equipment, e.g. full face respirator, air hood, or pressurized suit.

Classification of work areas

Work areas are classified according to the potential level of exposure:
- *Supervised area:* dose rate is less than 7.5µSv/h, but workers in that area may receive an effective dose of greater than 1mSv a year
- *Controlled area:* dose rate can exceed 7.5µSv/h and workers in that area may receive an effective dose of at least 6mSv a year.

Relevant legislation

- Ionizing Radiations Regulations (1999)
- Ionizing Radiation (Medical Exposure) Regulations (2000)
- Radiation (Emergency Preparedness and Public Information) Regulations (2001).

Further information

Cherrie J, Howie R, Sample S (2010). *Monitoring for health hazards at work*, 4th edn. Blackwell Science, Oxford.

HSE (2000). *Work with ionizing radiation. The Ionizing Radiations Regulations (1999)*, approved code of Practice and Guidance L121. HSE Books, Sudbury.

HSE (2011). Ionising radiation—radiation protection. HSE, Sudbury. Available at: ℘ http://www.hse.gov.uk/radiation/ionising/index.htm

Health Protection Agency (HPA) website. Available at: ℘ http://www.hpa.org.uk/ProductsServices/Radiation/

NRPB (1998). *Living with Radiation*, 5th edn. NRPB, Chilton.

Non-ionizing radiation 1: Electromagnetic fields

Electromagnetic fields (EMF) radiation does not have sufficient energy to break the bonds that hold molecules in cells together, and so it does not produce ionization of matter. Effects on the body depend on the frequency and magnitude of EMF. Static electric fields build up charge on the surface of the body. Magnetic fields can induce flows of electric current in the body. Radiofrequency (RF) radiation is partially absorbed, penetrating a short distance into tissues, and can give rise to localized heating.

Sources of exposure (occupational and environmental)

Static and extremely low-frequency fields (ELF)
- Electrical power lines
- Household electrical appliances
- Electrical transport
- Welding.

High-frequency or radiofrequency fields (RF)
- Radar
- Radio and television broadcast facilities
- Mobile telephones and their base stations
- Induction heaters
- Anti-theft devices.

Health effects of electromagnetic frequency

- ELF have been classified by the International Agency for Research on Cancer (IARC)[1] as a possible carcinogen for childhood leukaemia in humans, but have not been given a carcinogen notation for any other cancer. The evidence for childhood leukaemia is inconclusive and there could be other explanations for the association with ELF.
- While until recently the balance of evidence has suggested that there are no important health effects from RF, IARC has also classified this type of EMF as a possible human carcinogen (2B) for glioma.

💣 There is currently a high level of public interest and debate regarding exposure to RF (in particular mobile telephones and masts) and the focus of research is on the health effects of long-term low-level exposure. The Interphone study, co-ordinated by IARC, has yet to show any definite evidence of public health risk.

1 World Health Organization International Agency for Research on Cancer. Available at: 🔗 http://www.iarc.fr/

2 International Commission on Non-ionizing Radiation Protection. Available at: 🔗 http://www.icnirp.de/what.htm

Exposure guidelines

Countries set their own exposure standards for EMF, the majority of which are based on the International Commission on Non-ionizing Radiation Protection (ICNIRP).[2] These follow the precautionary principle in setting separate limits for occupational and public exposure. They cover frequencies in the range 0–300GHz and are based on short-term acute exposure. In the UK the National Radiological Protection Board (NRPB) (now part of the Health Protection Agency (HPA)) has defined exposure limits (see 📖 p. 25, Further reading and guidance).

Exposure control

Elimination is not usually possible. Control measures include:
- Effective enclosure and reflective screens
- Control by distance from source
- Personal protective equipment.

Relevant legislation

Directive 2004/40/EC on the minimum health and safety requirements regarding the exposure of workers to the risks arising from physical agents (electromagnetic fields). In 2006, it was decided to postpone this Directive until 2012 to permit further consultation. ℘ http://www.hse.gov.uk/radiation/nonionising/l184emf.pdf

Further reading and guidance

HPA (2004). *Advice on Limiting Exposure to Electromagnetic Field (0–300 GHz)*. Volume 15 No.2. Available at: ℘ http://www.hpa.org.uk/webc/HPAwebFile/HPAweb_C/1194947415497

Independent Expert Group on mobile phones (2000). *Mobile Phones and health*. IEGMP, c/o HPA, Chilton.

International Commission on Non-ionizing Radiation Protection (ICNIRP) (2012). ℘ http://www.icnirp.org/

World health Organization (2002). *Establishing a dialogue on risks from electromagnetic fields*. WHO, Geneva. ℘ http://www.who.int/peh-emf/publications/risk_hand/en/index.html

The International EMF Project has established a worldwide database of standards. ℘ http://www.who.int/peh-emf/standards/en/

Non-ionizing radiation 2: Optical radiation

Relevant legislation

The Control of Artificial Optical Radiation at Work Regulations (2010) aim to protect workers from risks from various sources, such as UV light (excluding sunlight) and lasers. The regulations distinguish between 'safe sources', such as most forms of visible light, and 'hazardous sources', such as high intensity ultra-violet and laser sources. There are requirements to consider alternative sources, undertake training and use control measures.

Hazardous light sources

Hazardous sources of light that present a risk of harming the eyes and skin of worker where control measures are needed include:

- *Metal working:* welding and plasma cutting
- *Hot processes:* furnaces, hot metals /glass
- *Motor vehicle repairs:* UV curing of paints and welding
- *Pharmaceutical and research:* UV sterilization and induced fluorescence
- *Printing:* UV curing of inks and paints
- *Medical and cosmetic treatment:* UV and blue light therapies, laser surgery (Class 3B and 4 lasers), intense pulsed light (IPL)
- *Industry and research:* use of Class 3B and Class 4 lasers as defined in BS EN 60825–1 (2007)
- Any Risk group 3 lamp or lamp systems as defined in BSEN 62471 (2008), e.g. professional projections systems.

Control measures

- Use alternative safer light sources
- *Engineering measures:* automation, controlled areas, remote control, screening, interlocks
- Use filters, remote viewing and time delays
- Protect others using screens/curtains/restricted access to hazardous areas
- Provide personal protective equipment, e.g. coveralls, goggles, face-shields, gloves
- Provide information and training on safe use and best practice
- Display safety and warning signs
- Monitor use of control measures.

▶ If any workers are over-exposed, e.g. damage to skin and eyes provide medical examination and follow-up health surveillance.

Ultraviolet

Subtypes

Ultraviolet light is divided into three types, according to wavelength. Only UVA and UVB from the sun affect humans as UVC is absorbed by the earth's atmosphere.

- *UVA*: 315–400nm
- *UVB*: 280–315nm
- *UVC*: 100–285nm.

Sources of exposure (occupational and environmental)

- Welding
- Printing
- Germicidal and mercury lamps
- Spectroscopy
- External work (sunlight).

Health effects

- Skin erythema/burn
- Premature skin ageing
- Cataract
- Photokeratitis
- Photosensitive and phototoxic reactions (associated with external or internal exposure to chemical agents, or skin or systemic diseases)
- Skin cancer (basal and squamous types are associated with prolonged sun exposure)
- Benefits, from Vitamin D production and improvement in some conditions, such as psoriasis.

Control measures

- Limit exposure time to sunlight, especially in the middle of the day
- Have shaded areas available for breaks
- Use suitable clothing and hats to protect the skin
- Use sun protection creams
- Provide training to workers including the above as well as on maintenance of hydration and observation of the skin for suspicious lesions.

Laser

See 📖 p. 28, Non-ionizing radiation 3: Laser.

Further information

HSE (2010). *Control of artificial optical radiation at work regulations.* HSE, Sudbury.
HSE (2010). *Guidance for employers on the control of artificial optical radiation at work regulations.* HSE, Sudbury. Available at: ℑ http://www.hse.gov.uk/radiation/nonionising/employers-aor.pdf

Non-ionizing radiation 3: Laser

Characteristics

- *Laser radiation has unique properties:* monochromatic, coherent, bright, high irradiance, and focused to deposit intense energy on small surfaces
- *Lasers can be operated in two major modes:* pulsed and continuous wave
- *Lasers are grouped into 7 classes:* the higher the class, the greater the potential for harm.

Health effects

- Visible and IR-A laser beams can be focused to create very high intensity exposures on the retina.
- The effects depend on a number of factors including the wavelength, power, and pulse duration and beam geometry
- Laser beams produce biological damage by thermal burns and photochemical injuries. Visible and IR-A lasers produce retinal damage
- The retina is most at risk; thermal and photochemical damage may also occur.
  - inadvertent reflections must be avoided so that beams are not redirected into safe zones
  - a classification system for lasers has been developed to ensure safe use (summary shown in Box 1.2)
  - training programmes are required for users of class 3 and 4 lasers. Medical surveillance is not required by legislation, although has been recommended with the use of class 3B and 4 lasers
  - the ACGIH publishes threshold limit values (TLV) standards for lasers emissions (ocular and skin exposures) for IR, UV and light exposure arising from viewing a laser beam.

Controls

Controls applied to different laser devices are shown in Box 1.2.

Engineering

The main engineering control is enclosure, often in the form of inter-locked rooms. Remote interlocks can make up safety chains covering a large area.

Administrative

Administrative controls are used during set up and maintenance. These include designated zones, authorization, and warning signs.

Personal protective equipment

Laser protective goggles must be selected to ensure that they are of appropriate optical density for the type (wavelength) of radiation encountered and its severity. Lenses are glass or plastic. Glass lenses are heavier, but offer more resistance to direct strikes and let through more light. Glass is often used when average laser power exceeds 100mW.

Box 1.2 Laser safety classification and required controls

Class 1
- Safe under reasonably foreseeable conditions of operation
- Protection measures not necessary, personal protective equipment (PPE) not required.

Class 1M
- Safe for naked eye, may be hazardous if the user employs optics
- Prevent use of magnifying, focusing, or collimating optics
- PPE not required.

Class 2
- Safe for short exposures, eye protection afforded by aversion response
- Follow manufactures instructions for safe use
- Do not stare in to beam
- PPE not required.

Class 2M
- Safe for naked eye for short exposures, may be hazardous if the user employs optics
- Do not stare in to beam, prevent use of magnifying, focusing or collimating optics
- Training recommended, PPE not required.

Class 3R
- Risk of injury is relatively low, but may be dangerous for improper use by trained by untrained person
- Enclosed
- Prevent direct eye exposure
- Training required
- PPE may be required subject to findings of risk assessment.

Class 3B
- Direct viewing is hazardous
- Enclosed and interlock protected
- Prevent eye and skin exposure to the beam.
- Training and PPE required.

Class 4
- Hazardous for eye and skin; fire hazard
- Enclosed and interlock protected
- Prevent eye and skin exposure from direct and diffuse reflection of the beam
- Training and PPE required.

Thermal environment 1: thermal balance and instrumentation

Heat stress

Heat stress occurs when the body's means of controlling internal temperature starts to fail. Operations involving high air temperatures, radiant heat sources, high humidity or strenuous physical activities have a high potential for inducing heat stress.

Heat balance

- The body core temperature must be regulated to remain typically at 37 ± 0.5°C. Below 31°C leads to loss of consciousness and death. Above 43°C leads to failure of the thermoregulation mechanism
- Heat balance between the human body and its surroundings can be expressed as the equation

$$M = \pm K \pm C \pm R - E$$

where M is the rate of metabolic heat production (see Table 1.3), K, C, and R are gain or loss of heat by conduction, convection, and radiation, respectively, and E is the evaporative heat loss from skin and respiratory tract.
- The heat balance is affected by work performed and the rate of change in the store of heat in the body.

Health effects

- *Exposure to high temperature:* heat stroke, heat syncope, heat exhaustion, heat fatigue and prickly heat, cataract, susceptibility to other disease (e.g. cardiovascular)
- *Exposure to low temperature:* hypothermia is a condition of low core temperature, and is clinically defined as a deep body temperature below 35°C.

Occupations at risk

Work activities that may lead to heat stress include: handling molten metal, metal refining, glass-making, boiler and furnace maintenance, mining and tunnelling, firefighting, and outdoor work in hot climates.

Parameters and instruments for heat stress

The following four environmental parameters must be assessed:
- air temperature
- air velocity
- radiant temperature
- relative humidity.

Instruments for measuring individual environmental parameters include:
- *Dry bulb thermometers or electric thermometers:* measure air temperature
- *Wet bulb thermometer:* dry bulb covered in a clean cotton wick wetted with distilled water
- *Psychrometers:* consist of wet and dry bulb thermometer mounted in a frame. There are two types—the sling and the aspirated. Used to determine the relative humidity
- *Globe thermometer (mercury-in-glass thermometer with its bulb in the centre of a matt black sphere or globe):* used to measure radiant temperature
- *Kata thermometer:* used for measuring air velocities less than 0.5m/s.

Integrating electronic heat stress monitors
- *Static instruments:* provide a single value for wet bulb globe temperatures (WBGT) and air velocities (Fig. 1.2)
- *Personal heat stress monitors (Fig. 1.3):* signals from various sensors including heart rate and temperature fed into a data logger, which calculates a strain index. The monitor can be set for different age ranges and clothing. An audible alarm, indicating if preset warning and action levels are exceeded, is usually fitted.

Table 1.3 Metabolic rates for activities

Class	Mean metabolic rate (Wm²)	Example
Resting	65	Resting
Low	100	Standing
Moderate	165	Sustained hand/arm work
High	230	Intense work
Very high	290	Very intense to maximum activity

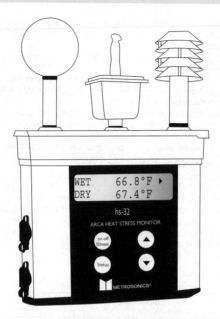

Fig. 1.2 Electronic integrating heat stress monitor.

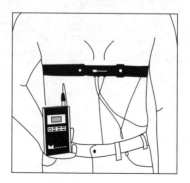

Fig. 1.3 Personal heat stress monitor.

Thermal environment 2: Assessment of the thermal environment

A number of heat stress indices have been developed for different industries, with the aim of preventing the deep body temperature from exceeding 38°C.

Classification of heat stress indices

Empirical and direct indices

Wet bulb temperature (WB), effective temperature (ET), corrected effective temperature (CET), WBGT.

Analytical indices

Required sweat rate, heat stress index, predicted 4h sweat rate.

Wet bulb globe temperature

The WBGT is the most widely accepted index for assessment of heat in industry and published as British Standard BS EN 27243 and also in the ACGIH threshold limits values.

WBGT (expressed in temperature units) is calculated as follows:

For indoor use, WBGT = 0.7 WB + 0.3 GT

For outdoor use, WBGT = 0.7 WB + 0.2 GT + 0.1 DB

where WB is natural wet bulb temperature); GT is the globe thermometer temperature (°C), and DB is the dry bulb temperature (°C).

Table 1.4 shows reference values of WBGT related to a maximum rectal temperature of 38°C for different metabolic rates and state of acclimatization. The reference values assume the individual is fit, normally clothed with adequate water and salt intake.

Example

In a foundry with still air, a worker is acclimatized and estimated to be working at 240W/m². Air temperature = 25°C, globe temperature = 27°C, natural wet bulb = 18°C,

WBGT = 0.7(18) + 0.3(25) = 20.1

The reference WBGT value of 25°C for this scenario is not exceeded, i.e. heat stress in not a risk in this environment.

When the WBGT reference values are exceeded a more accurate heat stress estimate can be obtained using, for example, the required sweat rate (BS EN12515). When performing physiological monitoring (core temperature, heart rate, sweat rat, etc.) use standard ISO 9886.

Acclimatization

Acclimatization is a set of physiological adaptations. Full heat acclimatization requires up to 3wks of physical activity under the heat stress conditions expected in the work environment. During acclimatization, the ability of the body to sweat is increased and amount of sweat produced is also increased. Salt content of sweat declines avoiding sodium deficiency.

Table 1.4 WBGT reference values from BS EN 27243

	Metabolic rate, M		WBGT reference value			
Metabolic Rate class	Related to a unit skin surface area (Wm^2)	Total (for a mean skin surface area of 1.8m^2) (W)	Person acclimatized to heat ($°$C)		Person not acclimatized to heat ($°$C)	
0 (resting)	M≤65	M≤117	33		32	
1	65<M≤130	117<M≤234	30		29	
2	130<M≤200	234<M≤360	28		26	
3	200<M≤260	360<M≤468	No sensible air movement	Sensible air movement	No Sensible air movement	Sensible air movement
			25	26	22	23
4	M>260	M>468	23	25	18	20

Note: BS EN ISO 27423 does not provide correction to WBGT values for different types of personal protective equipment (PPE). See ✇ http://www.hse.gov.uk/temperature/index.htm for estimated increase in metabolic when wearing personal protective equipment.

Risk control: reducing heat strain

- *Planning of work:* e.g. maintenance work
- *Modifying the environment:* reduce process heat, improve ventilation, evaporative cooling, shield radiant heat sources
- *Worker:* medical pre-selection, acclimatization, report symptoms
- *Managerial:* monitor heat stress conditions, develop work–rest regimes, training and supervision, selection of appropriate controls
- *Protective clothing:* ice-cooled jackets, air-cooled suits.

Relevant legislation

- Workplace (Health, Safety and Welfare) Regulations (1992)
- Management of Health and Safety at Work Regulations (1999).

Further information

American Conference of Industrial Hygienists (ACGIH) (2011). Threshold limit values for chemical substances and physical agents and biological exposure indices. ACGIH, Cincinnati.

British Occupational Hygiene Society (BOHS) (1996). The Thermal Environment, BOHS Technical Guide No.12, 2nd edn. BOHS, Derby.

Parsons KC (2003). Human thermal environment, 2nd edn. Taylor & Francis, London.

Youle A (2005). The thermal environment. In: Harrington JM, Gardener K, eds, Occupational Hygiene, 3rd edn. Blackwell Science, Oxford. Available at: ✇ http://www.hse.gov.uk/temperature/index.htm indices

Thermal environment 3: Assessment of cold workplaces

Health effects and occupations

- The 1° physiological responses to cold exposure are peripheral vasoconstriction and increase in metabolic heat production by shivering
- Effects of cold include hypothermia (below 35°C), localized tissue damage, and adverse effects on performance at work. Outdoor (construction, telecommunications, maintenance of electrical power lines, agricultural and forestry, fishing industry), indoor (cold stores, meat processing) also inland and offshore work.

Risk assessment

- ISO 1574 (2008) provides methodology and practical tool for assessing and managing cold risk in the workplace. It includes checklists and questionnaires to identify individuals at risk
- The main climate factors for cold stress are air temperature and air speed. As the difference between skin and ambient temperature increases and/or the air speed increases, the rate of heat loss from exposed skin increases
- A wind chill index (equivalent chill temperature) can be calculated has for different combinations of air temperature and speed (see 📖 p. 37, Calculating the Wind Chill Index and interpretation of values)
- The equivalent chill temperature is used when estimating the combined cooling effect of wind and low air temperature on exposed skin or when determining clothing insulation requirements to maintain core temperature above 36°C. The model is based on exposed flesh, but is a useful first approximation of cold stress.

Risk control

- For exposed skin, continuous exposure should not be permitted when the equivalent chill temperature is −32°C.
- If air temperature falls below 16°C for sedentary, 4°C for light, or −7°C for moderate work, gloves should be used by workers
- If fine work is performed with bare hands for more than 20min in an environment below 16°C, provision should be made to keep hands warm
- Total body protection is required if work is performed in an environment at or below 4°C
- The ACGIH recommends that protective measures should be introduced when air temperature is less than 5°C. The equation shown here can be used to estimate the amount of clothing insulation (1 clo) required for a specific task in a given air temperature (T in °C) and metabolic rate (M in W):

  $$clo = 11.5(33 - T)/M$$

- When cold surfaces below −7°C are within reach, a warning should be given to prevent inadvertent contact with bare hands.

Calculating the Wind Chill Index and interpretation of values

• The Wind Chill Index (Twc) can be calculated using the equation:

$$Twc = 13.12 + 0.6215.Ta - 11.37.v^{0.16} + 0.3965.Ta.v^{0.16}$$

where Ta is the air temperature (°C) and V air speed (km/h).

Example
If the dry temperature is −22°C at 16 km/h then the wind chill factor = −32°C

• Twc values (°C) −10 to −24 (uncomfortably cold), −25 to −34 (very cold, risk of skin freezing), −35 to −59 (exposed skin may freeze within 10min), below −60 (exposed skin may freeze in 2min).

Relevant legislation
• Workplace (Health, Safety and Welfare) Regulations (1992)
• Management of Health and Safety at Work Regulations (1999).

Further information
ISO 15743 (2008). *Ergonomics of the thermal environment—Cold workplaces—Risk assessment and management.*
ISO 11079 (2007). *Evaluation of the thermal environment—Determination of required clothing insulation (IREQ).*
BS EN 511 (2006). *Protective gloves against cold.*

Thermal environment 4: Thermal comfort

Definition

- Thermal comfort describes the person's psychological state of mind and is defined as 'that condition of mind which expresses satisfaction with the surrounding thermal environment' (BS EN ISO 7730).
- Thermal comfort depends on a range of environmental (air temperature, humidity, air movement, and radiant heat) and personal factors (clothing insulation and metabolic heat). In workplaces, thermal discomfort may only occur when heating ventilation and air conditioning systems either break down or do not work as intended.
- Thermal comfort can affect overall morale. Complaints may increase and productivity may fall. Most problems arise when individuals are not able to adapt to their work environment. Localized discomfort can also occur, e.g. due to vertical temperature gradients.

Assessment of thermal comfort

- International Standards (BS EN ISO 7730 and BS EN ISO 10551) provide methods for predicting the general thermal sensation and degree of discomfort (thermal dissatisfaction) in indoor environments. The methods for the objective assessment of the thermal environment included in these standards are based on those proposed by Fanger (1970)[1]
- Thermal comfort is determined using calculations of predicted mean vote (PMV) and predicted percentage dissatisfied (PPD)
- The PMV is an index that predicts the mean value of the votes of a large group of persons on the 7-point thermal sensation scale (Table 1.5) and can be calculated for different metabolic rates, air temperature, air velocity, clothing insulation, and air humidity. Combinations of these parameters, which on average will provide a thermally neutral sensation, can be determined
- The PPD establishes a quantitative prediction of the percentage of thermally dissatisfied people, i.e. those who will vote hot, warm, cool, or cold on the 7-point thermal sensation scale
- The 7-point thermal sensation scale can also be used to assess and compare the actual and desired thermal sensations.

Controlling the thermal environment

A combination of engineering and administrative are required:
- *Work planning:* location of work station and scheduling of work and breaks
- *Assess the type of heating system* (hot air based, combined heat and ventilation, under floor heating, overhead heating)
- *Air movement:* consider the type and location of fan(s), reduce draft discomfort by directing ventilation or air movement
- *Air conditioning:* determine whether the unit controls air movement and humidity as well lowering air temperature. Air distribution from units should be uniform throughout the workplace

- *Assess the need for thermal insulation:* insulation type present and its effectiveness
- Use mechanical aids for physically demanding jobs
- *Allow workers to make adaptation:* clothing, temperature, etc.
- Monitor the environment thermal conditions and staff who have special requirements, e.g. pregnancy.

Table 1.5 Seven point thermal sensation scale—American Society of Heating, Refrigerating and Air-conditioning Engineers Scale (ASHRAE) scale

−3	Cold
−2	Cool
−1	Slightly cool
0	Neutral
+1	Slightly warm
+2	Warm
+3	Hot

Relevant legislation
- Workplace (Health, Safety and Welfare) Regulations (1992).
- Management of Health and Safety at Work Regulations (1999).

Further information
BS EN ISO 7730 (2005). *Ergonomic of the thermal environment—analytical determination and interpretation of thermal comfort using calculation of the PMV and PPD indices and local thermal comfort criteria.*
BS EN ISO 10551 (2001). *Ergonomics of the thermal environment—assessment of the influence of the thermal environment using subjective judgment scales.*
ASHRAE (1992). *Standard 55—thermal environmental conditions for human occupancy.* ASHRAE Inc., Atlanta.
Fanger PO (1970). *Thermal comfort.* Danish Technical Press, Copenhagen.

Chemical hazards

Chemical hazards: classification and labelling

This chapter provides information on specific hazardous substances encountered in the workplace.

Relevant legislation

- The Chemical (Hazard Information and Packaging for Supply) Regulations 2009 (known as CHIP). CHIP requires that substances and mixtures placed on the market are classified, labelled and packaged appropriately. Under CHIP, information on hazards is communicated to users by means of *symbols* and *risk phrases*.

▶ CHIP is in the process of being replaced by a new European Regulation on Classification, Labelling and Packaging of Substances and Mixtures (CLP Regulation).

- The CLP Regulation was introduced in 2009; will fully replace CHIP in June 2015. The same classification and labelling system will be used worldwide. Information on hazards will be communicated to users by *hazard symbols* and *hazard statements* (see 📖 Appendix 1).

Classification and labelling of specific substances

- Agreed classification and labelling requirements for substances are contained in Annex VI of the CLP regulation.
- In the UK, substances hazardous to health are defined under the Control of Substances Hazardous to Health (COSHH) Regulations 2002. A substance hazardous to health need not be a single substance, but also includes mixtures of compounds, micro-organisms, allergens, etc.
- A new European Law on chemicals, Registration, Evaluation, Authorization and Restriction of Chemicals (REACH), came into force on 1 June 2007 (see 📖 p. 554). Under REACH it is a requirement for manufacturers or importers of substances to register with the Central European Chemical Agency (ECHA). REACH gives greater responsibility to industry to manage the risks from chemicals and to provide safety information on substances.

For each substance reported in the following pages of this chapter:

- Only the classification and labelling according to the CLP Regs is reported, comprising hazard class and category (e.g. carc 1B, See Table 2.1) and hazard statement (e.g. H350, See 📖 Appendix 1)
- Classification and labelling entries are for 'health effects' only. Those relating to 'physicochemical properties' and 'environmental effects' are not reported here, nor are precautionary statements.

Further information

🔊 http://www.hse.gov.uk/reach/index.htm
🔊 http://www.hse.gov.uk/chip/index.htm
🔊 http://echa.europa.eu/clp_En.asp
🔊 http://echa.europa.eu/reach_En.asp
All MDHS sampling and analysis methods are available at: 🔊 http://www.hse.gov.uk/pubns/mdhs/index.htm

Classification glossary

Table 2.1 CLP regulations

Acute tox.	Acute toxicity (category 1, 2, 3, or 4)
Corr.	Skin corrosion (category 1A, 1B, or 1C)
Irrit.	Skin irritation (category 2)
Eye dam.	Serious eye damage (category 1)
Eye irrit.	Serious eye irritation (category 2)
Resp. sens	Respiratory sensitization (category 1)
Skin sens	Skin sensitization (category 1)
Muta	Germ cell mutagenicity (category 1A, 1B, or 2)
Carc	Carcinogenicity (category 1A, 1B, or 2)
Repr	Reproductive toxicity (category 1A, 1B, or 2)
STOT/SE	Specific target organ toxicity—single exposure (category 1, 2, or 3)
STOT/RE	Specific target organ toxicity—repeated exposure (category 1, 2, or 3)

Chemical hazards: sampling and analysis methods

Pollutant types

Airborne chemical pollutant types can be categorized by their physical form e.g. fumes, fibres, vapours, etc. Table 2.2 shows definitions of chemical hazard types (physical form) together with processes that generate them.

Table 2.3 provides a summary of methods for sampling and analysing common chemical pollutants types. These sampling methods are based on the Methods for the Determination of Hazardous Substances (MDHS) published by the HSE.

Table 2.3 summarizes the methods for collecting different airborne chemicals. Examples of sampling devices are shown in Fig. 2.1.

Table 2.2 Aerosol types

Type (size range)	Description	Examples: processes/substances
Gases	Formless fluids that expand to occupy the space or enclosure in which they are confined	Gases arising from electrical arc welding, accidental chemical mixing of chemicals, combustion processes, biodegradation, e.g. carbon monoxide, hydrogen sulphide, methane
Vapours	Volatile forms of substances that are normally in the solid or liquid state at room temperature and pressure	Solvents used in degreasing, cleaning, paints, vanishes, plastics and rubber manufacture, e.g. toluene, xylene, acetone, n-hexane
Dusts (1.0 to >100.0µm)	Solid particles made airborne by the mechanical disintegration of bulk solid material	Generated by cutting, handling, grinding, crushing, abrasion, and transportation
Inhalable dust (0.05–200.0µm)	Fraction of total airborne particles that are inhaled through the nose and/or mouth	Wood dust, cement dust, flour dust
Respirable dust (0.05–10.0µm)	Fraction of airborne particles that penetrate the unciliated airways of the lung (alveolar region) where gas exchange occurs. Respirable particles have a median aerodynamic diameter of ~4µm with a cut-off of 10µm	Silica, coal dust, pulverized fuel ash, ferrous foundry particles
Fumes (0.01–1.0 µm)	Formed when material from a volatilized solid condenses in cool air. The solid particles formed are extremely fine (usually <1.0 µm in diameter). In most cases the hot vapour reacts with air to form oxides	Lead oxide, iron oxide, welding, soldering, diesel, and rubber fume
Fibres	Respirable fibre is defined as a fibre >5 µm in length, with a length to width ratio of at least 3:1 and a diameter <3 µm	Asbestos or machine-made sources including glass wool, rock wool, and ceramic fibre
Smoke (0.01–1.0µm)	Aerosol of solid or liquid particles, <0.1µm in size resulting from incomplete combustion of carbonaceous materials	Carbon or soot particles
Mists (0.01–20µm)	Suspended liquid droplets generated by condensation of liquids from the vapour back to the liquid state or by breaking up a liquid into dispersed state, e.g. splashing or atomization	Acid and alkali mists, metal working fluids, paint spraying mist

Table 2.3 Sampling and analysis methods for airborne pollutant types

Type	Substance	Substrate	Sampling device	Analysis	Comments
Mists	Chromic acid mist (electroplating)	GF Filter treated with sodium hydroxide	TI sampler e.g. multi-orifice sampler (Fig. 2.1a) or IOM sampler (Fig. 2.1b)	Spectrophotometry	
	Mineral oil mist from metal working fluids	GF filter	TI sampler	Gravimetric (weigh filter before and after oil extraction with cyclohexane)	Water mix metal working fluids are analysed by measuring a suitable marker (sodium, potassium or boron) in both the air sample and the circulating fluid.
Fibres	Asbestos, Man-made mineral fibres	Membrane filter	Open face Cowl sampling head	Fibre counting by phase contrast light microscopy	For counting, a fibre is defined as >5μm in length, <3μm in width and with an aspect ratio >3:1
Particulates	Dusts, e.g. wood, cement.	GF filter	TI sampler	Gravimetric analysis	Balance must be capable of weighing ±0.01mg
	Silica	Membrane filter	Cyclone (respirable dust sampler) (Fig. 2.1c)	IRS or XRD	Choice of filter for sampling depends on the analysis technique.
	Metals e.g. chromium, nickel, zinc, lead, cadmium, iron, copper	Mixed cellulose ester membrane filter	TI or respirable sampler	Filter dissolved in acids analysis by AAS or ICP-AES or XRFS	
	Welding fume	Mixed cellulose ester membrane filter	Open face sampler	Gravimetric followed by AAS or ICP for metals	
Fumes	Rubber fume	GF filter	TI sampler	Gravimetric analysis (cyclohexane extractable fraction of filter)	

	Solder fume (resin acids)	Mixed cellulose ester membrane filter	Solder fume sampler	GC analysis of resin acids (derivatised) extracted from filter.	Fix sampling head to the sidearm of a pair of safety spectacles (Fig. 2.1d).
Organic compounds	Volatile organic compounds e.g. solvents used in paints and glues.	Solid sorbent tubes	Glass tube containing a solid sorbent, e.g. charcoal	Desorption of solvents followed by GC analysis	The choice of sorbent depends on solvent type to be sampled. Sampling for VOCs may also be conducted using diffuse samplers
	Aldehydes, e.g., formaldehyde	Chemical coated filter		HPLC analysis of filter extracted in acetonitrile	Formaldehyde can also be sampled using a diffusion badge
	Isocyanates	Chemical coated GF filter	TI sampler	HPLC with UV and electrochemical detection	The sampler used depends on the form of the isocyanate. For vapours use an impinger. For a mixture of airborne particles and vapours use impinger and the impregnated filter in series
	Pesticides	GF filter with sorbent tube to collect the more volatile pesticides	TI sampler with sorbent tube	Filter and sorbent tube desorbed in a solvent. Analysis by GC with mass spectrometry	Dermal exposure samples collected using cotton gauze swabs (set at different positions on workers outer clothing) can also be analysed by this method

GF: glass fibre; TI: total inhalable; GC: gas chromatography; HPLC: high pressure liquid chromatography; IRS: infra-red spectrometry; AAS: atomic absorption spectrometry; XRD: X-ray diffraction; ICP-AES: induced coupled plasma-atomic emission spectrometry; XRFS: X-ray fluorescence spectrophotometry.

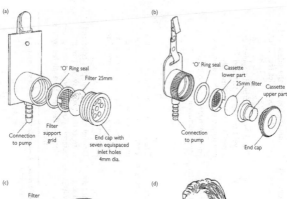

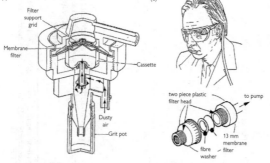

(a) Multi-orifice total inhalable sampler.
(b) IOM inhalable sampler.
(c) Cyclone respirable sampler.
(d) Sampler for rosin fume (resin acids).

Fig. 2.1 Sampling devices for collecting airborne chemical pollutants (from MDHS14/3 and MDHS 83/2, HSE Books). Material reproduced with permission from the Controller of HMSO.

Coal dust

General substance information
- Exposure to coal dust is regulated under the Coal Mines (Control of Inhalable Dust) Regulations (CIDR) 2007
- There is no allowance for the effect of respiratory protective equipment (RPE) to be taken in to account in deciding whether an exposure control limit has been exceeded
- CIDR requires control of inhalable dust exposure and compliance with exposure control limits (ECL) for respirable dust
- *ECL:* respirable dust averaged over a reference period of a working week of 40 h:
  - respirable dust 3.0mg/m³
  - quartz 0.3m/m³
- *Physical properties:* carbonaceous mineral dust with other minerals, notably crystalline silica (quartz). Quartz may comprise ≥10% of the respirable mass. Composition and physical properties (e.g. hardness) are highly variable.

CLP classification and labelling
Currently no classification.

Uses/occurrence
Exposure occurs during mining and processing of coal.

Key health effects
- *Pneumoconiosis:* the quartz content of freshly generated particles accelerates progression of the disease (see 📖 p. 54, Crystalline silica (quartz); 📖 p. 222, Silicosis)
- Emphysema and chronic bronchitis (see 📖 p. 212, Chronic obstructive pulmonary disease)
- Health surveillance is mandatory under CIDR for 'significantly exposed' workers and should include respiratory symptom questionnaires (including smoking history), spirometry and chest X-rays. Health records should be kept in a suitable form for 40yrs.

Measurement
- *MDHS 14/3* Pumped dust sample (total inhalable or respirable sampling head) on to filter, gravimetric analysis
- *MDHS 101* Pumped respirable dust sample on to filter, gravimetric analysis followed by assessment of quartz content by infrared radiation (IR) spectroscopy or X-ray diffraction (XRD)
- *Note:* need to determine the respirable quartz content of all samples unless the total respirable dust in the sample is less than the time-weighted average (TWA) exposure control limit for quartz.

HSE publications
EH59 Respirable crystalline silica. ISBN 0717614328.t
HSE L145 (2007). *The coal mines (control of inhalable dust) regulations 2007.* HSE, Sudbury. Available at: 🔗 http://www.hse.gov.uk/pubns/priced/l145.pdf
Ionizing Radiation (Medical Exposure) Regulations 2000. ISBN 0 11 099131 3.

Cotton dust

General substance information

- Cotton dust is defined by the HSE as 'the cellulose fibre that grows inside the seed pods (or bulbs) of the cotton plant'. For purposes of exposure monitoring, HSE defines cotton dust as 'the handling of raw and waste cotton including blends containing raw or waste cotton'
- The following are excluded:
  - dust from weaving, knitting, braiding, and subsequent processes
  - dust from bleached or dyed cotton
  - dust from finished articles, e.g. garments
- Occupational exposure limit (as inhalable dust): workplace exposure limit (WEL), 8h TWA of 2.5mg/m³
- Physical properties: organic fibrous matter.

CLP classification and labelling

Currently no classification.

Uses/occurrence

Manufacture of cotton and cotton-based products.

Key health effects

Byssinosis ('cotton worker's lung'), an asthma-like condition thought to be immunological in origin, although the causal agent is unknown (see 📖 p. 205, Byssinosis).

Measurement

MDHS 14/3 Pumped inhalable dust sample on to filter, gravimetric.

Flour dust

General substance information

- Defined by HSE as 'finely ground particles of cereals or pulses (including contaminants) that result from any grinding process and from any subsequent handling and use of that "flour". Any additives are included only where they have been added to the final product mix'
- Occupational exposure limit (as inhalable dust): WEL, 8h TWA of 10mg/m³; short-term exposure limit (STEL) of 30mg/m³
- Limit values are currently under review by HSE
- *Physical properties:* organic dust may be contaminated with bacterial debris.

CLP classification and labelling

Currently no classification.

Uses/occurrence

Exposure occurs widely across the food industry in bakeries and prepared foods. Key tasks include handling raw material (bagging, weighing, sieving, etc.) product mixing, production, and cleaning and maintenance.

Key health effects

Acute effects

- Eye irritation
- Irritation of mucous membranes
- *Asthma:* flour and grain dust currently account for 8% of the incidence of occupational asthma. Although not clearly understood, high short-term exposures are thought to be of significance (see 📖 p. 198).

Measurement

MDHS 14/3 Pumped inhalable dust sample on to filter, gravimetric analysis.

Grain dust

General substance information
- Defined by HSE as 'dust arising from the harvesting, drying, handling, storage or processing of wheat, oats, maize and rye, including contaminants'
- Occupational exposure limit (as inhalable dust): WEL, 8h TWA of 10mg/m^3
- *Physical properties:* organic dust may be contaminated with bacterial debris.

CLP classification and labelling
Currently no classification.

Uses/occurrence
Exposure occurs in flour mills, animal feed manufacture/handling, and the transport of bulk grain.

Key health effects
- *Acute effects:* eye irritation, irritation of mucous membranes
- *Asthma:* flour and grain dust currently account for 8% of the incidence of occupational asthma (see 📖 p. 198, Occupational asthma and rhinitis)
- Extrinsic allergic alveolitis (farmer's lung) may occur where fungal spores are present (see 📖 p. 206, Hypersensitivity pneumonitis).

Measurement
MDHS 14/3 Pumped inhalable dust sample on to filter, gravimetric analysis.

Further information
AIS3 Controlling Grain Dust on Farms. 🔊 http://www.hse.gov.uk/pubns/ais3.pdf
EH66 Grain Dust. ISBN 0717615359. 🔊 http://www.hse.gov.uk/pubns/priced/eh66.pdf
HSE (2007). The HSE Grain Dust Study workers' exposure to grain dust contaminants, immunological and clinical response. Research Report RR540.
HSE (2010). Current control standards for tasks with high exposure to grain dust. Research Report RR829.

Wood dust

General substance information

- Wood dust is designated as hardwood (from deciduous trees) or softwood (from coniferous trees)
- Occupational exposure limit, hardwood and softwood dust (as inhalable dust): WEL, 8h TWA of 5mg/m³
- Limit values are currently under review
- *Physical properties:* organic dust
- May contain other matter present in wood products, e.g. binders, coatings.

CLP classification and labelling

Currently no classification.

Uses/occurrence

Exposure may occur in any process involving the working of wood, chipboard, and fibreboard, including forestry, sawmilling, joinery, construction, and furniture making. The type of activity determines the nature of exposure (work intensity, type of dust, magnitude of exposure, and particle size distribution).

Key health effects

- *Dermatitis:* may cause contact or allergic dermatitis
- *Asthma:* many reports of asthmatic and other respiratory symptoms
- *Other respiratory effects from chronic exposure:*
  - alteration in nasal mucosa
  - reduced mucociliary clearance (furniture industry)
  - anosmia
- *Cancer:* carcinogenic risk appears to be confined to workers in the furniture industry with heavy use of hardwoods
  - excess adenocarcinoma of nose and sinus cavity
  - some evidence of excess lung cancer but confounding effects of
    (a) exposure to other occupational agents and cigarette smoke and
    (b) high historical exposures.

Measurement

MDHS 14/3 Pumped inhalable dust sample on to filter, gravimetric.

Further information

Free information Sheets including: WIS1, *Wood dust hazards and precautions*; WIS6, *COSHH and the woodworking industries*; WIS14, *Selection of respiratory protective equipment suitable for use with wood dust*; WIS24, *LEV dust capture at sawing machines*; WIS25, *LEV dust capture at fixed sanding machines*; WIS30, *Toxic woods*; WIS29, Occupational hygiene and health surveillance at industrial treatment plants. Available at: www.hse.gov.uk/pubns/

Crystalline silica (quartz)

General substance information

Occupational exposure limit
- Silica crystalline (respirable): WEL, 8h TWA of $0.1mg/m^3$. Limit to be kept under review by HSE
- Silica, amorphous, (inhalable): WEL, 8h TWA of $6.0mg/m^3$
- Silica, amorphous (respirable): WEL, 8h TWA of $2.4mg/m^3$.

CLP classification and labelling

Currently no classification.

Uses/occurrence

Most important sources of exposure are quarries, mines, ferrous foundries, construction, stone masonry, and the ceramics, heavy clay, and brick-making industries.

Key health effects

- *Silicosis:* usually slow onset over many years or 'acute silicosis' following high levels of exposure over 1–2yrs
- *Lung cancer:* IARC Group 1, carcinogenic to humans. Possible synergistic effect with smoking
- *Other respiratory effects:* some evidence that exposed workers may have an excess of tuberculosis, bronchitis, and emphysema. The role of smoking and the causal mechanisms are unclear
- *Other effects:* an excess of autoimmune, immunological, and renal disease has been reported.

Measurement

MDHS 101 Pumped respirable dust sample on to filter, analysis by IR spectroscopy or XRD.

Further information

EH75 /4. *Respirable crystalline silica: phase 1 hazard assessment*, document. ISBN 0717623747.
EH75/5. *Respirable crystalline silica: phase 2 carcinogenicity.* ISBN 0717621910.
COSHH essential in quarries. Available at: ℅ http://www.hse.gov.uk/pubns/guidance/qyseries.htm

Asbestos

General substance information

- Asbestos is a group of 'naturally occurring silicate minerals' comprising crocidolite, amosite, chrysotile, fibrous actinolite, fibrous anthophyllite, and fibrous tremolite, or mixtures containing these
- Exposure is regulated by the Control of Asbestos at Work Regulations (CAR) 2006 (see 📖 p. 540, Control of Asbestos Regulations 2006), and associated ACoPs. L143 and L127. CAR prohibits the importation, supply, and use of all form of asbestos
- *Control limits:*
  - control limit $0.1f/cm^3$ (equivalent to 0.1f/mL; all asbestos types).
  - STEL of 0.6f/mL over 10min
  - personal exposure (control) limits cover 10min and 4h periods. Exceeding a 12wk 'Action Level' triggers extra provisions under CAR including health surveillance
  - clearance sampling inside the enclosure is required after asbestos removal.

CLP classification and labelling

Carcinogen (Carc) (1A), STOT/RE (1); H350, 372.

Uses/occurrence

- Formerly lagging for pipes and boilers; cement pipes, sheets, and tiles
- Now mainly encountered in demolition and renovation operations.

Key health effects (see 📖 p. 214).

Asbestosis, mesothelioma, lung cancer.

Measurement

Surveys should be carried following the HSE guidelines
- *HSG 264:* covers survey planning, sampling, and assessment of asbestos containing materials, quality assurance, and survey reports
- *HSG248:* provides information on air and bulk asbestos sampling.

Pumped dust sample using specified cowled sampler onto filter, filter visualization by light microscopy and counting fibres of length >5μm, width <3μm, and a length/width ratio of at least 3:1.

Further information

HSE (2010). *Managing asbestos in premises: The survey guide*, HSG 264. Available at: ℘ http://www.hse.gov.uk/pubns/priced/hsg264.pdf

CAR (2006). *Work with materials containing asbestos*, ACoP and guidance L143 ISBN 978 0 7176 6206 7. (2009). *A short guide to managing asbestos in premises*, INDG223REV4. Available at: ℘ http://www.hse.gov.uk/pubns/indg223.pdf

CAR (2006). *The management of asbestos in non-domestic premises*, Reg. 4, ACOP and guidance L127, 2nd edn. ISBN 978 0 7176 6209 8. (2005). *Asbestos —The analyst's guide for sampling, analysis and clearance procedures*. Available at: ℘ http://www.hse.gov.uk/pubns/priced/hsg248.pdf

Machine-made mineral fibre

General substance information

- *Machine-made mineral fibre* (MMMF): machine-made vitreous (silicate) fibres, e.g. mineral wools (rock and glass wool) with alkaline oxide and alkali earth oxide content greater than 18% by weight. Refractory ceramic fibres and special purpose fibres have a separate WEL and classification
- *Occupational exposure limit*: WEL, 8h TWA of $5mg/m^3$ and 2 fibres/mL. except refractory ceramic fibres and special purpose fibres; WEL, 8h TWA of $5mg/m^3$ and 1 fibres/mL)
- *Physical properties*: individual fibres have a diameter of $\leq10\mu m$, with median diameter of $\sim3-4\mu m$. Majority of airborne MMMF clouds have a median diameter of $<1\mu m$

CLP classification and labelling

- MMMF: Carc (2), skin irrit (2); H351, 315
- Refractory ceramic fibres: Carc (1B), Skin irrit (2); H350i, 315.

Uses/occurrence

- MMMF materials have excellent thermal and acoustic insulation, as well as fireproofing, properties, and are widely used in commercial and residential property and in industry
- MMMF materials are highly workable, and exposure may occur during fitting or removal. Depending on the application, and whether materials are bonded or unbonded, preformed or applied *in situ*, exposure may be predominantly in the form of relatively coarse matted fragments or as respirable fibres; hence the dual WEL.

Key health effects

- *Irritant*: highly irritant to the eyes and skin
- *Cancer*: evidence for excess lung cancer is equivocal; may be partly dependent on particle size distribution.

Measurement

Gravimetric

- MDHS 14/3 Pumped inhalable or respirable dust sample on to filter, gravimetric
- Airborne fibre concentration
- MDHS 59 Pumped, non size-selective dust sample on to filter, filter visualization, fibre counting by phase- contrast light microscopy. Fibre defined as particles length $>5\mu m$, width $<3\mu m$, aspect ratio $>3:1$.

Diesel engine exhaust emissions

General substance information

- Diesel engine exhaust emissions (DEEE) are a complex mixture of gases, vapours and submicron particulate matter emitted from diesel engines
- Occupational exposure limit: none
- The German MAK value of 100µg/m^3 for elemental carbon may be useful as a guidance value
- *Physical properties:* gases include a wide range of compounds, including acrolein, formaldehyde, oxides of nitrogen, and sulphur dioxide (the latter much reduced by use of low sulphur fuel). Particulate matter is comprised of a carbonaceous core (elemental carbon) with adsorbed semi-volatile organics, including polycyclic aromatic hydrocarbons (PAHs) and hydrocarbon species (organic carbon).

CLP classification and labelling

- Currently no classification for DEEE under CLP Regulations. However, IARC classify diesel engine exhaust as carcinogenic to humans (Group 1), based on sufficient evidence that exposure is associated with an increased risk of lung cancer.
- Diesel fuel (liquid: CAS no.68334-30-5): Carc (2), Asp tox (1), Sk irrit (2), Acute tox 94). STOT RE(2); H351, 304, 325, 332, 373.

Uses/occurrence

Exposure arises from work with road vehicles (garages, test centres, bridge or motorway toll booths) and off-road vehicles (mines, manufacturing and distribution industry, construction).

Key health effects

- *Lung cancer:* plausible mechanistic basis for diesel fumes as a carcinogen, but epidemiological evidence is weak, confounded by poor exposure assessment and co-exposure to cigarette smoke and asbestos
- *Other respiratory effects:* some evidence of a cross-shift decrement in lung function
- Irritation of mucous membranes, particularly the throat.

Measurement

- It is difficult to determine which component should be measured to represent exposure to DEEE. One method favoured is to collect airborne diesel soot using a respirable cyclone sampler on to a quartz filter. The filter is then analysed for elemental carbon (EC), which is a good surrogate measure for DEEE
- Levels of carbon dioxide (CO_2) above 1000ppm 8-h TWA in the workplace, may indicate poorly maintained or faulty control systems
- Respirable dust levels can be measured to assess the particulate exposure. However, the levels measured will include particulates from all sources and not just the DEEEs. NIOSH 5040 pumped submicron sample on to filter in single-stage impactor, elemental carbon analysis.

Further information

HSE (2008). *Control of diesel engine exhaust emissions in the workplace,*, HSG187, 2nd edn. HSE, Sudbury. Available at: ✆ http://www.hse.gov.uk/pubns/priced/hsg187.pdf

Rubber process dust/fume

General substance information

- HSE have assigned functional definitions to rubber dust and fumes:
  - rubber dust—'dust arising in the stages of rubber manufacture where ingredients are handled, weighed, added to or mixed with uncured material or synthetic elastomers'
  - rubber fume is 'fume evolved in the mixing, milling and blending of natural rubber and rubber or synthetic elastomers, or of natural rubber and synthetic polymers combined with chemicals, and in the processes which convert the resultant blends into finished products or parts thereof, and including any inspection procedures where fume continues to be evolved'
- *Occupational exposure limit:*
  - *rubber process dust*—WEL, 8h TWA of 6mg/m^3
  - *rubber fume*—WEL, 8h TWA of 0.6mg/m^3; this limit relates to the cyclohexane soluble material
- Where other substances are present in the dust/fume, any WELs for such substances also applies.

CLP classification and labelling

Currently no classification for rubber fume.

Uses/occurrence

Exposure may occur in the production of vehicle tyres, components in the automotive industry and a range of other industries, footwear, and domestic appliances.

Key health effects

- *Cancer:* workers in rubber industry have a risk of excess cancers at a number of sites—bladder, lung, stomach, colon, prostate, liver, and oesophagus. There is a lack of epidemiological evidence to support a causal link at all sites. In particular, complex exposures occurring in the industry (solvents, plasticizers, accelerators, etc., in addition to polymers) are poorly characterized. Currently, IARC have concluded that 'sufficient' evidence exists only for leukaemia and bladder cancer
- *Respiratory effects:* emphysema, reduction in lung function, dyspnoea, and chest tightness have all been reported. Cases of respiratory sensitization are attributed to co-exposure to isocyanates
- *Dermatitis:* there are several reports of contact dermatitis among rubber workers. Eczema and vitiligo have also been reported
- *Reproductive effects:* studies of pregnancy outcome are inconclusive and are further limited by lack of exposure data.

Measurement

- *Rubber dust*—MDHS 14/3 Pumped inhalable dust sample on to filter, gravimetric analysis
- *Rubber fume*—MDHS 47/2 Pumped inhalable dust sample on to filter, cyclohexane extraction, gravimetric analysis.

Rosin-based solder flux fume

General substance information
- CAS No. 8050–09–7
- Occupational exposure limit. Rosin-based solder flux fume:
  - WEL, 8h TWA of $0.05mg/m^3$
  - STEL of $0.15mg/m^3$.

▶ *Note:* compliance with WELs for other components of the fume is required as appropriate (e.g. cadmium in silver soldering).

CLP classification and labelling
Currently no classification.

Uses/occurrence
Rosin (colophony) is widely used in solder fluxes in the electronics and other industries (also in paper products, adhesives, paints, varnishes, printing inks, plasticizers, cosmetics, and medical devices). Alternatives to rosin-based fluxes exist, and where these are used, the WEL is not applicable.

Key health effects
- *Asthma:* rosin is the third most common cause of occupational asthma in the UK (see 📖 p. 198, Occupational asthma and rhinitis)
- Other respiratory effects: evidence for reductions in respiratory function are equivocal
- Dermatitis (see 📖 p. 242, Dermatitis 1).

Measurement
MDHS 83/2 Measured volume of air drawn through a membrane filter in a sampling head (non-size selective). The filter is desorbed, the resin acids derivatized and then analysed by GC with FID.

Further information
INDG249 *Controlling health risks from rosin (colophony) based solder fluxes.* ISBN 0717613836. Available at: 🔗 http://www.hse.gov.uk/pubns/indg249.pdf
INDG248 REV *Solder Fume and You.* Available at: 🔗 http://www.hse.gov.uk/pubns/indg248.pdf
ES31. *Cadmium in silver soldering.* Available at: 🔗 http://www.hse.gov.uk/pubns/eis31.pdf
WL17. *Soldering: Hand-held with lead-based, rosin–cored solders.* 🔗 http://www.hse.gov.uk/pubns/guidance/wl17.pdf

Welding fume

General substance information

- CAS No. 8050-09-7
- *Occupational exposure limit:* none for total welding fume

▶ Compliance with WELs for components of the fume (metals and inorganic gases) is required as appropriate (e.g. Cr^{VI}, Ni, Mn, O3).
- Check WELs for fume components.

CLP classification and labelling

Currently no classification.

Uses/occurrence

- The most important substrates are mild and stainless steel, and their alloys, and aluminium and its alloys. The main types of welding are:
  - manual metal arc (MMA)
  - flux cored arc (FCA)
  - metal inert gas (MIG)
  - tungsten inert gas (TIG)
- The composition of fume is influenced by the many process factors including material to be welded, composition of the consumable electrode /flux and the welding technique. In general, MMA and FCA are more likely to produce high levels of fume than MIG or TIG welding. The most important applications are in engineering (e.g. boiler, tank, and vessel assembly), shipbuilding, and construction.

Key health effects

- *Lung cancer:* welding of stainless steel has been associated with an increased risk of lung cancer. However, HSE consider there is no significant risk under present conditions, i.e. in the absence of high historical exposures
- *Asthma:* mainly due to welding stainless steel (exposure to Cr^{VI})
- Chronic obstructive pulmonary disease
- *Acute effects:* irritation of eyes and throat, tightness in the chest at higher exposures, metal fume fever
- *Asphyxia:* asphyxiant properties of inert shield gases (Argon) in confined spaces should also be considered in MIG and TIG welding.

Measurement

BS EN ISO 10882–1:2011 Sampling of air borne particles (welding fume).

Further information

HSG204. *Health and safety in arc welding.* ISBN 0717618137.
INDG297. *Safety in gas welding, cutting and similar processes.* ISBN 9780717624737. Available at: ℘ http://www.hse.gov.uk/pubns/indg297.pdf
Guidance on welding techniques and control measures. Available at: ℘ http://www.hse.gov.uk/welding/guidance/index.htm

Oil mist (metal working fluids)

General substance information
- Metal working fluids (MWFs) are neat oils or water-based fluids used for lubrication and cooling when machining metals
- *Occupational exposure limit:* currently no classification
- *Physical properties:* variable composition and viscosity.

CLP classification and labelling
Currently no classification.

Uses/occurrence
Exposure to MWFs occurs via inhalation, through direct contact with unprotected skin, and through cuts and abrasions. The cutting operation may generate a mist from the fluid, and splashes may result in dermal exposure. Exposure to micro-organisms, including endotoxins, and anti-microbials may also occur.

Key health effects
- *Dermatitis:* irritant and allergic contact dermatitis have been widely reported in exposed workers (see 📖 p. 242, Dermatitis 1)
- *Cancer:* excess cancers of the larynx, rectum, pancreas, skin, scrotum, and bladder have been reported in exposed workers. However, high historical dermal and inhalation exposures have now been reduced because of improved control methods and the use of highly refined MWFs that are much reduced in carcinogenic substances (e.g. polycyclic aromatic hydrocarbons)
- *Respiratory conditions:* asthma, extrinsic allergic alveolitis, chronic bronchitis, and acute airway irritation have all been reported (see 📖 p. 198, Occupational asthma and rhinitis, 📖 p. 206, Hypersensitivity pneumonitis).

Measurement
- *Mineral oil-based MWFs of viscosity greater than 18mm2/s—MDHS 84* Pumped inhalable sample on to filter, gravimetric (after subtraction of cyclohexane soluble matter)
- *Water-mix MWFs—MDHS 95/2 (elemental marker method)* Airborne inhalable pumped sample (collected on a filter) and a sample of oil (from sump) are both analysed using a suitable marker (sodium, potassium or boron) by, atomic absorption spectroscopy (AAS) or inductively coupled plasma spectrometry (ICP).

Further information
INDG365 *Working Safely with Metalworking Fluids. A Guide for Employees.* Available at: ⅍ http://www.hse.gov.uk/pubns/indg365.pdf

Outbreak of respiratory disease at Power Train Ltd, Birmingham. Available at: ⅍ http://www.hse.gov.uk/metalworking/experience/powertrain.pdf

MW1. *Mist control-inhalation risk.* Available at: ⅍ http://www.hse.gov.uk/pubns/guidance/mw01.pdf

MW2. *Fluid control: skin risk.* Available at: ⅍ http://www.hse.gov.uk/pubns/guidance/mw02.pdf

Aluminium

General substance information
- CAS No. 7429–90–5
- Occupational exposure limit
  - *aluminium metal and oxides in inhalable dust*—WEL, 8h TWA of 10mg/m³
  - *aluminium metal and oxides in respirable dust*—WEL, 8h TWA of 4mg/m³
  - *aluminium alkyl compounds and soluble aluminium salts*—WEL, 8h TWA of 2mg/m³
- *Physical properties:* silver malleable metal, mp = 661°C, bp = 2467°C.

CLP classification and labelling
- Aluminum alkyl compounds: skin corr (1B); H314
- Aluminium powder (stabilized): no classification for health effects.

Uses/occurrence
- Occurs mainly as alumina or bauxite (Al_2O_3)
- Workers exposed during extraction and refining of ores and during electrolytic reduction of alumina
- Aluminum powder produced by atomization in air/ inert gas
- Used in manufacture of alloys, engine and aircraft components, window frames, roofs, food containers, and electrical wires and cables
- Also used as a powder in protective paints and coating. Aluminum can be electrically coated and dyed by anodic coating.

Key health effects
Aluminium metal Interstitial fibrosis of lungs associated with repeated exposure.

Measurement
- MDHS for other metals may be suitable
- *Alternative method*—NIOSH 7300 Pumped inhalable dust sample on to filter, acid digestion, ICPAES.

Arsenic

General substance information
- CAS No. arsenic metal 7440–38–2
- *Occupational exposure limit:* arsenic and its inorganic compounds, except arsine (as As)—WEL, 8h TWA of 0.1mg/m^3
- *Physical properties:*
  - occurs mostly in compounds of trivalent (e.g. As_2O_3) or pentavalent (As_2O_5) form
  - arsenic compounds occur in a range of physical forms (crystalline, powder, etc.)
  - pure arsenic sublimes at 613°C.

CLP classification and labelling
- Arsenic oxides: H350, 300, 314
- Arsenic and some other compounds: acute tox (3); H331, 301.

Uses/occurrence
- Impurity in ores of other metals, such as lead, zinc and copper
- Major use is as a wood preservative (e.g. chromated copper arsenate)
- Former use as a pesticide has now declined
- Used in lead (and some other) alloys
- Manufacture of semiconductors
- Contaminant in drinking water in many countries.

Key health effects
- Cancer of respiratory tract
- Cancer of skin and liver
- Irritant and allergic dermatitis
- Irritation of eyes and upper respiratory tract
- Perforation of nasal septum
- Severe haemorrhagic gastritis associated with ingestion of soluble arsenic compounds; may result in death.

Measurement
- *MDHS 41/2* Pumped inhalable dust sample on to filter and back-up pad, derivatization to hydride, analysis by AAS
- Pumped inhalable dust sample on to filter, analysis by X-ray fluorescence spectroscopy (XRF (MDHS 91) or by ICP-AES (MDHS 99))
- Arsenic in urine (sample at the end of work week).

Further information
EH73. *Arsenic and its compounds. health hazards and precautionary measures.* ISBN 0717613402.
MDHS 41/2. *Arsenic and inorganic compounds of arsenic (except arsine) in air.* ISBN 071761008X.
MSA8. *Arsenic and you* (free).

Beryllium

General substance information

- CAS No. 7440–41–7
- *Occupational exposure limit:* beryllium and beryllium compounds (as Be)—WEL, 8h; TWA, 0.002mg/m^3
- *Physical properties:* hard white metal; its utility arises from the combination of lightness and rigidity; mp = 1287 °C, bp = 2475 °C.

CLP classification and labelling

Carc (1B), acute tox (2), eye/skin irrit (2), skin sensitivity (Sen.) (1); H350i, 330, 301, 372, 319, 335, 315, 317.

Uses/occurrence

- Used in specialist structural and component applications in the aerospace and nuclear industries
- Hardening agent in alloys (copper, nickel)
- Electronics and computer industries.

Key health effects

- Pulmonary clearance of inhaled beryllium is slow (months to years for sparingly soluble compounds)
- Acute beryllium disease affecting lungs (pneumonitis, alveolitis, dyspnoea, fever), sometimes resulting in chronic fibrosis
- Chronic beryllium disease (CBD), a granulomatous disorder affecting lungs and skin, caused by cell-mediated sensitization to beryllium
- CBD symptoms include wheezing, dry cough, dyspnoea, fatigue and weight-loss
- Sub-clinical CBD can occur, with microscopic granulomas occurring in the lungs
- Possibility of cancer, based on animal evidence.

Measurement

- Pumped inhalable dust sample on to filter, acid digestion, analysis by flame and electrothermal AAS (MDHS 29/2, ICP-AES (MDHS 99)
- *Beryllium biomarker* Blood beryllium lymphocyte proliferation (BeLPT).

Further information

INDG311. *Beryllium and you* (free).

EH13. *Beryllium. health hazards and precautions.* ISBN 0717608247.

HSE (2011). *Beryllium. A review of the health effects and evidence for screening or surveillance in work-ers exposed to beryllium.* Research Report 873, HSE, Sudbury.

Cadmium

General substance information

- CAS No. Cadmium metal 7440–43–9
- *Occupational exposure limit:*
  - *cadmium and cadmium compounds* (as Cd), WEL, 8h; TWA of 0.025mg/m^3
  - *cadmium oxide fume* (as Cd)—WEL, 8h TWA of 0.025mg/m^3; STEL of 0.05mg/m^3
  - *cadmium sulphide and cadmium sulphide pigments* (as Cd)—WEL, 8h TWA of 0.03mg/m^3
- *Physical properties:* malleable and ductile soft white metal, mp = 321°C, bp=776°C.

CLP classification and labelling

Cadmium and cadmium oxide Carc (1B), Muta (2), reproductive toxin (Repr) (2), acute tox (2); H350, 341, 361fd, 330.

Uses/occurrence

- Nickel cadmium battery production
- Alloyed with other metals for use in electrical cables, solders, and fire-detection systems
- Metal coating, pigments, and stabilizers
- Exposure can occur during heating and welding of metals containing cadmium.

Key health effects

- Cadmium is excreted very slowly, accumulating in liver and kidneys
- Inhalation exposure causes metal fume fever and pulmonary oedema
- Kidney damage may be caused by repeated inhalation of all forms of cadmium (mainly tubular dysfunction, characterized by proteinuria; glomerular damage, glycosuria, aminoaciduria and renal stones)
- Repeated exposure to cadmium may cause severe lung damage (emphysema, loss of lung function and radiographic abnormalities)
- Possibility of cancer, based on animal evidence (for cadmium oxide, chloride, and sulphate)
- Impaired fertility and effects on foetus (for cadmium chloride).

Measurement

- Pumped inhalable dust sample on to filter, acid digestion, analysis by flame or electrothermal AAS(MDHS 10/2), or XRF (MDHS91) or inductively coupled plasma atomic emission spectrometry (ICP-AES (MDHS 99))
- Cadmium in blood or urine (sampling time not critical).

Further information

INDG391REV1 *Cadmium and You* (free) ISBN 9780717663972.
EIS31 *Cadmium in Silver Soldering and Brazing* (free).
EH1 *Cadmium health and safety precautions* (1995) ISBN 0717608255.

Chromium

General substance information

- CAS No. Chromium metal 7440–47–3
- *Occupational exposure limit:*
  - *chromium (VI) and compounds (as Cr)*—WEL, 8h TWA 0.05mg/m³
  - *chromium metal and chromium (II) and (III) compounds (as Cr)*—WEL, 8h TWA of 0.5mg/m³
- Biological monitoring guidance value: chromium (VI) (as Cr)—10μmol chromium/mol creatinine in urine (post shift)
- *Hazard classification and risk phrases:*
  - *chromium (VI)*—Carc, Sen
  - *chromium metal and chromium (II) and (III) compounds*—none
- *Physical properties:* hard brittle silver metal, extremely resistant to corrosion, mp = 1907°C, bp = 2671°C.

CLP classification and labelling

- Chromium (VI) trioxide: Carc (1A), Muta (1B), Repr (2), acute tox (2), skin corr (1A), resp/skin sens (1); H350, 340, 361f, 330, 311, 301, 372, 314, 334, 317
- Potassium dichromate: Carc (1B), Muta (1B), Repr (1B), acute tox (2), STOT/RE (1), skin corr (1B), resp/skin sen (1); H350, 340, 360FD, 330, 301, 372, 312, 314, 334, 317.

Uses/occurrence

- *Major use:* production of stainless steel with downstream users, particularly welders, potentially exposed
- Metallurgy is (as chromates) in electroplating
- Production of paint, pigments, corrosion inhibitors, and wood preservatives, and in the tanning and textile industries.

Key health effects

Adverse health effects are mainly from chromium (VI) compounds:
- *Acute:* irritation of upper respiratory tract, skin, eyes
- *Chronic:* lung cancer; skin and respiratory sensitization, nasal corrosion (septum perforation), kidney and lung damage, ↓ fertility, foetal toxicity.

Measurement

- Pumped inhalable dust sample on to filter, acid digestion, analysis by AAS (MDHS 12/2) or XRF (MDHS 91) or ICP-AES (MDHS99)
- Total chromium in urine (end of shift at end of work week) for soluble chromium compounds.

Further information

INDG346 *Chromium and you.* ℅http://www.hse.gov.uk/pubns/indg346.pdf

Cobalt

General substance information
- CAS No. Cobalt metal 7440–48–4
- *Occupational exposure limit.* Cobalt and cobalt compounds (as Co): WEL, 8h TWA of 0.1mg/m^3
- *Physical properties:* silver-white metal, mp = 1495°C, bp = 2870°C.

CLP classification and labelling
- Cobalt: resp/skin sens (1); H334, 317
- Cobalt dichloride and sulphate: Carc (1B), acute tox (4), resp/skin sens (1); H350i, 302, 334, 317.

Uses/occurrence
- Manufacture of hard alloys (super alloys) for heavy engineering and aerospace applications
- Production of ceramics, paint, glass magnets, and catalytic converters
- Production of hard metals (tools for cutting and grinding).

Key health effects
- *Skin sensitization:* humans with nickel sensitivity are predisposed to cobalt sensitivity
- *Respiratory sensitization:* leading to asthmatic response at very low exposure levels
- *Diffuse interstitial pulmonary fibrosis:* also associated with repeated exposure
- Short-term gastrointestinal (GI) effects following ingestion.

Measurement
- Pumped inhalable dust sample on to filter, acid digestion, analysis by AAS (MDHS 30/2) or XRF (MDHD 91) or ICP-AES (MDHS 99)
- Cobalt in urine or blood (end of shift at end of work week).

Further information
MSA17. *Cobalt and You* (free). Available at: ℞ http://www.hse.gov.uk/pubns/msa17.htm
EH68. *Cobalt. Health and Safety Precautions.* ISBN 0717608239.

Copper

General substance information

- CAS No. 7440–50–8
- *Occupational exposure limit:*
  - *in dust and mists (as Cu)*—WEL, 8h TWA of 1mg/m³; STEL of 2mg/m³
  - *copper fume*—WEL, 8h TWA of 0.2mg/m³
- *Physical properties:* reddish-brown, malleable, and ductile metal, mp = 1083°C, bp = 2595°C.

CLP classification and labelling

- Copper sulphate: acute tox (4), eye/skin irrit (2); H302, 319, 315
- Copper (I) chloride, oxide: acute tox (4); H302.

Uses/occurrence

- *Major uses:*
  - smelting and refining of copper
  - production of copper and copper alloy products for electrical cables
  - materials for the construction and water distribution industries.
- *Other uses:*
  - production of copper chemicals and powders
  - piping and plumbing
  - electroplating
  - coinage
  - antifouling agent on boat hulls
  - pigment in paints and glass.

Key health effects

- Copper is an essential element and effects may arise as a result of deficiency
- Acute oral toxicity characterized by GI symptoms, with nausea being the earliest symptom
- Eye irritation (copper (I) oxide and copper sulphate)
- Hepatotoxicity associated with long-term oral intake; also effects on kidney and GI tract
- Exposure to freshly-formed copper oxide fume has been linked to the occurrence of flu-like symptoms (metal fume fever).

Measurement

Pumped inhalable dust sample on to filter, analysis by XRF (MDHS 91) or ICP-AES (MDHS 99).

Iron

General substance information
- CAS No. Iron metal 7439–89–6
- *Occupational exposure limit:*
  - *iron oxide (Fe2O3) fume (as Fe)*—WEL, 8h; TWA of 5mg/m³; STEL of 10mg/m₃
  - *iron salts (as Fe)*—WEL, 8h; TWA, 1mg/m³; STEL 2mg/m³
  - *ferrous foundry particulate (FFP)*—WEL, 8h; TWA of 10mg/m³ (total inhalable dust) and 4mg/m³ (respirable dust). (*Note:* FFP is a surrogate for exposure in ferrous foundries, but components of FFP also have individual WELs)
- *Physical properties:* silver-white metal, mp = 1535°C, bp = 2750°C.

CLP classification and labelling
None.

Uses/occurrence
- Exposure may occur in smelting/refining of iron and production of steel and other alloys
- Exposure to iron oxide fume may arise during flame cutting of iron or its alloys
- Iron oxide is widely used as a pigment in paint, stains, plastics, construction materials, and ceramics
- In coarse form (rouge) it is used as a polishing material in the jewellery trade
- Iron salts are used as a flocculant in waste-water treatment, the dyeing of textiles, and the production of fertilizer and feed additives.

Key health effects
- Iron is an essential element and effects may arise as a result of deficiency
- Acute iron poisoning associated with accidental ingestion (vomiting, metabolic acidosis, liver and kidney damage); mainly in children
- Chronic iron toxicity associated with hereditary malabsorption condition (haemochromatosis) or excessive dietary intake (haemosiderosis in liver, spleen, heart, and endocrine organs)
- Effects on lungs (fibrosis) caused by long-term inhalation of iron oxide fumes or dust.

Measurement
Pumped dust sample on to filter, analysis by XRF (MDHS 91) or ICP-AES (MDHDS 99).

Lead

General substance information

- Exposure to lead is regulated under the Control of Lead at Work Regulations 2002 (CLAW). Statutory airborne exposure and biological monitoring values apply
- CAS No. 7439–92–1
- *Occupational exposure limit:* WEL, 8h TWA all lead (except lead alkyls), 0.15mg/m³; lead alkyls, 0.10mg/m³
- *Biological monitoring:* 3 threshold levels are indicated in the CLAW Regulations (see 📖 p. 538, Control of Lead at Work Regulations 2002):
  - a level at which health surveillance is required
  - 'action level': exposure should be reduced
  - 'suspension level': individual must be removed from exposure
- *Physical properties:* soft, malleable silver-grey metal, mp = 327°C, bp = 1740°C.

CLP classification and labelling

- Lead alkyls: Repr (1A), acute tox (1), STOT/RE (2); H360Df, 330, 310, 300, 373
- Other lead compounds (excluding azide, acetate and chromate): Repr (1A), acute tox (4), STOT/RE (2); H360Df, 332, 302, 373.

Uses/occurrence

- Extraction of lead from its ore (lead sulphide) and melting of scrap lead (2° smelting)
- Manufacture of lead acid batteries, lead compounds, and paints
- Production of solder, ceramics, glass, pigments, and ammunition
- Organic lead (alkyls) added to petrol as an anti-knocking agent
- Exposure during blast removal, stripping and burning of lead paint; hot cutting in demolition work; breaking and recycling lead batteries.

Key health effects

- *Haematological:* anaemia, reticulocytosis, basophilic stippled red cells
- Encephalopathy, peripheral neuropathy
- Renal toxicity (tubular damage and interstitial fibrosis)
- Effects on GI tract (colic)
- Reduced fecundity in males, impaired fetal neurological development.

Measurement

- Pumped inhalable dust sample on filter, acid digestion, analysis by flame or electrothermal AAS (MDHS 6/3) or XRF (91) or ICP-AES (99).
- *Biological monitoring:* lead (inorganic)—blood, zinc protoporphyrin (ZPP), ALA. Lead (organic)—urine (end of shift, end of working week).

Further information

L132. *Control of lead at work. Control of lead at Work Regulations 2002.* ACoP and guidance, (3rd edn. ISBN 9780717625659.

INDG305REV1. *Lead and you* (free). ISBN 9780717663873. Available at: 🔗 http://www.hse.gov.uk/pubns/indg305.pdf

Manganese

General substance information
- CAS No. Manganese metal 7439–96–5
- *Occupational exposure limit:* manganese and its inorganic compounds (as Mn)—WEL, 8h TWA of 0.5mg/m^3
- *Physical properties:* hard brittle grey-white metal found in mainly crystalline form, mp = 1244°C, bp = 1962°C.

CLP classification and labelling
- Manganese dioxide: acute tox (4); H332, 302.
- Manganese sulphate: STOT/RE (2); H373.

Uses/occurrence
- *Major use:* production of stainless and carbon steel
- Manganese compounds have various uses in the production of batteries, fertilizers, ceramics, and glass
- Exposure occurs during refining of ore, smelting and fabrication operations
- Welding (steel).

Key health effects
- Central nervous system effects associated with repeated exposure by inhalation; early signs include sleepiness and weakness in legs
- Historically, effects on lungs (pneumonitis) were associated with chronic exposure, although recent studies provide no evidence of this.

Measurement
Pumped inhalable dust sample on to filter, analysis by XRF MDHS91) or ICP-AES (MDHS 99).

Mercury

General substance information
- CAS No. 7439–97–6
- No WEL (EH40)
- Biological monitoring guidance value: 20µmol mercury/mol creatinine in urine (random sampling)
- *Physical properties:* silver coloured liquid metal, mp = −39°C, bp = 357°C.

CLP classification and labelling
- Mercury (elemental): acute tox (3), STOT/RE (2); H331, 373
- Some organic and inorganic mercury compounds: acute tox (1), STOT/RE (2); H330, 310, 300, 373.

Uses/occurrence
- Used as an electrode in the electrolytic production of chlorine from sodium hydroxide (chloro-alkali process).
- Widely used in thermometers, barometers, and batteries
- Use in dental amalgam is in decline
- Production of fungicides, biocides, and antifouling paints.

Key health effects
- Irritation of respiratory tract associated with short-term exposure to Hg vapours
- Effects on central nervous system (psychomotor effects)
- Renal toxicity (tubular damage).

Treatment
See 📖 p. 804, Mercury poisoning, for management of acute poisoning.

Measurement
- MDHS 16/2 Sampling:
  - *mercury vapour*—passive (badge) sampling *or* pumped sampling on to sorbent tube
  - *particulate mercury*—pumped sampling on to filter mounted in inhalable sampler; back-up sorbent tube if vapour also present
- Analysis by cold vapour atomic absorption spectroscopy
- *Biological monitoring:*
  - usually based on measuring total inorganic mercury in urine (cumulative exposure)
  - total inorganic mercury blood levels (acute exposure).

Nickel

General substance information

- CAS No. Nickel metal 7440–48–4
- *Occupational exposure limit:* nickel and its inorganic compounds.
  - water-soluble compounds (as Ni): WEL, 8h TWA of 0.1mg/m^3
  - metal and insoluble compounds (as Ni), 8h TWA of 0.5mg/m^3
- *Physical properties:* hard ductile silvery metal, resistant to corrosion, mp = 1453°C, bp = 2752°C
- Nickel tetracarbonyl is a gaseous metal compound.

CLP classification and labelling

- Nickel: H351, 317
- Nickel oxides and sulphides: H350, 317
- *Nickel sulphate:* H351, 302, 334, 317
- *Nickel tetracarbonyl:* Carc (2), Repr (1B), acute tox (3); H351, 360D, 330.

Uses/occurrence

- Used mainly in stainless steel alloys. Alloys with other metals include copper, aluminum and silver
- Also used in electroplating, as a catalyst and in the production of nickel compounds, rechargeable batteries, and coins
- Exposure occurs when welding and grinding nickel containing metal alloys.

Key health effects

- Nickel metal and insoluble salts are retained in the lung
- Soluble nickels salts may also be absorbed through the skin
- Skin and respiratory sensitization
- Cancer of the lungs and nasal sinuses
- Fibrosis of lungs, with loss of pulmonary function.

Measurement

Pumped inhalable dust sample on to filter, acid digestion, analysis by flame or electrothermal AAS (MDHS 42/2) or XRF (MDHS 91) or ICP-AES (MDHS 99).

Further information

INDG351. *Nickel and You* (free). Available at: 🔗 http:www.hse.gov.uk/pubns/indg351.pdf

Nickel and nickel alloy plating operations: controlling the risk of inhaling mist containing nickel. Available at: 🔗 www.hse.gov.uk/surfaceengineering/nickelinhalation.pdf

EH60. *Nickel and its inorganic compounds. health hazards and precautionary methods.* ISBN 0717613420.

Vanadium

- Vanadium is an essential element
- Inhalation is the main route of entry
- Vanadium compounds are poorly absorbed through the GI system and rapidly excreted in the urine.

General substance information

- CAS No. Vanadium pentoxide 1314–62–1
- Occupational exposure limit. Vanadium pentoxide: WEL, 8h TWA of $0.05mg/m^3$
- Physical properties: soft ductile gray-white metal; good resistance to corrosion by acids and alkalis.

CLP classification and labelling

Vanadium pentoxide Muta (2), Repr (2), STOT/RE (1), acute tox (4), STOT/ SE (3); H341, 361d, 372, 332, 302, 335.

Uses/occurrence

- Vanadium occurs in different minerals such as patronite (VS_4)
- Also present in carbon-containing deposits such as crude oil and oil shale. The ash from oils may be rich in vanadium and is a hazard for industrial furnace and boiler cleaners.
- Approximately 80% of vanadium produced is used as ferrovanadium, in the production of steel alloys
- Vanadium salts are used as catalysts in the manufacture of glass, dyes, inks, and pesticides
- Exposure also occurs during refining and manufacture of steel alloys.

Key health effects

- Effects include irritation of the eyes, skin, and respiratory tract, and GI disturbances
- Workers may complain of metallic taste and there may be a greenish discoloration of tongue (indication of exposure rather than toxicity)
- The key health effects of concern for vanadium pentoxide are mutagenicity and respiratory tract toxicity

Measurement

- Vanadium can be collected on a cellulose ester filter and analysed by ICP-AES (MDHS 99)
- Oxides of vanadium can be analysed by XRD after collection (total inhalable fraction) on a PVC membrane filter.

Zinc

General substance information

- CAS No. Zinc metal 7440–66–6
- *Occupational exposure limit:*
  - zinc chloride fume—WEL, 8h TWA of 1mg/m³; STEL of 2mg/m³
  - zinc distearate inhalable dust—WEL, 8h TWA, 10mg/m³; STEL, of 20mg/m³. Respirable dust: WEL 8h TWA, 4mg/m³
- *Physical properties:* hard, brittle, and lustrous bluish-white metal, mp = 420°C, bp = 907°C.

CLP classification and labelling

- Zinc powder (stabilized): no classification for health effects
- *Zinc chloride fume:* acute tox (4), skin corr (1B); H302, 314
- Zinc sulphate: acute tox (4), eye damage (1); H302, 318.

Uses/occurrence

- Major uses of zinc metal are in galvanizing and the production of batteries, die castings, and construction materials
- Many zinc alloys are of industrial importance, principally those with copper (brass), tin, lead, and aluminium
- Zinc chloride is used in soldering flux, as a battery electrolyte, and in textiles, wood preservatives, and medical products
- Uses of zinc distearate include the manufacture of plastics and pharmaceuticals.

Key health effects

- Zinc is an essential trace element and effects may arise as a result of deficiency
- Metal-fume fever, a transient acute condition associated with exposure to freshly formed fumes of zinc oxide (and some other metals); characterized by fever, chills, dyspnoea, nausea, and fatigue, which occur several hours after exposure.

Measurement

Pumped sampling on to filter in inhalable/respirable sampling head, analysis by ICP-AES (MDHS 99).

Acetone

General substance information
- CAS No. 67–64–1. Formula CH_3COCH_3
- Occupational exposure limit: WEL, 8h TWA of 1210mg/m³ (500ppm); STEL of 3620mg/m³ (1500ppm)
- Physical properties: colourless liquid, water-soluble liquid, mp = −94°C, bp = 56°C.

CLP classification and labelling
Eye irrit (2), STOT/SE (2); H319, 336.

Uses/occurrence
- Used in polymer synthesis in the plastics, textile, and pharmaceutical industries
- Widely used as a solvent in manufacturing, in paint, inks, varnishes, and other coatings, and in cleaning materials
- Some use in consumer products, e.g. nail varnish remover.

Key health effects
- Irritation of eyes and respiratory tract
- Central nervous system (CNS) effects.

Measurement
- *MDHS 96* Pumped solid sorbent tubes, solvent desorption, analysis by gas chromatography (GC)
- *MDHS 72* Pumped sorbent tubes, thermal desorption, GC
- *MDHS 88* Diffusive sorbent samplers, solvent desorption, GC
- Biological monitoring: acetone in urine (sampling time end of shift).

Acid anhydrides (cyclic anhydrides)

General substance information
- *Phthalic anhydride:*
  - *CAS No. 85–44–9*—formula $C_8H_4O_3$
  - *occupational exposure limit*—WEL, 8h TWA of 4mg/m³; STEL of 12mg/m³
  - *physical properties*—white crystalline solid, mp = 131°C, bp = 295°C
- *Trimellitic anhydride:*
  - *CAS No. 552–30–7*—formula $C_9H_4O_5$
  - *occupational exposure limit*—WEL, 8h TWA of 0.04mg/m³; STEL of 0.12mg/m³
  - *physical properties*—white crystalline solid, mp = 165–169°C
- *Acetic anhydride:*
  - *CAS No. 108–24–7*—formula $(CH_3CO)_2O$
  - *occupational exposure limit*—WEL, 8h TWA of 2.5mg/m³; STEL of 10mg/m³
  - *physical properties*—colourless liquid with a pungent odour, mp = −73°C, bp = 138–140°C.

CLP classification and labelling
- Phthalic anhydride: acute tox (4), STOT/SE (3), skin irrit (2), eye dam (1), resp/skin sens (1); H302, 335, 315, 318, 334, 317
- Trimellitic anhydride: STOT/SE (3), eye dam (1), resp/skin sens (1); H335, 318, 334, 317
- Acetic anhydride: acute tox (4), skin corr (1B); H332, 302, 314.

Uses/occurrence
Cyclic acid anhydrides are a group of reactive chemicals that are used as curing agents and plasticizers in the production of epoxy resins, a range of polymers, chemicals, dyes, and pesticides. At room temperature cyclic anhydrides are powders. The most abundant chemicals are listed here.

Key health effects
- Irritation of eyes and respiratory tract
- Occupational asthma and rhinitis
- Sensitization of the skin.

Measurement
MDHS 62 Carboxylic acid anhydrides in dust and fume measured by pumped sampling on to a glass fibre filter with a sorbent (tenax) back-up tube. During desorption, acid anhydrides are converted to the corresponding acids, analysis by high-performance liquid chromatography (HPLC).

Acrylamide

General substance information
- *CAS No. 79–06–1:* formula $H_2C=CHCON=H_2$
- *Occupational exposure limit:* WEL, 8h TWA of 0.3mg/m^3
- *Physical properties:* white crystalline solid, soluble, mp = 84–85°C, bp = 125°C.

CLP classification and labelling
Carc (1B), Muta (1B), Repr (2), acute tox (3), STOT/RE (1), eye/skin irrit (2), skin sens (1); H350, 340, 361f, 301, 372, 332, 312, 319, 315, 317.

Uses/occurrence
Used in the synthesis of polyacrylamides which are used in the treatment of drinking water and waste water, paper industry, metal ore processing, dye, adhesive and textile manufacturing, as an oil recovery agent in the oil industry, and in construction.

Health effects
- Irritation of the skin
- Neurotoxicity; symptoms include fatigue, muscle weakness, numbness of extremities, and other sensory effects
- Possibility of cancer, based on animal studies
- May cause adverse effects in offspring.

Measurement
MDHS 57 Acrylamide in air—collection of pumped sample into a Midget Impinger (containing water), analysis by HPLC.

Acrylonitrile

General substance information
- CAS No. 107–13–01. Formula $H_2C=CHCN$
- Occupational exposure limit: WEL, 8h TWA of 4.4mg/m^3 (2ppm). Limit values are currently under review by HSE
- Physical properties: colourless, soluble liquid, mp = −83°C, bp = 77°C.

CLP classification and labelling
Carc (1B), acute tox (3), STOT/SE (3), skin irrit (2), eye dam (1), skin sens (1); H350, 331, 311, 301, 335, 315, 318, 317.

Uses/occurrence
- Major use in the synthesis of acrylic co-polymers in the textile industry
- Used in the manufacture of acrylonitrile-butadiene-styrene (ABS) rubber, plastics, and in the production of acrylamide and other chemical intermediates.

Key health effects
- Acrylonitrile is a suspected carcinogen, based on animal studies
- Dermatitis may result from prolonged or repeated skin contact
- Central nervous system effects (headache, nausea, fatigue)
- Diarrhoea and jaundice
- Respiratory tract irritation
- Simultaneous exposure to some other organic solvents may enhance acrylonitrile toxicity.

Measurement
- Pumped sorbent tubes, followed by either thermal or solvent desorption, analysis by GC (MDHS 96, MDHS 72)
- Diffusive sorbent samplers, followed by solvent or thermal desorption, analysis by GC (MDHS 80 and 88).

Benzene

General substance information
- *CAS No. 71–43–2:* formula C_6H_6
- *Occupational exposure limit:* WEL, 8h TWA of 1ppm
- *Physical properties:* colourless liquid, slightly soluble in water, mp = −6°C, bp = 80°C. The main natural source of benzene is crude oil.

CLP classification and labelling
Carc (1A); Muta (1B), STOT/RE (1), Asp tox (1), eye/skin irrit (2); H350, 340, 372, 304, 319, 315.

Uses/occurrence
- Used in the synthesis of other organic compounds (e.g. styrene, phenol, aniline) and the synthesis of polymers used in the manufacture of plastics, resins, and textiles
- Also used in tyre and shoe manufacturing
- Exposure occurs mainly in petroleum industry
- Benzene also found in cigarette smoke

▶ Benzene is no longer used as a general solvent because of its high toxicity.

Key health effects
Effects on blood and blood-forming tissues (anaemia, leukaemia, and other blood disorders) (see 📖 p. 330, Haematological malignancies).

Measurement
Air monitoring
- Pumped sorbent tubes, followed by either thermal or solvent desorption, analysis by GC (MDHS 96, MDHS 72)
- Diffusive sorbent samplers, followed by solvent or thermal desorption, analysis by GC (MDHS 80 and 88).

Biological monitoring
S-phenylmercapturic acid in urine (sample end of week).

Further information
INDG329. *Benzene and You.* ✍ http://www.hse.gov.uk/pubns/indg329.pdf

Carbon disulphide

General substance information
- *CAS No. 75–15–0:* formula CS_2
- *Occupational exposure limit:* WEL, 8h of TWA of $32mg/m^3$ (10ppm). Physical properties: colourless liquid, mp = $-112°C$, bp = $47°C$.

CLP classification and labelling
- Repr (2), STOT/RE (1), eye/skin irrit (2); H361fd, 372, 319, 315.

Uses/occurrence
- Most important use is the production of viscose rayon and cellophane
- Also used in the production of carbon tetrachloride and as a pesticide and fungicide
- Solvent for oils, resins and phosphorous.

Key health effects
- Irritation of skin, eyes, and respiratory tract
- Repeated or prolonged skin contact may cause dermatitis (see 📖 p. 242, Dermatitis 1)
- Effects on nervous system (acute and chronic encephalopathy, peripheral and cranial polyneuropathy, central and peripheral nervous system dysfunction)
- Effects on cardiovascular system (coronary heart disease)
- Possible effects on reproduction, based on animal data.

Measurement

Environmental monitoring
- *MDHS 96* Pumped sorbent tubes, solvent desorption, analysis by GC
- *MDHS 88* Diffusive sorbent samplers, solvent or thermal desorption, analysis by GC (MDHS 80, 88).
- Biological monitoring: 2-thioxothia zolidine-4-carboxylic acid—end of shift.

Chloroform

General substance information
- *CAS No. 67–66–3:* formula $CHCl_3$
- *Occupational exposure limit:* WEL, 8h TWA of 9.9mg/m^3 (2ppm)
- *Physical properties:* colourless liquid, slightly soluble in water, volatile liquid mp = −64°C; bp = 62°C.

CLP classification and labelling
Carc (2), acute tox (4), STOT/RE (2), skin irrit (2); H351, 302, 373, 315.

Uses/occurrence
- Major use is in the production of fluorocarbon 22, a refrigerant and aerosol propellant
- Also used in the synthesis of polytetrafluoroethylene (PTFE) plastics and some dyes and pesticides.

Key health effects
- Brief exposure to high concentrations can result in CNS depression (dizziness, headaches, fatigue)
- Repeated exposure can cause renal toxicity and hepatotoxicity.

Measurement
MDHS96 Pumped sorbent tubes, solvent desorption, analysis by GC.
MDHS 80, 88 Diffusive sorbent samplers, solvent or thermal desorption, analysis by GC.

2, 2'-Dichloro-4, 4-methylene dianiline

General substance information

- *CAS No. 101–14–4:* formula $C_{(13)}H_{(12)}Cl_{(2)}N_{(2)}$
- *Occupational exposure limit:* WEL, 8h TWA of 0.005mg/m³; BMGV, 15 µmol total 2, 2'-dichloro-4, 4-methylene dianiline (MbOCA)/mol creatinine in urine (post-shift)
- *Physical properties:* colourless to tan, odourless solid, slightly soluble in water, mp = 110°C.

CLP classification and labelling

Carc (1B), acute tox (4); H350, 302.

Uses/occurrence

- MbOCA is used in the manufacture of polyurethane elastomers with many applications in industrial and consumer plastics
- Also used in adhesives.

Key health effects

- MbOCA is easily absorbed through the skin
- Bladder cancer following inhalation, skin absorption or ingestion via food, drink or cigarettes
- Acute effects on the blood (formation of methaemoglobin).

Measurement

- Environmental monitoring: collection on pumped acid coated filters, desorption and analysis by HPLC
- Biological monitoring: total MbOCA in urine (end of shift).

Further information

HSE Research Report 828 (2010). *Occupational exposure to MbOCA and isocyanates in polyurethane manufacture.* Available at: ✆ http://www.hse.gov.uk/research/rrpdf/rr828.pdf

HSL (2007). *Survey of MbOCA chemical exposure.* Available at: ✆ http://www.hse.gov.uk/research/hsl_pdf/2007/hsl0707.pdf

Formaldehyde

General substance information

- *CAS No. 50–00–0*: formula HCHO
- *Occupational exposure limit:* WEL, 8h and 15min TWA of 2.5mg/m^3 (2ppm)
- *Physical properties:* pungent colourless gas; soluble in water (formalin).

CLP classification and labelling

Carc (2), acute tox (3), skin corr (1B), skin sens (1); H351, 331, 311, 301, 314, 317.

Uses/occurrence

- Main use is the production of resins, principally urea-formaldehyde and phenol-formaldehyde, which are used to make cores and moulds for foundries; formaldehyde is given off when resins are heated
- Formaldehyde has various other uses in agriculture and medicine where it is used as a disinfectant, fungicide, fumigant, and preservative.

Key health effects

- Irritation of skin and upper respiratory tract
- Severe irritation of eyes
- Allergic contact dermatitis resulting from skin contact
- Suspected human carcinogen (nasopharyngeal cancer) based on animal and some human evidence
- Little evidence that formaldehyde induces asthma
- Formaldehyde mixed with hydrochloric acid can generate bis(chloromethyl)ether, a potent carcinogen.

Measurement

MDHS 102 Aldehydes in air (pumped sample) collected on to a chemical coated glass fibre filter contained in a personal inhalable dust sampler, sampler solvent desorbed (into acetonitrile), aldehydes derivatized and analysed using HPLC.

▶ Method is primarily intended for measurement of formaldehyde but also suitable for measurement of other aldehydes including glutaraldehyde. Not applicable where formaldehyde is partly in the particulate phase.

Further information

IAC (L) 88. *Formaldehyde—its safe use in foundries*. Available at: ℘ http://www.hse.gov.uk/pubns/iacl88.htm

Glutaraldehyde

General substance information
- *CAS No. 111–30–8:* formula $HCHO(CH_2)_3CHO$ (used in aqueous solution)
- *Occupational exposure limit:* WEL, 8h and STEL of $0.2mg/m^3$ (0.05ppm)
- *Physical properties:* colourless liquid.

CLP classification and labelling
Acute tox (3), skin corr (1B), resp/skin sens (1); H331, 301, 314, 334, 317.

Uses/occurrence
- Used as a sterilizing agent in medicine, mainly in endoscopy and other surgical procedures
- Used in leather tanning—leather softening and to improve resistance to water and moulds
- Minor uses in the production of resins and dyes
- Biocide in the pulp and paper industry
- Disinfect animal housing (sprays).

Key health effects
- Respiratory sensitization
- Skin sensitization
- Severe irritation of eyes
- Irritation of skin and upper respiratory tract.

Measurement
See 📖 p. 84, Formaldehyde MDHS 102.

Isocyanates

Definition

Isocyanates are a group of chemicals that contain the N=C=O group. Toluene 2,4-diisocyanate (TDI) and methylenebis(phenyl isocyanate) (MDI) are aromatic isocyanate monomers; 1,6-hexamethylenediisocynate (HDI) is an example of an aliphatic isocyanate.

General substance information

- *CAS No. TDI, 584–84–9; MDI, 101–68–8:* formula TDI, $CH_3C_6H_3(NCO)_2$; MDI, $CH_2(C_6H_4NCO)_2$
- *Occupational exposure limit:* WEL, 8h TWA of $0.02mg/m^3$ (total isocyanates as NCO)
- *Physical properties TDI:* colourless to yellow solid, mp = 20–22°C, bp = 251°C. MDI: yellow solid, mp = 37°C, bp = 196°C.

CLP classification and labelling

- TDI: Carc (2), acute tox (2), eye/skin irrit (2), resp/skin sens (1), STOT/SE (3); H351, 330, 319, 335, 315, 334, 317
- MDI: acute tox (4), eye/skin irrit (2), STOT/SE (3), resp/skin sens (1); H332, 319, 335, 315, 334, 317.

Uses/occurrence

- Used in the manufacture of polyurethane foams and for a range of coatings ('one-pack', i.e. pre-reacted, or 'two pack', formed in situ by the addition of a catalyst)
- *Motor vehicle coating:* spraying produces the highest exposure
- Released when heating polyurethane products.

Key health effects

- Respiratory and skin sensitization (see 📖 p. 198, Occupational asthma and rhinitis)
- Irritation of eyes and respiratory tract.

Measurement

- *MDHS 25/3* Pumped sampling train with reagent coated filters and absorbing solution, derivatization, HPLC
- Laboratories should compare total isocyanates with the WEL.
- Biological monitoring: urine sample (isocyanate derived diamine), at end of exposure.

Further information

INDG388 (REV1) *Safety in motor vehicle repair—working with isocyanate paints.* Available at: 🔊 http://www.hse.gov.uk/pubns/indg388.pdf

Controlling isocyanates exposure in spray booths and spray rooms. Available at: 🔊 http://www.hse.gov.uk/pubns/web36.pdf

Visiting premises spraying Isocyanates based paints—a checklist for HSE staff. Available at: 🔊 http://www.hse.gov.uk/mvr/priorities/isocyanates/checklist.pdf

Methyl ethyl ketone

General substance information
- CAS No. 78–93–3: formula C_2H_5COOH
- *Occupational exposure limit:*
  - WEL, 8h TWA of 600mg/m³ (200ppm)
  - STEL of 899mg/m³ (300ppm)
  - BMGV of 70 µmol/l in urine (post-shift)
- *Physical properties:* colourless volatile liquid with a faint odour, moderately soluble in water, mp = −86°C, bp = 80°C.

CLP classification and labelling
Eye irrit (2), STOT/SE (2); H319, 336.

Uses/occurrence
Widely used as a solvent in resins and coatings including paints, lacquers, varnishes, stains, and associated cleaning materials.

Key health effects
- Irritation of eyes and respiratory tract
- Acute central nervous system effects, with unconsciousness at high exposure levels
- Prolonged or repeated skin contact with liquid causes de-fatting of skin
- Possible effects on reproduction (based on animal data).

Measurement
Environmental monitoring
- MDHS 96, 72 Pumped sorbent tubes, solvent or thermal desorption, analysis by GC
- Diffusive sorbent samplers, solvent desorption, analysis by GC (88).
- Biological monitoring: MEK in urine (end of shift).

n-Hexane

General substance information
- *CAS No. 110–54–3:* formula $CH_6(CH_2)_4CH_3$
- *Occupational exposure limit:* WEL, 8h TWA of 72mg/m³ (20ppm)
- *Physical properties:* colourless volatile liquid insoluble in water, faint odour, mp = −95°C, bp = 69°C.

CLP classification, and labelling
Repr (2), Asp tox (1), STOT/RE (2), skin irrit (2), STOT/SE (3); H361f, 304, 373, 315, 336.

Uses/occurrence
- Main use is as a solvent in edible oil extraction and polymerization processes and as a starting material in the production of other organic chemicals
- Also used as a degreasing agent in various manufacturing processes and as a cleaning agent in printing.

Key health effects
- Peripheral neuropathy, including subclinical effects such as electrophysiological changes in peripheral nerves
- Depression of central nervous system (e.g. drowsiness and vertigo).

Measurement
- *MDHS 96, MDHS 72, NIOSH 1500* Pumped sorbent tubes, solvent or thermal desorption, analysis by GC
- *MDHS 80, MDHS 88* Diffusive sorbent samplers, solvent or thermal desorption, analysis by GC.

Pesticides

General substance information

- Broad spectrum of biocidal agents used in agricultural and non-agricultural industries. WELs (Tables 2.4 and 2.5).
- Biological monitoring value: lindane, 35nmol/l (10µg/l) in whole blood.

Uses/occurrence

- Main categories are organophosphate, organochlorine, and carbamate pesticides
- Exposure occurs mainly in agriculture, although pesticide use is very widespread
- Exposure arises through preparation (decanting, mixing, spillage), application (spraying, coating, dipping), and through persons not directly engaged in application entering affected areas.

Key health effects (see also ☐ p. 298, Organophosphate poisoning)

- Organochlorine pesticides cause a range of neurological effects.
  - acute effects include headache, dizziness, nausea, vomiting, fatigue, convulsions, stimulated respiration, tremors, ataxia
  - chronic effects include intermittent muscle twitching, muscle weakness, tremors, ataxia, in coordination, slurred speech, visual impairment, memory loss, irritation, and depression
- *Organophosphate* pesticides act by inhibiting acetylcholinesterase activity, resulting in a range of neurological effects
- *Bipyridylium* herbicides (e.g. paraquat) may cause the following effects following ingestion:
  - severe inflammation of mouth, throat, and GT tract
  - effects in the lungs (dyspnoea, anoxia, progressive fibrosis)
  - necrotic damage to liver, kidneys, and myocardial muscle
  - extensive haemorrhage, coma, and death

See ☐ Chapter 39 for management of acute contamination and poisoning.

Measurement

MDHS 94 Inhalable dust/mists sample on to filter with sorbent tube analysis by GC-MS. For dermal exposure use swabs (number and sites stipulated in MDHS), analysis by GC-MS.

Further information

Pesticides Safety Directorate. Available at: ℜ http://www.pesticides.gov.uk/home.asp

Guidance on storing pesticides for farmers and other professional users. Available at: ℜ http://www.hse.gov.uk/pubns/ais16.pdf

Sheep dipping—advice for farmers and others involved in dipping sheep. Available at: ℜ http://www.hse.gov.uk/pubns/as29.pdf

INDG141 *Reporting incidents of exposure to pesticides and veterinary medicines.* Available at: ℜ http://www.hse.gov.uk/pubns/indg141.pdf

HSE *Pesticides..* Available at: ℜ http://www.pesticides.gov.uk

Table 2.4 Risk phrases for pesticides in EH40/2005 (as amended 2007)

	CAS	CLP Reg	
		Class'n	H-statements
Captan	133-06-2	Carc (2), Acute tox (3), Eye dam (1), Skin sens (1)	H351, 331, 318, 317
Chlopyrifos	2921-88-2	Acute tox (3)	H301
Endosulfan	115-29-7	Acute tox (3), Eye irrit (2)	H311, 301, 319
Malathion	121-75-5	Acute tox (4)	H302
Paraquat dichloride	1910-42-5	Acute Tox. (2), STOT/RE (1), Eye irrit (2), STOT/SE (3), Skin irrit (2)	H330, 311, 301, 372, 319, 335, 315
Phorate	298-02-2	Acute tox (1)	H310, 300
Pichloram	1918-02-1		
Pyrethrum	8003-34-7		
Pyrethrin (I and II)	121-21-1 121-29-9	Acute tox (4)	H332, 312, 302
Rotenone	83-79-4	Acute tox (3), Eye irrit (2), STOT/SE (3), Skin irrit (2)	H301, 319, 335, 315
Sulfotep	3689-24-5	Acute tox (1)	H310, 300

Table 2.5 Workplace exposure limits (WELs) for pesticides in EH40/2005 (as amended 2007)

	Type	WEL (mg/m³)		
		8h	STEL	
Captan	OC	5.0	15.0	
Chlorpyrifos*	OP	0.2	0.6	Sk
Endsulfan*	OC	0.1	0.3	Sk
Malathion	OP	10.0	–	Sk
Paraquat e dichloride	Byp	0.08	–	
Phorate	OP	0.05	0.2	Sk
Picloram		10.0	20.0	
Rotenone	Bo	5.0	10.0	
Sulfotep	OP	0.1	–	Sk

OC, organochlorine; OP, organophosphate; Bot, botanical; Byp, bypiridylium; P, pyrethrin.

Phenol

General substance information
- *CAS No. 108–95–2:* formula C_6H_5OH
- *Occupational exposure limit:* WEL, 8h TWA of 2ppm
- *Physical properties:* colourless or white crystalline solid, slightly soluble in water, mp = 43°C, bp = 182°C.

CLP classification and labelling
Muta (2), acute tox (3), skin corr (1B), STOT/RE (2); H341, 311, 301, 373, 314.

Uses/occurrence
- Main use is in the manufacture of phenolic resins and plastics
- Also as intermediates in nylon and epoxy resins
- Phenol has a range of other uses in production of fertilizers, paints, rubber, textiles, drugs, paper, soap, and wood preservatives
- Also used as a disinfectant.

Key health effects
- Phenol can be absorbed through the skin
- Corrosive to eyes, skin, and respiratory tract
- Dermal exposure can lead to effects on the central nervous system (tremors, convulsions, nausea, circulatory failure, bowel cramps, and unconsciousness). Subsequent respiratory failure may result in death.

See 📖 p. 806, Phenol poisoning for acute poisoning with phenols.

Measurement
MDHS 96,72 Pumped sorbent tubes, solvent desorption, analysis by GC.

Styrene

General substance information

- *CAS No. 100–42–5:* formula $C_6H_5CH=CH_2$
- *Occupational exposure limit:* WEL, 8h TWA of 430mg/m³ (100ppm); STEL of 1080mg/m³ (250ppm). Limit values are currently under review by HSE
- *Physical properties:* colourless liquid with oily odour, slightly soluble in water, mp = −31°C, bp = 145°C.

CLP classification and labelling

Acute tox (4), eye/skin irrit (2); H332, 319, 315.

Uses/occurrence

- Major use is the production of polystyrene and as a copolymer in the production of styrene-butadiene rubber, styrene-acrylonitrile, and acrylonitrile-butadiene-styrene polymers and polyester resins
- Also used in the manufacture of reinforced plastics.

Key health effects

- Acute central nervous system depression
- Eye irritation following exposure to liquid or vapour
- Skin irritation following repeated exposure to liquid
- Nasal irritation
- Repeated exposure can result in central nervous system effects and ototoxicity.

Measurement

- *MDHS 72,96* Pumped sorbent tubes, solvent /thermal desorption, analysis by GC
- *MDHS 80,88* Diffusive sorbent samplers, solvent /thermal desorption, analysis by GC.

Further information

HSE (2003). *Assessing and controlling styrene levels during contact moulding of fibre-reinforced plastic (FRP) products.* Available at: ℜ http://www.hse.gov.uk/pubns/pps14.pdf

Tetrachloroethylene (perchloroethylene)

General substance information
- *CAS No. 127–18–4:* formula $Cl_2C=CCl_2$
- *Occupational exposure limit:* WEL, 8h TWA of 345mg/m^3 (50ppm); STEL of 689mg/m^3 (100ppm)
- *Physical properties:* colourless liquid practically insoluble in water with an ether odour, mp = −22°C, bp = 121°C.

CLP classification and labelling
Carc (2); H351.

Uses/occurrence
- Major use is as a dry cleaning agent
- Used as a cleaning/degreasing agent in the automotive and other industries.

Key health effects
- Acute central nervous system effects (drowsiness, dizziness, with unconsciousness at high exposures; very high exposures may be fatal)
- Irritation of skin and respiratory tract
- Liver and kidney toxicity
- Evidence from animal studies indicates that tetrachloroethylene may cause cancer.

Measurement
- *MDHS 72,96* Pumped sorbent tubes, solvent /thermal desorption, analysis by GC
- *MDHS 88* Diffusive sorbent samplers, solvent desorption analysis by GC.

Vinyl chloride

General substance information
- *CAS No. 75–01–4:* formula $H_2C=CHCl$
- *Occupational exposure limit:* WEL, 8h TWA of 3ppm
- *Physical properties:* colourless gas with a sweet odour, slightly soluble in water, mp = −154°C, bp = −14°C.

CLP classification and labelling
Carc (1A); H350.

Uses/occurrence
Used as chemical intermediate in the production of polymers, mainly poly-vinyl chloride (PVC) and copolymer resins.

Key health effects
- Liver cancer (angiosarcoma) (see 📖 p. 264, Hepatic angiosarcoma)
- Other chronic effects include liver and spleen toxicity, bone deterioration, circulatory disorders affecting feet and hands, and soft tissue lesions
- Acute central nervous system effects (e.g. dizziness and disorientation).

Measurement
- *MDHS 96* Pumped sorbent tubes, solvent desorption, GC
- *MDHS 88* Diffusive sorbent samplers, solvent desorption, GC
- *MDHS 80* Diffusive sorbent tubes, thermal desorption, GC.

Arsine

General substance information
- *CAS No. 7784-42-1:* formula AsH_3
- *Occupational exposure limit:* WEL, 8h TWA of $0.16mg/m^3$ (0.05ppm)
- *Physical properties:* colourless gas, garlic-like odour but odourless at low concentrations, slightly soluble in water, mp = $-117°C$, bp = $-63°C$.

CLP classification and labelling
Acute tox (2), STOT/RE (2); H330, 373.

Uses/occurrence
- Generated by the action of acid on arsenic
- Used as a doping agent in the semiconductor industry
- Minor use in the production of organic chemicals.

Key health effects
- Haemolysis is main acute effect, leading to haemolytic anaemia, possible kidney damage, and jaundice
- Renal failure may subsequently occur, sometimes leading to death.

Measurement
MDHS 34 Withdrawn.

Carbon monoxide

General substance information
- *CAS No. 630–08–0:* formula CO
- *Occupational exposure limit:* WEL, 8h TWA of 35mg/m³ (30ppm); STEL of 232mg/m³ (200ppm)
- *Physical properties:* colourless odourless gas, sparingly soluble in water, mp = −199°C, bp = −92°C.

CLP classification and labelling
Repr (1A), acute tox (3), STOT/RE (1); H360D, 331, 372.

Uses/occurrence
- Used in the production of hydrogen and acetic acid and in the production of hydrocarbons (Fischer–Tropsch process)
- Also used as an industrial reducing agent
- Produced as a ubiquitous by-product of incomplete combustion.

Key health effects
Acute effects resulting from formation of carboxyhaemoglobin:
- Asphyxiation
- Effects on the developing foetus
- Cardiovascular effects (effects in subjects with pre-existing cardiovascular disease; exacerbation of exercise-induced angina; ventricular arrhythmia; tachycardia)
- CNS effects (headache, dizziness, impaired fine manual dexterity, impaired mental capacity, fatigue, visual disturbance).

Treatment
See 📖 p. 794, Carbon monoxide poisoning for management of acute exposure.

Measurement
- *NIOSH 6604* Pumped sampling into inert sample bag, electrochemical detector
- Colorimetric methods commonly used. Pumped sampling on to proprietary tubes coated with reagent and pre-calibrated. (Also suitable for grab sampling.)
- BMGV 30ppm in end-tidal breath (post-shift).

Further information
EH43. *Carbon Monoxide. Health Hazards and Precautionary Measures.* Available at:: ⌕ http://www.hse.gov.uk/gas/domestic/co.htm

Hydrogen sulphide

General substance information

- *CAS No. 7783–06–04:* formula H_2S
- *Occupational exposure limit:* WEL, 8h TWA of $7mg/m^3$ (5ppm); STEL of $14mg/m^3$ (7ppm)
- *Physical properties:* colourless gas, odour of rotten eggs at low concentration but odourless at higher concentrations, mp = $-86°C$, bp = $-61°C$.

CLP classification and labelling

Acute tox (2); H330.

Uses/occurrence

- Used as a digesting agent in paper production and in the production of sulphide ores
- Encountered as a product of the decay of organic matter (e.g. sewage works, animal rendering) and desulphurization processes in the metal, oil, and gas industries.

Key health effects

- Irritation of eyes and upper respiratory tract
- Pulmonary oedema may occur with prolonged exposure
- CNS effects (headache, dizziness, staggering gait) may occur with high concentrations
- At higher concentrations, CNS effects can lead to paralysis of respiratory system, asphyxiation, and sometimes death.

Treatment

See 📖 p. 800, Hydrogen sulphide poisoning, for management of acute exposure.

Measurement

NIOSH 6013 Pumped sampling on to filter and sorbent tube, derivatization, ion chromatography.

HSE publications

Toxicology of Substances in Relation to Major Hazards. Hydrogen Sulphide. Available at: ℘ http://www.hse.gov.uk/offshore/infosheets/is6–2009.htm.

Nitrogen dioxide

General substance information
- *CAS No. 10102–44–0:* formula NO_2
- *Occupational exposure limit:* none
- *Physical properties:* reddish brown gas with irritating odour.

CLP classification and labelling
Acute tox (2), skin corr (1B); H330, 314.

Uses/occurrence
- Used in the production of nitric acid and nitrate fertilizers
- Produced as a reaction by-product during metal degreasing with nitric acid and during the breakdown of silage in agriculture
- Also produced during combustion processes.

Key health effects
- Irritation of the upper respiratory tract resulting from brief exposure to high concentrations
- Lung damage in the form of emphysema may be caused by repeated exposure

Measurement
- *No MDHS* Colorimetric methods commonly used although may be generic for NO_x. Pumped sampling on to proprietary tubes coated with reagent and pre-calibrated. (Also suitable for grab sampling)
- *OSHA ID-190/NIOSH 6014* Pumped sampling on to sorbent tube NO_2 converted to nitrite, analysis by IC or AS. May be used with three-stage sorbent/oxidation tubes for simultaneous determination of NO.

Ozone

General substance information
- CAS No. 10028–15–6.
- *Occupational exposure limit:* short-term exposure limit 0.2ppm (0.4mg/m^3)
- *Physical properties:* ozone is a liquid or gas, depending on temperature, appearing bluish in color. The gas has a pleasant odour at low concentrations (<2ppm); at higher concentrations the gas is pungent.

CLP classification and labelling
Currently no classification.

Uses/occurrence
- Generated during arc welding and from photochemical oxidation of automobile exhaust gases
- Used as a disinfectant for air and water, and for bleaching textiles, oils, and waxes
- Uses include water fumigant, bleaching and oxidizing agent.

Key health effects
- Respiratory tract and muscosal irritant
- High concentration leads to pulmonary oedema.

Measurement
Colorimetric detection tubes available.

Further information
EH38. *Ozone Health Hazards and Precautionary Measures.* Available at: ℘ . http://www.hse.gov.uk/pubns/priced/eh38.pdf

Sulphur dioxide (SO₂)

General substance information
- CAS No. 7446–09–5
- *Occupational exposure limit:* no WELs; TLV-TWA, 2ppm (5.2mg/m³); TLV-STEL, 5ppm (13mg/m³)
- *Physical properties:* colourless gas with pungent odour; density twice than of air.

CLP classification and labelling
Acute tox (3), skin corr (1B); H331, 314.

Uses/occurrence
- Formed when materials containing sulphur are burned. Important air pollutant, especially in the vicinity of smelters and electrical power plants burning soft coal or high sulphur oil
- Sulphur dioxide also used in paper industries as a bleaching, disinfecting, and fumigating agent.

Key health effects
- *Acute:* mucous membrane irritant. Prolonged high exposures may lead to pulmonary oedema and death. May trigger asthmatic attacks in more susceptible individuals. Eye irritant, if prolonged may lead to corneal ulceration
- *Chronic:* chronic bronchitis and diminution in olfactory and gustatory senses.

Measurement
- Sample on impregnated cellulose filter containing potassium hydroxide. An acetate pre-filter is used to collect particulate sulphates. The impregnated filter is extracted with water and extract analysed by chromatography
- Also sampled using a bubbler containing hydrogen peroxide
- Direct reading instruments and colorimetric tubes are also available.

Chapter 3

Biological hazards

Human tissue and body fluids

Sources of exposure/industries

See Table 3.1 for routes of exposure.

Respiratory infections

Those who undertake aerosol-generating procedures, e.g. post-mortem staff, physiotherapists (suction and expectoration), bronchoscopy staff.

Faecal–oral infections

Sewage workers, laboratory staff.

Factors affecting exposure and risk assessment

The risk of transmission is determined by:
- Dose or level of exposure depends on the details of the incident including route of exposure and body fluid involved
- Source infectivity.

Risk assessment for BBV exposure is described in detail on 📖 p. 816, Management of needlestick and contamination incidents.

Health effects

These are described for each organism: HBV (📖 p. 152, Hepatitis B); HCV (📖 p. 154, Hepatitis C); HIV 📖 p. 156), VHF (📖 p. 158, Viral haemorrhagic fevers); TB (📖 p. 166, Tuberculosis); SARS (📖 p. 172, Severe acute respiratory syndrome); influenza (📖 p. 174).

Risk controls

- Adherence to standard infection control procedures, including hand hygiene, use of PPE (gloves for procedures that involve a risk of contamination, double gloves for surgical procedures on patients known to be infected with BBV). Aprons, goggles, and mask are required where there is a risk of splashing, boots or overshoes if floor is contaminated. Other risk controls include:
  - use of safer sharps devices, avoidance of re-sheathing needles
  - correct disposal of sharps and infected waste
  - correct transport of specimens
  - filtering respiratory masks for aerosol-generating procedures
  - immunization against HBV, TB, influenza
  - appropriate decontamination procedures for spills
- Prompt management of sharps and contamination incidents (📖 p. 816, Management of needlestick and contamination incidents).

Relevant legislation

An EU Directive aimed at preventing sharps injuries in healthcare was issued in 2010. Member states must implement the directive by May 2013. HSE are currently considering the implication for UK law. For more information see 🔗 http://www.nhsemployers.org/EmploymentPolicyAndPractice/European_Employment_policy/Pages/Initiatives-On-Needlestick-Injuries.aspx

Table 3.1 Routes of exposure

Route	Examples
Through non-intact skin or intact mucous membranes (blood-borne transmission)	• Blood-borne viruses (BBV) • hepatitis B (HBV) • hepatitis C (HCV) • human immunodeficiency virus (HIV) • hepatitis D (HDV) • viral haemorrhagic fevers • Malaria
Inhalation (respiratory transmission)	• Tuberculosis • Influenza • SARS
Ingestion (faecal–oral transmission)	• Enteroviruses • Typhoid

Human biological material associated with transmission of BBV

- Blood
- Blood-stained fluid
- Pleural fluid
- Pericardial fluid
- Peritoneal fluid
- Cerebrospinal fluid
- Synovial fluid
- Amniotic fluid
- Breast milk
- Semen
- Vaginal secretions
- Unfixed tissues and organs

Occupations at increased risk from BBV

- Health care workers (HCWs), in particular:
  - surgeons, theatre nurses
  - dentists
  - midwives
  - dialysis technicians
  - ambulance technicians
  - mortuary technicians
  - laboratory workers
  - chiropodists
  - acupuncturists
- Police and firefighters
- Prison workers
- Social workers
- Military personnel

There is a lower, but significant, risk among:
- Embalmers and crematorium workers
- Cleaners

Specific guidance and further information

Guidance for clinical health care workers

Protection against infection with blood-borne viruses. ℘ http://www.dh.gov.uk/

Guidance on risk controls in hospitals and laboratory environments

HSE (2005). Biological agents: Managing the risks in laboratories and healthcare premises. Available at: ℘ http://www.hse.gov.uk/biosafety/biologagents.pdf

Controlling the risks of infection at work from human remains: a guide for those involved in funeral services (including embalmers) and those involved in exhumation. ℘ http://www.hse.gov.uk/pubns/web01.pdf

Safe working and the prevention of infection in the mortuary and post-mortem room. ℘ http://www.hse.gov.uk/pubns/priced/mortuary-infection.pdf; ℘ http://www.hpa.org.uk; ℘ http://www.hse.gov.uk/biosafety/infection.htm

Microbial pathogens (in laboratory settings)

Common sources

Exposure to dangerous pathogens through work occurs almost exclusively in the experimental or clinical laboratory setting, often in health care or veterinary science (see Table 3.2).

Table 3.2 Classification of microbial pathogens (according to COSHH Regulations)

Hazard group	
HG 1	Unlikely to cause human disease
HG 2	Can cause human disease, and likely to be a hazard to employees, but unlikely to spread in the community and is treatable
HG 3	A hazard to employees, and also likely to spread to the community, but is treatable
HG 4	Can cause severe disease in humans, a hazard to employees and the community, and no treatment or prophylaxis available

A full list of specific agents and their classification is published.[1]

Factors that affect the risk assessment

- Consequence of infection (serious human disease)
- *Potential for transmission:*
  - infect and harm employees
  - spread to the community
- Amenability to treatment.

Risk controls

These are defined in detail in guidance from the Health and Safety Commission (HSC) and Advisory Committee on Dangerous Pathogens (ACDP). In summary, risk controls include the following.

Exposure controls

- *Containment:* three levels of containment for Hazard Group 2–4 pathogens, including:
  - separation from other activities
  - −ve pressure ventilation
  - high-efficiency particulate absorption (HEPA) filtered air intake and output
  - restriction to authorized personnel (e.g. access controls)
  - safety cabinet
  - observation window to allow monitoring from outside.

1 HSE/ACDP (2004). *The approved list of biological agents.* ACDP. Available at: http://www.hse.gov.uk/pubns/misc208.pdf

Use of PPE including respiratory protective equipment
- Emergency/incident planning (handling accidents)
- Vector control (rats mainly)
- Display biohazard warnings
- Safe decontamination and disinfection procedures
- Safe waste management
- Safe transport of pathogens
- *Good hygiene:* separation of eating areas for staff, hand washing routines.

Occupational health input
- Immunization where available
- Health surveillance: in practice this consists mainly of education to be vigilant and report symptoms, record of immunity
- Advise on individual susceptibility, e.g. pregnancy, immunosuppression.

Specific legislation and guidance
- Mainly outlined in general legislation (COSHH, MHSWR) but with additional guidance
- Biological agents: managing the risks in laboratories and healthcare premises. ℘ http://www.hse.gov.uk/biosafety/biologagents.pdf
- Safe working and the prevention of infection in clinical laboratories and similar facilities. ℘ http://www.hse.gov.uk/pubns/priced/clinical-laboratories.pdf
- Immunization against infectious disease (The Green Book). Department of Health 2007.
  - ℘ http://www.dh.gov.uk/en/Publicationsandstatistics/Publications/PublicationsPolicyAndGuidance/DH_079917
  - *The Management, Design and Operation of Microbiological Containment Laboratories.* HSC, ACDP, 2001
  - *Vaccination of Laboratory Workers Handling Vaccinia and Related Poxviruses Infectious for Humans.* HSC, ACDP, Advisory Committee on Genetic Modification, 1990.

Genetically modified organisms

Genetic modification (GM) is the term given to deliberate manipulation of the genetic material (DNA or RNA) of organisms in a way that does not occur in nature. The aim of GM is to introduce new or altered characteristics into plants, animals or, most commonly, micro-organisms (bacteria, viruses, and fungi). These modified attributes can be transferred subsequently between cells or organisms.

Common sources/specific industries

- GM is carried out in laboratories, animal houses, and plant growth facilities (known as 'contained use').
- Those at risk of occupational exposure include:
  - laboratory workers
  - animal house workers
  - horticulturalists in experimental facilities.

Health effects

These mainly relate to genetically modified micro-organisms (GMMs) and include specific infections.

Risk assessment and control

This is governed by primary legislation (The GMO (Contained Use) Regulations 2000 (with subsequent amendments, most recently in 2010). The regulations (see 📖 p. 111, References) give a framework for the usual principles of risk assessment, risk reduction, monitoring, and review, requiring:

- Risk assessment of all activities involving genetically modified organisms (GMOs)
- A GM safety committee should be set up to advise on risk assessments
- Use of a four-level classification system based on the risk of the activity (this is based on the four levels of containment for microbial laboratories). See 📖 p. 108, Microbial pathogens (in laboratory settings), Table 3.2
- Notification of all premises to HSE before they are used for GM activities for the first time
- Notification of individual activities of Class 2 to Class 4 to the Competent Authority (administered by HSE)
- Maintenance of a public register of GM premises and certain activities.

In addition, laboratories should follow good laboratory and containment practice.

Relevant legislation
- The Genetically Modified Organisms (Contained Use) Regulations 2000. ℘ http://www.opsi.gov.uk/si/si2000/20002831.htm
- The Genetically Modified Organisms (Contained Use) (Amendment) Regulations 2002. ℘ http://www.legislation.gov.uk/uksi/2002/63/contents/made
- The Genetically Modified Organisms (Contained Use) (Amendment) Regulations 2005. ℘ http://www.legislation.gov.uk/uksi/2005/2466/contents/made.

Further information and guidance

HSE Contained use of genetically modified organisms. ℘ http://www.hse.gov.uk/pubns/indg86.pdf

Animals and animal products

Common sources and industries

Any industry that involves direct contact with animals (live or dead), their excreta, or products:

- Agriculture
- Veterinary medicine
- Meat processing (including abbatoirs), packing, and distribution.

Potential health effects

Zoonoses

These are a group of infections typically found in animals as the primary host, but which spread from animals to humans (see Table 3.3). Some can be transmitted from human to human. There are approximately 40 potential zoonoses in the UK and approximately 300,000 people in a variety of occupations are potentially exposed. Although most zoonoses are mild and self-limiting, some may cause long-term health effects.

Table 3.3 Zoonoses

Zoonotic infection	Animal host
Anthrax	Cows, sheep, others
Glanders	Horses, cats, dogs
Streptococcus suis	Pigs
Brucellosis	Cows, sheep, goats, pigs
Lyme disease	Deer
Chlamydia infections	Poultry, exotic birds, sheep
Q fever	Sheep, cows, goats
Orf	Sheep

The common zoonoses are covered in 📖 Occupational infections, pp. 149–96.

Allergic (immune-mediated) disease

Some organic antigens are animal products (e.g. rat urine), or found in association with animal products (e.g. bloom on bird feathers) see 📖 p. 114, Organic dusts and mists.

Risk assessment

- *Route of exposure:* high risk with skin contamination, inhalation of dusts and aerosols, and ingestion.

Prevention/exposure control

- *Good husbandry practices for livestock:*
  - good standards of hygiene in young-stock housing
  - low stocking densities
  - avoid contaminating animal drinking water with dung
  - keep animals as stress-free as possible

- *Education and awareness of zoonoses:*
  - warn employees and visitors about the risk of zoonoses and preventive measures
  - advise early consultation with a doctor and declaration of exposure to animals if suspicious symptoms occur
- *Identify those with individual susceptibility and restrict from exposure:*
  - pregnant women (avoid pregnant sheep)
  - immune compromised people
- Immunizing and treating livestock
- Good occupational hygiene practices (Table 3.4).

Table 3.4 Good occupational hygiene practices in agriculture and meat processing

Safe working practices	• Avoid tools that cause cuts and injuries
	• Safe use and disposal of sharps used to immunize/test animals
	• Avoid mouth-to-mouth resuscitation on newborn animals
	• Avoid handling birth fluids or placentae
	• Control or eliminate rats
	• Do not touch dead rats with unprotected skin
Personal protective equipment (PPE)	• Essential for birthing, handling infected stock, mouth or rectal examinations: gauntlets/gloves, apron, boots
	• Use face protection (mask and goggles) if there is a risk of splashing
	• Use respirator if risk of exposure to aerosols (hosing down) or organic dust
Personal hygiene	• Good washing facilities, separate eating areas
	• Wash hands and arms before eating or smoking
	• Cover wounds with waterproof dressing
	• Work wear should be retained and washed at the place of work (not taken home)

Relevant legislation

Brucellosis, anthrax, bovine tuberculosis, and bovine spongiform encephalopathy (BSE) in animals are notifiable to the Divisional Veterinary Manager of the Department for Environment, Food, and Rural Affairs (DEFRA).

Further information and guidance

HSE *Zoonoses* ℘ http://www.hse.gov.uk/biosafety/diseases/zoonoses.htm

Health protection agency. *Zoonoses (infections acquired from animals).* ℘ http://www.hpa.org.uk/Topics/InfectiousDiseases/InfectionsAZ/Zoonoses/

HSE *Common zoonoses in agriculture*, Agriculture information sheet No. 2 (revised) ℘ HSE http://www.hse.gov.uk/pubns/ais2.pdf

HSE/ACDP (1997). *Working Safely with Research Animals.* Available at: ℘ http://www.hse.gov.uk/pubns/priced/animal-research.pdf

Organic dusts and mists

These are a group of biological agents that have the potential to cause occupational disease, and are widespread in the workplace They are mainly high molecular weight proteins from plant and animal material and micro-organisms.

Common sources

Organic dusts

- *Animal proteins:*
  urine and dander from farm or laboratory animals (e.g. cows, rats)
- *Plant proteins:*
  - natural rubber latex
  - grain dust
  - flour dust
  - wood dusts
  - colophony
- *Microbial:*
  - moulds and spores that grow in vegetable matter (e.g. hay, mushroom compost)
  - enzymes.

Organic mists

- Proteinaceous mists from washing fish products, and surfaces or equipment contaminated with fish/animal proteins
- Bacterially infected metalworking fluids.

Specific industries

- Health care industry
- Rubber manufacturing
- Laboratories and animal houses/care facilities
- Farming
- Baking and flour milling
- Biological detergent manufacture
- Fish processing
- Engineering.

Health effects

- *Type I allergy (IgE-mediated):*
  - occupational asthma
  - allergic rhinitis
  - contact urticaria
  - anaphylaxis
- Hypersensitivity pneumonitis.

Factors affecting the risk assessment
- Exposure
- Potency of the specific allergen
- Individual susceptibility (e.g. atopy, previous sensitization, cross-reactivity to similar allergens).

Risk controls
- *Minimize exposure:* generic principles
  - good animal husbandry, including avoidance of overcrowding
  - *good hygiene*—regular cleaning of animal cages and housing, wood workshops, bakeries
  - general and local ventilation
  - dust abatement techniques: avoid dry sweeping or compressed air lines for cleaning; instead use an industrial vacuum cleaner or wet clean
- Detailed guidance on the following specific biological allergens is available at ℘ http://www.hse.gov.uk/asthma/index.htm
  - flour dust
  - grain dust
  - laboratory animals
  - natural rubber latex
  - wood dust.
- Use of PPE: can be used if a significant risk exists after appropriate efforts at exposure control, e.g. for intermittent dusty tasks.

☛ Some advocate the use of respiratory protective equipment (RPE) as a last resort in sensitized workers whose livelihood depends on working in 'at-risk' situations (e.g. farmers). If this approach is advised, it must be with extreme caution, and then only after all possible efforts have been made to reduce exposure. The individual must be monitored closely (health surveillance) for signs of deterioration.

Health surveillance
All those who are exposed to a significant risk of allergic disease must have health surveillance as required by the Management of Health and Safety at Work Regulations.
- Regular symptoms questionnaire and lung function
- Follow-up positive symptoms with further investigation:
  - serial peak flow tests
  - skin prick tests
  - skin patch tests
  - total IgE and specific IgE for suspect agent (e.g. latex).
- Exclude if exposure cannot be controlled adequately, or use PPE and monitor extremely closely.

Further information and guidance
Medical Aspects of Occupational Asthma. MS25, HSE ISBN 0717615472.
HSE (1994). *Preventing asthma at work: how to control respiratory sensitisers.* ISBN 0717606619.
HSE (1996). *Controlling grain dust on farms,* Agricultural information sheet No. 3. Available at: ℘ http://www.hse.gov.uk/pubns/ais3.pdf

Mechanical and ergonomics hazards

Ergonomics hazards: overview

Definitions

Ergonomics (or human factors) is the scientific discipline concerned with the understanding of interactions among humans and other elements of a system, and the profession that applies theory, principles, data, and methods to design in order to optimize human wellbeing and overall system performance.

International Ergonomics Association

Human factors refer to environmental, organizational and job factors, and human and individual characteristics, which influence behaviour at work in a way which can affect health and safety.

HSE

Industries

Ergonomics hazards to employees are ubiquitous, affecting almost every type of work. Ergonomics issues can also affect service users, the general public, and the environment. They are most important in safety-critical industries, e.g. transport and nuclear industries, and in the health services.

Specific ergonomics factors

The most important of these are covered separately in this chapter. However, ergonomics hazards often occur in combination with each other, and are commonly addressed together in designing risk controls. This list is not exhaustive.

Task-related (physical or cognitive)
- Loading (lifting and handling)
- Poor posture
- Repetition, particularly at high speed
- High forces
- Poor equipment and workplace design
- Task overload/under load
- Mental workload
- Poor system reliability
- Poor design of information, displays, controls.

Individual factors
- Anthropometry
- Social support
- Personality
- Attitude and behaviour
- Risk perception
- Human error.

Organizational factors
- Long working hours
- Shift work
- Short deadlines
- Poor staffing levels
- Lack of worker involvement in system design
- Control over work.

Adverse effects of poor ergonomics design (including health effects)

- Accidents
- Injuries
- Musculoskeletal disease (back, neck, and upper limb pain)
- Psychological morbidity (including stress)
- Critical incidents (including environmental disasters)
- Decreased efficiency, poor productivity
- Failure of complex systems
- Job dissatisfaction
- Low staff morale
- High job turnover.

Ergonomics risk management

Specific aspects of risk assessment and control are covered under each ergonomics hazard (see 📖 p. 120, Lifting and handling, 📖 p. 124, Posture, and 📖 p. 128, Repetitive work, and also 📖 p. 776, Carry out an ergonomics assessment and 📖 p. 780, Carry out a display screen assessment).

Relevant legislation

There is no specific legislation on ergonomics hazards, but some statutory instruments contain direction on ergonomics issues:
- Control of Major Accident Hazards Regulations 1999 (COMAH)
- Railways (Safety Critical Work) Regulations 1994
- The Manual Handling Operations Regulations 1992 (as amended)
- The Health and Safety (Display Screen Equipment) Regulations 1992
- Provision and Use of Work Equipment Regulations 1998 (PUWER)
- The Working Time Regulations.

Further information

International Ergonomics Association. Available at: 🔗 http://www.iea.cc/
Ergonomics society. Available at: 🔗 http://www.ergonomics.org.uk/
European Agency for Safety and Health at Work. Available at: 🔗 http://osha.europa.eu/en/front-page
Health and Safety Executive: human factors guidance. Available at: 🔗 http://hse.gov.uk/humanfactors/index.htm

Lifting and handling

Manual lifting or handling of loads constitutes one of the most common and important ergonomics hazards.

Definitions

The term manual handling comprises any non-mechanized (or incompletely mechanized) manipulation of a load, including lifting, pushing, pulling, sliding, or carrying. Loads may be inanimate or living (people and animals).

Specific industries

Manual handling is a ubiquitous exposure, which is common in a wide range of industries. However, of particular note are:
- Construction
- Warehousing and logistics
- Heavy engineering
- Airport baggage handling
- Agriculture
- Health care (patient-handling).

Risk assessment

See Table 4.1.

Risk controls

The following list is not exhaustive, but includes the most common examples of risk controls. Extensive guidance on risk controls (including industry-specific guidance) is readily available (references under Further information and guidance on p. 122).
- Divide load into smaller units, or scale loads up, and switch to bulk handling systems
- Ensure load is easy to grip and stable
- Arrange lifting environment free from obstacles and on level surface
- Address extremes of height, e.g. restrict transfers to levels below elbow and above knee height. Avoid lifting from the floor
- Mechanical lifting aids appropriate to the task. There are many examples for different purposes. More common examples include:
  - hoists, cranes, and vehicles
  - powered and non-powered trucks and trolleys
  - scissor lifts or other height-adjustable surfaces
  - tracks, conveyors, chutes, and rollers
  - specialized equipment for 'live' loads (patients), e.g. slide sheets.

Health effects

- Low back pain
- Neck/shoulder pain
- Osteoarthritis of the hip.

Table 4.1 Manual handling risk assessment

Factor	↑ Risk	↓ Risk
Load: weight shape stability others	15 kg or more Awkward shape, large size, poor grip Liable to shift or move Sharp edges, heavier than anticipated by the handler Centre of gravity of load eccentric	<15 kg Small, easy to grip Stable, predictable
Lever (distance from employee's centre of gravity)	Load held away from body	Load close to body, with arms vertical and parallel to trunk
Vertical distance (height)	Lifts above elbow height Lifts below knee height	Transfer at trunk height
Posture	Bent or twisted trunk Constrained posture	Straight trunk
Task	Long carrying distances (>4m = moderate risk) Frequent or repetitive lifting Prolonged lifting High effort (resistance)	Short distance Short duration
Environment	Limited space Steep slopes Slip or trip hazards Poor visibility Extremes of temperature	Level non-slip surface Comfortable temperature
Individual susceptibility	Previous history of back pain Pregnancy	
Work organization	Short deadlines Poor communication Lack of control Excessive demands	Reasonable pace of work Good support Good control and flexibility Reasonable volume of work

Specific legislative requirements

The Manual Handling Operations Regulations 1992 (amended) give a framework for the generic risk assessment, risk control, review cycle that is specifically relevant for hazards associated with manual handling.

Further information and guidance

Health and Safety Executive guidance and tools. *Manual handling.* Available at: ℘ http://www.hse.gov.uk/msd/manualhandling.htm

HSE (2004). *The Manual Handling Operations Regulations 1992.* Available at: ℘ http://www.hse.gov.uk/pubns/priced/l23.pdf

Posture

The main component of risk is non-neutral posture.

Definitions

Non-neutral means that the head, trunk, or limbs deviate from the normal anatomical (neutral) position.

Specific industries

Adverse posture is widespread across many industries, affecting workers in office environments as well as heavy manual occupations. In particular:
- Call centre operators
- Display screen equipment users
- Food industry, meat handlers
- Assembly line workers.

Potential health effects
- Low back pain
- Upper limb pain (neck–shoulder, elbow, forearm, and wrist pain).

Risk assessment
- Non-neutral posture is associated with ↑ risk of health effects if it is:
  - *persistent*—prolonged, constrained or awkward position of the trunk or limbs (e.g. sustained stooping)
  - *repetitive*—repeated adverse posture (e.g. bending up and down)
- Extreme deviation from the anatomical position increases risk:
  - head or trunk flexed or extended, especially ≥20°
  - *upper limbs*—extreme flexion or abduction of the shoulders (work with arms above shoulder height), elbows, or wrists; as a general rule, risk increases most with upper arm flexion ≥90°, elbows flexed ≥90°, and wrists flexed or extended ?15°
- Risk assessment tools are used for assessing posture (🕮 p. 776, Carry out an ergonomics assessment and 🕮 p. 780, Carry out a display screen assessment).

Risk control

Risk reduction is mainly by the application of good ergonomics principles to task and equipment design (see Fig. 4.1). Extensive guidance on risk controls is readily available (see 🕮 p. 126, Relevant legislation and guidance). Common examples include:
- Appropriate seating that is adjustable to allow for anthropometric variations between operators
- Controls that are within reach to avoid over-reaching or stretching
- Attention to the height at which tasks are carried out in order to minimize bending or stooping
- Task rotation, regular breaks, or variation in position in order to avoid prolonged constrained posture.

Fig. 4.1 Risk controls for poor posture

Common adverse posture	Example of control

Bent trunk

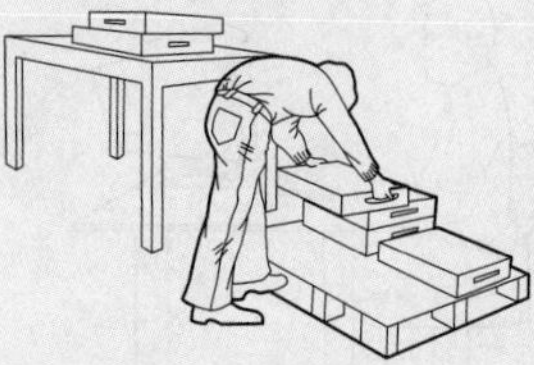

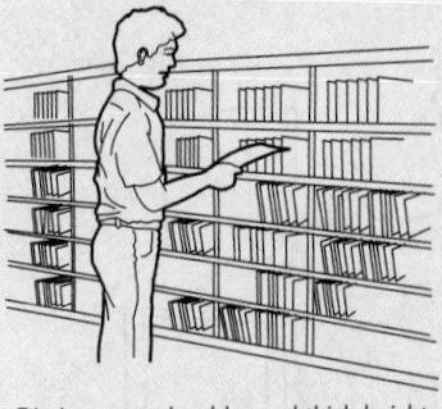

File between shoulder and thigh height

Scissor platform

Bent neck

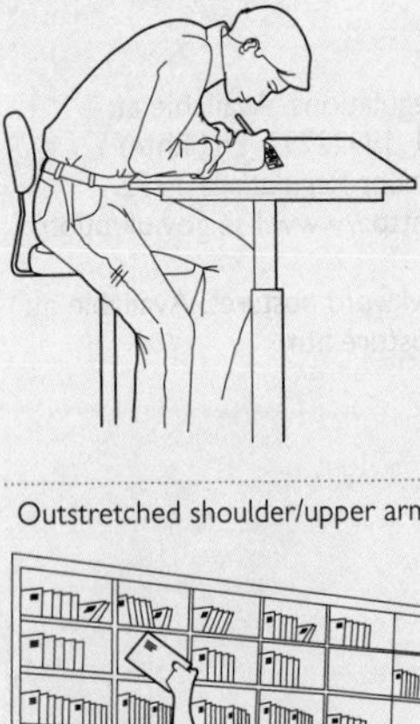

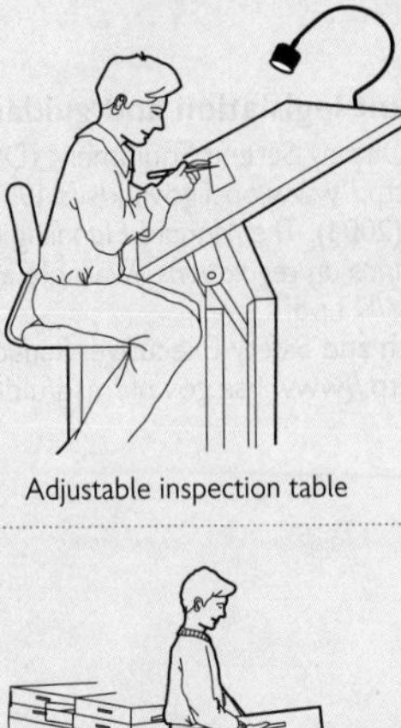

Adjustable inspection table

Outstretched shoulder/upper arm

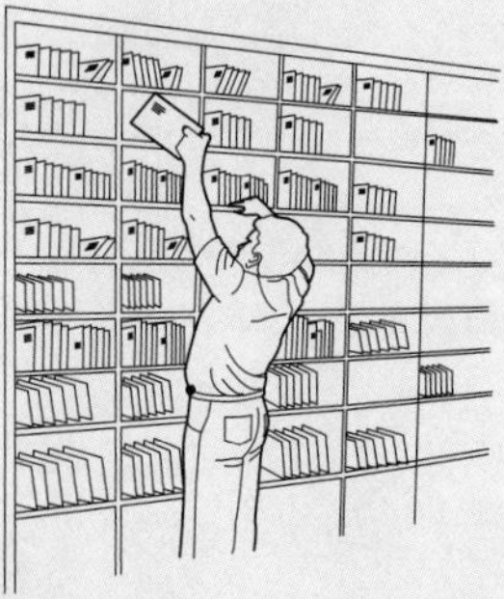

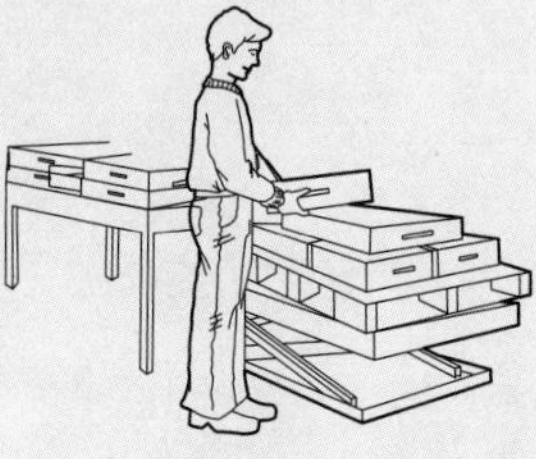

Scissor platform

File between shoulder and thigh height

(Continued)

Fig. 4.1 Risk controls for poor posture (*Cont'd*)

Common adverse posture	Example of control

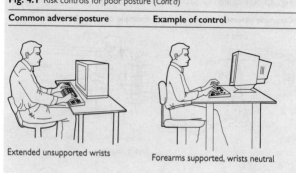

Extended unsupported wrists

Forearms supported, wrists neutral

Relevant legislation and guidance

- The Display Screen Equipment (DSE) Regulations. Available at: http://www.opsi.gov.uk/si/si1992/Uksl_19922792_En_1.htm
- HSE (2004). *The Manual Handling Operations Regulations 1992. Guidance on regulations* Available at: http://www.hse.gov.uk/pubns/priced/l23.pdf
- Health and Safety Executive. *Reducing awkward postures.* Available at: http://www.hse.gov.uk/msd/uld/art/posture.htm

Repetitive work

Definition
Repetitive work includes activities that are physically repetitive, or cognitively repetitive or monotonous. Physical and cognitive aspects of repetitiveness in work tasks often interact.

Specific industries/tasks
- Packaging
- Assembly lines
- Textile/garment production (sewing machine operators, cutting room)
- Poultry processing (plucking, evisceration)
- Fruit pickers
- Computer data entry operators.

Health effects
Musculoskeletal disorders
- Neck–shoulder pain
- Elbow, wrist pain
- Low back pain.

Risk assessment
See Table 4.2.

Table 4.2 Risk assessment for repetitive tasks

Risk factor	↑ Risk	↓ Risk
Cycle time	Rapid	Slow
Grip strength	Tight grip	Loose grip
Recovery time	Short	Long
Synergism with posture	Awkward posture	Supported neutral posture
Psychosocial factors	Lack of control over work (e.g. forced pacing)	Able to determine speed of work
	Excessive workload	Able to intersperse repetitive tasks with other activities (both physical and cognitive)

Risk controls
The following list is not exhaustive, but includes the most common examples of risk controls. Extensive guidance on risk controls is readily available (🕮 p. 129).
- Frequent rest breaks
- Task rotation
- Avoid forced pacing
- Job enrichment and variety

- Automation
- Mechanization
- Worker participation in job design and organization.

Further information

HSE (2002). *Upper limb disorders in the workplace*. HSG (60). ISBN 0717619788.

HSE (2003). *Work with Display Screen Equipment: Health and Safety (Display Screen Equipment) Regulations 1992 as amended by the Health and Safety (Miscellaneous Amendments) Regulations 2002*, L(26). ISBN 0717625826.

HSE (2003). *The law on VDUs: an easy guide*, HSG (90). ISBN 0717626024.

Health and Safety Executive. *Assessment of repetitive tasks (ART) tool*. ✍ http://www.hse.gov.uk/msd/uld/art/index.htm

Mechanical hazards

In the operation of machines a person may be injured as a result of:
- Machine movement
- Being trapped between the machinery and materials
- Being struck by materials ejected from the machinery.

Identification of machinery hazards

It is useful to consider three factors:
- *The different phases of the machine's life:*
  - design and construction
  - installation
  - commissioning
  - operation
  - cleaning
  - maintenance
  - disposal
- The circumstances giving rise to the injury
- The hazards that can cause the injury.

Types of machinery hazards

For the different types and range of machines used, their hazards can be summarized as follows:
- *Traps:*
  - reciprocating traps due to vertical or horizontal motion of machines
  - shearing traps produced by a moving part traversing a fixed part, and *in-running nips* where limbs are drawn in to a trap (e.g. where a moving belt or chain meets a roller or a tooth wheel).
- *Impact:* machinery parts, which can cause injuries by their speed or movement if the person gets in the way
- *Contact:* this may cause burns, lacerations, or injuries due to sharp, abrasive, hot, cold, or electrically live machine components
- *Entanglement:* limbs, hair, or clothing may become entangled with unguarded moving parts
- *Ejection:* machines may eject particles, metals, or actual parts of machines (e.g. grinding machines)
- *Injection:* machinery leaks may inject hydraulic fluid into the skin at high pressure.

Risk assessment

- Is the equipment fit for purpose?
- Is it suitable for use in the intended work conditions?
- Is it maintained in a safe condition?
- Some equipment should be regularly inspected to ensure it remains fit for use, e.g. power presses:
  - any inspection should be by a competent person
  - a record should be kept of the inspection.

Risk controls

- Mechanical hazards should be considered when purchasing equipment
- Machinery should be fitted with suitable safety devices, e.g.
  - machine guards
  - emergency stop buttons
  - interlocks to prevent operation if guards are removed
- Machinery should have appropriate warning signs
- Worker information, instruction, and training
- Safe systems of work including machine isolation before maintenance
- Personal protective equipment, e.g. safety goggles.

Relevant legislation and guidance

- HSE (2008). *Approved Code of Practice Safe use of work equipment. Provision and Use of Work Equipment Regulations 1998*, L22. HSE Books, Sudbury.
- HSE (1999). *Simple guide to the Provision and Use of Work Equipment Regulations 1998*, INDG 291. Available at: ℅ http://www.hse.gov.uk/pubns/indg291.pdf

Psychosocial hazards

Organizational psychosocial factors

Definition

The term 'psychosocial hazard' is used to describe any factor that may cause distress or psychological harm (see Table 5.1).

Table 5.1 Psychosocial hazards

Content of job	*Organization of work*
Work overload, deadlines, difficulty of work, time pressures, underloading (work too easy), safety critical work	Shift work, long working hours, unsociable hours, unpredictable working hours, organizational restructuring, non-consulted changes, time-zone changes
Workplace culture	*Work role*
Communication, involvement in decision making, feedback, resources, support	Clarity of job, conflict of interests and beliefs, lack of control over work
Structure	*Relationships*
Over-promotion (self/others), under-promotion (self/others), redundancy threats, pay structure/inequalities	Poor communication, harassment, bullying, verbal abuse, physical abuse/intimidation
Environment	*Home–work interface*
Noise, temperature, lighting, space, ergonomics, perceived hazard exposure	Childcare issues, transport problems, commuting, relocation, housing issues

Health effects

- Stress
- Musculoskeletal disorders
- Meta-analyses of the literature on stress show that many physical changes occur in stressed people, either directly or indirectly:
  - cardiovascular problems (direct physiological)
  - infections (direct physiological)
  - immunosuppression (direct physiological)
  - mental health problems; anxiety, depression (direct psychological)
  - cancers associated with increased use of drink, tobacco, and drugs (indirect physiological)
  - musculoskeletal problems (direct psychological).

Other adverse effects

- Low morale and job satisfaction
- Low productivity
- Increase in industrial disputes
- Increased accidents and injuries.

Further information and guidance
HSE *What are psychosocial risk factors?* Available at: ॐ http://www.hse.gov.uk/msd/mac/psychosocial.htm

Risk controls
These primary interventions decrease adverse organizational factors:

Workplace demands
- Ensure employees are able to cope with the demands of their jobs
- Provide achievable demands relative to the hours of work
- Match people's skills and abilities to the job demands
- Design jobs within the capabilities of employees
- Address employees' concerns about their work/environment.

Maintaining control
- Employees can have a say about how they do their work
- Employees have control over the pace of work
- Employee initiative and skills are encouraged
- Employees encouraged to develop new skills and remain challenged
- Employees can have a say when breaks are taken
- Employees are consulted over work issues whenever possible.

Workplace relationships
- Employees are not subjected to unacceptable behaviour, e.g. bullying
- Promote positive working and ensure fairness
- Avoid conflict and deal with unacceptable behaviour
- Employees share information relevant to their work
- Policies and procedures to address unacceptable behaviour
- Managers are able to deal with unacceptable behaviour
- Employees are able to report unacceptable behaviour.

Workplace roles
- Ensure clarity of roles within organizations and avoid role conflicts
- Employees understand their role and responsibilities
- Ensure different roles placed upon employees are compatible
- Check employees' understanding of their roles and responsibilities
- Employees can raise concerns about role uncertainties or conflicts.

Organizational change
- Engage employees frequently when undergoing organizational change
- Ensure adequate employee consultation on changes
- Make employees aware of the impact and time frames of changes
- Employees have access to relevant support during changes.

Employee support
- Employees receive adequate support from colleagues and superiors
- Policies and procedures to support employees
- Encourage managers to support their staff
- Encourage employees to support their colleagues
- Employees know what support is available and how to access it
- Employees know how to use any resources to do their job
- Employees receive regular and constructive feedback.

Violence and aggression

Definition

Any incident in which a person is abused, threatened, or assaulted in circumstances relating to their work, whether by colleagues or others. This can include verbal abuse or threats as well as physical attacks.

Incidence

- The British Crime Survey (2009/10) estimated the number of violent incidents experienced by workers in England and Wales to be 310,000 in 2009–2010
- For most workers the risk of threats of violence or actual violence at work is low (1.4%) and has been falling for some years
- Groups at high risk of experiencing threats or actual violence include:
  - protective services e.g. police officers (9%)
  - health care workers (3.8%)
- There were 6017 Reporting of Injuries, Diseases, and Dangerous Occurrence Regulations (RIDDOR) reported injuries, including one fatality, due to workplace violence in 2009/10
- Violence from colleagues represents only 5% of workplace violent incidents; 65% of physical and verbal attacks come from strangers and 18% from clients or customers.

Risk factors

Workplace violence can occur in different environments, including health care, public spaces, and commercial premises. Those most at risk from violence in the workplace include those who:

- Provide (medical/health/social) care for others
- Deliver/collect goods
- Control/schedule services
- Represent authority
- Provide a service
- Deliver education
- Transact cash or valuables.

Causes

Common causes of violence in workplaces include:

- Alcohol/drug intoxication
- Those wanting immediate attention
- Dissatisfaction with the (lack of) attention/treatment received
- Dissatisfaction with inappropriate or unsuccessful treatment received
- Robbery.

Behavioural markers of potential aggressors

- Previous history of violence
- Frustration (with the victim's organization)
- Emotional problems
- Social isolation with limited outlets
- Interpersonal problems

- Antagonistic relationships with others (e.g. victim or bully)
- Obsessive behaviour (e.g. romantic, political, religious, racial).

Risk control

Eliminating workplace violence should be a high priority for managers and team leaders.

▶ Organizations should not wait until violent events occur before preparing plans to combat violence and aggression, and should train their staff to prevent violence.

All organizations should have, and enforce, a zero-tolerance violence policy, which is communicated to both employees and non-employees. Actions that can reduce workplace violence include;
- Employee training
- Disciplinary or legal action when required
- Effective security measures.

See 📖 p. 388, Violence management policies, for specific guidance and examples of good practice.

Lone working

Definition

Lone working can be defined as 'any situation or location in which someone works without a colleague nearby; or when someone is working out of sight or earshot of another colleague'.[1] This definition includes those who are not obviously lone workers, e.g. school teachers working in isolated classrooms, remote from the assistance of colleagues.

Risk factors

Lone working of itself is not the issue—it is the lack of immediate assistance available to the worker. The main concerns are:
- Illness
- Accidents
- Personal safety (see also 📖 p. 134, Organizational psychosocial factors and 📖 p. 388, Violence management policies).

Exposed occupations

Many employers have staff who work alone.
- Those who work in the community, e.g.
  - social workers
  - traffic wardens
  - district nurses
  - lorry, bus, and taxi drivers
- Those who work in single-occupancy premises, e.g.
  - petrol stations
  - shops
  - those who work from home
- Those who work in isolated areas of large buildings, e.g.
  - reception staff
  - teachers
- Those who work in premises outside office hours, e.g.
  - cleaners
  - engineers
  - security staff.

Risk assessment

Factors to consider in a risk assessment include the following:
- *People:* the client group and the public
- Location
- Timing
- *Task:*
  - hazardous procedures
  - dealing with valuables or cash
  - enforcement activity (e.g. traffic wardens)
- Travel and accommodation.

1 NHS Security Management Service. (2009). *'Not alone': a guide for the better protection of lone workers in the NHS.* Available at:⅍ http://www.nhsbsa.nhs.uk/Documents/SecurityManagement/Lone_Working_Guidance_final.pdf

⚠ Where a risk assessment indicates inadequate controls, lone working should not proceed. Consider working in pairs, an alternative location for meeting, etc., to eliminate or reduce risk.

Control measures

- Employers of lone workers should have a lone-working policy
- Information, instruction, and training for lone workers and managers
- Access controls in buildings
- Internal alarm systems including panic buttons or fob-operated alarms are useful for premises (e.g. psychiatric hospitals)
- Lone-worker protection systems linked to a central control room (with or without a global positioning system) for mobile workers
- Personal attack alarm (although use may inflame difficult situations)
- *Mobile phone:* check that it is fully charged, has available credit, and that reception is adequate in that area
- Information sharing between public bodies regarding individuals with a history of violence towards staff
- *Visit log:* who is being visited, contact details, arrival/departure times, *but* this requires the co-operation of all staff to operate effectively.
- Lone worker details held in personal file. Include:
  - make, model, and registration of vehicle
  - next of kin
  - home and mobile phone numbers.
  ⚠ Do not place undue reliance on lone-worker protection systems.

Relevant legislation

- Under the Health and Safety at Work, etc., Act 1974 employers have a duty to protect worker's health and this would include lone workers
- Management of Health and Safety at Work Regulations 1999 requires that employers undertake a suitable and sufficient risk assessment of the risks to the health and safety of staff and others (regulation 3), which would include lone working.

Further information and guidance

Health and Safety at Work, etc., Act 1974, Chapter 37.

HSE *Management of Health and Safety at Work Regulations (1999) Approved Code of Practice and Guidance.* Available at: ✆ http://www.hse.gov.uk/pubns/books/l21.htm

NHS Security Management Service. (2009). *'Not alone': a guide for the better protection of lone workers in the NHS.* Available at: ✆ http://www.nhsbsa.nhs.uk/Documents/SecurityManagement/Lone_Working_Guidance_final.pdf

Shift and night work

Definition

Night work is defined as at least 3h of work taking place between 23.00 and 06.00 hours.

Epidemiology

- Approximately 14% of all employees in the UK usually work shifts
- A further 3% take part in shift work occasionally
- Shift work is only slightly more prevalent in men than women:
  - most common in personal protective services (45% men and 27% of women in the sector) and plant and machine operators (31% of men and 22% of women in the sector)
  - nurses are the most common group of female shift workers.

Health effects

- Fatigue and sleep deficits
- Anxiety/depression
- Increased substance use (eating, smoking, drinking)
- *GI disorders:* peptic ulcer, altered bowel habit
- CVD
- Neurological disorders
- Menstrual disorders
- Acute changes in cholesterol, uric acid, glucose, potassium, and lipids
- There is evidence of an association with miscarriage, preterm birth, and low birth weight, but it is not clear if the association is causal
- There is evidence of an association between long term night shift work and cancer, but it is not clear if the association is causal (see ℜ http://monographs.iarc.fr/ENG/Monographs/vol98/index.php)

Complications of night work

Much research has gone into determining whether or not night working imposes extra health effects. Evidence is inconclusive, but it seems likely that circadian disruption, fatigue, and sleep deficit will be exacerbated by a 12-h shift system. Other 2° factors affecting health and safety should be considered, such as exposure to toxic materials where occupational exposure limits appropriate for 8h would no longer be safe for 12h.

Effects on function

Risk of injury is 30% higher on night shifts than on morning shifts, and is usually highest in the first 2–3h, with the risk ↑ over successive nights. By the fourth night shift, there is 1.3 times greater risk of accident than on the first night. The use of sedatives to aid sleep at unusual times may lengthen reaction times and exacerbate the ↑ risk of accidents.

Risk factors

Factors associated with adverse effects of night/shift work include:
- Incomplete circadian adjustment
- Irregular food intake leading to stomach complaints
- Impairment of social or family life, and disrupted child-care.

Risk control

Employees should
- Drink coffee in the first half of the shift only
- Take short 'power naps'
- Take small breaks at least every hour
- Take a main meal break between midnight and 01.00 hours
- Take a smaller food break between 03.00 and 04.00 hours
- Be aware of subjective feelings of inertia for 15min after waking
- Avoid driving to and from work after prolonged periods of night shifts
- Eat healthily and keep fit/active
- Design and define their own shifts whenever possible
- Take up flexible working if possible
- Advice is available for shift workers on how to cope with the demands of night working. The HSE offers tips on dealing with sleep problems, eating, physical fitness, and social contact. (http://www.hse.gov.uk/humanfactors/topics/shift-workers.htm).

Employers should
- Minimize permanent nights
- Ensure safe travel to and from work at unusual hours
- Limit consecutive night shifts to no more than four
- If possible allow 24h between two night shifts
- Some weekends should be completely free of night shifts
- Consider making night shifts shorter than day shifts
- Avoid compressed working periods
- The length of night shifts should be related to the tasks performed
- Forward rotation of shifts is preferable to continuous night shifts
- Morning shifts should start later rather than sooner
- Rotas should be as regular as possible
- Allow opportunities to swap shifts and change handover times
- Avoid excessive short-term rota changes
- Good notice should be given of changes in shift patterns
- Allow return to day work without penalty (especially older workers)
- Ensure availability of hot food and drinks, rest areas, and first aid
- Night workers need the same access to training as other workers
- Allow access to union representation or daytime meetings
- Offer access to health checks for night workers.

▶ The ability to cope with changed sleep patterns varies considerably and should be considered when selecting night workers.

Relevant legislation
Workers who normally work at night (excluding those who only occasionally work nights) are protected under the Working Time Regulations (see 📖 p. 574, Working Time Regulations 1998). This includes provision of health checks for night workers.

Long working hours

Definition
'Long-hours' workers are those who work >48h/wk.

Epidemiology
- The average length of the European working week is decreasing. In the European member states, it has fallen from 40.5h in 1991 to 37.5h in 2010
- The proportion of the working population in Europe working longer than 48h has fallen from 15% in 2000 to 12% in 2010
- Long working hours are more common in men than women.

Health effects
- Generalized fatigue, both physical and psychological
- Anxiety/depression.

Effects on function
- Poor performance
- ↑ *Risk of accident or injury:*
  - *exponential increase with long hours*—by the twelfth hour of work risk is double that during the first 8h
  - *not taking a regular break linearly ↑ the risk of injury*—the risk of injury 1.5h after taking a break is twice that when resuming work immediately after the break.

Risk factors
A number of factors increase the likelihood of adverse effects from working longer hours:
- Female sex
- Older age
- Poor diet
- Little exercise
- *Pre-existing poor health:* examples of medical conditions that may be adversely affected include asthma, depression, and diabetes. These need to be considered before selecting individuals for long working hours duties (although they are not an absolute contraindication to long hours)
- Complex or demanding domestic situation.

Relevant legislation
The European Working Time Directive enforces standards on working time (see 📖 p. 574, Working Time Regulations 1998).

Further information and guidance
European Foundations for the Improvement of Living and Working Conditions. (2010). *Changes over time—First findings from the fifth European Working Conditions Survey.* Available at: ℘ http://www.eurofound.europa.eu/pubdocs/2010/74/en/3/EF1074EN.pdf

Time zone changes

Crossing time zones is commonly associated with jobs that require frequent international travel.

Health effects

Transmeridian displacement, or dysrhythmia (jet lag) is a disturbance of the internal circadian rhythm (body clock) caused by crossing international time zones. Crossing time zones when travelling east (travelling back in time) is usually worse than when travelling west (forward in time). Symptoms include:
- Tiredness
- Disorientation
- Lack of concentration
- Broken sleeping/night wakefulness
- Cognitive impairment
- Irritability
- GI upset.

Epidemiology of health effects

The impact of jet lag upon long-haul travellers is particularly high, with approximately 90–94% of travellers feeling some −ve effects after flying. Some surveys have shown that 96% of experienced flight attendants continue to feel jet-lagged after long-haul flights.

Risk factors

- Number of time zones crossed (≥ five time zones greatly ↑ risk)
- Cabin pressure
- Being a person of 'set routine'
- Pre-flight condition (e.g. tiredness, stressed, nervous, drunk/hung-over)
- Caffeine, alcohol, fruit juice
- Dehydration
- Poor fresh air supply
- Limited movement/stretching
- Flying at night time
- Older age.

Risk control

There are a number of preventive measures that travellers can take.

Pre-flight

- Ensure a good night's sleep before travel
- Be calm
- Exercise the day before the flight.

Flight factors

- Direction of flight (if possible)—may be a personal preference
- Daytime flights preferable to night time flights.

In-flight behaviour
- Drink plenty of water or other non-alcoholic fluids
- *Using sleeping aids:* pillows, neck-rests, blindfolds, earplugs
- Remove footwear
- Exercise as much as possible
- Take walks at stop-overs if possible
- Shower if available (refreshing, and activates muscles and circulation).

Management
Some research suggests that phototherapy and bright-light therapy can be useful in speeding up the circadian adaptation in those who are suffering ill effects. The efficacy of melatonin is uncertain.

Section 2

Occupational diseases

Occupational infections

Blood-borne viruses

An important group of occupational infections characterized by their blood-borne route of transmission.

The most common examples are:
- HBV
- HCV
- HIV.

Others include:
- HDV
- Viral haemorrhagic fevers (VHF).

Sources of exposure/industries

Transmission can occur after exposure to infected biological material (see 📖 p. 816, Management of needlestick and contamination incidents).

Epidemiology

3773 significant occupational exposures to infected blood and body fluids were reported to the Health Protection Agency surveillance scheme during 1996–2007. Among these were 15 seroconversions (12 HCV, 1 HIV, and 2 co-infections).

Factors affecting exposure and risk assessment

The risk of transmission is determined by:
- Details of incident including body fluid involved and exposure route
- Source patient infectivity.

Risk assessment is described in detail in 📖 p. 816, Management of needlestick and contamination incidents.

Biological material associated with transmission of BBV

- Blood
- Blood-stained fluid
- Pleural fluid
- Pericardial fluid
- Peritoneal fluid
- Cerebrospinal fluid

- Synovial fluid
- Amniotic fluid
- Breast milk
- Semen
- Vaginal secretions
- Unfixed tissues and organs

Health effects

These are described separately for each virus HBV, HCV, HIV, VHF (see 📖 p. 152, Hepatitis B; 📖 p. 154, Hepatitis C; 📖 p. 156, Human immunodeficiency virus; 📖 p. 158, Viral haemorrhagic virus).

Risk controls

- Reduce exposure to infected blood and body fluids by adherence to standard infection control precautions, e.g. hand hygiene, use of PPE

Occupations at risk from BBV

- HCWs, in particular :*
  - surgeons
  - theatre nurses
  - dentists
  - midwives
  - anaesthetists
  - dialysis technicians
  - ambulance technicians
  - mortuary technicians
  - laboratory workers
  - chiropodists
  - acupuncture practitioners

There is a lower, but significant, risk among:
- Embalmers
- Crematorium workers
- Cleaners
- Police
- Prison workers
- Social workers
- Military personnel
- Sewage workers
- Firefighters

* This list is not intended to be exhaustive

- Gloves should be worn for any procedures that involve a risk of contamination with infected material. Double gloves are recommended where surgical procedures are performed on patients known to be infected with BBV
- Aprons, goggles, and mask required where there is a risk of splashing
- Other risk controls include:
  - use of safer sharps devices
  - avoidance of re-sheathing needles
  - correct disposal of sharps
  - correct disposal of infected waste
  - correct transport of specimens
- Immunization against HBV
- Prompt management of sharps and contamination incidents in the workplace.

Specific guidance

- Guidance for Clinical Health Care Workers: Protection Against Infection with Blood-borne viruses. Recommendations of the Expert Advisory Group on AIDS and The Advisory Group on Hepatitis. ℘ http://www.dh.gov.uk/en/Publicationsandstatistics/Lettersandcirculars/Healthservicecirculars/DH_4003818/
- Guidance on risk controls in hospitals and laboratory environments is published by the HSE Health Services Advisory Committee (HSAC) and Advisory Committee on Dangerous Pathogens (ACDP). ℘ http://www.hse.gov.uk/biosafety/biologagents.pdf

Further information

℘ http://www.hpa.org.uk/Topics/InfectiousDiseases/InfectionsAZ/BloodborneVirusesAndOccupational Exposure/

℘ http://www.hse.gov.uk/biosafety/diseases/blood-borne-virus.htm

HPA (2008). Eye of the needle: UK surveillance of significant occupational exposure to blood-borne viruses in healthcare workers. Available at: ℘ http://www.hpa.org.uk/webc/HPAwebFile/HPAweb_C/1227688128096

Hepatitis B

Epidemiology
- HBV is a DNA virus
- 350 million people worldwide are chronically infected
- Endemic in many developing countries, where it affects up to 10% of the population; acquired mainly in childhood
- The epidemiology in westernized countries is quite different. In the UK, the prevalence of chronic HBV is 0.3%. Infection occurs mainly in young adulthood following sexual contact or intravenous drug misuse
- Occupational transmission to HCWs is well documented historically, but the incidence has reduced since the availability of vaccination. Among 296 occupational exposures to HBV reported to the HPA surveillance scheme 1996–2007, there were no HBV seroconversions.

Clinical features
- Incubation period 40–160 days
- *Acute illness:* malaise, fatigue, influenza-like symptoms, myalgia, nausea, vomiting, abdominal pain, and jaundice. About 30% of cases are asymptomatic
- Most patients clear the infection spontaneously
- 2–10% develops chronic carriage.

Causal exposures/industries
See 📖 p. 105.

Clinical assessment and diagnosis
In the occupational setting, cases of HBV infection are usually diagnosed:
- When a HCW fails to respond to hepatitis B vaccine
- Following pre-employment assessment of fitness for exposure prone procedures (EPPs)
- Rarely, infection might be detected following an exposure incident.

The main focus of investigation is to establish the degree of infectivity in order to assess the risk of transmission in the work setting. The OH professional should facilitate referral of active cases to a hepatologist for clinical management (if this has not already been done). Serological markers for HBV infection are shown in Table 6.1.

Medical management and prognosis
- HBV is treatable with interferon-alpha, leading to reversal of the carrier state in 40% of cases
- Untreated, 20–25% of chronic cases infected as adults will develop chronic liver disease, of whom 15–25% will die.

Prevention
- HBV is preventable by immunization:[1]
  - recombinant vaccines provide protection in >90% of recipients

1 Department of Health (2009). Hepatitis B. In: *Immunization against infectious disease.*. Available at: 🔗 http://www.dh.gov.uk/prod_consum_dh/groups/dh_digitalassets/@dh/@en/documents/digitalasset/dh_108820.pdf

Table 6.1 HBV serology

Serological markers	Interpretation
Anti-HBc (core antibody) +ve and HbsAg (surface antigen) +ve	Current infection or infectious carrier
Anti-HBc +ve, HbsAg +ve and HBeAg (e antigen) +ve	Current infection or infectious carrier with particularly high infectivity
Anti-HBc +ve and HBsAg −ve	Previous infection with natural immunity and non-infectious

- non-response to vaccine is associated with age >40yrs and immune suppression
- following immunization surface antibody levels (anti-Hbs) >100IU/L are protective, but those at continuing risk of occupational exposure should have a single booster dose after 5yrs. Poor responders (10–100IU/L) require an immediate booster and a reinforcing dose at 5yrs. Non-responders (<10IU/L) should be tested for previous HBV infection, and if negative receive a second course
- Reduce exposure (see 🕮 p. 150, Blood-borne viruses, Risk controls).

Fitness for work

Modifications to work are required to prevent occupational transmission. This is usually only required in the health care setting. Exposure prone procedures may only be carried out by infectious carriers of HBV under specifically defined circumstances and with appropriate ongoing monitoring of viral load (see 🕮 p. 150, Blood-borne viruses).

Compensation

- Viral hepatitis (including HBV) is a prescribed disease (B8) for Industrial Injuries Disablement Benefit among those who have worked with human blood or blood products, or a source of viral hepatitis
- NHS Injury Benefit (both temporary and permanent) would be payable to an NHS employee who lost remuneration because of HBV infection attributable to his or her NHS employment.

Relevant legislation

- HBV infection that is acquired occupationally (new case exposed to human blood or human blood products, or any source of HBV at work) is reportable to HSE under RIDDOR 1995
- Acute infectious hepatitis is notifiable (to Local Authority Proper Officers) under the Health Protection (Notification) Regulations 2010.

Further information

🕫 http://www.hpa.org.uk/Topics/InfectiousDiseases/InfectionsAZ/HepatitisB/

Hepatitis C

Epidemiology

- HCV is an RNA virus
- It is estimated that 170 million people worldwide are chronically infected (3% of the world's population)
- Prevalence rate for chronic HCV infection in England is estimated at 0.4%
- Most common in men, 25–44yr age group
- In the UK, >90% of cases are caused by intravenous drug use and 5% by blood transfusion or exposure to blood products. In contrast with other blood-borne viruses, sexual transmission is rare (2% of cases)
- Fewer than 1% of cases are acquired occupationally. Twelve cases of occupationally acquired HCV have been reported in the UK during the period 1996–2007.[1]

Clinical features

- Incubation period of 6–9wks
- Acute illness mild (malaise and jaundice)
- ▶ 80% asymptomatic.
- ▶ Only 20–40% of cases clear the virus spontaneously after acute infection.
- ▶ 80% go on to develop chronic infection.

Clinical assessment and diagnosis

- HCV antibodies (anti-HCV) are usually detectable 3mths after infection, but rarely may take up to 6mths to develop. The presence of anti-HCV indicates whether an individual has been infected, but does not distinguish between active and previous infection
- In the occupational setting, assessment of infectivity, on which advice about the likelihood of transmission to others is based, includes quantitative assessment of viral load (HCV RNA)
- New occupational cases should be referred to a hepatologist for clinical assessment (liver function tests (LFTs) ± liver biopsy) and treatment.

Prognosis

- Untreated, most chronic cases have a normal life expectancy
- 5–20% of chronic cases develop liver cirrhosis over 20yrs, and a small proportion of these develop liver cancer
- Risk factors for more rapid progression to severe liver disease (once infected) include >40yr age group, male gender, alcohol consumption, co-infection with HIV or HBV, and immunosuppression
- Combination antiviral therapy is successful in clearing HCV in around 50% of cases (range 45–80% depending on genotype).

1 HPA (2008). Eye of the needle—UK surveillance of significant occupational exposure to blood-borne viruses in health care workers. 2008 Health Protection Agency. Available at: ℘ http://www.hpa.org.uk/webc/HPAwebFile/HPAweb_C/1227688128096

Prevention

There is no vaccine or post-exposure prophylaxis for HCV. The mainstay of prevention is avoiding exposure (see 📖 p. 150, Blood-borne disease, Risk controls).

Medical management

- Treatment of chronic HCV infection is indicated for moderate to severe disease
- NICE guidelines recommend pegylated interferon-alpha (weekly subcutaneous injection) in combination with ribavirin (daily oral dose).

Fitness for work

Modifications to work are required to prevent occupational transmission. This is usually only required in the health care setting, where exposure prone procedures should not be carried out by infectious carriers of HCV (see 📖 p. 494, Fitness for exposure prone procedures).

Compensation

- Viral hepatitis (including HCV) is a prescribed disease (B8) for Industrial Injuries Disablement Benefit in occupations exposed to human blood and body fluids
- HCWs who acquire HCV infection occupationally, and lose remuneration as a result, are eligible for Temporary and Permanent NHS Injury Benefit.

Relevant legislation and benefits

- HCV infection that is acquired occupationally (new case exposed to human blood or human blood products, or any source of HCV at work) is reportable to HSE under RIDDOR 1995
- Acute infectious hepatitis is notifiable (to Local Authority Proper Officers) under the Health Protection (notification) Regulations 2010.

Further information

HPA (2012). Hepatitis C. Available at: ℜ http://www.hpa.org.uk/Topics/InfectiousDiseases/InfectionsAZ/HepatitisC/

Human immunodeficiency virus

Epidemiology

- HIV is an RNA virus
- Worldwide (2009) 33.3 million people are infected with HIV
- In the UK (2009) 86 500 adults have HIV, of which a quarter are unaware of their infection
- >90% of HIV infection is sexually acquired; 2% is associated with injecting drug use
- Occupationally acquired HIV is rare (see Table 6.2). Five definite cases have been recorded historically in the UK. However, only one new case of definite occupational transmission was documented in the UK between 1996 and 1999, and no new cases have occurred between 1999 and 2007.[1]

Clinical features

- *Seroconversion illness:* mild non-specific influenza-like symptoms and lymphandenopathy 2–4wks after infection
- Long asymptomatic phase (years) with gradually increasing immune suppression
- Acquired immune deficiency syndrome (AIDS) characterized by opportunistic infections.

Causal exposures/industries

Healthcare work

- Nurses and laboratory workers
- Surgeons
- Other doctors.

Clinical assessment and diagnosis

- Following acute infection HIV antibodies become positive
- The degree of immune suppression is assessed by measurement of CD4 count (normal range 500–1500 × 10^6 cells/mm^3):
  - bacterial infections, candida and mycobacterial infections arise when CD4 <500 (symptomatic phase)
  - AIDS is associated with CD4 <200 × 10^6 cells/mm^3, and infection with (e.g.) pneumocystis, toxoplasma, cryptosporidia.
- Infectivity is measured by HIV RNA viral load. Early in the illness, viral load can be several million copies/mL. This stabilizes during the chronic phase. HIV RNA is the best indicator of overall prognosis.

Medical management and prognosis

The advent of anti-retroviral therapy (ART) in HIV-positive patients has improved the prognosis of HIV infection dramatically. Current triple drug regimes (ART, and highly active ART (HAART)) aim to reduce viral load below detectable levels in the chronic phase. This is a rapidly changing field, with frequent introduction of new agents and combination regimens.

---

1 HPA (2008). Eye of the needle—UK surveillance of significant occupational exposure to blood-borne viruses in health care workers. Available at: ℛ http://www.hpa.org.uk/webc/HPAwebFile/HPAweb_C/1227688128096

Table 6.2 Occupationally acquired HIV

Location	Documented HIV seroconversion after occupational exposure	Possible occupational transmissions of HIV
Worldwide	106	238
UK	5	14

Data (up to 2002) collated by Health Protection Agency.

Fitness for work in HIV-infected employees

Modifications to work are sometimes appropriate:
- *To prevent occupational transmission to others:*
  - only important in a small number of special circumstances. HIV is not spread through casual contact at work
  - HIV-positive HCWs must not undertake exposure prone procedures (see 📖 p. 494, Fitness for exposure prone procedures 1)
- *To accommodate impairment in function:*
  - usually only necessary in the late symptomatic stages (AIDS)
  - most HIV +ve employees in the clinical latent phase can work normally.

Adjustments to work in AIDS

- *If fatigue is a problem:* part-time or flexible work, or ↓ physical work
- Restrict from activities where exposure to infection is a risk, e.g. care of patients who are sputum-positive for multi-drug-resistant TB
- HIV-positive employees should not be given live vaccines (including bacillus Calmette–Guérin (BCG)), but can be immunized with recombinant or killed vaccines.

Compensation

- HIV is not a prescribed disease, but HIV acquired through discrete accidental exposure at work might be eligible as an industrial injury
- HCWs who acquire HIV infection occupationally, and lose remuneration as a result, are eligible for Temporary and Permanent NHS Injury Benefit.

Relevant legislation HIV infection that is acquired occupationally (new case exposed to human blood or human blood products, or any source of HIV at work) is reportable to HSE under RIDDOR 1995.

Further information

Department of Health. *Sexual health and HIV.* Available at: ℘ http://www.dh.gov.uk/ PolicyAndGuidance/HealthAndSocialCareTopics/HIV/fs/en

HPA (2012). HIV. Available at: ℘ http://www.hpa.org.uk/Topics/InfectiousDiseases/InfectionsAZ/HIV/

Viral haemorrhagic fevers

The viral haemorrhagic fevers are a group of zoonotic infections caused by various families of viruses. They are all transmitted from primary wild animal hosts, none of which are natural residents in the UK. The diseases vary in severity and clinical picture. However, a number of VHFs are important in occupational medicine because of the following key features:
- High transmissibility from human to human
- High case fatality rate
- Difficulty in diagnosis in the early stages.

Disease	Virus family
• Lassa fever	• Arenavirus
• Marburg virus	• Filovirus
• Ebola virus	• Filovirus
• Crimean/Congo haemorrhagic fever (CCHF)	• Bunyavirus

There are many more VHFs, but these are the most important with respect to occupational transmission.

Epidemiology
- These diseases are endemic in parts of Africa, South America, and Asia. Primary cases in the UK are exceedingly rare, and can only arise from imported animals or laboratory sources
- There have been eight cases of imported (i.e. acquired abroad) Lassa fever in the UK between 1980 and 2010. No cases of Ebola or Marburg virus had been imported to the UK up to 2010
- There have been no cases of transmission to HCWs in the UK
- One case of Ebola virus and two cases of Marburg virus infection in the UK have resulted from laboratory accidents.

Clinical features
Some cases are mild or subclinical. The hallmarks of severe infection are:
- Fever
- Multi-system failure
- Bleeding in the terminal stages.

Causal exposures/industries
- Transmission in the UK is usually secondary (human to human rather than animal host to human). Infection occurs through exposure to blood and body fluids, and transmission to HCWs is well described in West Africa
- There is no evidence of transmission through the respiratory route
- VHFs have potential to be used in bioterrorism.[1]

1 Health Protection Agency (2012). Deliberate and accidental releases. Available at: ℜ http://www.hpa.org.uk/infections/topics_az/deliberate_release/VHF/Homepage.asp?Source=Professional&Agent=VHF&Document=Homepage

At-risk occupations include:
• Clinical HCWs caring for infected cases
• Laboratory workers handling viral material
• Mortuary staff handling infected bodies.

Clinical management and prognosis

Management is very specialized, and suspected cases must be notified and isolated in a high-security infectious diseases unit. Treatment is with the antiviral agent ribavirin. The overall fatality of Lassa fever is 1%, although 15–20% of those who are hospitalized will die.

▶ There is no evidence to support the use of ribavirin as post-exposure prophylaxis.

Prevention

• Specialized guidance is available from the Advisory Committee on Dangerous Pathogens covering:
  • risk assessment
  • isolation facilities
  • containment requirements
  • handling infected bodies
  • handling specimens
  • laboratory facilities
• There is no vaccine for VHFs.

Relevant legislation

• VHFs are notifiable (to Local Authority Proper Officers) under the Health Protection (Notification) Regulations 2010
• VHFs that are reliably attributable to occupation are reportable under RIDDOR
• An incident or accident that resulted in exposure to VHFs at work would be reportable as a dangerous occurrence under RIDDOR.

Further information and guidance

Health Protection Agency (2012). Viral haemorrhagic fever. Available at: ℘ http://www.hpa.org.uk/infections/topics_az/VHF/menu.htm

Centre for Disease Control guidance (2011). Viral hemorrhagic fevers. Available at: ℘ http://www.cdc.gov/ncidod/dvrd/spb/mnpages/dispages/vhf.htm

Variant Creutzfeldt–Jakob disease

Epidemiology

Approximately 85% cases of Creutzfelt-Jakob Disease (CJD) are sporadic with no known cause and 10–15% of cases are inherited. Variant CJD (vCJD) was first identified in 1996. It has affected younger patients (mean age 27yrs vs. 65yrs), with a longer course (median of 14 vs. 4.5mths). The epidemic of vCJD peaked in mid-2000. It is strongly linked to exposure, probably through food, to a transmissible spongiform encephalopathy (TSE) of cattle called bovine spongiform encephalopathy (BSE). There is compelling scientific evidence that BSE and vCJD are caused by the same infectious agent, suggesting that BSE in cattle is the source of the human disease. All TSEs are caused by infectious proteins called prions.

Clinical features

- Initially psychiatric or behavioural symptoms:
  - predominantly depression
  - less often, a schizophrenia-like psychosis
- Unusual sensory symptoms, such as 'stickiness' of the skin
- Unsteadiness, difficulty walking, and involuntary movements
- By the time of death, patients become completely immobile and mute.

Causal exposures/industries

There is a *theoretical* risk of transmission through occupational exposure to infected tissues. Occupations at risk include:

- Abbatoir workers
- Mortuary workers, neurosurgeons, and neuropathologists
- ▶▶ No occupationally acquired infections have been reported
- ▶▶ There are no reported cases of transmission to humans as a result of a surgical or dental procedure.

Clinical assessment and diagnosis

- The clinical presentation, progressive nature of the disease, and failure to find any other diagnosis are the hallmarks of vCJD
- Magnetic resonance imaging (MRI) brain scan may show a characteristic abnormality in the posterior thalamic region (pulvinar sign)
- Tonsillar biopsy and cerebrospinal fluid tests may be helpful
- The brainwave pattern observed on electroencephalogram is usually abnormal, but waveforms characteristic of sporadic CJD do not occur
- Currently, the diagnosis of vCJD can only be confirmed following pathological examination of brain tissue, usually at post-mortem.

Treatment and prognosis

- vCJD is a progressive and ultimately fatal disease
- There is currently no proven treatment for the underlying process.

Risk control

Careful adherence to standard infection control procedures should prevent occupational exposure.

Surveillance

The Health Protection Agency and the National CJD Research and Surveillance Unit have set up a registry to find out more about the risk from exposures to CJD and other TSEs to health care and laboratory workers. In these occupational groups, percutaneous or mucocutaneous inoculation of tissues or blood from probable or confirmed cases of all types of human prion diseases including CJD or TSE infected animals or tissues must be reported to the registry. Details on how to report an exposure are available on the Health Protection Agency website. The registry will provide long-term monitoring of the exposed workers.

Further information

HSE (2007). BSE occupational guidance, Advisory Committee on Dangerous Pathogens. Available at: ℗ http://www.hse.gov.uk/pubns/web22.pdf

Department of Health (2003). Guidance from the ACDP TSE Risk Management Subgroup (formerly TSE Working Group). Available at: ℗ http://www.dh.gov.uk/ab/ACDP/TSEguidance/index.htm

Health Protection Agency (2012). *Creutzfeldt-Jakob Disease (CJD)*. Available at: ℗ http://www.hpa.org.uk/Topics/InfectiousDiseases/InfectionsAZ/CreutzfeldtJakobDisease/

Bovine spongiform encephalopathy

BSE is a transmissible prion disease of cattle.

Epidemiology

A major problem with infection in UK cattle herds in the 1990s was associated with transmission to humans (as the human variant Creutzfeldt–Jakob disease) via the food chain. In theory, the disease can also be acquired occupationally, although occupational cases have not been described in the UK.

Statutory controls on animal feeding should have eliminated BSE in cattle born after 1 August 1996. Therefore, the incidence of the disease in cattle coming to slaughter should have decreased year on year to exceedingly low levels.

Clinical features

See 📖 p. 160, Variant Creutzfeld–Jakob disease.

Causal exposures/industries

Transmission to humans could occur from exposure to the neural tissue of infected cattle through the percutaneous or mucocutaneous route (through breach of the skin, or direct contact with non-intact skin or intact mucous membranes):
• Farmers
• Abbatoir workers
• Meat processors.

Prevention

Prevention is through good hygiene practices in agriculture and meat processing (including abbatoirs). This is covered in detail in 📖 p. 112, Animals and animal products (animals and animal products).

Relevant legislation

• BSE in animals is notifiable to the Department for the Environment, Food, and Rural Affairs (DEFRA)
• Any infection reliably attributable to work would be notifiable to HSE under RIDDOR.

Further information and guidance

HSE (2007). *BSE occupational guidance, Advisory Committee on Dangerous Pathogens.* Available at: ℠ http://www.hse.gov.uk/pubns/web22.pdf

HSE *Controlling the risk of exposure to bovine spongiform encephalopathy (BSE).* Available at: ℠ http://www.hse.gov.uk/biosafety/diseases/bovine.htm

Meningococcal infection

These infections are a collection of systemic disorders caused by the bacterium *Neisseria meningitidis*. Humans are the only known reservoir for the organism.

Epidemiology

- 10% of the population (and up to 25% of 15–19-yr-olds) carry *N. meningitidis* asymptomatically in the nasopharyx. It only causes disease in a small proportion
- Most cases are sporadic, but <5% occur as clusters
- Strong seasonal variation; highest incidence in winter
- Most cases in the UK are caused by subtypes B and C
- Occupational cases are very rare.

Clinical features

- Early features non-specific: fever, malaise, vomiting
- Characteristic petechial rash
- Progression from onset to death can be extremely rapid (few hours)
- Septicaemia (can be complicated by multi-organ failure)
- Meningitis.

Causal exposures/industries

- *Transmission is through very close contact:* inhaling respiratory secretions from the mouth or kissing
- *HCWs (documented case in ambulance technician): only* if very close contact with aerosolized respiratory secretions
- *University students:* OH professionals who provide services to universities may be asked to advise
- Occupational travellers to endemic countries (sub-Saharan Africa, Middle East).

Clinical assessment

Blood cultures.

Treatment and prognosis

- Penicillin or third-generation cephalosporins intravenously (IV). In view of the risk of rapid progression, GPs are guided to treat with a bolus of IV benzylpenicillin (1.2g intramuscular (IM)/IV) prior to admission if the diagnosis is suspected. Intensive support is needed for severe cases
- 90% recover, 10% fatal.

Prevention

Post-exposure prophylaxis

- Ciprofloxacin 500mg single oral dose (unlicensed indication) OR rifampicin 600mg bd for 2 days for:
  - HCWs who have taken part in resuscitation, endotracheal intubation, suctioning, or post-mortem without wearing appropriate respiratory protection
  - students who are prolonged close contacts of cases

Vaccination
- Subgroup C vaccination (MenC) in students living in halls of residence
- A+C vaccine for travellers where indicated by advisory sources (see 📖 p. 418)
- There is no vaccine for subgroup B.

Education

OH departments may be involved in informing HCWs/students to report suspicious symptoms early.

Compensation

A HCW who contracted meningococcal infection at work, and lost pay as a result, would be eligible for NHS Injury Benefit.

Relevant legislation

- Meningococcal septicaemia is notifiable (to Local Authority Proper Officers) under the Health Protection (Notification) Regulations 2010
- Meningococcal infection that is readily attributable to work is reportable to HSE under RIDDOR.

Further information

HPA (2006). *Guidance for public health management of meningococcal disease in the UK.* Health Protection Agency. Available at: ℛ http://www.hpa.org.uk/infections/topics_az/meningo/meningococcalguidelines.pdf

Managing meningococcal disease (meningitis or septicaemia in higher educational institutions. Available at: ℛ http://www.universitiesuk.ac.uk/Publications/Pages/Publication-218.aspx

Tuberculosis

Epidemiology

TB notifications declined in the UK until the mid-1980s. Subsequently, there have been small increases in annual incidence. The incidence is highest in people of Indian subcontinent and black African origin. Around 9000 cases of TB are currently reported each year in the UK. Most cases occur in major cities, particularly in London.

Clinical features

TB can affect many body sites; therefore, the range of presenting symptoms may be wide and non-specific. TB may be asymptomatic (latent).
- Consider TB in anyone with intermittent fever and weight loss
- *Symptoms:* chronic cough, night sweats, and haemoptysis.

Causal exposures/industries

Transmission is by inhalation of droplets following close personal contact with a sputum-positive case. At risk occupations include:
- HCWs having contact with patients or clinical specimens, especially if involved in aerosol-generating procedures (bronchoscopy, nebulization)
- Veterinary staff who handle animal species that are susceptible to TB
- Staff of prisons, old people's homes, and hostels for the homeless or refugees.

Individual susceptibility

- Contacts, including people from the same household sharing kitchen facilities, boy- or girlfriend, and frequent visitors to the home of the index case. A contact at work may be close enough to be equivalent to a household contact; therefore, a risk assessment is imperative
- Those who have lived in, who travel to, or receive visitors from places where TB is 'common' (incidence >40 per 100,000 per year)
- HIV infection, children and elderly, homeless, drug or alcohol dependency
- Hostel dwellers, and those living in poor or crowded housing
- Individuals who are immunocompromised.

Clinical assessment and diagnosis

- *Diagnosis of latent TB:* tuberculin skin test (TST), i.e. Mantoux or interferon-gamma testing if available locally. Those with a positive TST or gamma-interferon test should be assessed for active infection and if not actively infected they should be considered for treatment for latent TB
- *Respiratory TB:* CXR, multiple sputum samples, or bronchial washings for microscopy and culture
- *Non-respiratory TB:* biopsy for culture or needle aspiration for cytology, computed tomography (CT)/MRI/ultrasound/echocardiogram depending on suspected site. CXR to exclude co-existing respiratory TB.

Treatment and prognosis

Sputum +ve respiratory TB is usually rendered non-infectious after 2wks treatment with quadruple therapy. However, individuals with multidrug resistant TB (MDR-TB) may be intermittently sputum +ve for long periods. British HIV Association Guidelines should be consulted when caring for any patient who is or might be co-infected with HIV. All TB should be managed by a specialist, usually a respiratory physician.

Management of occupational risk

NICE guidance covers the assessment of the contacts of aircraft crew, school teachers, and childcare workers who are diagnosed with TB. Workplace contacts are at low risk of contracting TB from an infected individual, but a risk assessment is imperative. HCWs (including students and temporary staff) and prison staff should have the same pre-employment screening for TB. New staff should be screened according to the NICE clinical algorithm. HCWs should not work with patients or clinical specimens until an occupational health (OH) assessment has been undertaken or documented within the past 12mths.

Assessment should include:

- Symptoms and signs enquiry
- Documentary evidence of a BCG scar checked by an occupational health professional
- TST or interferon-gamma result within the last 5yrs, if available.

All staff should be reminded to report symptoms suggestive of TB promptly to their OH department. HIV positive staff are at increased risk of TB and may require modifications to their work. A tuberculin or interferon-gamma negative HCW who declines BCG vaccination should have the risks explained and supplemented by written advice, which should be signed by the individual. They should not work where there is a known risk of exposure to TB.

Personal protective equipment

HCWs caring for people with TB need not use PPE unless MDR-TB is suspected or aerosol or cough-inducing procedures are being performed. For the latter, filtering respirator masks (FFP3) are required.

Relevant legislation and guidance

- TB is notifiable (to Local Authority Proper Officers) under the Health Protection (Notification) Regulations 2010
- Occupationally acquired TB is prescribed (B5) for Industrial Injuries Disablement Benefit
- Additional information from Health Protection Agency and World Health Organization. See ℘ http://www.hpa.org.uk/Topics/ InfectiousDiseases/InfectionsAZ/Tuberculosis/ and http://www.who.int/ topics/tuberculosis/en/
- NICE guideline: NICE guideline: Clinical diagnosis and management of tuberculosis, and measures for its prevention and control. Available at: ℘ http://guidance.nice.org.uk/CG117/Guidance

Legionnaires' disease

Legionnaires' disease is an uncommon bacterial infection caused by the bacterium *Legionella pneumophila*. The organism is found living naturally in environmental water sources.

Epidemiology

The majority of cases are sporadic (single), but outbreaks can occur. There are approximately 300–400 reported cases in England annually, of which 30–50% are acquired abroad.

Clinical features

- Incubation 2–19 days (median 6–7 days)
- Influenza-like illness with fatigue, myalgia, fever, headache, and dry cough
- Diarrhoea and confusion
- Atypical pneumonia.

Causal exposures/industries

Transmission is by inhalation of infected aerosols. In workplaces, *L. pneumophila* is found in air-conditioning units, cooling towers, and showers. Any occupation working in air-conditioned buildings might be affected. Occupational travellers who stay in hotels can be exposed to infected droplets in showers.

Individual susceptibility

- Age > 50yrs
- Men are three times more likely than women to be affected
- Smoking
- Underlying chronic disease
- Immunosuppressive treatment.

Clinical assessment

- Rapid urine antigen test
- Culture of respiratory secretions
- Serology.

Treatment and prognosis

Treatment is with antibiotics, particularly erythromycin. Most cases recover, but 10–15% are fatal (higher in susceptible groups).

Prevention

Prevention is through treating water systems, and detailed specific guidance is available from HSE (see 📖 p. 168, Relevant legislation and guidance).

Relevant legislation and guidance

- Legionnaires' disease is notifiable (to Local Authority Proper Officers) under the Health Protection (Notification) Regulations 2010
- Legionellosis that is readily attributable to work is reportable to HSE under RIDDOR

- Legionnaires disease: The Control of Legionella Bacteria in Water Systems. Approved Code of Practice and Guidance. HSE, 2000. ✍ http://www.hpa.org.uk/webc/HPAwebFile/HPAweb_C/1263812807228

Tetanus

Tetanus is caused by neurotoxin produced by *Clostridium tetani*, an anaerobic spore-forming bacillus. *C. tetani* is present in the GI tract of horses and other animals. It is widespread in the environment, including soil, where it can survive for long periods. Transmission from human to human does not occur.

Epidemiology

Tetanus infection in humans is rare. Up to 7 cases per year were notified in the UK between 2005 and 2010. The majority of cases are non-occupational.

Clinical features

- Localized muscle spasm
- Generalized tetany (lockjaw).

Causal exposures/industries

Transmission is through non-intact skin following contamination with soil or other infected material. Outdoor workers who might sustain skin cuts or abrasions are at risk:

- Forestry workers
- Farm workers
- Veterinary practitioners.

Clinical assessment

Usually a clinical diagnosis, but the following confirmatory tests may help:

- Tetanus toxin in serum
- Isolation of *C. tetani* from the wound
- Tetanus toxin antibodies in serum.

Treatment and prognosis

- IV TIG
- Wound debridement
- Metronidazole
- 29% fatality rate.

Prevention

- Tetanus is preventable by immunization, for which there is a national programme (in childhood). A reinforcing dose of vaccine is not likely to boost immunity sufficiently quickly after a tetanus-prone wound. Therefore for high risk wounds, human TIG should be given irrespective of vaccination history.[1]
- Cover cuts and abrasions if working with soil or outdoors
- Individuals who are exposed to tetanus organisms at work (e.g. in microbiology laboratories) must be protected by immunization.

1 Department of Health *Immunization against Infectious Disease* (The Green Book). Available at: http://www.dh.gov.uk/prod_consum_dh/groups/dh_digitalassets/@dh/@en/documents/digitalasset/dh_103982.pdf

Relevant legislation
- Tetanus is notifiable (to Local Authority Proper Officers) under the Health Protection (Notification) Regulations 2010
- Tetanus that is readily attributable to work is reportable to HSE under RIDDOR.

Severe acute respiratory syndrome

Epidemiology

The first known case of severe acute respiratory syndrome (SARS) occurred in Guangdong province, China, in November 2002 and was recognized as a global threat in March 2003. The aetiological agent, the SARS coronovirus (SARS-CoV) is believed to be an animal virus that crossed the species barrier to humans. By the end of the epidemic in July 2003, SARS CoV had resulted in 8098 SARS cases in 26 countries, with 774 deaths. HCWs accounted for 1707 (21%) of the reported cases. Since then, the few sporadic cases have been mainly due to exposure in laboratories. During the epidemic four probable cases of SARS were reported in the UK and the risk of infection in the UK remains very low. The possibility of SARS re-emergence remains and there is a need for continuing vigilance.

Clinical features

SARS-CoV causes a spectrum of clinical illness from severe respiratory disease to mild or atypical presentations. When transmission has occurred from a single point source, the incubation period has been 2–10 days.

Symptoms include:
- Fever ≥38°C
- Cough, difficulty in breathing, and shortness of breath
- *Non-specific symptoms:* malaise, headache, myalgia
- Profuse watery diarrhoea.

Caution should be exercised in diagnosing non-specific viral pneumonia without detailed inquiry to ascertain risk factors for SARS in the 10 days before the onset of the illness.

Causal exposures/industries

Transmission occurs through inhalation of droplets following close person-to-person contact. At-risk occupations include:
- HCWs in clinical contact with SARS-CoV
- Workers in laboratories where the virus is stored
- Contacts including those who have cared for, lived with, or had direct contact with the respiratory secretions, body fluids, and/or excretions of cases of SARS
- Travellers to an area at risk of SARS-CoV transmission from animal reservoirs or a recent outbreak of SARS.

Clinical assessment and diagnosis

- For definitions of probable, confirmed, and discarded cases of SARS see the British Thoracic Society website (ℜ http://www.brit-thoracic. org.uk/guidelines/severe-acute-respiratory-syndrome-guideline.aspx)
- Specimens must only be sent for laboratory testing after the Communicable Disease Surveillance Centre (CDSC) has been

informed of the suspected case. All specimens should be double bagged and labelled as biohazard.

Health surveillance

- Maintain a list of all staff who have had contact with SARS-CoV
- All staff should be vigilant for symptoms of SARS in the 10 days following exposure and should not come to work if they have a fever
- Inform CDSC of any contacts and their details to ensure follow-up.

Risk controls in the health care industry

Full infection control precautions, including use of personal protective equipment (gloves, gowns, and masks), should be instituted, and HCWs must strictly adhere to these.

- The patient should be admitted to a designated isolation unit in a negative pressure room
- Visitors should be kept to a minimum and all entrants to the isolation room must be logged
- Those who deliver clinical care must wear an FFP3
- Aerosol-generating procedures (nebulizers, bronchoscopy) constitute a particular risk, and the minimum number of personnel should be present when these are carried out.

Contingency planning

Guidance from the World Health Organization on contingency planning is available on 🖰 http://www.who.int/csr/sars/en/index.html

Relevant legislation and guidance

- SARS is notifiable (to Local Authority Proper Officers) under the Health Protection (Notification) Regulations 2010
- Detailed guidance, including advice on risk controls when managing a suspected case of SARS, is available on the HPA website. 🖰 http://www.hpa.org.uk/infections/topics_az/SARS/Guidelines.htm

Influenza

Influenza is a virus that is found in animals and humans. Many strains are recognized, and these tend to infect different species. An important characteristic of the organism is the propensity to undergo minor or major changes in antigenic profile (antigenic drift or shift, respectively). Influenza is transmitted from human to human. Moreover, transmission between species has been described (although is still uncommon).

Epidemiology

Seasonal influenza

Influenza infection in the general population shows strong seasonal variation with highest incidence in the winter (December–March in the northern hemisphere). WHO figures suggest that worldwide 7500,000 people die of influenza each year in non-pandemic years. In England, influenza activity is measured according to new GP consultations for influenza and influenza-like illness (ILI), and normal winter seasonal levels are 30–200 cases per 100 000 population per week .[1] A very small proportion of cases of seasonal influenza are acquired occupationally.

Epidemic influenza Normal seasonal activity crosses threshold (>200 new cases per 100 000 per week in England) into severe 'epidemic' activity unpredictably.

Pandemic influenza

Pandemics, with high rates of transmission worldwide, have occurred when new strains emerge which have high transmissibility against a background of absent herd resistance. Previous pandemics in 1918–1919, 1957, and 1968 resulted in high global mortality (40–50 million in 1918–1919), particularly among susceptible groups. The H5N1 strain, which infects birds (avian influenza), has been transmitted to small numbers of humans, but has not transmitted easily between humans. The most recent pandemic influenza virus (H1N1 'swine flu') emerged in Mexico in 2009. Swine flu was transmitted between humans, but in most cases the disease was mild. Severe illness and death did occur in a small proportion of cases, particularly among pregnant women and young adults. There is currently global concern about the possibility of a future influenza pandemic and the UK has a preparedness strategy for this event.

Clinical features

- Fever >38°C
- Headache
- Myalgia
- Severe malaise
- Complications include pneumonia.

---

1 HPA. (2012). *Definitions and rates vary in Wales and Scotland because of different reporting methods*. Available at: ℘ http://www.hpa.org.uk/infections/topics_az/influenza/seasonal/uk_data_sources.htm

Causal exposures/industries

Most occupations do not have a greater risk than the general population. The following groups are at increased risk:

- HCWs who:
  - look after infected patients
  - handle influenza organisms in the laboratory
- Teachers and care workers in institutions.

Individual susceptibility The working age population is at increased risk if they have chronic disease (e.g. diabetes mellitus, renal failure, cancer, chronic respiratory illness).

Clinical assessment

- Serology
- Near patient test can be useful for instant diagnosis.

Treatment and prognosis

Treatment is with anti-viral agents (oseltamivir, zanamivir, or amantadine).[2] Prognosis varies according to the strain and the level of herd immunity.

Prevention

Influenza immunization

- The Chief Medical Officer has recommended annual immunization against seasonal influenza for fit HCWs (i.e. in the absence of specific medical indications). As well as protecting HCWs from occupational transmission, there is reasonable evidence that immunization reduces mortality in their elderly patients
- Many OH providers offer influenza immunization to staff outside the health care sector, even in the absence of increased occupational risk. This is usually justified on the basis that it might reduce sickness absence, although the evidence base for this assumption is incomplete.

Preventing exposure

In the health care industry, exposure to staff is minimized by:

- Wearing masks for close clinical contact
- Observing infection control procedures
- Wearing filtering respirators, gowns, and goggles for aerosol-inducing procedures (bronchoscopy, post-mortems, intubation, chest physiotherapy, nebulization).

Pandemic planning OH professionals who provide services to health care or emergency services (fire, police, and ambulance) have a major role in advising about pandemic preparedness. Detailed guidance is given on the HPA website.

Further information

HPA (2012). *Influenza*. Available at: ℘ http://www.hpa.org.uk/Topics/InfectiousDiseases/InfectionsAZ/Influenza/

2 NICE (2003). *Flu prevention—amantadine and oseltamivir (TA67)*. Available at: ℘ http://www.nice.org.uk/page.aspx?o=86770

Anthrax

Anthrax is a rare zoonosis caused by *Bacillus anthracis*, a spore-forming Gram +ve bacterium that can survive in soil for long periods.

Epidemiology

Anthrax occurs mainly in herbivores and is endemic in the Middle East, Africa, and Asia. It is transmitted to humans from infected animal products, but not human-to-human spread. Nineteen confirmed cases were notified in England and Wales 1981–2009 (most were occupational). Since 2009 large outbreaks have occurred in drug users from infected heroin.

Clinical features

There are three clinical forms of anthrax; cutaneous anthrax is the most common. Occupationally acquired anthrax is usually cutaneous. Inhalational anthrax in non-endemic areas raises the possibility of bioterrorism.

Cutaneous anthrax

Skin lesion appears days or weeks after exposure, usually on the head, neck, arms, or hands. The lesion is surrounded by oedema and develops into a characteristic painless ulcer with a black centre (eschar). Cutaneous anthrax can be complicated by septicaemia.

Gastrointestinal anthrax

Acquired by consuming undercooked infected meat.

Inhalational anthrax

Much rarer than cutaneous anthrax but i mortality. Characterized by influenza-like illness; onset up to 48h after exposure.

Causal exposures/industries

- Laboratory staff handling anthrax spores or infected material
- Workers handling infected hides, e.g. leather tanners
- Workers handling infected animals, e.g. abbatoir workers, veterinary practitioners
- Postal workers (deliberate release) (see 📖 p. 830, Biological weapons).

Clinical assessment and diagnosis

Suspected cases should be investigated in liaison with the Special Pathogens Reference Unit (SPRU)[1] which offers diagnostic services for rare pathogenic organisms. Investigation includes:

- Detailed exposure history
- Serology
- Blood cultures
- Swab of lesion fluid for stain and culture
- *Biopsy lesion*: polymerase chain reaction (PCR) for *b. Anthracis* DNA
- Additionally, for inhalational anthrax, CXR, CT scan of thorax, LFTs.

---

1 🔗 http://www.hpa.org.uk/ProductsServices/InfectiousDiseases/SpecialPathogensReferenceUnit/

Prognosis Untreated, 5–20% of cutaneous anthrax cases are fatal. Inhalational anthrax is often fatal (775% despite optimal treatment).

Prevention Inactivated acellular vaccine available from the HPA. Vaccination only offered to occupational groups at i risk of exposure (laboratory staff handling spores/infected material). Vaccine not indicated in the public unless exposed.

Medical management Undertaken in liaison with the HPA Centre for Infections. Cutaneous anthrax is treatable with oral antibiotics; ciprofloxacin is the drug of choice. Management of inhalational anthrax is very specialized, involving IV ciprofloxacin plus two other antibiotics.

Post-exposure prophylaxis

Following exposure, antibiotic treatment ± vaccination is indicated.
- *Antibiotics for 60 days:*
  - initial 3 days—oral ciprofloxacin 500mg bd
  - remaining 57 days—oral ciprofloxacin 500mg bd OR oral doxycycline 100mg bd
- *Immunization:*
  - three doses at 0, 3, and 6wks after exposure
  - given with vaccine, duration of post-exposure prophylaxis (PEP) antibiotics can be ↓ to 4wks
  - further doses at 6mths and 1yr, if continuing exposure
  - PEP not required for case's contacts unless exposed to original source.

Compensation

- In the UK anthrax is a prescribed disease (B1) for Industrial Injuries Disablement Benefit in workers who have contact with anthrax spores, including contact with animals infected by anthrax, or those involved in handling, loading, unloading, or transport of a type susceptible to infection with anthrax or of the products or residues of such animals
- HCWs are eligible for NHS Injury Benefit if they contract anthrax at work and lose pay as a result.

Relevant legislation

- Anthrax is notifiable (to Local Authority Proper Officers) under the Health Protection (Notification) Regulations 2010
- Anthrax that is readily attributable to exposure to B. anthracis at work is notifiable to HSE under RIDDOR
- An exposure in the workplace would be notifiable to HSE under RIDDOR as a dangerous occurrence.

Further information

HPA (2012). Anthrax. Available at: ℘ http://www.hpa.org.uk/infections/topics_az/anthrax/menu.htm
CDC. *Emergency preparedness and response.* Available at: ℘ http://www.bt.cdc.gov/agent/anthrax/faq/
HPA (2012). *Deliberate and accidental release.* Available at: ℘ http://www.hpa.org.uk/infections/topics_az/deliberate_release/Anthrax/Homepage.asp?Source=Professional&Agent=Anthrax&Document=Homepage

Glanders

Glanders is a zoonotic infection, caused by the bacterium *Burkholderia mallei*. It is essentially a disease of equine species, including horses, donkeys, and mules. It is rarely found in dogs, cats, and goats.

Epidemiology

Glanders has been eradicated in the UK, but still occurs in Europe and the Far East.

Clinical features

The incubation period is 10–14 days, but long latency (up to 30yrs) has been described. Presentation depends on the route of infection, which can be through non-intact skin or mucous membranes, inhalation, and potentially ingestion. Once infected, it can affect any organ system.
- *Acute infection:*
  - skin infection, with ulceration and local lymphadenopathy
  - mucosal upper respiratory tract infection, with bloody nasal discharge
  - pneumonia, with pleural effusion and lung abscess
  - septicaemia
- *Chronic infection:* with abscess formation in skin, muscle, liver, and spleen.

Causal exposures/industries

Glanders does not occur in the environment. It can only be acquired through prolonged contact with infected animals, although the infectivity of secretions is extremely low. Realistically, the only occupational cases in the West are likely to be laboratory workers:
- Laboratory workers handling *B. mallei*
- Veterinary practitioners
- Horse handlers, grooms, and breeders.

Treatment and prognosis

Glanders can be treated with antibiotics. Historically, treatment was with sulphonamides, but newer antibiotics including co-trimoxazole may be effective (the disease disappeared before these could be evaluated). Untreated, it is rapidly fatal in >90% of cases (particularly if acquired through the inhalational route). For this reason, it is a potential candidate for bioterrorism (see 📖 p. 830, Biological weapons), although no incidents have occurred to date.

Prevention

There is currently no vaccine for glanders.

Compensation

Glanders is a prescribed disease for Industrial Injuries Disablement Benefit in workers who have contact with equine animals or their carcasses.

Relevant legislation

Glanders that is readily attributable to work would be reportable to HSE under RIDDOR.

Leptospirosis

Leptospirosis is a zoonotic disease caused by a spirochaete bacterium of the genus *Leptospira*. There are many different pathogenic varieties that use different animal hosts. Common carriers in the UK are rats (*L. ictohaemhorrhagica*), cattle (*L. hardjo*), and pigs. Person to person transfer is rare, if it occurs at all.

Epidemiology

Leptospirosis is uncommon. Between 28 and 81 cases per year have been notified in the UK over the past 10yrs. Some of these are acquired during leisure activities or overseas. In 2010, 42 cases were notified in the UK, including 10 of occupational origin.

Clinical features

- Incubation most commonly 7–14 days (range 2–30 days)
- Biphasic clinical illness.

Acute bacteraemic phase

Bacteria are disseminated to every organ system. Characterized by influenza-like symptoms, headache, chills, and myalgia. Most cases are mild and resolve without treatment, but rarely severe illness occurs (Weil's disease).

Immune phase

Follows acute phase in some cases. Recurrence of fever, associated with jaundice, conjunctivitis, abdominal pain, and rash. Can be complicated by multi-organ failure.

Causal exposures/industries

Transmission is by direct or indirect contact with infected animal urine or contaminated water. This usually occurs through intact mucous membranes or non-intact skin:

- Farm workers
- Sewerage workers
- Dog handlers
- Abbatoir workers
- Veterinary practitioners.

Clinical assessment and diagnosis

Serological tests are available through the Leptospira Reference Unit (LRU).[1]

Treatment and prognosis

Oral penicillin or doxycycline. IV antibiotics, and intensive support are required for severe cases. Prognosis is good if the diagnosis is made early and appropriate treatment started. Emergency and Intensive Care Units in rural areas should be aware of the possibility of leptospirosis in febrile icteric illnesses.

---

1 HPA (2012). Leptospira Reference Unit (LRU). ℰ http://www.hpa.org.uk/ProductsServices/InfectiousDiseases/LaboratoriesAndReferenceFacilities/LeptospiraReferenceUnit/

Prevention
- There is no vaccine for humans
- Prophylactic doxycycline (200mg weekly) can be given for high-risk occupational tasks
- Reduce rodent populations by avoiding rubbish accumulation and culling
- Infected farm animals can be immunized and treated
- PPE (especially waterproof gloves and footwear) for jobs that entail splashing or immersion in rivers, puddles, or sewage
- Advise workers of risk and symptoms; information cards are often used for this purpose
- Cover cuts and abrasions with waterproof dressings. Wash new cuts thoroughly if acquired near potentially contaminated water.

Compensation
Leptospirosis is prescribed (B3) for Industrial Injuries Disablement Benefit for those who work in places which might be infested by rats, field mice, voles, or other small mammals, in dog kennels or the care or handling of dogs, or in contact with bovine animals or their meat products, or pigs or their meat products.

Relevant legislation
- Since 2010, leptospirosis is no longer notifiable under public health legislation
- Leptospirosis that is reliably attributable to work is reportable to HSE under RIDDOR.

Streptococcus suis

Strep. suis is a zoonotic infection, of which 35 subtypes have been identified. The organism is an important pathogen in pigs, but can occur in cattle and other animals.

Epidemiology

Transmission to humans is rare, but it is probably under-diagnosed. Only a few hundred human cases have been reported worldwide, and the annual incidence in England and Wales is around two cases.

Clinical features

Severe febrile illness, with systemic disease:
- Meningitis
- Septicaemia
- Endocarditis
- Deafness.

Causal exposures/industries

Transmission is through non-intact skin from infected pig products, although overall the risk of infection is low. There have been no reported cases of transmission through inhalation:
- Abbatoir workers
- Butchers
- Farmers
- Veterinary practitioners.

Individual susceptibility

Immunosuppressed (particularly asplenic) individuals are at increased risk.

Medical management

Penicillin is the treatment of choice.

Prevention

- There is no human vaccine
- The mainstay of prevention is good hygiene practice in slaughterhouses and butchers. Thorough washing of hands and arms before and after touching pig products is essential
- Exposed workers must be educated about hygiene, and should report suspicious symptoms (febrile illness) immediately, declaring their exposure to the treating doctor.

Compensation

Strep. suis is a prescribed disease (B9) for Industrial Injuries Disablement Benefit among those who are in contact with pigs infected by *Strep. suis*, or with infected carcasses, pig products, or residues.

Relevant legislation

- *Strep. suis* is *not* reportable under public health legislation
- *Strep. suis* that is readily attributable to work is reportable to HSE under RIDDOR.

Further information and guidance

HSE (2008). *Common zoonoses in agriculture.* Agriculture Information Sheet No.2 (rev). Available at: ✎ http://www.hse.gov.uk/pubns/ais2.pdf

Brucellosis

A group of zoonoses caused by the bacterial species *Brucella*:
- *B. melitensis*: sheep and goats
- *B. abortus*: cattle
- *B. suis*: pigs.

The main source of non-occupational brucellosis is unpasteurized milk products.Epidemiology

Brucellosis is rare in the UK. The 10 cases per year seen in the UK are almost always acquired abroad (the disease is still endemic in Africa, the Middle East, Asia, and South America). There is likely to be under-reporting of laboratory –acquired occupational infection.

Clinical features
- 2–8wks incubation
- *Non-specific ILI:*
  - fever and malaise
  - arthralgia
  - can affect any organ system.

Causal exposures/industries

Occupational transmission is through direct contact with non-intact skin, inhalation, or ingestion. Direct skin exposure occurs in occupations that handle raw meat and unpasteurized dairy products. Respiratory exposure is through washing down farm or slaughterhouse buildings.
- Farm workers
- Abbatoir workers
- Meat packers (raw products)
- Veterinary practitioners
- Animal laboratory workers
- Laboratory workers handling *Brucella* species or infected material.
  Brucella is a potential candidate for bioterrorism in view of its high infectivity on inhalation (see 📖 p. 854).

Clinical assessment

Diagnosis is by serology and culture of blood and body fluids in liaison with the Brucella Reference Unit.[1]

Treatment and prognosis
- Treatment is with antibiotics, usually combination of tetracycline-streptomycin or tetracycline-rifampicin
- Brucellosis is rarely fatal, but it can cause prolonged debilitating illness.

---

1 HPA (2012). *Brucella Reference Unit (BRU) Liverpool.* Available at: 🔗 http://www.hpa.org.uk/ProductsServices/InfectiousDiseases/LaboratoriesAndReferenceFacilities/BrucellaReferenceUnit/

Prevention

- There is no human vaccine
- Prevention is through good hygiene practice in slaughterhouses and farms, including handwashing and wearing respiratory protection for aerosol-generating procedures.

Compensation

Brucellosis is a prescribed disease (B7) for Industrial Injuries Disablement Benefit in those who handle animals infected by *Brucella*, or their carcasses or their untreated products, or laboratory specimens containing *Brucella*.

Relevant legislation

- Brucellosis is notifiable (to Local Authority Proper Officers) under the Health Protection (Notification) Regulations 2010
- Brucellosis that is readily attributable to work is reportable to HSE under RIDDOR.

Further information and guidance

HSE (2008). *Common zoonoses in agriculture*. Agriculture Information Sheet No.2 (rev). Available at: ℘ http://www.hse.gov.uk/pubns/ais2.pdf

Lyme disease

Lyme disease is a bacterial infection of birds and mammals caused by the spirochaete *Borrelia burgdorferi*. It is spread to humans from the animal reservoir (commonly deer) by a tick vector (*Ixodes* species).

Epidemiology

The reported incidence of Lyme disease has been increasing in the UK over the past 10yrs, reaching a level of 1.79 cases per 100,000 population in 2009. Most cases are non-occupational. Infections tend to be seasonal, with over half of all cases occurring between July and September.

Clinical features

Erythema migrans, a spreading rash, is the most common manifestation and often the only symptom. However, untreated cases can develop the following complications:

- Transverse myelitis
- Cranial nerve palsies
- Meningitis
- Arthritis
- Encephalitis (rare)
- Post-viral syndrome.

Causal exposures/industries

- Forestry workers
- Gamekeepers
- Farmers.

Clinical assessment

- Do not discount the possibility of Lyme disease in the absence of a history of tick bite as many sufferers cannot recollect a tick bite
- Diagnosis is by serology, but antibodies are often not detectable within the first few weeks of appearance of the rash.

Treatment and prognosis

Treatment is with antibiotics (doxycycline or amoxycillin). The rash responds promptly, but established neurological symptoms can be slow to improve.

Prevention

- There is no vaccine
- The mainstay of prevention is tick avoidance:
  - cover skin if working in infested areas
  - use insect repellants
  - daily skin checks (particularly skin folds, axillae, and groins) and removal of ticks. the risk of transmission is low in the first 24hrs, and so risk is greatly reduced by vigilant tick removal
  - education among at-risk groups to report rashes and seek early treatment.

Compensation

Lyme disease is prescribed (B14) for Industrial Injuries Disablement Benefit in those who are exposed to deer or other mammals of a type liable to harbour ticks carrying *Borrelia* bacteria.

Relevant legislation

- Lyme disease is NOT reportable by clinicians under public health legislation but, since 2010, PHLS microbiology laboratories are required to report all serologically confirmed cases to the Health Protection Agency
- Lyme disease that is reliably attributable to work is reportable to HSE under RIDDOR.

Chlamydia infections

Chlamydiosis is a bacterial zoonosis caused by the organism *Chlamydia psittaci*. There are two main types: avian chlamydiosis (psittacosis or ornithosis) and ovine chlamydiosis. Human-to-human spread is rare.

Epidemiology

Most cases of chlamydiosis are non-occupational, occurring in pet owners.

Clinical features

Incubation 1–2wks.

Avian chlamydiosis

- Fever, cough, myalgia
- Delirium in severe cases
- Pericarditis, myocarditis, endocarditis
- Atypical pneumonia
- Hepatitis.

Ovine chlamydiosis

Abortion/stillbirth.

Causal exposures

Avian chlamydiosis

C. psittaci is excreted in the faeces and nasal discharges of infected birds. A range of bird species are susceptible. The most important sources for occupational transmission are ducks and other poultry, pigeons, and psittacines (exotic birds, e.g. parrots, cockatiels, macaws). The organism is resistant to dessication and can remain infectious for months. Transmission to humans is by inhalation of dust containing excreta of infected birds or by direct handling of birds, plumage, and tissues.

Ovine chlamydiosis

Transmission is through handling infected sheep placentas at lambing. Clothing soiled with sheep products of conception are also infectious.

Industries

- Pet shop workers
- Poultry farm workers
- Feather-processing workers
- Abbatoir workers
- Poultry meat inspectors
- Pigeons nesting in buildings that are used as workplaces can lead to exposure in a wide range of occupations
- Sheep farm workers
- Veterinary practitioners.

Individual susceptibility

Pregnant women are at risk of ovine chlamydiosis and must avoid contact with pregnant sheep.

Clinical assessment and treatment

Diagnosis is by serology and treatment is with tetracycline.

Prevention

Avian chlamydiosis

The mainstay of prevention is good animal husbandry, and avoidance of build-up of bird excreta in any area where people are at work.

- Screen breeding stock and treat with medicated seed
- Good flock husbandry (avoidance of overcrowding and stress among caged birds)
- Avoid dry sweeping of bird excreta
- Good general ventilation where birds are housed
- Local exhaust ventilation for de-feathering and evisceration tasks
- *PPE:* respirator with protection factor of at least 20 for dust-generating tasks.

Ovine chlamydiosis

- Vaccinate breeding ewes
- *PPE:* waterproof overalls and gloves for lambing
- Segregation and decontamination of soiled PPE: must not be taken home to be washed.

Compensation

Chlamydiosis is prescribed (B10(a) Avian, B10(b) Ovine) for Industrial Injuries Disablement Benefit.

Relevant legislation

- Chlamydiosis is NOT reportable under public health legislation
- Chlamydiosis that is reliably attributable to work is reportable to HSE under RIDDOR.

Further information and guidance

HSE (2008). *Common zoonoses in agriculture.* Agriculture Information Sheet No.2 (rev). Available at: ℘ http://www.hse.gov.uk/pubns/ais2.pdf

Q fever

Q fever is a highly infectious zoonosis caused by the bacterium *Coxiella burnetii*. The organism is widespread in animals, but the most common sources of transmission to humans are cattle, sheep, and goats. Human-to-human spread does not generally occur.

Epidemiology

It is difficult to estimate the true incidence of Q fever, as cases are often mild and may go unreported. Therefore the 50–100 cases per year reported in the UK are probably an underestimate. The peak incidence in the UK is in the spring, associated with the lambing season.

Clinical features

- Incubation period 7–30 days
- *Acute infection:* 50% experience an acute influenza-like illness with pneumonia. Symptoms are often mild and only 5% need hospital treatment
- *Chronic infection:* develops in a small proportion up to 18mths after the acute event. Complicated by endocarditis. Chronic infection has a high fatality rate if untreated.

Causal exposures/industries

Transmission is through inhalation of infected dusts or aerosols comprising infected animal products. Direct transmission can occur through non-intact skin. The most common source of infected material is products of conception at lambing:
- Sheep farmers
- Abbatoir workers
- Meat packers (raw)
- Veterinary practitioners.

Individual susceptibility

Those with chronic diseases are most at risk (chronic renal disease, cancer, prosthetic heart valve, and transplant recipients).

Treatment and prognosis

Treatment of acute Q fever is with antibiotics (doxycycline or tetracycline) for 7–14 days. Chronic disease is difficult to treat, and 50% relapse despite combination therapy. Therefore, antibiotics for chronic cases must be continued for 3yrs.

Prevention

- There is no vaccine for Q fever
- Mainstay of prevention is minimizing exposure to animal products, including good animal husbandry and hygiene. Use of PPE (gloves, waterproof overalls) at lambing reduces skin exposure (see 🕮 p. 112, Animals and animal products).

Compensation

Q fever is a prescribed disease (B11) for Industrial Injuries Disablement Benefit among those who are in contact with infected animals, their remains, or untreated products.

Relevant legislation

- Q fever is NOT reportable under public health legislation
- Q fever that is readily attributable to work is reportable to HSE under the RIDDOR.

Enteric zoonoses

A number of organisms colonize the GI tract of farm and domestic animals, and can be transmitted to humans.

Causal exposures/industries

Infection occurs after contact with animal dung, usually after putting hands or fingers in the mouth without washing:

- Farm workers
- Veterinary practitioners
- Abbatoir workers
- Meat packers (raw).

Clinical features

These are similar for a number of organisms.

Escherichia coli 0157 (E.coli 0157)

A bacterium that inhabits the gut of cattle, sheep, deer, goats, pets, and wild birds. It produces a toxin that causes illness in humans ranging from diarrhoea to renal failure. Can be fatal in humans (but rarely). Few organisms are required to infect humans. There is no specific treatment.

Salmonella

Salmonellosis is caused by *Salmonella* bacteria, and is characterized by fever, diarrhoea, vomiting, and abdominal pain. As well as the more familiar food-borne transmission to humans, infection can be acquired directly from farm animals that carry the organism. An important mode of transmission is hand-to-hand contact in farm workers. Treatment is with oral ciprofloxacin.

Cryptosporidium

Cryptosporidiosis is caused by the protozoan *Cryptosporidium parvum* which is carried by calves, sheep, lambs, deer, and goats. It presents as an influenza-like illness with diarrhoea and abdominal pain.

Prevention

Risk controls are outlined in detail on 📖 p.112, Animals and animal products. *Salmonella* is treatable in herds using medicated feed.

Relevant legislation

Any infection that is readily attributable to work is reportable to HSE under RIDDOR.

Further information and guidance

HSE *Zoonoses*. Available at: ℗ http://www.hse.gov.uk/biosafety/diseases/zoonoses.htm

HPA (2012). *Escherichia coli*. Available at: ℗ http://www.hpa.org.uk/infections/topics_az/ecoli/O157/facts.htm

Zoonotic skin infections

Causal exposures/industries

Transmitted by direct skin contact with infected animal lesions:
- Shepherds
- Farmers
- Veterinary practitioners
- Abbatoir workers
- Meat inspectors.

Orf

Orf is a viral zoonosis caused by the parapoxvirus. It causes contagious pustular dermatitis (ecthyema contagiosum or 'scabby mouth') in sheep (mainly lambs) and goats. Human-to-human transmission has not been recorded.

Epidemiology

The frequency of orf in the general population is extremely low. Virtually all cases are occupational. Because the disorder is mostly trivial in humans, it is difficult to obtain accurate incidence data because of under-reporting. Only 8 cases per year on average were reported to the HPA during 1991–2006, and just 2 cases per year since 2005.

Clinical features, diagnosis, and treatment
- 1-wk incubation period
- Rapidly developing red papule, typically on the finger; usually up to 5cm in diameter, and can ulcerate
- Can be complicated by fever, lymphadenopathy, erythema multiforme, and (rarely) bullous pemphigoid
- Diagnosis is by electron microscopy of a lesion biopsy
- Self-limiting; infection usually confers immunity
- Antibiotics for 2° bacterial infection.

Individual susceptibility

Immunocompromised (particularly haematological malignancy) may develop large fungating granuloma or tumour-like lesion.

Ringworm

Ringworm is a dermatophyte (fungal) infection.

Clinical features, diagnosis, and treatment
- Characteristic annular plaque with raised edge and central clearing
- Scaling and pruritis common
- Diagnosis by microscopy and culture of skin scales
- Treatment with topical antifungals
- Oral griseofulvin only for severe cases
- Treat secondary bacterial infection with antibiotics.

Others
- Viral warts (papillomavirus) in butchers and fishermen
- Erysipeloid (erysipelothrix) in fish processors

- Cutaneous granulomata (*Mycobacterium marinum*) in tropical fish dealers.

Prevention of zoonotic dermatoses
- Live vaccine for affected flocks
- Use PPE (gloves) when examining the months of sheep and lambs
- See 📖 p. 112, Animals and animal products, for specific guidance.

Compensation
Orf is prescribed (B12) for Industrial Injuries Disablement Benefit in those who have contact with sheep or goats, or with the carcasses of sheep or goats.

Relevant legislation
Orf or ringworm that is reliably attributable to occupation is reportable to HSE under RIDDOR.

Respiratory and cardiovascular disorders

Occupational asthma and rhinitis

Occupational asthma and rhinitis are caused by immunological sensitization to agents in the workplace. Once an individual is sensitized, symptoms can occur after very low level re-exposure.

Epidemiology

- Around 9–15% of asthma in adults of working age is occupational.
- The number of new cases of occupational asthma in the UK has been falling over the past 10yrs.
- The estimated rate of occupational asthma is 45–75 cases per 100,000 workers per year (based on a European population-based study).

Clinical features and aetiology

- *Asthma:* wheeze, chest tightness, dyspnoea. Classically, symptoms are worse at work or soon after work, and better at weekends or during holidays. This pattern can be lost in the later stages of the disease. Late reactions can occur at night or early morning after a day at work
- *Rhinitis and conjunctivitis:* rhinorrhea, nasal stuffiness and itching of the eyes/nose, sneezing. These are often associated with asthma and may precede chest symptoms
- When the individual is sensitized, symptoms can be precipitated by non-specific irritation (e.g. cigarette smoke or cold air).

Causal exposures/industries

See Table 7.1. Allergens can be divided broadly into:
- High molecular weight proteins (e.g. animal and plant proteins)
- Low molecular weight substances that act as haptens (e.g. isocyanates, acid anhydrides).

Individual susceptibility

- Atopy
- Cigarette smoking

Atopy is common (30% of the population); it is not usually appropriate to screen out atopics from exposure to sensitizing agents at pre-employment.

Clinical assessment and diagnosis of occupational asthma

- Initial investigation with lung function tests (FEV_1, forced vital capacity (FVC), and peak flow) to explore the diagnosis of asthma (reversible airways obstruction).
- Exposure assessment (pattern of exposure and specific allergens and relationship to symptoms, use of respiratory protective equipment):
  - a full history should include current and previous exposures
  - be aware of the possibility of late reactions
  - the lack of a clear temporal relationship to work does not exclude the diagnosis of occupational asthma

Table 7.1 Causal exposures/industries

Exposure	Industry/uses
Isocyanates	Car body shops
Flour, grain dust	Bakeries, agriculture
Acid anhydrides	Manufacturing, use of epoxy resins/varnishes
Rosin flux	Electronics (soldering)
Proteolytic enzymes	Manufacture of biological washing powders
Animal proteins (urine/dander)	Laboratory animal research
Platinum salts	Platinum industry
Antibiotics, cimetidine, ispaghula	Pharmaceutical manufacturing
Glutaraldehyde, natural rubber latex	Health care
Wood dust	Construction, forestry, carpentry
Persulphate salts or henna	Hairdressing
Fish proteins, soya bean, tea dust	Fish preparation, food industry
Reactive dyes	Cosmetic and rubber manufacture
Metal working fluids	Manufacturing

Serial peak flow recording (see 📖 p. 762, Serial peak flow testing)

- *Bronchial provocation challenge tests:*
  - should be carried out in a specialist centre (contact your local consultant respiratory physician for advice)
  - individuals can be sensitized to more than one asthmagen
- Specific IgE, skin prick testing (if specific test reagents are available).

Prognosis

Symptoms usually resolve after removal from exposure, but the practical constraints of exposure control can be a real threat to employment.

👉 Where exposure cannot be controlled completely, individuals are sometimes allowed to continue working whilst wearing PPE. However, they must be informed about risk and have frequent health surveillance.

Compensation

Occupationally acquired asthma and allergic rhinitis are both prescribed for Industrial Injuries Disablement Benefit (D7 and D4, respectively) in those who are exposed to a known sensitizing agent at work.

Health surveillance

Individuals who are exposed to respiratory sensitizers must undergo health surveillance (Management of Health and Safety at Work (MHSW) and COSHH Regulations). The surveillance programme depends on the likelihood of sensitization, and is outlined in specific guidance from HSE.[1]

Relevant legislation and guidance

- Occupational asthma is reportable under RIDDOR. Asthmagen? *Critical Assessments of the Evidence for Agents Implicated in Occupational asthma*
- Occupational asthma: a guide for occupational physicians and occupational health physicians. http://www.bohrf.org.uk/downloads/asthlop.pdf

---

1 *MS 25. Medical Aspects of Occupational Asthma.* HSE, Sudbury.

Latex allergy

Latex allergy may manifest as:
- A type I immediate hypersensitivity reaction due to a reaction to natural rubber latex (NRL) proteins
- More commonly as a type IV delayed hypersensitivity reaction in response to the chemical additives in latex products.

Epidemiology

During the past 20yrs, latex allergy has become a major occupational hazard in the rubber processing and healthcare industries. In the healthcare industry the use of disposable powdered NRL gloves, many dusted with corn starch to aid donning, increased exponentially after 1987 until the mid-1990s. However, the apparent prevalence of latex allergy has been steadily decreasing since 1998. The prevalence of type I allergy (based on skin-prick testing) in HCWs is currently estimated to be up to 12%. Around 1% of the general population are sensitized to NRL, but not all sensitized individuals develop symptoms.

Clinical features

- *Type I:* urticaria, rhinitis, conjunctivitis, occasionally asthma or very rarely anaphylaxis. Onset is usually within 20min of exposure.
- *Type IV:* dermatitis, characterized by a red, itchy, scaly rash often localized to the area of use, i.e. wrists and forearms with glove use, but may spread to other areas. Onset is usually >12h after exposure

Causal exposures/industries

- Health care workers
- Individuals exposed to NRL regularly, e.g. food handlers, hairdressers and construction workers
- Latex product manufacturing workers.

Individual susceptibility

- Patients with spina bifida and congenital genitourinary abnormalities
- A history of certain food allergies, such as banana, avocado, kiwi and chestnut
- Individuals with atopic allergic disease may be at increased risk.

Clinical assessment and diagnosis

- The clinical history is essential in establishing the diagnosis of type 1 allergy:
  - supporting tests include a positive skin prick test to latex allergens and a serological test for specific IgE; not all individuals with a positive skin or serological test manifest allergic disease
  - consider referring the individual for specialist advice and a latex challenge or use test
- Type IV allergy is diagnosed by a positive patch testing

Prognosis

Reducing exposure to latex may lead to a reduction in type 1 allergic symptoms in sensitized individuals.

Management

Latex policy

All health care organizations should have a latex policy outlining the hazards of NRL, how to identify and manage individuals with NRL allergy, and how to reduce exposure in the workplace. Organizations should be moving towards a latex free environment.

Adjustments to work

If NRL allergy is diagnosed, a risk assessment of the individual's workplace must be made to ensure a safe working environment. If the individual has a history of severe type I allergy or anaphylaxis, they must work in a latex free environment. Redeployment may be necessary. They should be advised to wear a medic alert bracelet, carry an epipen, and inform healthcare providers of their NRL allergy.

For non-life threatening allergies the following are recommended:
• Avoid contact with NRL gloves or products
• Avoid areas where there is a risk of inhalation of powder from NRL gloves worn by others
• Substitute to other glove materials where appropriate, e.g. nitrile, PVC, or neoprene.
• If use of NRL gloves is necessary they should be single use disposable gloves and be low-protein (<50µg/g) and powder-free.

Relevant legislation

Employers and employees need to comply with the COSHH Regulations 2002 (as amended) (see 📖 p. 532, Control of Substances Hazardous to Health). This includes assessing and reducing risks and providing health surveillance in appropriate cases (see 📖 p. 426, Skin surveillance and 📖 p. 428, Respiratory health surveillance).

Further information and guidance

HSE *Latex allergy*. Available at: 🖰 http://www.hse.gov.uk/skin/employ/latex.htm
NHS. Latex allergy: occupational aspects of management. Available at: 🖰 http://www.nhsplus.nhs.uk/providers/images/library/files/guidelines/Latex_allergy_guidelines.pdf
HSE (1998). *Medical aspects of occupational skin disease*, MS24. HSE, Sudbury.

Byssinosis

Epidemiology and pathogenesis

This disease has been associated historically with exposure to cotton dust. It is thought that the disease is caused by an endotoxin, which is produced by bacteria within raw cotton, but the precise pathology is unclear. Byssinosis is rare, having largely been eliminated by good exposure controls in the textile industry. In the UK, the disease was most common in Lancashire and Northern Ireland; both are areas that have local textile mills. The condition is more prevalent in developing countries with large textile industries (e.g. India and China) where poor control of exposure may result in extremely high exposures, in some cases >100mg/m³.

Clinical features

- Wheezing and chest tightness
- Typically worse after a break from work (Mondays), improving with return to exposure (better towards the end of the working week)
- Temporal relationship can be obscured after prolonged exposure.

Causal exposures/industries

- Raw cotton, flax, or hemp
- Development of byssinosis within 10yrs of exposure is rare; usually symptoms are associated with >20yrs of exposure
- Textile and rope-making industry.

Individual susceptibility

Cigarette smokers develop more severe disease.

Clinical assessment and treatment

- *Lung function:* cross-shift decline in FEV$_1$
- There are no specific radiological abnormalities associated with byssinosis
- Treatment is with bronchodilators and antihistamines.

Prevention

Exposure controls include enclosure of carding operations and steaming of raw cotton to reduce particle formation.

Compensation

Byssinosis is a prescribed disease (D2) for Industrial Injuries Disablement Benefit in those who work with raw cotton or flax.

Relevant legislation

Byssinosis is reportable under RIDDOR.

Organic dust toxic syndrome

The syndrome known as organic dust toxic syndrome (ODTS) is an acute inflammatory disorder of the lower respiratory system. Precise pathology is unclear, but is thought to be caused by a toxic reaction to organic dusts. It occurs in the absence of immunological sensitization.

Epidemiology

ODTS is primarily a disorder of agricultural workers. It does not feature in routinely collected statistics, but surveys of farming populations suggest a prevalence of around 6%.

Clinical features

- Fever, chills, malaise, dry cough, dyspnoea
- Acute onset 4–6h after exposure
- Brief duration (<36h)
- Transient decrease in lung function (FEV_1, FVC, and peak expiratory flow (PEF)).

Causal exposures/industries

- Mouldy grain and vegetable material
- Agricultural workers
- Clusters of cases are typically associated with very heavy exposures (e.g. emptying silos).

Differential diagnosis and clinical assessment

ODTS shares many features with acute hypersensitivity pneumonitis (farmer's lung (farmer's hypersensitivity pneumonitis, FHP)), including exposure, a similar clinical presentation, and the presence of neutrophils in alveolar lavage fluid. However, the prognosis and treatment are different, and differentiation is important. ODTS is distinguished from FHP by:

- Short duration of symptoms
- Benign natural history, with absence of progressive lung damage
- Absence of immunological hypersensitivity
- Absence of lung infiltrates on CXR
- Absence of hypoxaemia.

Treatment and prognosis

- Self-limiting
- No specific medical intervention required.

Prevention

- Reduction of exposure to mouldy organic material (see 📖 p. 114, Organic dusts and mists).
- PPE for high exposure activities
- Because of the link to heavy exposures, education of farm workers is particularly important.

Hypersensitivity pneumonitis

Also known as extrinsic allergic alveolitis (EAA), this inflammatory disorder of the lower respiratory system results from an immunological reaction to specific allergens (particularly thermophilic *Actinomycetes* and *Aspergillus* spp.) in mouldy organic material. The classical pathological feature is lymphocytic interstitial pneumonitis. Pathogenesis is not fully understood, but it is likely to result from a type III (immune complex) or type IV (cell-mediated) reaction. It is not an IgE-mediated (type I) allergic condition.

Epidemiology

- In the UK, an average of 47 cases of allergic alveolitis per year (2006–2010) were reported to the Surveillance of Work-related and Occupational Respiratory Disease (SWORD) reporting scheme by respiratory and occupational physicians. There have been fewer than 5 cases per year assessed for Industrial Injuries Disablement Benefit over the same period. These figures are likely to be an underestimate of the number of new cases
- Data from death certificates in the UK shows attribution of death to occupational allergic alveolitis of <10 cases per year
- The most prevalent form is farmer's hypersensitivity pneumonitis (FHP) or farmer's lung, but a number of other forms are recognized, each with a specific causal antigen (Table 7.2). Up to 5% of farmers report symptoms. HSE has reported a recent increase of cases related to metal working and wash fluids in the engineering sector. There is some evidence of EAA in association with exposure to hard metals (nickel).

Table 7.2 Forms of EAA, causal antigens, and source

Disorder	Antigen	Antigen source
Farmer's lung (FHP)	Thermophyllic actinomycetes including *Saccharopolyspora rectivergula* *Aspergillus species.*	Mouldy hay, grain, straw
Bird fanciers lung	Avian proteins	Bird excreta and bloom
Mushroom workers lung	*Aspergillus fumigatus*, *Aspergillus umbrosis*	Mushroom compost
Bagassosis	*Thermoactinomyces sacchari*	Bagasse (fibrous residue of sugar cane)
Malt workers lung	*Aspergillus clavatus*	Mouldy barley in whisky distilling
Ventilation pneumonitis	Thermophilic actinomycetes species	Water reservoirs in air-conditioning systems

This list is not intended to be exhaustive.

Clinical features

Acute form
- Fever, chills, cough, dyspnoea, myalgia, headache
- Onset 4–8h after exposure to antigen
- Resolution after 1–3 days.

Subacute/chronic form
- Gradual onset of dyspnoea over months or years
- Recurrent acute attacks may be distinguished in some cases
- Chronic productive cough.

Causal exposures/industries
- Agricultural workers
- Forestry workers
- Mushroom workers
- Bird handlers
- Sugar cane processors
- Distillery workers.

Clinical assessment
- ↑ Erythrocyte sedimentation rate (ESR) and neutrophil count (peripheral blood eosinophilia does not occur)
- Lung function (d FEV$_1$, FVC, typically with restrictive pattern, although mild obstructive changes may occur)
- Impaired gas transfer (↓ transfer factor for carbon monoxide); hypoxia may occur
- Chest X-ray (CXR) shows diffuse pulmonary infiltrates (acute) or upper and mid-zone interstitial fibrosis (chronic); 20% of CXRs in acute cases are normal
- Serum precipitins to causal allergens.

Treatment and prognosis
- Low-dose oral steroids
- Avoidance of exposure
- Prognosis is highly variable. Can be progressive, with lung fibrosis. If fibrosis develops, the main functional consequences for work are reduced stamina and physical capability.

Prevention
- Reduction of exposure to mouldy organic material (see 📖 p. 114, Organic dust and mists)
- PPE for high exposure activities.

Compensation
EAA is prescribed for Industrial Injuries Disablement Benefit (B6) in those who are exposed to moulds, fungal spores, or heterologous proteins.

Relevant legislation
EAA is reportable under RIDDOR 1995.

Humidifier fever

Humidifier fever is a self-limiting illness that is associated with exposure to humidified air from air-conditioning systems. The pathophysiology is incompletely understood. However, the disorder is distinct from hypersensitivity pneumonitis (ventilation pneumonitis), which can result from the same exposure. It is currently thought that humidifier fever is caused by either a direct effect of organisms in contaminated humidifier reservoirs, or a product of such organisms (e.g. endotoxin).

Epidemiology

Because of the self-limiting nature of this condition, prevalence estimates are neither readily available nor likely to be accurate.

Clinical features

- Usually non-specific: fever, chills, myalgia
- Dyspnoea and wheezing can occur
- Onset 6–8h after exposure
- Rapid and complete recovery
- Usually occurs after a break from work (e.g. on Mondays).

Differential diagnosis

- Can develop mild hypoxia, ↓ gas transfer, and audible crackles at the lung bases.
- Distinguished from hypersensitivity pneumonitis (HP) by an invariably normal CXR.
- Serum precipitins to organisms that are present in humidifier fluid are often positive. However, these do not bear any relation to disease activity, and are only useful as a marker of exposure. The presence of serum precipitins cannot help to distinguish from HP, as they are positive in both disorders.

Treatment and prognosis

Self-limiting; medical intervention is not indicated.

Causal exposures

- Recirculated air from air-conditioning units, particularly where the aim is to achieve high humidity
- Long list of possible causative organisms in humidifier fluid include many species of bacteria, fungi, and protozoa
- Ubiquitous exposure in many office environments
- Highest risk in textile industry where high humidity is desirable as this makes fibres pliable and easier to work.

Prevention

Guidance on the selection, maintenance, and cleaning of humidifiers and air-conditioning systems to minimize the risk of humidifier fever and other disorders is available from HSE.

Metal fume fever

This benign disease results from deposition of fine metal particulates in the alveoli. The precise pathological mechanism is unknown. No epidemiological information is available, as the mild symptoms are often overlooked and tolerated by metal workers.

Causal exposures and industries

- Primarily caused by zinc oxide fume generated by cutting, welding, or brazing galvanized steel
- Similar effects can be caused by other metal fumes. However, although these metals have been implicated, there is little evidence in the literature. Moreover, the nature of work activities is such that exposure is often to a mixture of metal oxides:
  - iron
  - copper
  - aluminium
  - tin
  - magnesium
- Found in a wide range of jobs involving metal working:
  - welders
  - oxy-fuel gas cutters
- Typically in heavy engineering industries:
  - shipbuilding
  - foundries
  - scrap metal industry
  - demolition
  - motor vehicle repair.

Factors affecting exposure

Exposure is increased by:
- increasing thickness of metal in cutting operations
- speed of metal cutting and arcing (welding) time
- automated cutting
- poor ventilation.

Clinical features

- Influenza-like illness with fever, chills, headache, and myalgia
- Dyspnoea and cough
- Metallic taste in the mouth
- Tolerance over the working week, with recurrence after break from exposure ('Monday fever')
- Onset 4–12h after exposure
- Benign illness, self-limiting after 1–2 days.

⚠ Must not be confused with exposure to cadmium fume, which can cause a severe toxic reaction in lungs and kidneys.

Prevention

- It is difficult to avoid metal cutting completely in demolition and shipbuilding

- Alternative cutting methods (thermal and non-thermal) are available. However, they are not suitable for all purposes, and all have associated hazards to health. Specialized advice on use of cutting tools is required
- Using the correct nozzle for cutting
- Turning off the torch during pauses in activity
- Fume capture methods including local exhaust ventilation
- Use of appropriate respiratory protective equipment
- Training and information, including advice on hygiene (hand washing and avoiding eating or smoking in the work area) and other risk controls.

Further information

HSE *Oxy-fuel cutting: control of fume, gases and noise*, HSE 668/30. Available at: ℘ http://www.hse.gov.uk/fod/infodocs/668_30.pdf#search=%22metal%20fume%20%22

Chronic obstructive pulmonary disease

This is a group of chronic lung disorders comprising chronic bronchitis and emphysema. They are characterized by irreversible airflow limitation, with impairment of lung function and debility in severe cases.

Epidemiology

- The main risk factor is smoking
- Population studies have estimated the burden of COPD that is attributable to occupational causes, with a population attributable risk percent of 15% (median).[1] This equates to around 4000 deaths per year
- 145 cases of chronic bronchitis and emphysema were prescribed for Industrial Injuries Disablement Benefit during 2010.

Clinical features

- Exertional dyspnoea
- Wheeze
- Chronic productive cough for >3mths of the year.

Causal exposures/industries

An increased risk of COPD has been associated with the following:

- *Mineral dusts:*
  - coal mining
  - manmade vitreous fibres
  - oil mists
  - cement (construction)
  - silica
- *Organic dusts:*
  - *Farming*—animal confinement (especially pigs), grain dust
  - flour mill work and baking
  - cotton textile work
  - wood (paper milling)
- *Chemicals:*
  - cadmium
  - welding fumes
  - vanadium
  - polycyclic aromatic hydrocarbons
  - isocyanates.

Clinical assessment

- Lung function declines progressively: FEV_1 <80% of predicted values, FEV_1/FVC <70% (obstructive pattern). The pattern of lung function in occupational cases can be complicated by dual pathology (e.g. pneumoconiosis), and restrictive patterns may be seen in coal miners and silica-exposed workers
- CXR is not necessary for diagnosis.

---

1 HSE (2011). *Chronic Obstructive Pulmonary Disease (COPD): COPD in Great Britain*. Available at: ℡ http://www.hse.gov.uk/statistics/causdis/copd/copd.pdf

Treatment and prognosis
- Removal from occupational exposure
- Advise smoking cessation
- Inhaled bronchodilators
- Inhaled corticosteroids
- Oral corticosteroids and antibiotics for acute infective exacerbations
- Supportive treatment for advanced disease
- Prognosis is variable; severe disease can result in respiratory failure.

Prevention
See (📖 p. 114, Organic dust and mists, 📖 p. 218, Coal worker's pneumoconiosis) for preventive measures and exposure control.

Compensation
- Chronic bronchitis and emphysema have recently been added to the list of prescribed diseases for Industrial Injuries Disablement Benefit (IIDB) (D1), but only for coal miners who have spent >20yrs working underground. FEV_1 must be reduced by 1L to qualify for benefit
- Emphysema is prescribed for IIDB (C18) for those exposed to cadmium fumes for a cumulative period of ≥20yrs.

Relevant legislation and further information
See 📖 p. 218, Coal worker's pneumoconiosis for legislation and guidance relevant to dust control in the mining industry.

Asbestos-related diseases

A number of medical conditions are related to asbestos exposure:
- Asbestosis
- *Pleural disorders:*
  - mesothelioma
  - diffuse pleural thickening
  - benign pleural effusion
  - pleural plaques
- Lung cancer
- Laryngeal cancer.

Details of epidemiology, clinical features and management are covered under each condition (Asbestosis, Lung cancer, Pleural disorders, and Laryngeal cancer). Aspects that are common to all asbestos-related disease (exposure, prevention, compensation and legislation) are covered here.

Causal exposures/industries

- Historically, asbestos has been widely used for fire protection and insulation. In the past (before the danger of asbestos was recognized) controls were poor, and exposures in some industries were very high.
  - *dockyards*—shipbuilders, ship breakers, and fitters
  - railway engineering
  - asbestos textile industry
  - construction
  - plumbing
  - pipe lagging and thermal insulation/pipe fitters
  - asbestos mining and distribution
  - engineering (brake linings and clutch faces)
- Currently, exposure mainly occurs during the demolition or renovation of old buildings (asbestos insulation, lagging, and roof tiles).

Prevention

- Mainly by elimination (replacement of asbestos with other materials)
- *UK legislation:*
  - prohibits import, supply, and use of most asbestos products
  - defines exposure limits for asbestos
  - controls the identification and removal of asbestos in buildings.

Health surveillance

- Employees who are currently exposed to asbestos above a defined action level must undergo regular health surveillance (2-yearly lung function) by a doctor who has been appointed by HSE CXRs are not required as part of health surveillance.
- Individuals who have been exposed previously need not undergo surveillance. However, it is important to :
  - Document previous exposure carefully, including historical hygiene measurements where available. It is appropriate to inform the GP with the individual's consent, so that the exposure is noted in the event of future asbestos-related disease.

- Counsel the individual about the risk of asbestos-related disease and the availability of compensation
▶ Counsel the individual about smoking cessation, as the risk of lung cancer from smoking and asbestos is multiplicative.

Compensation

It can be difficult to clarify the source and extent of exposure after >20yrs latency. It is essential to take an exhaustive occupational history to ensure that affected patients have appropriate access to benefits.

Industrial injuries disablement benefit

Some asbestos-related disorders are prescribed:
- Asbestosis (D1)
- Mesothelioma (D3)
- Primary carcinoma of the lung ± accompanying evidence of asbestosis (D8, D8A)
- Diffuse pleural thickening (D9).

Specific details of prescription according to exposure activities are outlined in the List of Prescribed Diseases.[1] Surviving next of kin can claim up to 6mths posthumously.

War Pensions Scheme

Those who develop asbestos-related disease as a result of exposure whilst working in HM Forces may be eligible for compensation.

Civil compensation

If an employee can prove negligence on the part of his/her employer, he/she may be successful in seeking compensation through the civil courts. Claims must be declared within 3yrs of the diagnosis of asbestos-related disease, including pleural plaques.

Relevant legislation

- Asbestosis is reportable under RIDDOR 1995
- Control of Asbestos Regulations 2006
- Asbestos (Licensing) Regulations 1983
- Asbestos (Prohibitions) Regulations 1992.

Further information

HSE *Asbestos health and safety*. Available at: ℘ http://www.hse.gov.uk/asbestos/index.htm

---

1 DWP. *Appendix 1: List of diseases covered by Industrial Injuries Disablement Benefit*. Available at: ℘ http://www.dwp.gov.uk/advisers/db1/appendix/appendix1.asp

The pneumoconioses

Pneumoconioses are a group of chronic lung diseases caused by long-term exposure to respirable particles (<5 μm diameter) of mineral dust (see Table 7.3).

Epidemiology

In the UK, an average of 167 cases of pneumoconiosis per year (2005–2010) were reported to the SWORD reporting scheme by respiratory and occupational physicians. This is likely to be an underestimate of the number of new cases.

Pathophysiology

The classical features of pneumoconiosis are as follows:
- Deposition of mineral dust in the alveoli
- Mineral particles are phagocytosed by alveolar macrophages
- Localized inflammatory reaction leads to long-term changes in the histology of the lung:
  - fibrotic reaction in the surrounding lung parenchyma, with reticulin formation and collagen deposition
  - necrosis and cavitation of the fibrotic nodules can occur in the later stages of the disease
  - progressive disease leads to coalescence of fibrotic areas into large parenchymal masses (progressive massive fibrosis (PMF))
- Gas diffusion is affected, leading to ↓ transfer factor
- Lung volumes are ↓ (FEV_1 and FVC), classically a restrictive pattern.

Table 7.3 The pneumoconiosis

Disease	Exposure	Cross reference
Coal worker's pneumoconiosis	Coal dust	📖 p. 218, Coal worker's pneumoconiosis
Asbestosis	Asbestos fibres	📖 p. 220, Asbestosis
Silicosis	Quartz (crystalline silica)	📖 p. 222, Silicosis
Kaolin pneumoconiosis	Kaolin (china clay)	📖 p. 225, Kaolin pneumoconiosis
Berylliosis	Beryllium	📖 p. 224, Berylliosis
Stannosis	Tin ore	📖 p. 226, The 'simple' pneumoconiosis
Siderosis	Iron oxide	📖 p. 226, The 'simple' pneumoconosis
Baritosis	Barium sulphate	📖 p. 226, The 'simple' pneumoconiosis
Bauxite worker's lung, Shaver's disease	Aluminium	

Radiological features

CXR shows small nodular opacities in the lung parenchyma. Distribution depends on the specific disease, but tends to affect the upper lobes first.

- PMF is associated with large areas of confluent shadowing, usually starting in the upper zones
- The International Labour Organization (ILO) has devised a classification system for the CXR features of all pneumoconioses.[1] This classification is used to determine severity of disease for compensation purposes, and is based on the size, shape, and distribution of the opacities:
    - *size*—small round opacities *p* (up to 1.5mm), *q* (1.5–3mm), or *r* (3–10mm). Irregular small opacities are classified by width as *s*, *t*, or *u* (same sizes as for small rounded opacities)
    - profusion (frequency) of small opacities is classified on a four-point major category scale (0–3), with each major category divided into three, giving a 12-point scale between 0/– and 3/+
    - large opacities are defined as any opacity >1cm that is present in a film. Large opacities are classified as category A (for one or more large opacities not exceeding a combined diameter of 5cm), category B (large opacities with combined diameter >5cm, but not exceeding the equivalent of the right upper zone), or category C (larger than B).

Natural history

Natural history, clinical features, and radiological appearance vary according to the specific mineral exposure. Some conditions always follow a benign course (stannosis, siderosis), others are often aggressive (asbestosis), and CWP can follow either a benign or a progressive pattern.

Management

There is usually no specific treatment. Management is to remove from exposure, and treatment of advanced disease is supportive.

Compensation

Pneumoconiosis is prescribed for Industrial Injuries Benefit (D1) in those who have been exposed to the appropriate mineral at work. In general, pneumoconiosis would have to be at least ILO category 2 on CXR for an employee to be eligible for benefits.

Relevant legislation

Pneumoconiosis is reportable under RIDDOR 1995 if it complies with categories 1, 2, 3 on the ILO classification, whether simple or with PMF categories A, B and C. There is no requirement to report a case that is assigned to category 0.

---

1 International Labour Office (ILO) (2011). *Guidelines for the use of the ILO International Classification of radiographs of pneumoconioses*, rev edn. ℛ http://www.ilo.org/safework/info/publications/WCMS_168260/lang – en/index.htm

Coal worker's pneumoconiosis

Coal worker's pneumoconiosis (CWP) is a form of pneumoconiosis caused by exposure to coal dust, characterized pathologically by collections of coal-laden macrophages in the lung parenchyma, surrounded by fibrosis and localized emphysema.

Epidemiology

- The onset of CWP lags behind exposure by >10yrs, and so incidence and mortality reflect past exposures and working conditions
- *Mortality is declining in developed countries:*
  - new cases are uncommon in the UK because of improved dust control and the decline in coal mining
  - cases are still common in China and there is a low, but significant incidence in India.
- *In the UK:*
  - more than 65% of new cases occur in those who have reached retirement age (>65yrs), although in the past miners would develop symptoms in their thirties and forties
  - published incidence data are based on claims for Industrial Injuries Benefit. Compensation is well established in the industry. An average of 251 cases/yr prescribed for IIDB 2005–2010.

Clinical features

Severity of disease varies according to local conditions, including composition of the coal (proportional content of silica and other minerals) and its surrounding strata. It is also related to total cumulative respirable dust exposure.

Simple CWP

- Often asymptomatic
- Minor impairment in ventilatory capacity is difficult to distinguish from the effects of cigarette smoking.

Complicated CWP

- *Progressive massive fibrosis (PMF):* development of large or confluent solid fibrotic nodules in the lung parenchyma. Cavitation and necrosis can occur in larger lesions, leading to expectoration of tarry black sputum (melanoptysis). Local emphysema can develop
- Dyspnoea and productive cough.

Comorbidity

It is accepted that COPD develops in parallel with fibrosis in coal miners. They are also at risk of silicosis. It can be difficult to distinguish silicosis other than at autopsy, as the radiological features are similar.

Causal exposures/industries

- *Coal mining:* the dustiest jobs give rise to the highest risk (face work, roof bolting, drilling holes for shot placement)
- Coal trimming and transportation.

Individual susceptibility

A rare complication of CWP is described in miners who are rheumatoid factor +ve. Large cavitating parenchymal nodules develop at relatively low dust exposure levels (Caplan's syndrome).

Diagnosis

- History of chronic exposure to coal dust
- *Lung function:*
  - *Simple CWP*—normal FEV_1 and FVC, but transfer factor can be reduced
  - *PMF*—↓FEV_1 and FVC with restrictive pattern, or obstruction if widespread emphysema has developed; transfer factor ↓
- *X-ray findings:* nodular opacities, predominantly in the upper zones (see 📖 p. 216, The pneumoconiosis for ILO classification of radiographic changes).

Prognosis

- Simple CWP is benign in most cases
- Prognosis in complicated CWP is variable. Severe disease can be debilitating. Life expectancy can be normal, but some develop life-limiting cor pulmonale
- There is no increased risk of lung cancer or emphysema with CWP
- The effect of exposure to cigarette smoke is additive.

Prevention

Exposure controls in the mining industry including ventilation, dust reduction measures, and use of PPE.

Health surveillance

Miners must undergo regular CXRs at 4-yearly intervals. Those in whom early signs of CWP are detected should be removed from exposure.

Compensation

CWP is prescribed (D1) for Industrial Injuries Disablement Benefit (see 📖 p. 218, Coal worker's pneumoconiosis) in those who have been exposed chronically to coal dust in mining or above ground.

Relevant legislation

- CWP is reportable to HSE as a pneumoconiosis under RIDDOR 1995.
- The Coal Mines (Control of Inhalable Dust) Regulations 2007. Available at: ℘ http://www.legislation.gov.uk/uksi/2007/1894/contents/

Asbestosis

This disease is characterized by chronic pulmonary interstitial fibrosis, resulting from exposure to asbestos (in particular amphibole fibres).

Epidemiology

- The disease develops after a long latent period of 25–40yrs following exposure
- There is a clear dose–response relationship, and asbestosis tends to occur in those who have been exposed heavily
- *In Great Britain:*
  - although exposures have improved, the incidence is still increasing due to historical exposure. Claims for Industrial Injuries Disablement Benefit (IIDB) rose from 405 in 1999 to 1015 in 2010
  - industries most commonly cited in IIDB claims are construction, extraction, energy, and water supply industry, and manufacturing
  - 189 deaths due to asbestosis were recorded in 2009.[1]

Clinical features

- Gradual onset of dyspnoea and cough
- Basal crepitations on auscultation
- Finger clubbing in 40% of cases.

Individual susceptibility

Smoking is associated with ↑ severity and rate of deterioration of asbestosis.

Clinical assessment and diagnosis

- Lung function typically shows ↓ FEV₁ and FVC with a restrictive pattern, although obstructive or mixed patterns can occur
- d Transfer factor
- *Radiographic investigations:*
  - CXR shows fine nodular shadowing predominantly in the lower zones. Other hallmarks of asbestos exposure (pleural plaques) may be present
  - because CXR is relatively insensitive for early disease, high-resolution CT scanning is often used to confirm the diagnosis.
- Lung biopsy is the gold standard for diagnosis, showing interstitial fibrosis and asbestos bodies.

Treatment and prognosis

- No specific intervention can halt the disease
- Patients should be advised to stop smoking
- Treatment is supportive in the later stages
- Up to 40% of patients progress after removal from exposure
- The correlation between CXR findings, lung function, and clinical progression is poor
- The risk of lung cancer is increased.

---

1 Based on death certificates, where asbestosis was the main cause of death.

Other aspects

For causal exposures/industries, prevention, compensation, legislation, and further sources of information see 📖 p. 214, Asbestos-related diseases.

Further information

Further information on the epidemiology of asbestosis can be found on the HSE statistics website. See HSE (2011). *Asbestosis: asbestosis mortality in Great Britain 1978–2009*. Available at: ℘ http://www.hse.gov.uk/statistics/causdis/asbestosis/asbestosis.pdf

Silicosis

This is a pneumoconiosis associated with exposure to respirable crystalline silica. Silica is encountered mainly as crystalline quartz, a component of igneous rocks.

Epidemiology

- There is a long latent period between exposure to silica and onset of disease
- The risk of disease varies according to level of exposure
- Silicosis is now rare because of substitution and controls in mining.

Clinical features

There are three recognized types of silicosis:

- *Acute:* early onset of dyspnoea and dry cough within a few months of heavy exposure to fine dusts (e.g. sand-blasting). CXR shows patchy small airway consolidation (appearance similar to pulmonary oedema). Progression over 1–2yrs, with respiratory failure
- *Subacute:* gradual onset of dyspnoea and dry cough over years after moderate exposure. CXR shows upper- and mid-zone nodular fibrosis, with classical feature of 'egg-shell' calcification of the hilar lymph nodes. PMF can occur, with coalescence of the fibrotic nodules. Restrictive pattern of impaired lung function
- *Chronic:* slow development of nodules on CXR over many years after low level exposure.

Silicosis is associated with larger nodules on CXR and more rapid progression than coal worker's pneumoconiosis with which it may co-exist. However, with the exception of egg shell calcification, silicosis can be difficult to distinguish from CWP clinically and radiologically in dual exposed cases.

↑ Risk of infection with tuberculosis (TB) (thought to be due to impairment of phagocytosis in the lung). Characterized by cavitation on CXR.

Causal exposures/industries

- *Mining:* silica is often contained in surrounding strata in coal and other mineral mines. Tunnel drillers/blasters, roof bolters, transportation crew are at highest risk (although face workers and others are also exposed)
- *Quarries:* workers who blast, cut, and transport stone
- *Stone-working:*
  - stone-masonry (granite dressing and grinding)
  - flint-knapping
- *Heavy engineering and manufacture:*
  - shot blasting
  - preparation and use of grinding wheels/stones (historically, cutlers)
  - use of compressed airlines to clean off silica-containing material

- *Foundries:*
  - sand-moulding
  - shot-blasting
  - compressed air cleaning of moulded items
  - fettling
- Ceramics and pottery making
- Brick-making.

Prognosis and treatment

- No specific intervention halts progression
- Remove from further exposure
- Regular examination of sputum for tubercle bacilli; confirmed infection is treated with standard anti-tuberculous chemotherapy
- 10–30% of silicosis cases progress after removal from exposure.

Health surveillance

Health surveillance (respiratory questionnaire, lung function tests, and CXR) is required for those who are exposed above a defined threshold exposure (despite control measures). See 📖 p. 223, Further information, for sources of specific guidance from HSE.

Prevention

Control of exposure is through substitution with low-silica sand for moulding and shot-blasting, dust control measures (ventilation, suppression), and use of RPE. See 📖 p. 40 for workplace exposure limit (WEL).

Compensation

Silicosis is prescribed (D1) for Industrial Injuries Disablement Benefit (see 📖 p. 216, The pneumoconiosis) in those who have been mining, quarrying, or working with silica rock or dust (sand).

Relevant legislation

Silicosis is reportable to HSE as a pneumoconiosis under RIDDOR 1995.

Further information

HSE (2004). *Silica,* Construction Information Sheet No 36 Revision 1. ℘ http://www.hse.gov.uk/pubns/cis36.pdf

HSE (2002). *Control of exposure to silica dust in small potteries.* ℘ http://www.hse.gov.uk/pubns/ceis2.pdf

Berylliosis

Beryl is a hard crystalline ore (aluminium beryllium silicate), found in the strata of mines dug for other purposes. Beryllium is an extremely hard metal, producing useful alloys when mixed with copper and other metals. The metal, oxide, and soluble salts are all extremely toxic.

Epidemiology Berylliosis is extremely rare (because of elimination from industrial use).

Causal exposures/industries

- Because of its extreme toxicity, the previous widespread use in fluorescent light tubes and the ceramic industry has been eliminated
- However, it is still used:
  - in the nuclear industry
  - in the production of X-ray tubes.

Clinical features

There are two main forms of disease.

Acute

- Follows inhalational exposure to high levels of the dust of soluble beryllium compounds
- Severe bronchoalveolitis with tissue necrosis
- High fatality rate within a few days
- Progression to subacute phase, with tissue scarring, in the survivors.

Subacute/chronic

- Only a proportion of those exposed (<5%) develop the disease
- Florid non-caseating granulomata heal by fibrosis, with disruption of the normal lung architecture
- Progression to diffuse interstitial fibrosis, leading to respiratory failure, is usual
- CXR shows fine nodular shadowing and hilar lymphadenopathy
- Lung function tests show a restrictive deficit
- ↓ Transfer factor.

Differential diagnosis is from sarcoidosis, which has similar clinical and CXR features.

Treatment and prognosis

Treatment is with high-dose oral corticosteroids. Treatment can be tailed off, but needs to be prolonged for many months in chronic cases. Relapse can follow early cessation of therapy.

Prevention

Prevention is by elimination, or by containment, ventilation (with filtering of discharged air), and fastidious use of PPE.

Compensation

Chronic beryllium disease is prescribed for Industrial Injuries Disablement Benefit (C17) in those who are exposed to beryllium and its compounds.

Kaolin pneumoconiosis

Kaolin (china clay) is a multilayered particulate containing aluminium hydroxide and silicon oxide. Formed from the action of water on granite, and commonly contaminated by silica-containing compounds.

Epidemiology

- Historically, this was variable in different kaolin mining regions because of differing levels of contamination and extraction methods
- Generally low incidence in the exposed populations gave rise to a belief that contaminating silica was responsible for lung disease in kaolin workers
- It is now accepted that kaolin itself can cause pneumoconiosis.

Clinical features

- Asymptomatic, or mild exertional dyspnoea
- Mild ↓ FVC
- CXR shows small nodular opacities consistent with interstitial fibrosis
- Progressive massive fibrosis can occur
- No specific treatment.

Causal exposures/industries China clay mining.

Prevention Prevention is by dust abatement measures.

The 'simple' pneumoconioses

These disorders are all relatively uncommon.

Exposures

- *Siderosis:*
  - exposure to iron ore (haematite)
  - iron ore mining
  - welding (mild steel)
  - classic finding of red lungs at autopsy
- *Stannosis:* exposure to tin ore
- *Fuller's earth pneumoconiosis:*
  - occurs in workers who extract clay material
  - traditional use of fuller's earth to clean wool
  - results from exposure to a mixture of silicates of sodium, potassium, aluminium, and magnesium.
- *Baritosis:* exposure to barites in mining, processing, or handling
- *Gypsum pneumoconiosis:* exposure in open-cast or deep mining, and production of plasterboard.

Clinical features

- Asymptomatic
- Benign course
- Normal lung function
- Small rounded opacities on CXR (appearance similar to coal worker's pneumoconiosis).

Prevention

Prevention is by dust suppression and ventilation, and use of PPE.

Lung cancer

Epidemiology

- 90% of lung cancers are related to smoking
- The proportion of lung cancer that can be attributed to occupation (based on 2004/05 data) is 14.5%, but (like most other occupational cancers) is higher in men than women:
  - attributable fraction men 21.2%
  - attributable fraction women 5.3%
- 4749 lung cancer deaths were attributable to occupation in 2005
- 150 new cases of lung cancer were associated with applications for Industrial Injuries Disablement Benefit in 2010
- The interaction between smoking and both asbestos and nickel are multiplicative (or between additive and multiplicative).

Clinical features

Clinical presentation is very variable, and some patients present with metastatic features rather than the effects of local disease. The most common features are:
- Weight loss
- Cough with haemoptysis
- Dyspnoea
- Chest pain
- Unresolving pneumonia.

Causal exposures/industries

- *Crystalline silica:*
  - mining
  - quarrying
  - stone masonry
  - glass manufacture
  - foundries
  - shot-blasting and grinding
  - ceramic and pottery manufacture
- *Asbestos fibres:*
  - shipbuilding and fitting
  - mining
  - asbestos textile industry
  - construction
  - engineering (particularly railway works)
- *Radon daughters:* tin mining
- Arsenic
- Nickel (nickel refining)
- Bis-chloromethyl ether (BCME)
- Polycyclic aromatic hydrocarbons
  - aluminium smelting
  - coke production
- Chromates (zinc, calcium, strontium)
- Passive smoking, e.g. in the entertainment and catering industry.

Clinical management and prognosis
- Definitive investigation is with CXR or CT, bronchoscopy, and biopsy
- Surgical resection
- Chemotherapy
- Radiotherapy
- Prognosis is variable, and depends on the stage at diagnosis.

Prevention
Prevention is mainly through exposure control.

Compensation
Primary carcinoma of the lung is prescribed for Industrial Injuries Disablement Benefit in those who have:
- Worked underground in a tin mine
- Been exposed to BCME, or zinc, calcium, or strontium chromates (D10)
- Worked with asbestos in defined circumstances (D8)
- Been exposed to crystalline silica in defined industries (D11)
- Worked before 1950 in the refining of nickel (C22(b))
- Been exposed to fumes, dust, or vapour of arsenic or arsenic-containing compounds (C4).

Relevant legislation
Asbestos-related lung cancer is reportable to HSE under RIDDOR 1995.

Further information
HSE *Index of data tables*. Available at: ℜ http://www.hse.gov.uk/statistics/tables/index.htm

Pleural disorders

Benign pleural disorders

Pleural plaques

These are the most common sequelae of asbestos exposure, occurring in up to 50% of an exposed population:
- Can occur after low-level exposure
- Discrete areas of pleural thickening ± calcification
- Latent period of 20–30yrs after exposure
- No evidence that the plaque lesions are pre-malignant
- Usually asymptomatic; rarely mild dyspnoea if sufficiently extensive to restrict expansion of the underlying lung
- Lung function usually normal.

Diffuse pleural thickening
- Dose-related, usually after heavier exposures
- Extensive poorly circumscribed areas of adhesion in the parietal pleura and fibrosis in the visceral pleura
- Often symptomatic (chest pain and exertional dyspnoea), and can be associated with restrictive lung function tests
- CXR shows extensive shadowing (>25% of chest wall affected) ± obliteration of the costophrenic angles
- Surgical treatment is difficult, and the results are often unsatisfactory
- Important differential diagnosis is mesothelioma; investigation (biopsy) is required in an attempt to exclude malignancy.

Benign pleural effusion
- Dose-related, usually after heavier exposures
- Usually develops within 10yrs of exposure
- Typically asymptomatic
- Pleural aspiration and biopsy to exclude malignancy
- No evidence of progression to mesothelioma.

Mesothelioma

Mesothelioma is a diffuse malignant tumour that arises in the pleural, peritoneal, or (rarely) pericardial lining.

Epidemiology
- Asbestos exposure is the single major cause (>90% mesotheliomas)
- Any asbestos type can cause the disease, but the risk is highest with amphibole fibres
- Long latency between exposure and disease of 15–60 (mean 40) years.

▶ Unlike asbestosis, there is no dose–response relationship. There is no threshold below which there is no risk, but the risk is very small at low exposure levels. Mesothelioma has occurred in workers' spouses who have washed contaminated work clothes.

In Great Britain
- Applications for Industrial Injuries Disablement Benefit have risen steadily in the past 10yrs (640 in 1996 to 1895 in 2010) and continue to rise

- Deaths due to mesothelioma have ↑ steadily from 153 in 1968 to 2321 in the year 2009.[1] It has been estimated that annual deaths will peak in the year 2016, with 2100 per annum. The highest mortality occurs in geographical areas where shipbuilding or railway engineering were common (Dumbartonshire and Clyde, Tyne and Wear, Portsmouth, Southampton, and Plymouth, and Eastleigh, Doncaster, and Crewe, respectively).

Clinical features
- Usually presents with pleural effusion
- Chest wall pain and dyspnoea
- Rarely presents with ascites, pericardial effusion, or encasement syndromes
- CXR (or CT) shows:
  - pleural effusion
  - pleural mass or thickening ± free fluid
  - local invasion of chest wall, heart, or mediastinum
  - concomitant pleural plaques or pulmonary fibrosis (minority).

Treatment and prognosis
- Surgical intervention (pleurectomy) is offered in some cases
- Palliative treatment: drain effusions, pleurodesis
- Typically fatal over 1–2yrs.

Other aspects

Causal exposures/industries, prevention, compensation, legislation, and further sources of information are covered in 📖 p. 214, Asbestos-related diseases.

---

1 Mesothelioma age standardized death rates per million by region, time period, and sex.

Nasal disorders

Nasal cancer

Cancer of the nasal passages has been noted to have an occupational association since early descriptions in nickel workers in the 1920s, furniture makers in the 1960s, and workers in the boot and shoe manufacturing industry in the 1970s.

Epidemiology

- The proportion of sinonasal cancer attributable to occupation in 2004 was:
  - 46% in men
  - 20% in women
- In the years 2005 and 2004, respectively, occupational sinonasal cancer gave rise to 39 deaths and 133 cancer registrations
- Approximately 5 cases per year are awarded Industrial Injuries Disablement benefit due to cancer of the nasal cavity
- Adenocarcinoma of the ethmoids and middle turbinates are the most common tumours (although still very rare).

Clinical features

- Blood-stained nasal discharge
- Unilateral nasal stuffiness/obstruction
- Facial pain
- Facial numbness.

Causal exposures/industries

- Leather and wood dust in:
  - boot and shoe manufacture
  - furniture and cabinet making
- Isopropyl alcohol manufacture
- Nickel and nickel compounds.

Compensation

Primary cancer of the nose or paranasal sinuses is prescribed for Industrial Injuries Disablement Benefit:

- In those who worked before 1950 in the refining of nickel (exposure to oxides, sulphides, or water-soluble compounds of nickel) (C22 (a))
- In those working in the repair and manufacture of wooden goods or footwear (D6).

Other nasal disorders

- Chronic hypertrophic rhinitis, nasal mucosal atrophy, and nasal polyps have been associated with woodworking
- Nasal septal ulceration associated with long-term exposure to chromates (work with dyes, tanning agents and chromium plating tanks).

Prevention

Prevention is through exposure control:

- enclosure with exhaust ventilation
- portable tools with dust extraction
- use of respiratory PPE.

Further information

HSE (2007). *COSHH and the woodworking industries*. Available at: ℘ http://www.hse.gov.uk/pubns/ wis6.pdf

HSE (1997). *Wood dust: hazards and precautions*, Woodworking sheet No. 1, revised. Available at: ℘ http://www.hse.gov.uk/pubns/wis1.pdf

Laryngeal cancer

Laryngeal cancer has been associated with a number of carcinogens that are used in occupational settings. The disease is rare.
- 2.6% of laryngeal cancer cases are attributable to occupation
- 20 deaths were attributable to occupation in 2005

Causal exposures/industries
- Asbestos (see 📖 p. 214, Asbestos-related diseases for list of industries)
- Mustard gas (also carcinoma of the pharynx)
- Nickel and nickel compounds (nickel refining)
- Strong inorganic acid mists (e.g. sulphuric acid) (these are used widely in industry).

Clinical features and management
- Hoarse voice, dysphagia
- Surgical treatment, but prognosis poor.

Prevention
Generic exposure control measures.

Relevant legislation
- See 📖 p. 214, Asbestos-related diseases.

Occupational voice loss

Occupational voice loss

Epidemiology

- US statistics suggest that 25% of employees critically rely on their voice for their work. There are no comparable UK statistics available
- Voice disorders are common in the general population, with prevalence rates of:
- 13.5% of men and 21.5% of women having a 'dry throat'
- 15.1% of men and 18.6% of women reporting a 'sore throat'
- In some occupations having common respiratory symptoms can impair ability to undertake the task requirements of the job, but does not mean that the job causes the voice disorder.

Clinical features

Voice disorders, whether caused or impacting on occupation, produce the same symptoms, i.e. hoarseness, dry throat, repeated clearing of the throat, weak voice, and a lack of vocal projection.

Occupational causes

The following general features of work increase the risk of voice disorders:

- Excessive voice use, e.g. frequently shouting
- Poor upper body posture
- Work in contaminated environments (such as those involving exposure to dusts, vapours and fumes).

The literature contains many studies linking voice disorders to specific occupations, but most are cross-sectional and do not prove causation. Teachers are over-represented in outpatient attendances for voice disorders.

▶▶This is not evidence that voice disorders are *caused* by teaching as it may indicate that if there is a voice condition then the job of teaching is more difficult and prompts access for medical advice.

Prevention

Prevention involves:

- *Work design*: e.g. ensuring shorter scripts for call centre workers
- *Workplace design*:
  - reduce ambient noise to prevent the need to talk-over colleagues in offices
  - classroom design
  - adequate humidity and ventilation
- *Education and information*: individuals who rely on their voice for their job need to be provided with advice on prevention:
  - avoid shouting and highly charged explosive speech
  - ensure adequate hydration
  - use aids such as microphones.

Clinical assessment and diagnosis

An individual who has had a hoarse voice for longer than 2–3wks should be referred to a multi-disciplinary service to primarily exclude malignancy. Usually an ENT specialist will carry out an initial assessment, but once malignancy is excluded, follow up is with a speech therapist. The cornerstone of management is education about:

- Vocal hygiene
- Exercises
- Advice on breathing.

Compensation/legal aspects

Civil litigation has been pursued and been successful in some jobs, e.g. call centre workers, but a review by the Industrial Injuries Advisory Committee (IIAC) found insufficient evidence for inclusion as an industrial injury.

Further information

Williams N, Carding P (2005) *Occupational voice loss.* Taylor & Francis, Boca Raton.

Coronary heart disease

Ischaemic heart disease (IHD) is one of the most common causes of death in industrialized nations. Interest in occupational risk factors for coronary heart disease has grown with increasing research into the role of job strain as a risk factor for hypertension, acute coronary syndromes, and sudden death. Research suggests that workers in jobs with low decision latitude and high psychological demands are at increased risk of cardiovascular disease.

Epidemiology

- Shift work is associated with 40% ↑ risk of heart disease. However, confounding by social class has been suggested as an explanation for this finding
- Major organizational downsizing (>18% of staff laid off) doubled the risk of cardiovascular deaths among workers in one prospective Finnish study.

Individual susceptibility

- It was once thought that type A behaviour was a risk factor for coronary vascular disease. Type A behaviour is characterized by excessive competitiveness, impatience and anger/hostility. However, the evidence of ↑ risk of IHD is stronger for one component of type A behaviour, namely hostility, than type A behaviour overall
- Depression and anxiety are associated with an increased risk of coronary vascular disease and a poorer prognosis. The ↑ risk attributable to psychosocial factors such as depression is of a similar scale to risk factors such as smoking, ↑ cholesterol, and hypertension.

Clinical assessment

The investigation of coronary heart disease is the same whether occupational risk factors are suspected or not. However, where chemical exposures are implicated, an exposure history is indicated.

Possible causal exposures/industries

- *Solvents:*
  - dichloromethane (methylene chloride, CH_2Cl_2)
  - carbon disulphide (CS_2)
- Job strain (low job control and high workload)
- Shift work
- Long working hours
- *Low organizational justice:* unfair inconsistent treatment of workers
- Effort/reward imbalance.

Historically, workers in the viscose rayon industry were heavily exposed to CS_2 and may have had an increased risk of IHD. Painters may be exposed to CH_2Cl_2 in confined spaces. Metabolism of CH_2Cl_2 leads to production of carbon monoxide and thus angina.

Health surveillance

No health surveillance is currently recommended in the UK for workers exposed to job strain or shift work.

Prevention

- Some organizations offer their senior executives periodic health checks which often include screening for cardiac risk factors. The inverse care law, which states that those least in need are most likely to receive care, appears to operate here
- National workplace health promotion initiatives (e.g. Healthy Working Lives) seek to address such health inequalities by addressing lifestyle risk factors, such as smoking, obesity, and lack of exercise.

Prevention

-
-

Skin disorders

Dermatitis 1

Epidemiology

Prevalence data[1] suggest that 20 000 people in the UK have skin problems that are caused or made worse by work. Occupational dermatitis (OD) makes up the greatest proportion of these. Data come from two main sources:

- Voluntary reporting schemes for occupational physicians and dermatologists: the incidence of OD is falling steadily.[2] Of 2055 new cases of occupational skin disease reported in 2010, 1497 (73%) were due to dermatitis. However, this is likely to be an underestimate as mild cases might not present to a dermatologist and many workplaces do not have access to OH services
- *Industrial Injuries Disablement Benefit:* 55 awards in Great Britain in 2009/10, but these are a small proportion of the most severe OD.

Classification

Endogenous eczema

An inherited disorder often associated with other atopic conditions, such as rhinitis. Not primarily caused by work that may be exacerbated by exposures at work.

Acquired occupational contact dermatitis

- *Irritant contact dermatitis (IrCD):* skin irritation from direct contact with irritant agents, e.g. chemicals or plants. Reversible impairment of the barrier properties and local inflammation of skin is dose related for mild (chronic) irritants
- *Allergic contact dermatitis (ACD):* has an immune-mediated mechanism due to a type IV (cell-mediated) reaction. Sensitization can occur within 7–10 days of exposure; usually develops after months or years. Once sensitized, the individual can react to very low level exposures.

Clinical features

The clinical appearance of dermatitis derives from oedema of the epidermis and inflammatory infiltration in the dermis. Typically, onset is slow and >24h after exposure. There may be a temporal relationship to work, with improvement during holidays. IrCD is classically confined to areas of contact, usually the face and hands. With ACD, involvement of eyelids and spread to secondary sites, not directly exposed, is common. See HSE website for colour pictures of dermatitis is available at: ℘ http://www.hse.gov.uk/skin/imagelibrary.htm

Acute features

- Redness
- Pruritis
- Vesiculation, exudation, and crusting
- Dryness, cracking, and fissuring.

Chronic features

- Cracking
- Lichenification.

Complications
2° bacterial infection.

Causal exposures/industries

Exposures
▶▶ Causal exposures often occur in combination
- *Chemicals or biological agents:*
    - irritants (common examples include weak acids and alkalis, soaps and detergents, oxidizing and reducing agents, solvents)
    - sensitizing agents
- Frequent hand washing (wet work)
- Gloves and other PPE
- Mechanical trauma
- Radiation and UV light.

Jobs
Dermatitis can occur in any job, but is particularly common in:
- Health care work
- Cleaning
- Engineering (cutting oils)
- Hairdressing
- Catering
- Printing
- Agriculture
- Chemical manufacture.

Individual susceptibility
- The response of normal skin to physical and mechanical damage and to irritant agents varies widely in the population
- The risk of sensitization ↑ if the barrier integrity of skin is impaired, e.g. pre-existing skin conditions which lead to ↑ antigen presentation
- Risk of irritation and sensitization ↑ in those with a history of atopy.

Compensation
Non-infective dermatitis is prescribed for Industrial Injuries Disablement Benefit (D5) in workers whose skin is exposed to irritants. Dermatitis and skin ulceration (C30) is prescribed in those exposed to chromic acid, chromates, or dichromates.

Relevant legislation and further information
- Occupational dermatitis is reportable under RIDDOR. A list of agents for which associated dermatitis would be reportable is given in the guidance document (see 📖 Appendix 3), but exposure to any known irritant or sensitizing agent would qualify
- HSE (2011). Statistics on work-related skin disease. Available at: ℘ http://www.hse.gov.uk/statistics/causdis/dermatitis/skin.pdf

1 Self-reported work-related illness survey 2010–11.

2 The Health and Occupation Reporting Network (THOR) scheme (see 📖 p. 692, Routine health statistics).

Dermatitis 2: management

Clinical investigation and treatment

Differential diagnosis

It can be difficult to distinguish IrCD and ACD from history and examination alone. Clues include exposure to a known irritant or sensitizing agent. However, always consider whether a previously unknown sensitizer might be responsible. Careful enquiry into exposures at home and work is important, but it can be difficult to identify the cause. A history of childhood eczema indicates endogenous dermatitis, but exacerbation by irritants or sensitizers at work should still be considered.

▶▶ *Skin patch testing* is crucial in making a diagnosis. This should include common allergens, medicaments, and agents that are present at work. Patch testing is a specialized procedure. It should be carried out by an experienced dermatologist, particularly when investigating rare or possible new sensitizers, as standardized skin patch test reagents may not be available commercially. Care is needed in the standardization of tests in this context, and the interpretation of results. The occupational health team has an important role in:

- Providing dermatologist with a list of possible workplace exposures
- Ensuring that samples of products, excipients, and other potential causative agents are supplied to the investigating clinic.

Treatment The treatment of occupational dermatitis is the same as for endogenous eczema. Topical emollients and topical steroids.

Occupational health input

Advise the employer about primary prevention

- Substitution of known sensitizing agents with suitable alternatives
- Engineering controls (e.g. enclose computerized cutting operations to reduce contact between cutting oils and the skin of operators)
- Use of PPE (gloves). ⚠ Some components of gloves (typically carbamates and thiurams used as preservatives and accelerants) can themselves cause sensitization
- Education about the risks and good hand care (see Box 8.1).

Manage individual cases

- Facilitate careful clinical investigation and diagnosis
- Reinforce education about good hand care (see Box 8.1)
- Advise about adjustments to work to reduce direct skin contact with irritants or allergens.

Epidemiological surveys

Sometimes it can be difficult to determine if a single case of dermatitis is occupational. It is useful to ascertain whether there is a higher incidence of dermatitis among the population of employees who have similar dermal exposures. Surveys are also useful for investigating unexplained clusters of cases. It is important to undertake epidemiological investigations ethically, and to involve the employees' representatives.

Box 8.1 Good hand care: measures to ↓ risk of irritant dermatitis

- Ensure hands are not wet for >2h/day or >20 times each day. For potent irritants ↓ these exposure limits
- Avoid wearing gloves for >4h/day
- Use tools that avoid wet-work or contact with irritants
- Wash hands in warm (not cold or hot) water and dry thoroughly
- Use protective gloves from the start of wet-work
- Minimize glove use—induces dermatitis by occluding skin surface
- If protective gloves used for >10min wear cotton gloves underneath
- Keep gloves intact and dry inside
- Avoid introducing irritants into the gloves
- Do not wear rings at work—they trap water and contaminants
- Use lipid-rich moisturizing creams at and after work.

Health surveillance

Skin surveillance is required under the COSHH Regulations where there is a significant risk of dermatitis. The detail of skin surveillance programmes is covered on 📖 p. 426, Skin surveillance. OH has a role in:

- Advising employers about the need for and format of surveillance
- Training competent persons
- Follow-up of cases identified by routine surveillance.

Prognosis

- Because irritant contact dermatitis is dose related, it is usually possible to manage by attention to exposure controls outlined here
- Allergic contact dermatitis can be much more difficult to manage:
  - once an individual is sensitized, he/she reacts to very low levels of exposure; elimination of the allergen is not always possible
  - redeployment is sometimes required as a last resort if symptoms cannot be controlled by other means, but the risks of dermatitis need to be weighed carefully against the (often greater) health risks of losing employment completely
  - if the allergen is common in the environment outside work, symptom control is more difficult to achieve.

Further information and guidance

HSE (2004). *Medical aspects of occupational skin disease*, guidance note MS24, 2nd edn. Available at: 🖰 http://hse.gov.uk/pubns/ms24.pdf

HSE *Skin at work*. Available at: 🖰 http://www.hse.gov.uk/skin/index.htm

Concise guidance to good practice: diagnosis, management, and prevention of occupational contact dermatitis. Available at: 🖰 http://www.nhsplus.nhs.uk/providers/images/library/files/guidelines/Dermatitis_concise_guideline.pdf

Dermatitis: occupational aspects of management—a national guideline. (Full guideline and associated leaflets). Available at: 🖰 http://www.nhsplus.nhs.uk/providers/clinicaleffectiveness-guidelines-evidencebased.asp

BOHRF (2012). *Occupational contact dermatitis: evidence review*. Avaialble at: 🖰 http://www.bohrf.org.uk/projects/dermatitis.html

Contact urticaria

Epidemiology

Data from the specialist physicians reporting **schemes**[1] show that the annual incidence of reported new cases of occupational contact urticaria is declining; 56 cases were reported in 2010.

Clinical features

- *Wheal and flare:* 'nettle rash', itchy skin lumps with erythema:
  - rapid onset within 20min of exposure
  - subsides within hours of exposure
  - see HSE website for colour pictures of urticarial. Available at: ℘ http://www.hse.gov.uk/skin/imagelibrary.htm
- *Associated with systemic features:* asthma, GI symptoms, anaphylaxis.

Non-allergic contact urticaria

Tends not to have systemic features and is probably due to local release of histamines and bradykinins in response to direct stimulus.

Causal exposures

- Certain arthropods, jellyfish, algae
- Nettles and certain seaweeds
- Benzoic acid, ascorbic acid.

Allergic contact urticaria

This is a classical type I (IgE-mediated) hypersensitivity reaction. It occurs when an individual who has been previously sensitized to an allergen is re-exposed.

Causal exposures/industries

- *Exposures:*
  - latex (see 📖 p. 202, Latex allergy)
  - protein allergens, e.g. animal products
  - foods, spices, herbs, food additives (benzoic acid, cinamic acid)
  - resins
  - disinfectants
- *Industries:*
  - health care
  - rubber manufacture
  - veterinary practitioners
  - food handlers
  - horticulture.

Investigation

- Skin-prick testing
- Total and specific IgE.

Management Allergen avoidance.

---

1 Under The Health and Occupation Reporting Network, (THOR) scheme (see 📖 p. 692, Routine health statistics).

Skin cancers

Epidemiology

- Skin neoplasia is the second most commonly reported form of occupational skin disease, comprising 20% of all reported cases[1]
- Data from the specialist physicians reporting schemes[2] show that 390 new cases of occupational skin neoplasia were reported in 2010.

Types

- Squamous cell carcinoma
- Basal cell carcinoma
- Melanoma.

Causal exposures/industries

- *UVA and UVB radiation:* any occupation where work is predominantly outdoors, e.g. agricultural and construction workers
- Ionizing radiation
- *PAHs:* historically an important cause of skin cancer, but now rare because of good hygiene controls
- Arsenic and arsenicals.

Clinical features and management

- Skin nodule; itching or colour change in existing naevi
- Surgical excision.

Prevention

- Education and protection against the sun for outside workers
- Reducing exposure to tar, pitch, and mineral oils through substitution and engineering controls
- Control of ionizing radiation (see p. 20, Ionizing radiation 3: exposure control).

Compensation

Primary carcinoma of the skin is prescribed for Industrial Injuries Disablement Benefit (C21) in those who are exposed to arsenic or arsenic compounds, tar, pitch, bitumen, mineral oil (including paraffin), or soot.

Relevant legislation

- Skin cancer that is attributable to occupational exposure is reportable under RIDDOR The EU directive on optical radiation requires health surveillance for workers who are exposed to optical radiation and are likely to have health effects.

---

1 Self-reported Work-related Illness Survey 2010–2011.
2 Under The Health and Occupation Reporting Network (THOR) scheme (see p. 692, Routine health statistics).

Skin pigmentation disorders

Altered skin colour

Causal exposures

- Silver and silver salts produces blue-grey skin pigmentation: *argyria*
- Trinitrotoluene (TNT) causes orange staining of skin
- A number of other chemicals can cause skin staining:
  - potassium permanganate
  - fluorescein, etc.

Hyperpigmentation

Causal exposures

- Pitch, tars; associated with photosensitivity
- Mercury compounds
- Arsenic and arsenicals.

Hypopigmentation (vitiligo)

Can be localized or generalized, and is indistinguishable from naturally occurring vitiligo.

Causal exposures

- Hydroquinones
- Phenols
- Catechols.

Screening

Using a Woods lamp, loss of melanin can be detected before it is apparent in white skin. This method is useful for detection of occupational vitiligo in exposed workers.

Compensation

Vitiligo is prescribed for Industrial Injuries Disablement Benefit (C25) in those exposed to paratertiarybutylphenol, paratertiarybutylcatechol, para-amylphenol, hydroquinone, monobenzyl ether of hydroquinone, or monobutyl ether of hydroquinone.

Folliculitis and acne

Epidemiology

Data from the specialist physicians reporting schemes[1] show that reported new cases of occupational folliculitis and acne are declining. Three cases were reported in 2009 and no cases in 2010.

Clinical features

Oil folliculitis
- Papules and pustular lesions
- Discoloration of the hair follicles
- Comedone formation with marked inflammatory component
- Typically occurs on thighs and forearms, where prolonged contact with oil saturates clothing.

Chloracne
- Pale comedones and cysts (unlike the inflamed lesions of oil acne)
- *Typically on the face:* cheeks, forehead, and neck
- Less commonly on the trunk, limbs, and genitalia
- Larger inflammatory lesions in chronic cases.

Coal tar acne
- Comedone formation
- Photosensitivity
- Skin pigmentation.

Causal exposures

Oil folliculitis
- Cutting oils
- Lubricants.

Chloracne
- Chlorinated naphthalenes (used as a synthetic insulating wax)
- Polychlorinated biphenyls (PCBs), e.g. chlorinated dibenzodioxins and dibenzofurans (used as heat insulator in electric transformers and capacitors).

Coal tar acne
Coal tar and products (used in roofing and civil engineering).

Prevention

The incidence of oil acne has reduced drastically because of exposure controls, particularly the decrease in use of cutting oils, use of safer products, and better hygiene. The use of PCBs has been greatly restricted in the UK.

Compensation Oil folliculitis and acne are prescribed for Industrial Injuries Disablement Benefit under D5 (non-infective dermatitis).

---

1 Under The Health and Occupation Reporting Network (THOR) scheme (see 🕮 p. 692, Routine health statistics).

Photodermatitis

Some occupational exposures can give rise to skin damage through interaction with UV light.

Polycyclic aromatic hydrocarbons

- Coal tar
- Pitch
- Creosote
- *Industries:*
  - gas production
  - coke oven work
  - roofing
  - production of graphite from pitch.

Plants

Many plants cause dermatitis that is triggered by sunlight.

- *Compositae*
- *Umbelliferae:*
  - giant hogweed
  - celery, etc.
- Some lichens
- Gardeners and grounds men are at risk when handling plants, but particularly when using lawn strimmers to cut verges, etc.

Others

Methylene blue causes dermatitis through a phototoxic reaction.

Scleroderma

Occupational scleroderma is rare.

Causal exposures

Inhalation of vinyl chloride monomer (VCM)

Scleroderma-like changes have been reported in association with exposure to the following:

- Pesticides
- Epoxy resins
- Perchlorethylene and trichloroethylene
- Silica.

Clinical features

Thickened shiny skin on the fingers.

VCM disease

Occurs as part of a syndrome which includes the following:

- *Acro-osteolysis:* resorption of the terminal phalanges on X-ray
- *Raynaud's phenomenon:* digital vascular spasm giving rise to blanching in cold conditions
- *Associated features of VCM exposure include:*
  - hepatic fibrosis
  - angiosarcoma of the liver.

Prevention

VCM disease has been virtually eliminated by good hygiene controls (enclosure) in the PVC manufacturing industry.

Compensation

Sclerodermatous thickening of the skin of the hands is prescribed for Industrial Injuries Disablement Benefit (C24b (iii)) in those who are exposed to vinyl chloride monomer in the manufacture of PVC.

Occupational skin infections

Occupation can be a risk factor for skin infection because of either association with environmental conditions that favour microbial overgrowth or exposure to specific organisms.

Epidemiology

Data from the specialist physicians reporting schemes[1] show that new cases of infective skin disease due to occupation have been declining over the past decade—26 cases were reported in 2010.

Saturation diving

Divers who live for prolonged periods in dive chambers are susceptible to infections of the skin and ear because of the persistently warm humid conditions. *Pseudomonas species* are a particular problem. Prevention of otitis externa requires meticulous aural toilet.

Zoonotic skin infections

These are a hazard for agricultural workers, veterinary practitioners, abbatoir, and fish-processing workers. They include Orf, Herpes Simplex, Anthrax, Scabies, Lyme Disease.

Multi-resistant *Staphylococcus aureus*

Persistent carriage of MRSA has been described in HCWs. This has mainly been described as nasal colonization on repeated swabbing, and is mostly asymptomatic. It usually clears with topical antibiotic treatment for the nose and chlorhexidine body washes. However, true infections (e.g. of skin lesions) are potentially serious and difficult to treat. Those who are at increased risk of multi-resistant *Staphylococcus aureus* (MRSA) carriage include HCWs with hand eczema or persistent respiratory tract infection (e.g. sinusitis or bronchiectasis).

🖝 There is no definitive guidance on exclusion of HCWs who are at risk of MRSA colonization or infection, or those who are chronically colonized. Decisions to restrict from work where there is a high risk of acquiring MRSA, or transmitting infection to patients (e.g. care of surgical wounds) should be made on an individual basis. There is little hard evidence to guide such decisions, and the risk of legal challenge in the event of loss of employment is significant.

Compensation

Certain occupational zoonoses that affect skin are prescribed for Industrial Injuries Disablement Benefit.
- Cutaneous anthrax (B1)
- Glanders (B2)
- Orf (B12).

Relevant legislation Any infection that is clearly attributable to occupation is reportable under RIDDOR.

---

1 Under The Health and Occupation Reporting Network (THOR) scheme (see 📖 p. 692, Routine health statistics).

Chapter 9

Musculoskeletal disorders

Low back pain

Epidemiology

- LBP has a lifetime prevalence of 60–80%, point prevalence of 15–40%, and annual incidence of 5%. It is:
  - the second most common cause of work-related ill health (prevalence 207 000, annual incidence 51 000)[1]
  - the second most common cause of absence from work (7.6 million days/year lost)[1]
  - the second most common reason for claiming incapacity benefit
  - There has been a reduction in the prevalence and incidence of work-related back pain since 2001/02.

Causal exposures/industries

- *Exposures:*
  - physical (lifting, bending, twisting, whole-body vibration)
  - psychosocial (high demand, low control, low job satisfaction)
- *Industries:* exposures are ubiquitous, but LBP most common in:
  - transport and logistics
  - construction
  - agriculture
  - clinical health care.

Features and investigation

- Pain radiating to the thigh is common (~40% of cases)
- In most cases, pathology is not defined (non-specific or mechanical LBP)
- <10% of cases have identifiable pathology, e.g. nerve root compression
- X-rays and MRI are not useful in most cases of mechanical back pain.
- Investigations aim to distinguish cases of serious spinal pathology. This is mainly done on the basis of clinical markers (red flags, see Box 9.1)
- Conceptual models of LBP recognize the importance of psychological and social factors (biopsychosocial theme).

Prevention Ergonomic risk controls (covered on 📖 p. 8, Vibration 1: whole body vibration, 📖 p. 120, Lifting and handling, 📖 p. 124, Posture).

Prognosis

- *Natural history:* most episodes of mechanical LBP are self-limiting.
  - more than 50% of episodes resolve completely within 4 weeks, but up to 20% have some symptoms for a year
  - there is a marked tendency to recurrence, 70% of those with back pain go on to experience three or more attacks
  - 20% of those with LBP develop chronic symptoms
- Probability of return to work ↓ with ↑ duration of sickness absence
- Clinical examination and investigations are poor predictors of disability
- Outcome is strongly influenced by individual psychological, workplace and cultural factors (see Box 9.1; 📖 p. 256, Work-related upper limb disorders 1).

---

1 2010/11 Labour Force Survey.

Box 9.1 Red flags indicate possible of serious spinal pathology

Thoracic pain, fever, weight loss, bladder or bowel dysfunction, carcinoma, other illness, progressive neurological deficit, disturbed gait, saddle anaesthesia, age <20yrs or >55yrs, structural deformity, systemic steroid therapy

Yellow, blue and black flags are risk factors for chronicity and disability

Yellow flags are psychological and behavioural

• A –ve attitude that back pain is harmful or severely disabling
• Fear avoidance behaviour and reduced activity levels
• Expectation that passive, rather than active, treatment will be beneficial
• A tendency to depression, low morale, and social withdrawal
• Social or financial problems.

Blue flags are occupational psychological factors

• Poor job satisfaction
• Blaming working conditions
• Adverse job characteristics (heavy work, poor relationships).

Black flags are organizational and social factors

• Health benefits or insurance
• Litigation
• Sickness policies.

Management

• Refer those with red flags for urgent clinical assessment
• *Rehabilitation comprises:*
    • encouragement to stay active; early physical therapy; reassurance
    • advise early return to work, ↓ risk by adjustments and job redesign
    • rarely, restriction from work or redeployment
• Early rehabilitation and job redesign ↓ employment costs and litigation.

Relevant legislation

HSE (2009). *The Manual Handling Operations Regulations 1992* (amended). Available at: ℘ http://www.hse.gov.uk/pubns/priced/l23.pdf

HSE (2009). *Work with display screen equipment: Health and Safety (Display Screen Equipment) Regulations 1992 as amended by the Health and Safety (Miscellaneous Amendments) Regulations 2002.* Available at: ℘ http://www.hse.gov.uk/pubns/priced/l26.pdf

Further information and guidance

Waddell, G, Burton, AK (2000). *Occupational Health Guidelines for the management of low back pain. Evidence review and recommendations.* Faculty of Occupational Medicine, London. Available at: ℘ http://www.fom.ac.uk/publications-policy-guidance-and-consultations/publications/faculty-publications

NICE (2009). *Low back pain: early management of persistent non-specific back pain*, NICE clinical guideline 88. Available at: ℘ http://www.nice.org.uk/nicemedia/pdf/CG88NICEGuideline.pdf

HSE *Back pain.* Available at: ℘ http://hse.gov.uk/msd/backpain/index.htm

Work-related upper limb disorders 1

Epidemiology

- Upper limb and neck pain are common. In some surveys, up to 17–20% of people complain of neck–shoulder pain and 20% of hand–wrist pain during the past 7 days
- Many have pain in the absence of clearly defined clinical pathology, but distinct disorders (e.g. epicondylitis, carpal tunnel syndrome (CTS)) each affect 1–3% of older subjects. Such symptoms are often attributed to work
- The HSE estimates an incidence of work-attributed upper limb and neck complaints in Britain of 280/100,000 adults/year with 3.6 million lost working days per annum.

Clinical features

According to NIOSH, some 165 ICD disease codes should be considered under the umbrella definition of 'Work-related upper limb disorders' (WRULD). Classification is contentious and complex. The surveillance criteria for 9 of the commoner upper limb disorders (ULDs), as agreed at a UK expert workshop, are listed in the table (see Table 9.1).

Clinical assessment and diagnosis

- Diagnosis is based on history and clinical examination
- Median nerve conduction is used if CTS is suspected
- Table 9.1 provides a short guide on diagnostic criteria
- Assessment should cover co-morbid non-occupational factors, e.g. trauma, diabetes, rheumatoid arthritis, acromegaly, hypothyroidism

Medical management

- *For all disorders:* non-steroid anti-inflammatory agents (although there is some evidence of non-effectiveness in epicondylitis and possibly other ULDs), analgesics
- *Shoulder disorders:* physical therapy, corticosteroid injection, exercise programmes
- *Neck disorders:* soft cervical collar, physical therapy (heat pad, exercises, ultrasound/short-wave diathermy, massage, transcutaneous electrical nerve stimulation (TENS), manipulation, acupuncture)
- *Elbow disorders:* corticosteroid injection, pulsed ultrasound, wrist splint (to prevent wrist dorsiflexion)
- *Tenosynovitis/peritendinitis:* local heat, corticosteroid injection, splinting, surgical decompression of the first extensor compartment +/– tenosynovectomy (chronic cases)
- *CTS:* splinting, local corticosteroid injection, surgical release.

Prognosis

- Acute florid tenosynovitis tends to settle quickly if thoroughly rested
- Frozen shoulder lasts 12–18mths and is resistant to treatment
- Epicondylitis is said to resolve in 8–12mths, but often lasts longer
- Symptoms of CTS can improve if the causal factor is removed, but otherwise tend to become chronic

Table 9.1 Diagnostic criteria for ULDs proposed by an HSE-convened expert workshop

Disorder	Diagnostic criteria
Rotator cuff tendinitis	Pain in deltoid region + pain on resisted active movement (abduction—supraspinatus; external rotation—infraspinatus; internal rotation—subscapularis)
Bicipital tendinitis	Anterior shoulder pain + pain on resisted active flexion or supination of forearm
Shoulder capsulitis (frozen shoulder)	Pain in deltoid area + equal restriction of active and passive glenohumeral movement with capsular pattern (external rotation > abduction > internal rotation)
Lateral epicondylitis	Epicondylar pain + epicondylar tenderness + pain on resisted extension of the wrist
Medial epicondylitis	Epicondylar pain + epicondylar tenderness + pain on resisted flexion of the wrist
De Quervain's disease of the wrist	Pain over radial styloid + tender swelling of first extensor compartment + either pain reproduced by resisted thumb extension or positive Finkelstein's test
Tenosynovitis of wrist	Pain on movement localized to the tendon sheaths in the wrist + reproduction of pain by resisted active movement
Carpal tunnel syndrome	Pain or paraesthesia or sensory loss in the median nerve distribution + one of: Tinel's test positive, Phalen's test positive, nocturnal exacerbation of symptoms, motor loss with wasting of abductor pollicis brevis, slowed nerve conduction
Non-specific diffuse forearm pain	Pain in the forearm in the absence of a specific diagnosis or pathology

• According to one systematic review only a half of new shoulder episodes end in complete recovery within 6mths
• In general, ULDs tend to persist if causal or aggravating factors remain in place. Persistence is more frequent if 'yellow flag' (see Box 9.1) –ve psychological factors are also present.

Work-related upper limb disorders 2

Causal exposures and industries

- ULDs may be caused (or aggravated) by undesirable permutations of force, repetition, duration and posture, with insufficient recovery time (see Table 9.2) (see also 📖 p. 120, Lifting and handling, 📖 p. 124, Posture, 📖 p. 128, Repetitive work)
- Occupations in which high rates of ULD have been reported include packing, assembly and food processing
- Psychological risk factors (e.g. low mood, somatizing tendency, job dissatisfaction, negative perceptions about the work environment) are also associated with disease reporting and 'yellow flag' risk factors for persistence.

⚠ All of the ULDs labelled as 'work-related' also have non-occupational risk factors. The clinical pattern may be indistinguishable in occupationally and non-occupationally related cases, making attribution problematic in the individual case.

Prevention

Depending on the risk assessment and context, preventive measures at work may include:

- *Better design of tools, equipment, and work layout:* to make the work easier, the posture better, the forces lower, etc.
- *Advice & training:* to promote risk awareness and better working practices
- *An induction period:* to allow new employees to start out at a slower pace
- *Job rotation/job enlargement:* to provide respite from repetitive monotonous work
- *Rest breaks:* to allow recovery time
- *A rehabilitation programme:* to ease affected workers back into productive work
- *Redeployment:* as a last resort in recalcitrant cases.

Relevant legislation and guidance

There are no legal provisions in the UK specific to the prevention of WRULDs. HSE provides useful advice on good practice and prevention including:

- Upper limb disorders in the workplace (HSG60)
- Working with VDUs (INDG36)
- Aching arms (or RSI) in small businesses (INDG171rev1)
- The Assessment of Repetitive Tasks (ART) tool. Available at: ℘ http://www.hse.gov.uk/pubns/indg438.pdf
- A task rotation worksheet. Available at: ℘ http://www.hse.gov.uk/msd/uld/art/resources.htm

Table 9.2 Associations between mechanical factors and ULDs

Anatomic site	Strong evidence of effect	Some evidence of effect	Insufficient evidence of effect
Neck and neck/shoulder			
Repetition		+	
Force		+	
Posture	+		
Vibration			+
Shoulder			
Posture		+	
Force			+
Repetition		+	
Vibration			+
Elbow			
Repetition			+
Force		+	
Posture			+
Several of these 3 exposures	+		
Tendonitis of the hand/wrist			
Repetition		+	
Force		+	
Posture		+	
Several of these exposures	+		
Carpal tunnel syndrome			
Repetition	+/-	+/-	
Force		+	
Posture			+
Vibration		+	
Several of these exposures	+		

Source: NIOSH Publication No. 97–141 (1997).

Osteoarthritis of the hip

Epidemiology

- As with osteoarthritis in other joints, the prevalence of hip osteoarthritis (hip OA) rises steeply with age
- In Britain, approximately 5% of the elderly population are affected, with slightly higher rates in men than women
- Hip OA is the main reason for the more than 40,000 total hip replacements that are carried out each year.

Clinical features

- Pain around the hip (in the groin, buttock or lateral to the joint), with radiation to the knee in some patients
- Stiffness of the hip after immobility (e.g. on getting up in the morning and after prolonged sitting)
- Limitation of hip movement, especially internal rotation and flexion
- In severe cases there may be fixed flexion of the joint.

Occupational causes

Epidemiological studies have consistently demonstrated an increased incidence in agricultural workers, with relative risks generally in excess of two. There is still some debate about the aspects of agricultural work that are responsible, but the strongest evidence is for a role of frequent, heavy lifting. Several studies have indicated an elevated risk also in other occupations that entail heavy lifting.

Individual susceptibility

A number of non-occupational factors are also associated with an increased risk of hip osteoarthritis, and are likely to make individuals more susceptible to relevant occupational exposures. These include:

- Developmental deformities of the hip (congenital dislocation, Perthes disease, slipped femoral epiphysis)
- Genetically-determined susceptibility to osteoarthritis in multiple joints
- Obesity.

Clinical assessment and diagnosis

- History of relevant symptoms and associated disability
- Clinical examination of the hip, looking particularly for limitation of movement and fixed flexion deformity
- Radiology (plain radiograph of the hip), looking for narrowing of the joint space, osteophytes, and subchondral thickening of bone with cyst formation
- Additional tests may sometimes be appropriate to exclude other types of arthritis.

Prognosis

Tends to progress, but at a variable rate. Spontaneous improvement in symptoms occasionally occurs.

Health surveillance
This is not currently practised in the occupational setting.

Compensation
In Britain, hip osteoarthritis is prescribed for Industrial Injuries Disablement Benefit (A13) in people who have worked in agriculture as a farmer or farm worker for at least 10yrs in total.

Bursitis

The beat conditions are a group of disorders that comprise bursitis or subcutaneous cellulitis overlying pressure points in the palm, elbow, or knee.

Clinical features

- *Beat hand:* bruising or tenderness in the palm
- *Beat elbow/knee:* painful localized swelling, with inflammation and sometimes effusion in the bursa (olecranon or infrapatellar).

Causal exposures/industries

Sustained exposure to friction, pressure, or impact
- *Prolonged use of picks or shovels:*
  - miners
  - road workers
- *Prolonged kneeling:*
  - carpet fitters
  - joiners/carpenters.

Treatment and prognosis

- Usually self-limiting
- Occasionally require antibiotics (if infected) or local steroid injection.

Prevention

The mainstay of prevention is in improving the ergonomics of physical tasks. Solutions might include attention to working posture, tool redesign, task rotation, frequent rest breaks (see 📖 p. 118, Ergonomics hazards: overview), and appropriate use of personal protective equipment (e.g. kneeling pads, padded clothing).

Compensation

Bursitis or subcutaneous cellulitis is prescribed for Industrial Injuries Disablement Benefit (A5, A6, A7) in manual workers who sustain severe or prolonged pressure or friction over the hand, knee, or elbow.

Relevant legislation

Bursitis or subcutaneous cellulitis of the hand, knee, or elbow that is attributable to manual work is reportable under RIDDOR.

Gastrointestinal and urinary tract disorders

Hepatic angiosarcoma

Epidemiology

This otherwise very rare hepatic cancer occurs among workers exposed to VCM and, less frequently, pesticide-exposed agricultural workers. Reactor (autoclave) cleaners may be highly exposed to VCM, a genotoxic carcinogen. When this association was first recognized, VCM production workers showed 400× expected incidence of hepatic angiosarcoma. However, owing to improved exposure control, the disease is now very rare in developed countries.

Clinical features

- Fatigue
- Abdominal pain
- Weight loss
- Pyrexia
- Jaundice
- Ascites
- Hepatosplenomegaly
- Oesophageal varices.

Causal exposure/industries

- Vinyl chloride monomer production in the plastics industry
- Arsenic-containing pesticides used in vineyards.

Clinical assessment/diagnosis

- Thrombocytopenia, anaemia, on full blood count
- Abnormal liver function tests
- *CT/MRI scan:*
    - CT scan may show a multifocal tumour with hypo-attenuation; hyper-attenuation to liver suggests haemorrhage into the tumour
    - angiosarcoma is hypo-intense to normal liver on T_1-weighted MRI images
- *Liver biopsy:* histology variable within a tumour. Vascular spaces, lined with tumour cells, may or may not be obvious.

Prognosis

Untreated, death occurs within months from hepatic encephalopathy or intra-abdominal bleeding.

Health surveillance

- Long latent interval between exposure and presentation
- Liver function tests (alanine aminotransferase (ALT), aspartate aminotransferase (AST)) identify hepatic impairment in VCM exposed workers
- Hepatic ultrasound has been used to identify pre-symptomatic angiosarcoma.

Medical management

Hepatic resection and/or chemotherapy may prolong life in those with an operable tumour.

Prevention
Prevent by limiting exposure to VCM.

Compensation
Angiosarcoma of the liver is a prescribed disease (C24) for Industrial Injuries Disablement Benefit in those exposed to VCM in the manufacture of PVC.

Relevant legislation
- *COSHH Schedule 5:* monitor employee breathing zone VCM exposure
- *COSHH Schedule 6:* annual health surveillance by HSE appointed doctor
- *EH 40/2005* VCM, WEL 3ppm (8h TWA)
- *RIDDOR Regulations 1995:* Angiosarcoma of the liver is a reportable disease among those exposed to VCM.

Hepatic cirrhosis

Epidemiology

Common causes of liver cirrhosis worldwide include HBV, HCV, and alcohol. Most cases of cirrhosis due to these agents are not work-related, but a small proportion may be due to occupational exposure. Other rare causes of cirrhosis include work with halogenated hydrocarbons.

Clinical features

- Fatigue
- Anorexia
- Nausea
- Spider naevi
- Jaundice
- Pruritus
- Ascites
- Bleeding/bruising
- Finger clubbing
- Portal hypertension
- Oesophageal varices
- Hepatocellular cancer
- Hepatic encephalopathy.

Causal exposures/industries

- *Hepatitis B:*
  - HCWs
- *Hepatitis C:*
  - HCWs
- *Alcohol:*
  - transport industry
  - publicans and bar staff
- *Organic solvents:*
  - carbon tetrachloride
  - 1,1,1-trichloroethane.

Clinical assessment/diagnosis

- LFTs
- Full blood count and clotting studies
- Hepatitis B surface antigen
- Hepatitis C antibody
- Hepatic ultrasound
- Liver biopsy.

Prognosis

Depends on the disease stage; once complications such as hepatic encephalopathy supervene, the prognosis is generally poor. A small proportion will develop primary carcinoma of the liver as a complication of cirrhosis.

Health surveillance

- Biological monitoring of solvent-exposed workers using urinary metabolites or exhaled breath sampling may be indicated dependent on the risk assessment
- HCWs and others at risk of hepatitis B should be immunized and their immune status confirmed by measuring hepatitis B surface antibody levels.

Medical management

- See 📖 p. 152, Hepatitis B ; 📖 p. 154, Hepatitis C
- Abstinence from alcohol in alcoholic cirrhosis
- *Liver transplant:*
    - employment rates pre-operatively are lower for alcoholic liver disease than other indications for liver transplant. However, return to work rates post-transplant are similar
    - 45–70% of transplant recipients will return to work
    - poor physical functioning and fatigue influence employment status post-transplant
    - some centres employ living donor hepatic lobe transplants. Limited evidence suggests donors have a mean work absence of about 3mths.

Prevention

Preventing exposure to human blood and body fluids—see 📖 p. 104, Human tissue and body fluids.

Compensation

Liver fibrosis is a prescribed disease for Industrial Injuries Disablement Benefit in those who have been exposed to VCM in the manufacture of PVC (C24d). Cirrhosis is prescribed in those who have been exposed to chlorinated naphthalenes (C13).

Acute hepatotoxicity

A number of chemicals are recognized as causing acute hepatotoxicity, although some of them are no longer used in the way that once led to workers suffering adverse effects. Hepatotoxicity due to occupational chemical exposure is now rarely reported in the UK.

Epidemiology

Common causes of hepatic insult

- Alcohol
- Metabolic syndrome
- Drug reactions.

Clinical features

- Fatigue
- Weight loss
- Right upper quadrant abdominal pain
- Anorexia
- Nausea
- Jaundice
- Impaired clotting.

▶ Mild steatosis may be asymptomatic

Causal exposures/industries

- *Chemical industry including:*
  - carbon tetrachloride (CCl₄)
  - chlorinated napthalenes
  - dimethylformamide
  - chlordecone (kepone)
  - methylene dianiline
  - polychlorinated biphenyls
  - phosphorus
  - trinitrotoluene
- *Painting:*
  - 2-nitropropane
- *Dry cleaning:*
  - perchloroethylene.

Mechanism of hepatotoxicity

Acute chemical hepatotoxicity may manifest itself in a number of ways:
- *Steatosis (fatty liver):*
  - steatohepatitis if hepatic inflammation present
- *Acute hepatocellular injury (necrosis):*
  - direct toxicity
  - idiosyncratic reaction (e.g. halothane)
- Cholestasis (impaired bile flow).

Clinical assessment and diagnosis

- Clinical examination looking for stigmata of chronic liver disease or alcohol misuse

- Liver enzymes:
  - alkaline phosphatase (AlkPhos)
  - alanine aminotransferase (ALT)
  - gamma glutamyl transpeptidase (GGT)
- Bilirubin
- *Carbohydrate deficient transferrin (CDT)*: in suspected alcohol misuse
- Albumin
- Full blood count
- Clotting screen—prothrombin time
- Hepatitis B surface antigen and core antibody
- Hepatitis C antibodies
- *Liver ultrasound +/− biopsy*: findings are dependent on the nature of the hepatic insult.

Prognosis
Dependent on the degree of hepatic injury but some cases will progress to cirrhosis.

Health surveillance
Biological monitoring may be indicated for some agents (e.g. solvents).

Medical management
- Withdraw from exposure to hepatotoxin
- *Lifestyle changes:*
  - abstinence from alcohol
  - weight loss if obese

- Review workplace risk assessment—further controls may be required.

Compensation
Liver toxicity is prescribed for Industrial Injuries Disablement Benefit in those who are exposed to carbon tetrachloride (C26(a)) or trichloromethane (C27).

Relevant legislation
Hepatotoxicity is reportable under RIDDOR where it is due to poisoning by any of the chemicals listed in Schedule 3, part 1.

Gastrointestinal cancers

Epidemiology
Gastric cancer is the fourth most common cancer.
- Adenocarcinoma is the most common gastric cancer
- Gastric cancer is much more common in Asia (Japan and China) than in Europe
- The annual incidence of gastric cancer is falling and is presently estimated at 870 000 cases/year worldwide
- Men are at twice the risk of gastric cancer as women
- Occupational exposures have been linked to an increased risk of gastric cancer
- Most studies of pancreatic cancer have not found a link to occupation.

Clinical features
Gastric cancer
- Weight loss
- Abdominal pain
- Dyspepsia
- Dsyphagia
- Anorexia.

Causal exposures
- Nitrosamines (gastric cancer)
- Phenoxy herbicides

Industries at risk
- *Industries at high risk:*
  - tin mining
  - steel works
  - carpentry
- *Industries at increased risk:*
  - chemical industry
  - coal mining
  - coke works
  - rubber industry
  - oil refining.

Clinical assessment and diagnosis
Investigation of gastric cancer includes endoscopy and biopsy. CT scan may be used to identify metastases.

Prognosis
The prognosis of gastric cancer is generally poor as many patients present with advanced disease. Among those with operable disease 5yr survival is about 45%.

Health surveillance
No health surveillance has yet been proven to be beneficial in occupational groups. Screening for gastric cancer in at-risk groups may be appropriate, but further evaluation is necessary.

Medical management and prevention

The treatment of gastric cancer is partial or total gastrectomy. Prevention relies on control of exposure to carcinogens.

Relevant legislation

COSHH Regulations 2002 (as amended).

Renal failure

Acute renal failure

Occupational exposures that can cause acute renal failure (ARF)
- Cadmium (see 📖 p. 65, Cadmium)
- Mercury (see 📖 p. 72, Mercury)
- Organic solvents
- Occupationally acquired infections (e.g. leptospirosis).

Clinical features of ARF
- Oliguria or anuria
- Nocturia
- Ankle oedema
- Fluid retention
- Impaired appetite
- Tremor
- Fatigue
- Hypertension.

Clinical assessment of renal failure
- Urinalysis
- Urea, electrolytes, and creatinine
- Blood lipids
- Full blood count
- Renal ultrasound
- IVP.

Health surveillance
Health surveillance for nephropathy is only likely to be undertaken in chronic exposure to cadmium. Cadmium workers should wear appropriate protective equipment and have regular biological monitoring of blood and urinary cadmium levels, with retinol binding protein (RBP) if levels are persistently elevated.

Compensation
Kidney toxicity is prescribed (C26(b)) for Industrial Injuries Disablement Benefit in those who are exposed to carbon tetrachloride.

Bladder cancer

Epidemiology

- Bladder cancer is the seventh most common cancer in the UK
- About 5–10% of bladder cancer in Europe may be due to occupational exposures
- Smoking is the major risk factor and may account for up to 80% of cases. However, where smokers are exposed to carcinogens it is not possible to distinguish between occupational and non-occupational causes
- Bladder cancer is most common in the elderly and rare under age 40. Therefore, bladder cancer occurring at a young age is a red flag for possible occupational aetiology.

Clinical features

- Microscopic haematuria
- Frank haematuria
- Dysuria
- Urinary frequency.

Causal exposures

- Polycyclic aromatic hydrocarbons (PAHs)
- *Aromatic amines:*
  - benzidine
  - β-napthylamine
  - ortho-toluidine
  - auramine
  - magenta.
- MbOCA
- Arsenic.

Industries at risk

- Historically, due to β-napthylamine—withdrawn in 1949:
  - chemical industry (dyestuffs)
  - rubber industry
- Currently:
  - coke works/coal gas works
  - printing
  - metal working
  - aluminium smelting (Soderberg process)
  - painting
  - truck drivers
  - leather industry
  - hairdressers.

Individual susceptibility

Family history of bladder cancer.

Clinical assessment and diagnosis

- Physical examination including rectal examination
- Urinalysis

- Intravenous pyelogram (IVP)
- Cystoscopy and tumour biopsy
- Urine cytology
- *Disease staging:* CT scan, CXR, bone scan.

Prognosis

Five-year survival is ~60% although this is influenced by the presence of multiple tumours, tumour bulk, and tumour stage.

Health surveillance

- Workers should remain subject to follow-up after exposure ceases
- Once diagnosed, patients with superficial bladder cancer are followed up with regular cystoscopy at 3–6-monthly intervals.

Medical management

- Transurethral resection +/– chemotherapy, radiotherapy
- Cystectomy for more extensive disease.

Prevention

- Improved control of chemical exposures has ↓ incidence of occupational bladder cancer
- Most agents associated with bladder cancer are now banned in the UK (e.g. benzidine)
- Substitution of carcinogenic agents with less hazardous agents.

Compensation

- Primary neoplasm of the epithelial lining of the urinary tract is a prescribed disease (C23) for Industrial Injuries Disablement Benefit in those who are exposed to:
  - aromatic amines
  - MbOCA for ≥12mths
  - orthotoluidine, 4-chloro-2-methylaniline
- Coal tar pitch volatiles produced in aluminium smelting involving the Soderberg process for ≥5yrs.

Relevant legislation

Bladder cancer is a reportable condition under RIDDOR 1995 where there has been work with any of the agents listed in Schedule 3.

Eye disorders

Eye injuries

Epidemiology

Occupational eye injuries are common. Men suffer >80% of eye injuries with young men at highest risk. Those using power tools in engineering, construction, and farming are at particular risk.

Causes

Trauma

Leading to:
- Subtarsal foreign body
- Corneal abrasion
- Corneal foreign body
- Intra-ocular foreign body
- *Contusion:*
  - hyphaema
  - lens dislocation
  - retinal tear
  - commotio retinae
  - globe rupture.

Non-ionizing radiation
- Ultraviolet radiation B (UV-B) 280–315 nm
- Arc welding: 'arc eye' or 'welder's flash'
- Lasers
- High-intensity discharge lamps (HIDL).

Chemicals
- Acids
- Alkalis.

Industries/occupations at greatest risk
- Construction
- Agriculture
- Metalworking, especially welding, grinding, shot-blasting
- Woodworking
- Transport.

Prevention
- Safe systems of work
- Machinery guards, interlocks
- Dust suppression
- Enforce use of appropriate eye protection: goggles, glasses, masks
- Information, instruction, and training.

Clinical assessment and diagnosis
- Visual inspection: evert eyelids to identify sub-tarsal foreign body
- Fundoscopy
- Slit-lamp microscopy
- Fluorescein staining for suspected corneal abrasions: fluoresce under blue light

- Test visual acuity: near and distance vision
- X-ray globe to identify retained foreign body.

Medical management

- Chemical exposures: irrigate eye thoroughly using normal saline or sterile water. Exposure to strong alkali or acid can be sight threatening (see 📖 pp. 792, 793, General principles, Management of chemical exposures to the eye)
- It is important that appropriate first aid facilities including eye-wash stations are present in high-risk work areas.

Relevant legislation

Temporary or permanent loss of sight, penetrating eye injury, chemical or hot metal burns to the eye are all reportable under RIDDOR as major injuries.

Conjunctivitis and keratitis

Conjunctivitis may be due to exposure to physical, chemical, or biological agents (e.g. bacteria, viruses).

Epidemiology

Data from an American workers compensation scheme found:
- Annual incidence of allergic conjunctivitis, 731/100,000 workers
- Annual incidence of keratitis, 723/100,000 workers.

Clinical features

- Severe photophobia
- Lacrimation
- Conjunctival injection
- Headache.

Causal industries and exposures

- Arc welding: intense UV-B light from the arc
- Inappropriate use of UV-C lights instead of the required UV-A lights in electric fly killers used in food industry and commercial kitchens: such incidents may affect several workers who develop keratitis and facial erythema. Diagnosis is often delayed by several months
- Acid mists

Hydrogen sulphide (H_2S) conjunctivitis: occurs at 750 ppm H_2S (see 🔲 p. 99, Hydrogen sulphide and 🔲 p. 800, Hydrogen sulphide poisoning)
- Vanadium pentoxide
- Some organic solvents

Allergens: e.g. laboratory animals such as rats and mice, in association with rhinitis: *rhinoconjunctivitis*
- Ophthalmology: exposure when examining infected patients may lead to the clinician developing bacterial or viral conjunctivitis
- Sharing microscopes: e.g. in electronics factories, may lead to outbreaks of infectious conjunctivitis.

Diagnosis

Welder's flash

History of unprotected eye exposure to arc welding
- *Symptoms develop 6–12h post-exposure:*
  - severe photophobia
  - lacrimation
  - headache
- The typical patient is an apprentice who, through ignorance or carelessness, is close to a welder when an arc is struck.

Allergic conjunctivitis

Based on history of exposure to allergen and ↑ specific IgE.

Infectious conjunctivitis

Diagnosis by swabs for microscopy, culture, and sensitivity.

Prognosis
Welder's flash: full recovery.

Health surveillance
None appropriate.

Medical management
- 'Arc eye' (kerato-conjunctivitis) is treated with topical local anaesthetic drops and a mydriatic
- Bacterial conjunctivitis is treated with topical antibiotics
- There is no consensus as to whether ophthalmologists should work when suffering from conjunctivitis, given the potential to cross-infect patients.

Relevant legislation
An injury at work that caused conjunctivitis, and was associated with 7 days' work loss or temporary loss of sight, would be reportable under RIDDOR.

Cataract

Epidemiology
- Worldwide cataract is the most common cause of blindness
- A number of occupational exposures contribute to this burden
- Penetrating eye injuries are most common in young men and may lead to traumatic cataract.

Causes
- Non-ionizing radiation:
  - UV-B (cortical cataract)
  - IR
- Lasers (medical, industrial)
- Electrocution
- Penetrating eye injuries
- Inorganic lead
- Chemicals, e.g. trinitrotoluene, ethylene oxide, methyl isocyanate.

Industries at risk
- Metal foundries
- Arc welding
- Glass blowing
- Printing with use of HIDL.

Investigations
In the event of a disease cluster, an occupational hygiene survey may be undertaken to monitor workplace exposures.

Health surveillance

There is no regulatory requirement for health surveillance.

Medical management and prevention
- *Engineering controls:*
  - interlocks
  - shielding
- *Administrative controls:*
  - information, instruction, and training
  - access controls
- *Personal protective equipment:*
  - safety goggles.

Compensation
Cataract is a prescribed disease (A2) for Industrial Injuries Disablement Benefit in those who have frequent or prolonged exposure to radiation from red-hot or white-hot material.

Relevant legislation
Cataract due to electromagnetic radiation (including radiant heat) is reportable under RIDDOR.

Retinal burns

Epidemiology

Retinal burns may occur in the workplace because of the use of high-power lasers (the acronym laser stands for light amplification by the stimulated emission of radiation) or, less commonly, arc welding equipment. Intense exposure to solar radiation (e.g. on snowfields) may also lead to retinal burns.

Lasers are very widely used (e.g. consumer electronics, telecommunications, engineering). However, estimates suggest there are <15 occupational laser injuries per year worldwide, mostly due to exposure to powerful Q-switched industrial or military lasers (see 📖 p.28, Non-ionizing radiation 3: laser).

Lasers can cause photomechanical and photochemical eye injuries, as well as retinal burns. Most laser incidents involve damage to the macula; an affected worker will be immediately aware of altered vision and will present to an optician or doctor.

Clinical features
- Blurred vision
- Usually painless.

Causal exposures/industries
- Research, e.g. nuclear physics
- *Military:*
  - laser rangefinders
  - target designators
- *Health care:* ophthalmology.

Clinical assessment and diagnosis
- Visual acuity: Snellen chart
- Test visual fields
- Fundoscopy
- Retinal photography
- Fluorescein angiography.

Prognosis
- Retinal damage due to lasers is permanent
- Outcome depends on the location and size of the burn
- Foveal burns may have a severe effect on visual acuity.

Health surveillance

In the UK, HSE does not currently recommend routine health surveillance for laser workers.

Medical management

Refer on to an ophthalmologist with expertise in the management of retinal burns for assessment.

Relevant legislation
- Maximum permissible exposure values (MPEs) for lasers are specified by the International Commission on Non-ionizing Radiation Protection, and are set at levels where no harm is likely to occur
  ⚠ Risk assessments under the Management of Health and Safety at Work Regulations 1999 should also consider non-beam hazards such as the use of high-voltage power sources.
- The Private and Voluntary Health Care (England) Regulations 2001 govern the use of lasers in the private health sector in England.

Neurological disorders

Brain cancer

Epidemiology

Primary brain cancers are relatively rare with an annual incidence in UK adults of 7/100,000 population.

- Although relatively rare, 1° brain tumour is the eighth most common tumour in people of working age
- Most adult 1° brain tumours are supratentorial and are gliomas (85%)
- The incidence of 1° brain tumour increases with increasing age
- Epidemiological findings regarding possible risk factors for primary brain tumour have been inconsistent
- Several occupations (e.g. firefighters) and chemical exposures (e.g. pesticides) have been associated with ↑ risk of 1° brain tumour, but studies are inconclusive
- Metastatic brain tumour is much more common than 1° brain tumour:
  - up to 40% of adult cancer sufferers develop brain metastases.

Clinical features

Patients with a primary brain tumour may present with:

- Headache
- Seizure
- Focal neurological deficits:
  - diplopia
  - dysphasia
  - hemiparesis
  - hemisensory deficits
- Non-focal neurological deficits:
  - confusion/memory problems
  - visual symptoms
  - ataxia
  - personality change.

Causal exposures/industries

- Few occupational risk factors for primary brain tumour have been identified
- Some studies suggest an increased risk in the petroleum industry.

Clinical assessment and diagnosis

- CT scan with contrast or an MRI scan
- Tumour excision or biopsy will permit histological diagnosis.

Prognosis

Survival for those adults with malignant brain tumour remains poor with 64% mortality in 12mths and 85% mortality by 5yrs.

Medical management

- Surgical excision or biopsy, with/without subsequent local radiotherapy
- Corticosteroids to reduce brain swelling
- Chemotherapy such as vincristine, lomustine, and procarbazine

- During the immediate phase of diagnosis and management most patients will not be fit for work.

Legislation/guidance

DVLA. *At a glance guide to the current medical standards of fitness to drive.* Available at: M http://www.dft.gov.uk/dvla/medical/ataglance.aspx

Acute narcosis

Acute narcosis occurs in those workers exposed to solvent vapour or to gases with narcotic action.

Epidemiology

There is little information regarding the incidence of acute narcosis in the workplace in the UK.

Clinical features

The features of acute narcosis are those of anaesthesia. If sufficiently heavily exposed, workers will go through the four stages of anaesthesia unless exposure ceases. Signs and symptoms of narcosis include:

• Euphoria
• Disinhibition
• Aggression
• Dizziness
• Ataxia
• Loss of consciousness
• Apnoea
• Death.

Causal exposures

Exposure to narcotic agents may occur during normal work, or following spills or accidents. Rarely, volatile substance abuse may present in the workplace with narcosis.

• *Organic solvents*:
  • glues and adhesives
  • polishes
  • paint or varnish
  • degreasants (e.g. trichloroethylene)
  • printing inks
  • dry cleaning fluids (e.g. perchloroethylene)
• Nitrogen dioxide
• Nitrogen (air divers below 30m)
• VCM.

Clinical assessment and diagnosis

The diagnosis may be made by workmates or the emergency services responding to a reported collapse. History of exposure to narcotic agents such as organic solvents (especially in confined spaces) should alert you to the diagnosis.

Prognosis

Most make a full recovery. Those workers who suffer hypoxia may sustain long-term damage (e.g. cognitive impairment).

Emergency medical management

See 📖 p. 792, General principles and contact details for specialist advice, Immediate management of poisoning in the workplace)
- The affected worker, if conscious, may appear drunk
- *If it is safe to do so:*
  - withdraw from exposure
  - remove contaminated clothing
- If respiratory depression is present, administer oxygen.

Relevant legislation

Acute narcosis leading to unconsciousness is reportable under RIDDOR 1995.
⚠ A serious incident, such as acute narcosis, demands that the risk assessment for that work activity be reviewed; it is likely that further controls are necessary.

Parkinsonism

Parkinsonism is the term for a group of movement disorders, the best known of which is Parkinson's disease (PD). Degeneration of the dopaminergic neurons of the substantia nigra occurs in PD. The neuropathological hallmark of PD is the presence of Lewy bodies, although this is not unique to PD.

PD epidemiology

- Peak age at disease onset 65yrs
- Incidence 17/100,000 population/year
- Prevalence 1 in 1000 of population
- Prevalence 1 in 100 of population aged >65yrs
- No figures exist regarding the number of cases of PD that may be due to occupational exposures.

PD clinical features

- Tremor
- Rigidity
- Bradykinesia (slow movements)
- Postural instability
- Half of patients show unilateral onset
- Expressionless face
- Shuffling gait
- Cognitive impairment later in illness
- Speech becomes soft and indistinct as disease progresses
- Drooling
- Sleep problems
- 'On–off' phenomenon.

Causal exposures

- Repeated head trauma
- *Pesticides:* no single agent identified as causal
- *Manganese:* parkinsonism, not PD
- Carbon disulphide (CS_2)
- 1-methyl-4-phenyl-1,2,3,6-tetrahydropyridine (MPTP), very rare.

Industries at risk

- Boxing
- Farming
- Manganese mining, smelting
- Industrial chemistry.

Individual susceptibility

- Tobacco smoking halves the risk of PD
- Familial forms of PD are recognized.

Clinical assessment and diagnosis

- On clinical features and response to L-dopa-containing drugs
- Exclude vascular parkinsonism (stepwise progression) or drug-induced parkinsonism.

Prognosis

Progressive deterioration in neurological and cognitive function occurs over several years. Working life may be curtailed by disease progression. The main functional consequences are reduced mobility, dexterity, and stamina.

Medical management

- Optimize drug regime
- Patients do best when cared for by a neurologist with an interest in movement disorders
- Support from a specialist PD nurse is helpful for patients
- Depression is common and may go unrecognized.

Compensation

Central nervous system toxicity characterized by parkinsonism is prescribed (C2) for Industrial Injuries Disablement Benefit in those who are exposed to the fumes, dust, or vapour of manganese, or a compound of manganese, or a substance containing manganese.

Relevant legislation

Parkinsonism due to occupational poisoning by manganese (or one of its compounds) or CS_2 is reportable under RIDDOR.

Compression neuropathies

Compression neuropathies may occur in jobs where local pressure, high force, or repetition leads to peripheral nerve entrapment. They include the following:

- *Carpal tunnel syndrome (CTS):* compression of the median nerve within the carpal tunnel at the wrist
- *Cubital tunnel syndrome:* compression of the ulnar nerve at the medial humeral epicondyle or more distally as it goes between the two heads of flexor carpi ulnaris in the forearm
- *Guyon's canal syndrome:* compression of the ulnar nerve at the wrist
- *Radial tunnel syndrome:* compression of the posterior interosseous branch of the radial nerve in the forearm without motor symptoms. Where motor weakness occurs, it is termed posterior interosseous nerve syndrome.

Epidemiology

- CTS is the most common entrapment neuropathy in the upper limb; cubital tunnel syndrome is the second most common
- Radial tunnel syndrome is uncommon
- Twin studies suggest that genetic factors may explain up to half of CTS cases among women
- Prevalence estimates of CTS vary widely, reflecting differing case definitions between studies
- Occupational exposures are only one among a number of risk factors for these conditions.

Clinical features

Carpal tunnel syndrome

- Tingling or burning of the thumb, index, middle fingers, and lateral border of the ring finger
- Pain in the hand and wrist, sometimes spreading up the forearm
- Symptoms often worse at night
- Symptomatic relief by shaking the affected limb in the air—'flick sign'
- Thenar wasting
- ↓ Grip strength.

Cubital tunnel syndrome/Guyon's canal syndrome

- Tingling of the little and ring fingers and medial border of the hand
- ↓ Grip strength.

Radial tunnel syndrome

- May be confused with lateral epicondylitis (tennis elbow)
- Maximal tenderness approximately 4cm below the lateral epicondyle
- Forearm pain without objective weakness
- Pain ↑ by extending the middle finger against resistance.

Causal exposures

- Awkward posture
- High force
- Frequent repetition
- Hand-transmitted vibration.

Individual susceptibility for CTS

- Female gender
- Pregnancy
- Diabetes mellitus
- Obesity
- Hypothyroidism
- Rheumatoid arthritis
- Acromegaly.

Clinical assessment and diagnosis

- A good history is central to the diagnosis of CTS
- *Tinel's test:* pain on percussing the median nerve in the carpal tunnel
- *Phalen's test:* pain reproduced by holding the forearm upright and flexing the wrist for 1min
- Nerve conduction studies may be helpful in confirming the diagnosis
- Neither a negative Tinel's test nor normal nerve conduction studies excludes CTS.

Prognosis

- Following surgery to divide the flexor retinaculum the majority of CTS sufferers will make an excellent recovery
- Time to return to normal work following open or endoscopic CTS surgery is about 7–14 days for sedentary work and 42–70 days for heavy work. Where workplace modifications are available, return to work can be earlier
- Dependent on underlying cause, CTS may develop in the other wrist
- An important differential diagnosis of CTS is hand–arm vibration syndrome (HAVS). Surgery for CTS in a worker with HAVS and symptoms consistent with CTS is unlikely to give complete resolution of CTS symptoms because of digital nerve damage.

Health surveillance

None appropriate.

Medical management

- Clinical care includes physiotherapy, splinting, and surgical decompression
- Workplace interventions should focus on occupational risk factors
- Task redesign may be required because of ↓ grip strength and dexterity; the advice of an ergonomist may be required.

Prevention

- Task rotation and ↑ automation may be indicated
- Consider tool redesign.

Compensation

CTS is prescribed (A12) for Industrial Injuries Disablement Benefit in those who are exposed to hand-transmitted vibration.

Relevant legislation

CTS that is reliably attributable to work is reportable under RIDDOR.

Peripheral neuropathy

Peripheral neuropathies may occur because of occupational exposure to physical agents, neurotoxic chemicals, or zoonoses (e.g. Lyme disease). Physical factors include local pressure leading to compression of a peripheral nerve. Peripheral neuropathy may affect the sensory, motor, or autonomic nerves. A mixed sensory–motor neuropathy is usual, but some agents such as inorganic lead may cause a pure motor neuropathy.

Epidemiology

Most peripheral neuropathy is not due to occupation—common causes of peripheral neuropathy include diabetes mellitus and connective tissue diseases.

Clinical features

Sensory neuropathy

- Altered sensation (paraesthesia) or anaesthesia
- Patient may describe a *glove and stocking* pattern of altered sensation—as if wearing gloves and stockings
- Typically, the feet are affected first; with continued exposure the neuropathy may ascend the legs before affecting the hands and arms
- ↓ Vibration perception
- ↓ Thermal sensation
- ↓ Proprioception
- Loss of reflexes
- *Neuropathic pain:* burning pain (worse at night)
- *Allodynia:* non-painful stimuli (e.g. light touch) are perceived as painful
- *Altered skin appearance:* skin becomes shiny, with loss of hair.

Motor neuropathy

- Muscle wasting
- Paralysis
- Fasciculation
- Cramps.

Autonomic neuropathy

Symptoms depend on affected organ:
- Postural hypotension
- Loss of sweating
- Diarrhoea or constipation
- Incontinence (faecal or urinary).

Causal exposures

- Radiation
- Lead
- Mercury
- Arsenic
- Thallium
- Tellurium (rare)
- Methyl bromide (CH_3Br)

- Acrylamide monomer
- Organic solvents:
  - n-hexane
  - methyl n-butyl ketone
- Organophosphates:
  - tri-orthocresyl phosphate (TOCP)
  - organophosphate insecticides (see 🕮 p. 90, Pesticides; 🕮 p. 298, Organophosphate poisoning).

Clinical assessment and diagnosis

- A good history is important in the diagnosis of occupationally acquired peripheral neuropathy
- Neurological examination
- Nerve conduction studies to confirm the diagnosis
- Electromyography (EMG) to distinguish between muscle and nerve disease
- Nerve biopsy, if taken, may show demyelination, but an axonopathy is more usual in occupational toxic neuropathy. Some agents may cause axonopathy and demyelination.

Prognosis

- After withdrawal from exposure some patients continue to deteriorate for several months
- Over many months recovery generally occurs (assuming the neurons have survived), but may be incomplete.

Health surveillance

Depends on the agent implicated. For lead, see 🕮 p. 434, Inorganic lead.

Medical management

- Substitute a less hazardous agent in the workplace
- Withdraw the worker from further exposure to the neurotoxin.

Compensation

Peripheral neuropathy is a prescribed disease (C29) for Industrial Injuries Disablement Benefit in those exposed to n-hexane or methyl *n*-butyl ketone.

Relevant legislation

- Peripheral neuropathy reliably attributable to work is reportable under RIDDOR in work with n-hexane or methyl n-butyl ketone
- Lyme disease in work involving tick exposure is reportable under RIDDOR
- Poisoning by acrylamide monomer, arsenic, lead, or methyl bromide is reportable under RIDDOR.

Organophosphate poisoning

Organophosphates (OPs) are used widely as insecticides.

Epidemiology

- Most cases of acute OP poisoning occur in developing countries
- A systematic review in 2007[1] estimated that there were ~260 000 deaths/year from pesticide self-poisoning worldwide with OPs accounting for 2/3 of cases in Asia.

Clinical features

Three patterns of illness are associated with OP poisoning.

Acute OP poisoning

Acute poisoning presents with the symptoms of cholinergic toxicity due to inhibition of acetylcholinesterase (AChE), leading to a failure to break down acetylcholine post-synaptically. 'Ageing' of the enzyme may occur, resulting in irreversible inhibition. Main clinical features of OP poisoning;

- Bronchospasm
- Diarrhoea
- Meiosis (constricted pupils)
- Nausea and vomiting
- Lacrimation
- Profuse salivation
- Urinary incontinence.

Other effects include:

- Psychomotor effects: increasing confusion, anxiety, sleep problems
- Cardiac arrhythmia: bradycardia (dizziness, fainting) or tachycardia
- Tremor, muscle fasciculation
- Sweating
- Seizures
- Coma
- Death may occur because of respiratory paralysis or cardiac arrhythmias.

Intermediate syndrome

- Develops ~12–96h after exposure
- Proximal muscle weakness
- Cranial nerve palsies
- Respiratory muscle paralysis
- Death due to respiratory paralysis.

OP-induced delayed neuropathy (OPIDN)

- OPIDN occurs with OPs that inhibit neuropathy target esterase (NTE), e.g. TOCP. Nowadays this is only seen following severe OP poisoning
- Gradual onset over several days after acute OP poisoning
- Paraesthesia
- Distal muscle wasting: feet > hands
- Ataxia
- Spasticity.

❧ Chronic OP poisoning in the absence of previous acute poisoning is a condition that some attribute to exposure to OPs, e.g. in sheep dipping or aviation. The symptoms reported are similar to chronic fatigue syndrome. However, a causal association with OPs remains unproven.

Causal exposures/industries

The main route of exposure is dermal.
- Agriculture:
  - pesticide applicators
  - cotton growers
  - market gardening
  - sheep dippers
  - crop-dusting pilots, pesticide loaders
- Agrochemical manufacture
- Terrorism, chemical warfare (sarin, tabun, VX) (see 📖 p. 829, Chemical weapons).

Clinical assessment and diagnosis

- 5mL of blood in EDTA tube for measurement of both red cell and plasma cholinesterase in suspected poisoning
- Nerve conduction tests in suspected OPIDN.
- ▶ AChE level within the normal range does not exclude poisoning.
- ▶ The emergency treatment of OP poisoning is covered in 📖 p. 802, Organophosphate poisoning.

Prognosis

- *Acute poisoning:* resolves over 3–4 days
- *Intermediate syndrome:* resolves over 14 days
- *OPIDN:* depends on severity. Recovery takes place over 6–12mths, but deficits are lifelong if severe.

Health surveillance

- Pre-exposure red cell and plasma AChE level
- Monthly AChE testing during use of OPs
- Absolute level of AChE is less important than change in level
- Multiple exposures may lead to cumulative depression of cholinesterase levels and presentation with acute poisoning after apparently low-level exposure
- If AChE ↓ 30% from pre-exposure level, examine worker and consider suspension from OP exposure.

Relevant legislation/guidance

- OP poisoning is reportable under RIDDOR
- HSE Biological monitoring of workers exposed to organo-phosphorus pesticides. MS 17. Health and Safety Executive, Sudbury.
- HSE (1999). Reporting incidents of exposure to pesticides and veterinary medicines ℘ http://www.hse.gov.uk/pubns/indg141.pdf

1 Gunnell D, Eddleston M, Phillips MR, Konradsen F (2007). The global distribution of fatal pesticide self-poisoning: Systematic review. *BMC Public Health* **7**, 357.

Hand–arm vibration syndrome

The term 'hand–arm vibration syndrome' has been used to collectively define the disorders thought to be associated with exposure to hand-transmitted vibration.

Clinical features

- *Vibration white finger (VWF)*: episodic finger blanching, usually marble-white (but occasionally cyanotic) and cold-induced. Classically:
  - is sharply demarcated and distal in initial development (only rarely affecting the thumbs)
  - affects the areas most in contact with vibrating parts
  - is associated (during the attack) with numbness/coldness and (in recovery) with parasthesiae and a reactive hyperaemia
- Vibration-induced sensorineural disease (peripheral neuropathy and carpal tunnel syndrome)
- Effects on hand function (weakness of grip, poor manual dexterity) that may have a neuropathic or myopathic origin
- Hand-arm pains, osteoarthritis of the wrist or elbow, specific musculoskeletal disorders of the upper limb and Dupuytren's contracture may also be commoner in workers exposed to hand-transmitted vibration
- Dysfunction of the autonomic nervous system (with protean non-specific symptoms) is a proposed but not a well accepted effect.

Epidemiology

HAVS is common. According to one population survey there are more than 220,000 cases in the UK; while claims assessed among ex-miners from British Coal exceeded 90,000.

Causal exposures and industries

See 📖 p. 10, hand-transmitted vibration.

Clinical assessment and diagnosis

Diagnosis usually rests on a careful clinical history in a worker with symptoms post-dating substantial exposure. Episodic attacks of VWF are seldom witnessed, while crude cold challenge tests lack sensitivity.

- *More complicated procedures exist for specialist legal assessment of HAVS, including:* measurement of finger systolic blood pressure during cooling, skin temperature and skin re-warming rates after cold challenge, thermal aesthesiometry, vibrotactile thresholds and tests of dexterity
- Vascular and sensory effects are normally graded separately, according to two three-point scales proposed in 1986 by an expert Stockholm Workshop (see 📖 p. 768, clinical assessment of HAVS). Some assessors now combine these clinical features with the output from objective tests.

Medical management

There is no well-established and really satisfactory treatment. Most efforts are directed against blanching attacks.

- Conservative measures are often advocated (e.g. the wearing of thermal gloves and warm clothing, avoidance of draughts and exposure to cold, wet, windy conditions), but such advice cannot always be followed in the work situation
- Evidence on efficacy of other forms of treatment is relatively weak; benefits have been claimed from:
  - physical therapy (exercises, compresses, hot packs, paraffin baths, massage, traction, infrared treatment)
  - adrenergic receptor blockers
  - antiplatelet and antithrombotic agents
  - *calcium-channel blockers*—oral nifedipine and diltiazem may offer some promise.

Prognosis
- Until the 1960s VWF was considered irreversible, but more recent studies show vascular symptoms can improve on withdrawal from exposure, albeit slowly, over several years. Workers with advanced disease are less likely to recover
- The neurological effects do not improve with time; stage 3SN disease can be seriously disabling, in terms of impaired hand function, and is the most important avoidable morbidity (the aim should be to prevent progression from early- to late-stage 2SN).

Prevention
See 📖 p. 10, Hand-transmitted vibration.

Health surveillance
- This is required for workers who remain regularly exposed above the EAV A(8) of 2.5m/s^2 despite controls
- The aims are:
  - to aid early detection and counselling/job modification
  - to provide a check of workplace control measures
- The main element is periodic symptom inquiries. Health records need to be maintained.

Compensation
- In the UK, HAVS (A11) is prescribed for Industrial Injuries Benefit in employed earners, provided that it occurs the year round, is extensive, and occurs in a scheduled occupation[1]
- Many other European countries compensate VWF on a similar basis.

Relevant legislation
Employers are required to notify cases to the appropriate enforcing authority (HSE or local authority) under the RIDDOR Regulations.

---

1 Social Security (Industrial Injuries) (Prescribed Diseases) Regulations 1985, Schedule 1: http://www.dwp.gov.uk/docs/a4-3851.pdf

Noise-induced hearing loss

Hearing loss due to occupational noise exposure is, in theory, preventable, but noise-induced hearing loss (NIHL) remains common.

Epidemiology
- Hearing loss affects 2% of adults of working age in Britain
- Prevalence ↑ from 1% among ♂ aged 16–24yrs to 8% among those aged 55–64yrs
- British estimates[1] suggest that 153,000 men and 26,000 women have deafness due to occupational noise exposure.

Clinical features
- Reduced auditory acuity
- Tinnitus
- Increasing social isolation as hearing decreases.

Causal industries
- Quarrying and mining
- Food industry
- Agriculture
- Entertainment industry (pubs, clubs, discos)
- Armed forces and security services
- Construction industry
- Metal working
- Aviation.

Individual susceptibility
Some individuals with 'tender ears' appear to be especially sensitive to the adverse effects of noise exposure. Others, despite significant noise exposure, have apparently normal hearing.

Clinical assessment and diagnosis
Noise exposure history: both occupational and hobby exposures
- DIY
- Music
- Motor sport
- Hunting/target shooting.

Medical history seeking risk factors for hearing loss
- Meningitis
- Congenital infections: rubella, CMV
- Head injury (fracture of base of skull)
- Ototoxic medication including
- Aminoglycosides (e.g. gentamicin):
  - quinine
  - salicylates
  - furosemide
- Ménière's disease (tinnitus, deafness, vertigo)
- Family history of deafness
- Otitis media

- Otosclerosis
- Perforated tympanic membrane.

Examination

- *Examine external ear:* scars (previous surgery)
- Otoscopy:
  - tympanic scars
  - tympanic perforation
  - mastoid surgery
- Tuning fork testing (512 Hz tuning fork):
  - Rinne's test—
  - – air conduction > bone conduction (Rinne positive) in sensorineural loss or normal hearing
  - – bone conduction > air conduction (Rinne negative) in conductive hearing loss (e.g. otosclerosis)
  - *Weber's test*—lateralizes to affected ear in conductive loss
- *Pure tone audiometry:* classical pattern in NIHL is a 4kHz dip with recovery although peak loss can be anywhere between 3 and 6kHz (📖 p. 430, Classification of hearing loss and 📖 p. 432, Patterns of hearing loss)
- Auditory evoked response (AER).

Prognosis

NIHL does not progress after withdrawal from exposure. However, the combination of established NIHL and age-related hearing loss (presbyacusis) means that even after withdrawal from exposure the affected worker's hearing will continue to decline.

Health surveillance

- Pre-employment audiometry (identifies existing losses) (see 📖 p. 764, Screening audiometry)
- Annual testing for first 2yrs of employment
- Three-yearly testing after first 2yrs.

Medical management

NIHL suggests that the hearing conservation programme has not protected worker's hearing. Exclude other causes of hearing loss.

Compensation

NIHL is prescribed (A10) for Industrial Injuries Disablement Benefit for those involved in specified activities. Hearing loss must be at least 50dB in each ear to qualify.

Relevant legislation/guidance

HMSO (2005). *The Control of Noise at Work Regulations.* Stationery Office, London. Available at: ℘ http://www.legislation.gov.uk/uksi/2005/1643/contents/made

---

1 Palmer KT *et al.* (2002). Occupational exposure to noise and the attributable burden of hearing difficulties in Great Britain. *Occup Environ Med* **59**, 634–9.

Psychiatric disorders

Psychoses due to occupational exposures

Epidemiology

Organic psychosis due to occupational exposures is thankfully unusual, but its very rarity means that the diagnosis may be missed. Historically, exposures in certain industries put workers at risk of organic psychoses or psychiatric effects:

- Mirror silvering (mercury)
- Manganese mining
- Cold vulcanization of rubber (CS_2)
- Manufacture of organoleads for leaded petrol.

Clinical features

Manganese madness

A syndrome of hallucinations, nervousness, insomnia, emotional lability, (especially inappropriate laughter), compulsive behavior, and altered libido.

Organolead

Insomnia, anxiety, emotional lability, delusions and mania. If exposure is severe, death due to encephalopathy may occur.

Methylmercury

Depression, emotional lability (including inappropriate laughter), and increased response to stimuli (erethism). Neurological deficits, including coarse tremor, dysarthria, ataxia, visual field losses, and peripheral neuropathy, may co-exist.

Carbon disulphide

Irritability, agitation, hallucinations, and bipolar illness.

Causal exposures/industries

- Organolead (tetraethyl lead, triethyl lead)
- Methylmercury
- *Manganese*: chronic exposure in manganese mining
- Aluminium?
- Tin (triethyl tin, trimethyl tin)
- *Organic solvents*: e.g. in glues, paints, degreasants
  - carbon disulphide (CS_2)
  - *styrene*—boat building
  - *lacquers, varnishes*—furniture making
  - microelectronics industry.

Individual susceptibility

Manganese: adverse effects generally present in susceptible individuals after 6mths exposure. The young appear more susceptible.

Clinical assessment and diagnosis

A history of exposure to any of these agents should alert the treating doctor to the possibility of an organic cause for the patient's illness. Manganese intoxication may present with both psychiatric symptoms and parkinsonian features (see 📖 p. 292, Parkinsonism).

Prognosis

The psychiatric effects of manganese may be reversible if identified early and exposure ceases.

Health surveillance

See 📖 p. 436, Organic lead for details of organic lead surveillance.

Medical management

Withdraw from exposure.

Compensation

CNS toxicity characterized by tremor and neuropsychiatric disease is prescribed (C5(a)) for Industrial Injuries Disablement Benefit in those who have been exposed to mercury for >10yrs.

Relevant legislation

Control of Lead at Work Regulations 2002 Approved Code of Practice.

Stress 1: recognition and assessment

Definition

The emotional and physiological state of disequilibrium that pertains when the perceived demands of life exceed one's perceived ability to cope. It is:

- Not a mental illness
- Not listed in the International Classification of Diseases (ICD) or the Diagnostic and Statistical Manual of Mental Disorders, 4th edition (DSM IV)
- Natural response to range of challenges or life events
- Not necessarily harmful; can improve performance in some situations
- In some individuals may be a risk factor for poor mental ill health.

Epidemiology

- 435,000 people in the UK reported work related stress, anxiety, or depression in 2006/7. See ℬ http://www.hse.gov.uk/statistics/overall/hssh0910.pdf
- 20% of the UK working population 'very' or 'extremely' stressed
- More than 9.3 million working days are lost each year in the UK from work-related mental ill health or 'stress'
- Individual, local, organizational, and cultural factors affect the level of reported stress
- The sharp rise in cases of reported stress contrasts with the relatively minor secular changes in prevalence of mental illness.

Clinical features

Individual symptoms

- Reduced self-confidence
- Feelings of tension and nervousness
- Self-doubt
- Indecisiveness
- Increased irritability
- Fluctuations of mood
- Sleep difficulties
- Poor concentration
- 'Burn-out'

Behavioural changes

- Increased irritability
- Impulsive behaviour
- Social withdrawal
- Less able to relax at home
- Working more than usual
- Increased use of caffeine, cigarettes or alcohol, addictive drugs or other substances

⚠ Remember stress is not an illness and all these symptoms are non-specific

Adjustment disorders

- Mainly anxiety ± depressive symptoms
- Temporal association with an apparent stressor
- Significant impairment of social and occupational functioning is required to establish the diagnosis

Causal exposures/industries

The Management Standards

HSE describes a system to identify risk factors at work (see 📖 p. 134, Organizational psychosocial factors)

- Demand
- Change
- Relationships
- Control
- Role
- Support

Workers in several sectors report higher levels of stress, but that does not mean these sectors are more stressful:
- Secondary school teachers
- HCWs
- Call centre operatives
- Emergency service workers (police in particular).

Sector-specific guidance on risk management is available on the HSE website. ✍ http://www.hse.gov.uk/stress/information.htm

Individual susceptibility

- Previous history of work-related stress
- Co-existing non-work-related stress (e.g. domestic upheavals)
- Previous history of mental health problems
- High alcohol intake
- Excessive personal expectations, Type A personality.

Diagnostic assessment

- *Exclusion of psychiatric disorder:* e.g. major depressive illness, generalized anxiety disorder, obsessive–compulsive disorder (OCD)
- *Identification of potential occupational stressors:* including interpersonal conflict, bullying, harassment, or grievances, by risk assessment
- Identification of non-work stressors
- *Identify current coping strategies:* are they helpful, can they be influenced by individual mentors or training?
- 'Post-traumatic stress disorder' has very specific diagnostic criteria and the term should not be used if these are not met.

Prognosis

- In general, excellent
- Early intervention critical to successful outcome (see 📖 p. 311, Stress 2: interventions/risk controls).

Time off work
- Can be detrimental to recovery of the employee unless the condition interferes significantly with performance at work. As far as possible, with adequate support and adjustments, it is advisable to keep the employee at work
- If time off work is needed, there should be clarity about reason for absence, return to work process, and how progress will be monitored.

Relevant legislation and guidance
- Protection from Harassment Act 1997
- Tackling stress: The Management Standards Approach (1997).
  ℘ http://www.hse.gov.uk/stress/standards/

Stress 2: interventions/risk controls

Primary (preventing stress in the workforce)

See 📖 p. 134, Organizational psychosocial factors, Risk controls.

- Stressor identification and risk assessment
- Attention to job design
- Skills and leadership training at all levels in the organization
- Flexible working as part of work–life balance programme.

Secondary (preventing recurrence or exacerbation in an individual with work-related stress)

- Attentive and compassionate management
- Cognitive behavioural therapy (CBT)
- Change management
- Assertiveness training
- Time management
- Interpersonal skills training.

Interventions for the individual with work-related stress

Psychological support through occupational health (OH) and employee support programme:

- Confidential self-referral service available to all employees
- Access to clinical psychology
- Therapy techniques aimed at problem-solving
- Highly focused individualized approach
- Emphasis on therapeutic benefits of work.

Including round-table discussions

- Involving employee, OH +/– treating psychologist, patient's manager, and HR taking a shared problem-solving approach to deal with stress issues
- Particularly useful if patient is off work and where interpersonal conflict has complicated the situation
- Enabling early agreement on a graduated rehabilitation programme back to work, establishing job definition, hours and days of work, etc.
- Educating managers on nature of stress-related difficulties and ensuring their commitment to the rehabilitation programme, including preparation of the rest of the team for the employee's return from sickness absence.

Further information and guidance

Health and Safety Executive. (1999). *Managing Stress at Work*. HSE, Sudbury.
Health and Safety Executive. (2001). *Tackling work-related stress: a manager's guide to improving and maintaining employee health and wellbeing*. HSE, Sudbury.
Health and Safety Executive. (2004). *Stress Management Standards*. HSE, Sudbury.
Calnan M, Wainwright D (2002) *Work stress: the making of a modern epidemic*. Open University Press, London. Available at: ℘ http://www.hse.gov.uk/stress/index.htm

Post-traumatic stress disorder 1: diagnosis and risk factors

Effects of severe stress

Extremely disturbing events can have marked and sustained emotional effects. Warfare has provided most evidence and it has generated many diagnoses, including Da Costa's syndrome, soldier's heart, and shell shock. The Vietnam War led to post-traumatic stress disorder (PTSD) entering the Diagnostic and Statistical Manual of Mental Disorders (DSM III) (American Psychiatric Association, 1980). The current revision is the DSM-IV (1994 American Psychiatric Association, 1994). The nosology used most frequently in the UK is the ICD-10 (WHO, 1992).[1]

Epidemiology

- *Community samples:* no community-based survey of PTSD has been conducted in the UK and most data derive from the USA. Note the obvious sociocultural differences, including availability of firearms.
  - lifetime prevalence for adult exposure to trauma 3.9–89.6%
  - lifetime PTSD prevalence rates 1.0–11.2%
  - risk of PTSD is greater for ♀ than ♂ (20.4% vs. 8.1%)
  - younger urban populations report higher incidence (up to 30.2% for ♀ and 13% for ♂)
- *Selected samples:*
  - 4% of UK Armed Forces deployed to Iraq and Afghanistan
  - 20% of those who have experienced physical assault.

Diagnosis and assessment (ICD-10 criteria)

- Stressor criterion: victim must have been exposed to a stressful event or situation (either short- or long-lasting) of an exceptionally threatening or catastrophic nature, which is likely to cause pervasive distress in almost anyone.
- *Symptoms:*
  - repetitive, intrusive recollection or re-enactment in memories, daytime imagery or dreams
  - commonly fear and avoidance (i.e. reminders of the event)
  - usually hyperarousal, such as an exaggerated acoustic startle response and hypervigilance.

⚠ Do not use the term PTSD loosely.

Acute, chronic, and delayed PTSD

- The ICD-10 is not very specific: The onset [of PTSD] follows the trauma with a latency, which may range from a few weeks to months (but rarely exceeds 6mths)
- *DSM-IV subclassification:* 1–3mths (acute); >3mths (chronic), and onset after 6mths (delayed)
- Delayed onset is uncommon; delayed reporting is more common.

---

1 http://www.who.int/classifications/icd/en/WHO (1992).

Assessment
- Victims may be reluctant to admit to symptoms for fear of being seen as weak (especially military and emergency service personnel)
- Victims may find it too disturbing to talk about the event
- Insensitive and premature assessment may lead to re-traumatization
- Relatives' observations can be helpful.

In addition to clinical interview and mental state examination, there are standardized psychiatric measures:

- *Clinician Administered Assessment Scale for PTSD (CAPS):* highly structured interview gives a measure of lifetime and current PTSD severity and functional impairment. Regarded as the gold standard
- *Impact of Event Scale–Revised (IES–R):* a 22-item self-report scale, which assesses frequency of the core symptoms; intrusive phenomena (e.g. flashbacks), avoidance, and hyperarousal (not diagnostic measure)
- *Davidson Trauma Scale (DTS):* a 17-item self-report scale that provides a measure of the severity and frequency of each DSM-IV symptom.

Risk factors for PTSD

No single event will cause PTSD in all exposed individuals. Risk factors include the following:
- *Pre-trauma factors:*
  - anxious personality
  - previous and/or familial psychiatric history
  - lower education and sociocultural status
  - genetic predisposition, ↑ concordance in monozygotes
  - female gender, except among the military
  - younger age, especially in males
- Concurrent life stressors
- *Trauma and peritraumatic factors:*
  - severity—generally, there is a dose–response curve
  - *physical injury*—the meaning of an injury is as important as its objective severity
  - (perceived) threat of serious injury or to life (of self and/or others)
  - *dissociation*—depersonalization, derealization
  - extended exposure, such as being taken hostage and being trapped
  - elevated autonomic arousal, especially heart rate.
- *Post-trauma factors:*
  - adverse reactions of others: criticism, rejection, blame
  - 2° life stressors
  - lack of support.

Occupations at risk

Sectors likely to expose employees to work-related trauma.
- Military
- Heavy industry
- Emergency services
- Offshore oil and gas industry
- Construction
- Sea fishing
- Farming.

Post-traumatic stress disorder 2: management

The National Institute for Health and Clinical Excellence (NICE) has published guidelines on the management of PTSD.

- Psychological first aid is a widely agreed paradigm for helping individuals and communities after major calamity, including:
  - attending to basic needs for food, safety, etc.
  - outreach and dissemination of information
  - strengthening community, social, and family structures
  - *psycho-education*—normal reactions and coping methods
  - *triage*—identify those requiring psychiatric care
- *Watchful waiting*:. most individuals do not develop PTSD; thus do not subject all victims to psychiatric treatment or even counselling. Instead, monitor progress and provide treatment for those whose symptoms last ~1mth
- Facilitate peer, family, and community support
- *Critical incident stress debriefing (CISD)*:
  - mandatory debriefs should not be conducted
  - single-session debriefs are neutral or occasionally harmful.

Formal treatments

PTSD mostly occurs in the context of comorbidity, especially depression, anxiety, and alcohol abuse. The NICE guidelines endorse the following treatments:

- *Psychological therapies should be tried first:*
  - trauma-focused cognitive behavioural therapy (TFCBT)
  - eye movement desensitization and reprocessing (EMDR)
- *Pharmacotherapy:*
  - paroxetine and mirtazapine for general use
  - amitriptyline hydrochloride and phenelzine for specialist use
- Medication is appropriate if the patient has not responded to TFCBT or EMDR, or is unwilling and/or unable to undergo such psychotherapy
- Patients should be advised of side effects and discontinuation/ withdrawal symptoms (particularly paroxetine)
- A hypnotic may be used in the short term for sleep problems
- Antidepressants are preferred for chronic sleep difficulties to avoid dependence
- Propranolol and hydrocortisone may have psychoprophylactic properties, but routine use *cannot* be justified.

Prognosis

- Most spontaneous recovery is within the first few weeks
- There may be a re-emergence of symptoms 12mths after the event—the anniversary reaction
- If persistent or recurrent after 12mths, symptoms may run a lengthy chronic course.

PTSD and the law

- *Civil proceedings:* concerns about feigning and exaggeration of PTSD symptoms are common, but evidence suggests that this is not a widespread problem. Symptoms tend not to remit after claim settlement
- *Criminal proceedings:* PTSD can mitigate or explain the conduct of the accused. However, merely suffering from PTSD does not mean that there is any causal connection between the individual's mental state and the alleged offence
- *False vs. genuine claimants:* rigorous assessment is essential and should include:
  - clinical interview
  - standardized measures
  - GP and hospital records
  - information from others (e.g. spouse).

Distinguishing false from genuine symptoms

Genuine claimants display consistent accounts across different settings and at different times. Caution should be exercised when individuals do not describe their symptoms and experiences in spontaneous and lay terms. Pseudo-technical language may suggest coaching. In most genuine cases, descriptions of dramatic events are accompanied by appropriate emotional displays (e.g. distress, disgust, anxiety). Reporting of symptoms (e.g. hallucinations and delusions), rarely associated with PTSD, should raise suspicion, as should the reporting of unremitting symptoms: PTSD is a phasic condition with spells of remission and relapse. Genuine claimants do not tend to be uncooperative or suspicious of the examiner. Most genuine claimants minimize their suffering and distress, and do not blame all their difficulties on PTSD.

Further information

National Institute for Health and Clinical Excellence (2005). *Post-traumatic stress disorder. the management of PTSD in adults and children in primary and secondary care.* Royal College of Psychiatrists, London/British Psychological Society, Leicester. Available at: ℳ http://www.nice.org.uk/CG26

Meze G (2006). Post-traumatic stress disorder and the law. *Psychiatry,* **5**, 243–7.

Klein S, Alexander DA (2009). Epidemiology and presentation of post-traumatic disorders. *Psychiatry,* **8(8)**, 282–7.

Klein S, Alexander DA (2011). The impact of trauma within organisations. In: Tehrani N., ed., *Managing trauma in the workplace,* pp. 117–38. Routledge, Abingdon.

Reproductive disorders

Impaired fertility

Infertility is defined as a failure to conceive after 12mths of attempting to conceive:

- Many factors which can lead to delayed time to pregnancy are not due to reduced fecundity
- Occupational factors which may interfere with reproduction by reducing the opportunity for sexual intercourse include:
  - shift working
  - long working hours
  - prolonged absences from home
- Relatively few occupational exposures have been associated with impaired fertility and usually only in the most exposed. Improved workplace control measures mean that some exposures, such as anaesthetic gases (when used without a scavenging system), are only of historical interest in this regard
- Some have linked environmental oestrogens (PCBs, phthalates, dioxin, etc.) to recent reductions in male sperm counts.

Epidemiology

- Infertility now affects ~15% of couples in developed countries and has almost doubled in the last 20yrs
- The ratio of ♀ to ♂ causes of infertility is approximately 2:1
- One difficulty in identifying occupational risk factors is that only a proportion of workers are seeking to conceive at any given time. Therefore detecting reproductive hazards can be difficult
- As sensitive pregnancy tests have become available, it has become apparent that a significant proportion of conceptions do not lead to successful pregnancy.

Clinical factors

Males

- *Azoospermia:* no detectable spermatozoa
- Low sperm count
- Reduced or absent libido.

Females

- Anovulation
- Reduced or absent libido
- Implantation failure
- Abortion.

Causal exposures

The following have been associated with reduced fecundity in those exposed in an occupational setting. Evidence is usually based on cross-sectional surveys and case-control studies.

- Metals:
  - lead
  - mercury
  - chromium

- *Pesticides:* dibromochloropropane (DBCP), carbaryl
- *Organic solvents:* carbon disulphide, glycol ethers
- Anaesthetic gases
- Sex hormones
- Ionizing and non-ionizing radiation
- Heat stress.

Industries at risk
- Chemical industry
- Lead smelting
- Farming
- Industrial painting.

Clinical assessment and diagnosis
- Reproductive history: establish whether either partner has previously had children to distinguish primary infertility from secondary infertility
- Confirm that the couple are sexually active (shift work, overseas postings, etc.) and that the woman is menstruating
- The occupational history should focus on work with known reproductive hazards, taking into account likely exposure intensity
- It may be difficult to establish whether workplace factors are responsible for delayed conception, although in ♂ an improved sperm count on exposure reduction would support an occupational aetiology
- ♂ Semen analyses should be done on two samples
- ♀ Menstruation suggests ovulation, but check mid-luteal (day 22–26) serum progesterone
- Referral to an infertility clinic for further investigation
- Hysterosalpingogram or diagnostic laparoscopy
- Ultrasound to confirm ovulation may be useful.

Prognosis
Depends on cause. Withdrawal from exposure may allow recovery in some cases.

Health surveillance
None.

Medical management
- Women contemplating pregnancy may seek advice from an OH professional
- Many couples finding difficulty in conceiving will do so within 12mths of presentation without intervention
- Age and family history of early menopause may dictate early investigation
- Assisted reproduction may be necessary in some cases.

Relevant legislation
- HSE (2002). *Control of Lead at Work Regulations*, 3rd edn. *Approved Code of Practice and Guidance*, L132. HSE Books, Sudbury.
- HSE (1999). *Ionizing Radiation Regulations 1999. Approved Code of Practice and Guidance*, L121. HSE Books, Sudbury.

Adverse pregnancy outcomes

Adverse pregnancy outcomes include:
- Spontaneous abortion
- Low birth weight (<2500g)
- Pre-term delivery (<37wks gestation)
- Birth defects.

Epidemiology
- Over half of pregnant women are in paid employment
- 15% of pregnancies end in a spontaneous miscarriage
- 60% of congenital malformations have no identified cause
- Attention has focused on maternal factors, but paternal pre-conceptual exposures may be relevant. Further studies are required
- A large number of studies have examined occupations and occupational exposures and pregnancy outcomes.

Causal exposures
Chemical hazards
- *Metals:*
  - lead
  - mercury
- Organic solvents
- Pesticides?

Physical hazards
- Lifting
- Heavy physical work
- Prolonged standing
- Ionizing radiation
- Heat
- Physical violence.

Biological hazards
Infections:
- Rubella
- Toxoplasma
- *Chlamydia psittaci* (enzootic abortion)
- *Coxiella burnetti* (Q fever)
- Parvovirus B19 (fifth disease).

Industries at risk
Several industries have been associated with adverse pregnancy outcomes but the evidence is inconsistent. Industries implicated include:
- Agriculture
- Healthcare
- Painting
- Printing
- Firefighting

- *Security services (risk of violence):*
  - police
  - prison service.

Health surveillance
None appropriate.

Medical management
The issue of adverse pregnancy outcomes may arise when an employee is pregnant, and the question is asked whether it is safe for her to continue her current role. This is a difficult area as an anxious worker's fears may be realized even where there is no association between her work and adverse pregnancy outcomes. For many work exposures there is insufficient evidence to offer definitive advice regarding the likely risks.

HSE advises against a number of work activities during pregnancy:
- Diving
- Work at pressure
- Lead (Pb) work
- Preparation of cytotoxic drugs.

Evidence-based guidelines on 'Physical and shift work in pregnancy' found consistent evidence for some adverse pregnancy outcomes in relation to prolonged standing, heavy lifting, and prolonged hours (>40h), but the risk was low. On precautionary grounds they advised employers should reduce pregnant workers' exposure to prolonged standing, heavy physical work, and lifting.

Measures to control exposures should be taken for women potentially exposed to ionizing radiation or hazardous chemicals. If adequate control cannot be achieved, the pregnant worker should be allocated alternative duties or, if this is not possible, should be suspended from work. Note that as pregnancy progresses the hazards may change (e.g. ergonomic factors in office workers) and the risk assessment should be kept under regular review (see p. 524, New and expectant mothers and p. 557, Employment law).

Relevant legislation and guidance
- HSE (1999). *Management of Health and Safety at Work Regulations 1999*. Available at: http://www.hse.gov.uk/pubns/books/l21.htm
- HSE (2002). *New and expectant mothers at work*, 2nd edn. HSE Books, Sudbury.
- NHS Plus, Royal College of Physicians, Faculty of Occupational Medicine. (2009). *Physical and shift work in pregnancy: occupational aspects of management. A national guideline*. RCP, London.

Gynaecomastia

- Gynaecomastia is the most common benign breast condition in men
- Breast enlargement may be painless or associated with discomfort
- Galactorrhoea may also occur.

Epidemiology

- The most common causes of gynaecomastia are puberty, obesity, and drugs, including anabolic steroid abuse, and medication for HIV
- Rarely, gynaecomastia in ♂ may be due to breast cancer
- Gynaecomastia is present in up to a third of adolescent ♂.

Clinical features

Gynaecomastia may be bilateral or unilateral.

Causal exposures

- *Gynaecomastia:*
  - female sex hormone manufacture
  - anabolic steroids (bodybuilders)
- *Pseudo-gynaecomastia:*
  - obesity
  - work requiring repetitive force on chest (rare).

Industries at risk

- Pharmaceutical industry. Sex hormone manufacture
- Professional sports especially 'power' sports where misuse of anabolic steroids may be prevalent.

Clinical assessment and diagnosis

Palpable gynaecomastia is common in otherwise healthy males but the palpable breast tissue is generally <5cm in diameter.

Prognosis

Most cases settle with withdrawal from exposure.

Health surveillance

Periodic medical examination is indicated where pharmaceutical workers may be exposed to sex hormones despite workplace control measures.

Medical management

- If occupationally acquired withdraw from exposure
- If gynaecomastia fails to settle following withdrawal from exposure to drugs, surgery may be necessary.

Chapter 15

Haematological disorders

Bone marrow aplasia

Causal exposures/industries

- *Ionizing radiation:* acute (usually accidental) exposure to a dose of ionizing radiation above ~0.2Sv produces marrow hypoplasia/aplasia as a deterministic (dose-related) effect.
  - nuclear industry
  - medical radiography and nuclear medicine
  - industrial radiography
- *Benzene:* chronic exposure above approximately 50ppm produces a range of haematotoxic effects including marrow suppression.
  - rubber and shoe industries
  - plastics production
  - explosives production
  - motor vehicle repair.

Clinical features

Haematopoietic stem cell hypoplasia leads to peripheral blood cytopenias. The clinical features vary according to the severity of stem cell suppression, and the cell lines that are affected (erythrocytes, leucocytes, and platelets), but include combinations of:

- *Anaemia:*
  - fatigue
  - dyspnoea
- Neutropenia/lymphopenia: ↑ incidence of bacterial infections
- *Thrombocytopenia:*
  - petechiae and ecchymoses
  - gingival bleeding
  - ↑ risk of serious bleeds, e.g. renal or GI.

Radiation exposure

- Following acute exposures, the peripheral blood lymphocyte count falls within 24–48h (because of rapid cell death). Other cell lines are not destroyed immediately. Although unable to divide, damaged neutrophils and platelets can survive for up to 2–3wks, and red cells for up to 100 days. Therefore, there is a delay of 1–3wks before pancytopenia develops because of failure of replacement from marrow stem cells
- Treatment for victims of serious exposures is intensive multi-system support, transfusions of red cells and platelets, and management of acute infection with appropriate antibiotics. In severe cases, erythropoietin and colony-stimulating factors (e.g. granulocyte-colony stimulating factor (G-CSF), granulocyte-macrophage colony-stimulating factor (GM-CSF)) are used to facilitate stem cell function. Bone marrow transplantation is possible, but the success rate is very low
- Prognosis depends on the dose:
  - dose of ≥1Sv has a fatality rate of at least 10%; at <1Sv recovery from a nadir in peripheral blood counts at 4–6wks is usual. Normal blood counts re-established 2–3mths after the exposure incident
  - dose of 3–4Sv has a 50% fatality rate at 30 days post-exposure.

Prevention

Prevention is through fastidious regulatory control of exposure, including control of the working environment and work practices, and workplace exposure limits (see 📖 p. 22, Ionizing radiation 4: exposure control; 📖 p. 542, Ionizing Radiation Regulations 1999).

Health surveillance

- *Ionizing radiation:* 'classified' workers under the Ionizing Radiation Regulations (personal exposure >6mSv or 3/10ths of any other exposure limit) require baseline medical assessment plus periodic reviews (usually annual) of dosimetry results and sickness absence records (see 📖 p. 542, Ionizing Radiation Regulations).
- *Benzene:* appropriate health surveillance for benzene would be a health record, as described in the COSHH Regulations. Routine periodic screening of haematological indices is probably inappropriate with adequate risk controls.

Relevant legislation

- The following are reportable under RIDDOR:
  - blood dyscrasias that are attributable to ionizing radiation
  - benzene poisoning
- The approved dosimetry service should be informed in the event of a radiation accident.

Anaemia

Anaemia can be caused by a number of (acute or chronic) occupational exposures, and by a number of different mechanisms including impairment of haem synthesis, marrow suppression, and haemolysis. Marrow suppression and haemolysis are covered separately in 📖 p. 324, Bone marrow aplasia and 📖 p. 329, Haemolysis.

Impaired haemoglobin synthesis

Exposures/industries

- Lead is the classical occupational exposure associated with impaired haemoglobin synthesis
- Industries:
  - lead smelting
  - battery manufacture
  - demolition
  - glass making.

Mechanism

Lead, through its high affinity for binding to sulphydryl groups, inhibits important enzymes in the haem synthesis pathway (see Fig. 15.1).

Clinical features

- Mild anaemia, which may play little or no part in the fatigue that is commonly associated with lead poisoning
- Associated features include palsies due to peripheral neuropathy, arthralgia, and (rarely) confusion due to encephalopathy
- The characteristic finding on investigation is basophilic stippling of erythrocytes on a peripheral blood film
- Blood lead levels >80 g/dL.

Prevention

Prevention is by substitution and exposure control (see 📖 p. 538, Control of Lead at Work Regulations 2002).

Health surveillance

Statutory surveillance includes baseline and periodic screening (intervals are specified by individual susceptibility (e.g. women and young people) and exposure level). For health surveillance for inorganic lead, see 📖 p. 434, Inorganic lead.

Compensation

Anaemia with haemoglobin ≤9g/dL and a blood film showing punctate basophilia is prescribed (C1(a)) for Industrial Injuries Disablement Benefit in those who are exposed to lead.

Relevant legislation

Lead poisoning is reportable under RIDDOR.

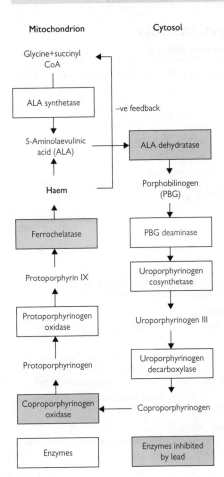

Fig. 15.1 Haem synthesis.

Methaemoglobinaemia

Methaemoglobinaemia arises when the ferrous iron moiety in haem is oxidized into the ferric form. The consequence is a decreased oxygen-carrying capacity of haemoglobin. It can be caused by a number of acute occupational exposures.

Causative agents

- Ferricyanide
- Bivalent copper
- Chromates
- Chlorates
- Quinones
- Dyes with a high oxidation–reduction potential
- Nitrite, often used as a preservative, is one of the most common methaemoglobin-forming agents
- Aniline dye derivatives.

Clinical features

- Cyanosis
- Dyspnoea
- Headaches and dizziness
- Muscle weakness
- Peripheral blood film shows mild anaemia and erythrocyte abnormalities (Heinz bodies and punctate polychromasia).

Individual susceptibility

Hereditary methaemoglobin reductase deficiency.

Treatment

Acute treatment is with methylene blue (methylthioninium chloride), administered by slow IV infusion. Management of acute poisoning is covered in detail on 🕮 p. 808, Methaemoglobinaemia (acute treatment).

⚠ Methylthioninium chloride may cause brisk haemolysis in those with glucose-6-phosphate dehydrogenase (G6PD) deficiency.

Relevant legislation

Acute poisoning with a nitro-, chloro-, or amino- derivative of benzene is reportable under RIDDOR .

Haemolysis

Haemolysis is the process of premature red blood cell destruction.

Clinical features and treatment

- *Acute:*
  - haemoglobinuria, jaundice, and abdominal pain
  - methaemoglobinaemia and methaemoglobinuria
  - complicated by anuric renal failure
  - exchange blood transfusion is life-saving in severe cases
- *Chronic:*
  - anaemia
  - reticulocytosis due to ↑ red cell production is the hallmark of haemolysis.

Exposures

- *Arsine gas:*
  - *industries*—micro-electronics industry (semiconductor manufacture), metal smelting, plating, galvanizing, and soldering
  - effects occur with acute poisoning at exposures >3ppm for several hours, or >20ppm for <1h
  - chronic low-level exposure can cause anaemia with mild ↑ bilirubin
  - diagnosis is based on history of exposure and ↑ urinary arsenic
- *Naphthalene:*
  - *industries*—manufacture of plastics and dyestuffs, mothballs, biocides for the wood industry
  - can precipitate haemolysis in individuals with G6PD deficiency
- *Rare occupational exposures associated with haemolysis include:*
  - potassium chlorate
  - pyrogallic acid
  - stibine gas (rare accidental exposure).

Prevention

Prevention is by substitution and exposure control.

Haematological malignancies

Leukaemias

Exposures

Two exposures have a well-established association with leukaemia.

- *Ionizing radiation:* leukaemogenesis is a late stochastic effect of ionizing radiation (no dose threshold for the effect). The following have been noted in excess among radiation workers:
  - acute myeloid leukaemia (AML)
  - acute lymphoblastic leukaemia (ALL)
  - chronic myeloid leukaemia (CML)
- *Benzene:* AML.

Other exposures (or job/industry used as a marker, but with the exact exposure unclear) have been implicated with small increases in leukaemia risk. Most studies have been small, and in many there is a problem with confounding by benzene exposure.

- *Possible ↑ leukaemia risk:*
  - 1,3-butadiene
  - ethylene oxide.

Clinical features

Presents with a combination of anaemia, bleeding, and infection.

Compensation

Acute non-lymphatic leukaemia is prescribed (C7) for Industrial Injuries Disablement Benefit in those who are exposed to benzene.

Lymphoproliferative disorders

Exposures

- *Ionizing radiation:* the following have been noted in excess among radiation workers, and are late stochastic effects:
  - multiple myeloma
  - non-Hodgkin's lymphoma.

Clinical features

Presents with anaemia or local mass.

Treatment and prognosis of haematological malignancies

Treatment is complex and beyond the scope of this book. However, the usual approach includes chemotherapy regimes +/− radiotherapy +/− bone marrow transplant. The prognosis for treated acute leukaemias has improved significantly in the past 10yrs.

Prevention

Prevention is through exposure control. See 📖 p. 542, Ionizing Radiation Regulations 1999.

Medically unexplained occupational disorders

Post-conflict illness in military personnel

In the aftermath of every major conflict over the past century, some returning personnel have complained of ill health. Some have symptoms of physical origin, others psychiatric disorder including post-traumatic stress disorder (PTSD). However, there is a third group characterized by vague and non-specific symptoms, for which (despite extensive investigation) no cause is found. Different names have been ascribed to this third group, including Agent Orange syndrome and Gulf War illness. These syndromes share many common features. There are also similarities with other medically unexplained symptoms, including chronic fatigue syndrome, multiple chemical sensitivity syndrome and neurasthenia. All groups have definitive health care needs.

Gulf War illness

Gulf War illness affecting the veterans of the Arabian Gulf Conflict of 1991 has been extensively investigated, with over $300 million of funds from the US and UK governments. Despite extensive study into possible links with vaccinations, depleted uranium exposure, oil well fires, and exposure to pesticides or other chemical agents; no definitive cause has been found. However, the following lessons have emerged, and are pertinent to other post-deployment conditions:

- In general, military populations are healthier than civilians—the healthy warrior effect
- More than a decade after deployment, some Gulf War veterans still suffer ill health. However, the same symptoms and groupings are seen in non-Gulf Veterans control groups. There appears to be no unique Gulf War syndrome
- Although the condition persists two decades after exposure and many veterans remain ill, in general they appear to be getting better gradually
- Gulf veterans are 2 or 3 times more likely to have symptom complexes including multi-focal pain, fatigue, cognitive or memory problems, and psychological distress. Most of these individuals do not meet criteria for established psychiatric illness
- Although there is a raised incidence of PTSD in Gulf War veterans as in other conflicts, it is not elevated to the degree that could explain the overall increase in ill health. Common symptoms include tiredness, headaches, lack of concentration, memory loss, and numbness
- Thorough medical examination including physical, physiological, and psychological testing have revealed no major abnormalities
- Reported health is worse the lower the rank and after retirement
- In contrast to control groups, Gulf War veterans report more of every hazard and recall exposure to more of these over time. Those who are in good health recall fewer exposures
- There is no evidence of an excess of malignancy, birth defects, or increased mortality.

Management of post-conflict illness

- A detailed history, examination, and investigation should be taken to detect the presence of any organic disease. Treatment should be appropriate to the findings, and any patient with a known clinical disorder should be referred promptly to the appropriate 2° care consultant
- Enquiries about stress-related symptoms should be handled with care, to avoid any impression that the individual's symptoms are being dismissed as psychological. However, it is worthwhile exploring patient's beliefs with regard to the aetiology of the condition
- If necessary, a follow-up appointment should be used to:
  - discuss investigation results
  - give the physician an opportunity to review the literature
  - counsel the patient over any subjective concerns

Within the UK, the Medical Assessment Programme provides a specialized referral facility for investigation of any deployment-related problems in respect of the 1991 and 2003 Gulf Conflicts and subsequent operations in Iraq and Afghanistan. All regular and reserve service men, servicewomen, and MOD civilians who participated in these operations are eligible to attend.

Further information and guidance

Ministry of Defence. *Medical Assessment Programme*: Available at: ℛ http://www.mod.uk/
DefenceInternet/FactSheets/PersonnelFactsheets/MedicalAssessmentProgramme.htm
Post-conflict illness in military personnel

Sick building syndrome

The term sick building syndrome (SBS) was first used in the mid-1980s to describe an ill-defined collection of symptoms that are typically reported by workers located in the same building. Despite substantial research, the cause of the syndrome has not been fully explained.

Epidemiology
- More common in women
- More common at lower end of the organizational hierarchy.

Reported symptoms
Usually mild, but can lead to significant impairment of performance:
- Headache
- Fatigue
- Dizziness
- Nausea
- Eye soreness and dryness
- Upper respiratory tract (nose, throat) symptoms
- Skin rash/redness
- Generalized pruritis
- ↑ Rate of respiratory infections.

Possible causative factors
Many causal factors have been proposed. Among the factors listed here, some have been associated with SBS in epidemiological studies. Most have a plausible link to some of the common symptoms, but none have been proven to be the cause of the syndrome at low-level exposure.

Physical and environmental factors
- *Humidity:* either excessively high (encouraging mould formation), or excessively low (leading to drying of the mucous membranes)
- Excessively high temperature
- *Air conditioning:* associated with microbial contamination, exotoxins produced by contaminating organisms, biocides
- Poor lighting
- Nuisance dusts.

Chemicals
- Formaldehyde is ubiquitous in office environments due to 'off-gasping' from furniture, carpet adhesive and other fixtures made of particle board
- *Volatile organic compounds (VOCs):* many are known irritants at high exposure levels. Some have low odour thresholds, thus contributing to the perception of poor air quality (irrespective of actual health effects)
- Nitrogen dioxide
- *Cigarette smoke:* passive smoking may have been a factor in the past, but smoking in public buildings is no longer permissible by law in the UK.

Bio-aerosols

Airborne particles comprising or contaminated with bacteria, fungi, or mites.

Psychosocial factors

- Low control over work
- Insufficient or excessive demands
- Low job satisfaction
- Poor support.

The syndrome is likely to have a multifactorial aetiology with contributions from more than one of the factors listed here. Mechanisms are unclear, but might include allergic (immune-mediated) or non-allergic (non-specific inflammatory or directly toxic) reactions.

Management

- Optimize physical environment
  - attention to standards of lighting, temperature, humidity
  - allow adequate personal space to work
  - regular cleaning to minimize nuisance dust
- Address known risk factors for stress (see 📖 p. 134, Organizational psychosocial factors):
  - promote good industrial relations and communication
  - increase control—demand ratio where possible
- Investigate specific issues, e.g. odours.

Further information and guidance

HSE (1995). *How to Deal with sick building syndrome*, HSG132. HSE, Sudbury.

Karoshi: death from overwork

The concept of '*karoshi*' or death from overwork originates in Japan and refers to sudden death in workers believed to have been caused by very long working hours. There is limited research evidence to support this belief, at least in those suffering acute myocardial infarction (MI).

The family of a worker whose death has been accepted by the Worker's Compensation Bureau (part of Japan's Ministry of Labour) as being due to karoshi is eligible for compensation. These deaths may be due to a number of conditions as listed here.

Karoshi is not a concept widely recognized in the West. However, there are overlaps between the beliefs that sudden death may be due to over-work and the increasing body of research that suggests a link between work demands and cardiovascular mortality.

Epidemiology

Japan's Ministry of Labour compensates about 20–60 deaths from *karoshi* each year. Some authors estimate that up to 10,000 deaths in the 20–59-yr-old age group may be due to *karoshi*. Robust estimates of incidence are lacking. Two Japanese case-control studies have shown increased odds ratios for acute MI in workers working >11h/day or >60h/wk, respectively.

Causes of death

- Subarachnoid haemorrhage
- Cerebral infarction
- Cerebral haemorrhage
- Heart failure
- Myocardial infarction.

Relevant legislation

In an effort to prevent Karoshi, the Japanese government issued guidance in 2002 that employees should not work more than 45h overtime per month.

Section 3

Occupational health practice

Operational issues

General principles of occupational health services

Aims

Occupational medicine is preventative medicine practiced in the workplace; promoting health and fostering wellness within the workforce. Although services must be reactive to unforeseen problems, the aim is to proactively prevent work-related ill-health wherever possible.

OH is concerned with the interaction between work and health, and is concerned with the health and welfare of four (overlapping) groups:

- The workforce as a group or population
- *Individual* workers or prospective employees
- The employer's customers or clients (product or service safety)
- The local population (environmental issues).

▶ The population perspective is central to understanding OH practice.

Status of occupational health advice

In health and safety law, the ultimate responsibility for protecting the health and welfare of employees and the public rests with the employer. Managers may choose whether to take and how to implement OH advice. Therefore, rather than *instructing* the employer, the OH professional seeks to *influence* key decision-makers (management and trade unions) regarding health and safety issues. This is best achieved by seeking 'buy-in' from the top of the organization downwards. The approach will be most effective if the OH professional is well respected by all parties.

🖋 OH professionals should remain impartial (preserving good relationships even if managers ignore advice), but should ensure that the responsibility for accepting risk has been taken at an appropriately high level in the organization.

> ### Impartiality
>
> OH professionals advise *both* employee(s) and the employer. This fundamental difference between occupational medicine and other specialties, in which the health professional is primarily responsible for providing care, is often misunderstood. In an environment where employer, employees, and their representatives may be adversarial, the OH professional must remain impartial to be effective.
>
> ▶ This dual responsibility must be understood and respected by all. Its importance in effective OH practice cannot be overemphasized.

Trade unions

- Trade union support can be crucial in developing OH services
- Trade unions have a legitimate interest in their members' welfare
- The principles of medical confidentiality hold whether or not a union representative is involved in issues concerning individual members.

Traditionally, OH activities have been classified under two main headings:
- The effect of work on health
- The effect of health on work.

The effect of work on health: preventing work-related illness

▶ Occupational illness is prevented by a proactive cycle of risk assessment, risk reduction, and review.

- The classical occupational diseases of the industrial age are becoming less common in the developed world due to improved health and safety practice, increasing mechanization, and reduced exposure to hazards. However, these diseases remain in developing countries
- Work-related illnesses still represent a significant proportion of sickness absence in developed countries
- The workplace is often one of a number of interacting factors. Many musculoskeletal or mental health problems are multifactorial and may have a substantial psychosocial component. It can be difficult to disentangle the contribution of workplace and non-work factors
- Occupational demands may aggravate or sustain existing illness.

The effect of health on work: fitness for work

▶ The important underpinning principle is that most work is 'healthy', and is a positive aspect of overall health and wellbeing.

Advice about fitness for work can be divided conceptually as follows.

Context
- Pre-employment or pre-placement
- *Intra-employment:*
  - following an episode of ill health
  - following a change to job or exposures
  - following/during long term sickness absence
  - to inform the management of short term sickness absence.

Timescale
- *Short-term:* temporary rehabilitation programme with the finite endpoint of achieving a return to *normal* work (hours and tasks)
- *Long-term: permanent adjustments* to hours or tasks

Context and timescale are not mutually exclusive, but are important dimensions in a conceptual framework for fitness for work. This framework emphasizes the important hierarchy of advice, the broad aims of which are:
- To maximize the potential for maintaining gainful employment
- To minimize any health risks to the employee
- To view ill-health retirement as a last resort after all options for maintaining employment have been explored.

The occupational health team

Roles and overlap

- Occupational health is a multidisciplinary specialty
- Each professional group has different expertise and may have different approaches influenced by background and training
- However, there is substantial commonality of experience between professional groups, and potential overlap between roles
- There is no fixed or typical configuration for an OH team.
- Provided role definitions are clear, and overlaps and gaps are managed sensitively, any model can be successful.

The occupational health team

The make-up of the OH team is likely to be influenced by;
- The model of service delivery (see 🔲 p. 344, Models of OH services)
- The service requirements of client organization(s)
- Prevailing hazards, and the knowledge to assess them
- Availability of manpower in the various OH professions
- Local, historical or industry precedent
- Individual personalities and attributes
- Legal requirements
- The prevailing OH market.

Occupational physician

- In a small OH service the occupational physician (OHP) may act as part-time medical support to a nurse-led service
- In other services the OHP may be the service manager, with overall responsibility for occupational health and (sometimes) safety
- An OHP's clinical work includes sickness absence assessments, health surveillance, and giving advice on adjustments and rehabilitation for ill, injured, or disabled workers
- In the broader clinical context, workplace visits, advice on risk management, attendance at safety meetings, meetings with managers and trade unions, and policy writing may be undertaken
- Some OHPs have a managerial function. They manage an occupational health service, provide clinical governance, set overall strategy, policy, and procedures for others to follow. This role may cross national boundaries and involve the management of health professionals from varying backgrounds
- All OHPs should have input to audit and quality assurance.

Occupational health nurse

- Occupational health nurses (OHNs) may work in isolation in single-handed services, or within a larger occupational health service
- Trained OHNs, often called occupational health advisers (OHAs), may be involved in an extended range of professional activities, including pre-employment and sickness absence assessments, health surveillance

(e.g. screening audiometry, skin inspections), drug and alcohol screening, workplace monitoring (e.g. noise, chemicals), advisory role in risk management, health promotion, counselling, and first aid training
- Some OHNs have a managerial role and lead OH departments
- Some nurses in industry may have had no formal training in occupational health and can be professionally isolated. Such nurses may fill a limited role, providing a treatment room service, immunizations, and basic (non-statutory) health and pre-employment screening.

Occupational hygienist
- Specialists in assessing and monitoring workplace exposures. Their role is described in detail in 📖 p. 598, Role and function of occupational hygienists
- Relatively few organizations employ a full-time occupational hygienist
- Many hygienists work in consultancies or as independent contractors.

Counsellor
- Many occupational health services provide in-house staff counselling or have contracted with an employee assistance programme (EAP) that employs counsellors and occupational psychologists
- While some counsellors may be qualified psychologists, this is not an occupational requirement.

Ergonomist
- Specializes in fitting the task to the human, and may be involved in assessing and advising on processes, products, and work systems
- Ideally an ergonomist's advice should be sought at the process or plant design stage in an effort to design out potential problems
- As with occupational hygienists, ergonomists are generally found in large organizations or working on a consultancy basis.

Case manager
- Case managers are employed by some OH services to manage sickness absence. They can come from various health professional backgrounds
- Their role focuses on identifying and overcoming, in conjunction with the ill or injured employee and their employer, barriers to an early, sustained return to work
- Their approach to sickness absence follows a non-medical model.

Other occupational health team members
- Health and safety adviser or manager
- Fire safety specialist
- Manual handling adviser
- Physical therapist
- Health promotion specialist
- Business/finance adviser
- Clerical support (including specialist medical secretaries)
- Screening technicians (non-medically qualified)
- Environment specialists.

Models of OH services

Models of OH provision are influenced by many changing factors, including legal requirements, the economy, the nature of risks, and political priorities (see Table 17.1).

- In 1998 the World Health Organization defined the purpose of OH services as the 'promotion of health and maintenance of workability'
- In Scotland the Healthy Working Lives and Health Works strategies 'maximize the functional capacity (physical, mental, social, spiritual) of the working age population', and help the unemployed find work
- In The Netherlands, the political initiative to move the responsibility for sickness absence benefits to employers led to models that were focused on the evaluation and control of sickness absence. In the UK it has been proposed that employers should commission a functional capacity assessment after 4wks sickness absence.

Factors that influence occupational health service models

- *Legal:* in some countries the model may be prescribed (e.g. Germany, Italy, Austria)
- *Risks and type of industry:* treatment and primary care will be included in countries or locations with poor access to health services. The services that are needed by an office population in a large city will require a different skill mix to those in a steel foundry or shipyard
- *Priorities of the service purchaser:* these may include health surveillance, sickness absence control and rehabilitation, and workplace health promotion depending on priorities and profitability
- *Resources and manpower availability:* in some countries the discipline of OH nursing is not well developed or recognized; in others there may be few OH physicians
- *Extent of multidisciplinary working:* services may be monodisciplinary (e.g. a doctor or nurse working independently) or, more commonly, two disciplines, when a team consists of OH physicians and nurses
- *Internal services:* OH professionals are employed by the enterprise
- *External contracted services:* the enterprise buys in services from a commercial provider or local group service
- *Government-funded services:* for small and medium enterprises, self-employed, home workers, micro-enterprises, the unemployed, e.g. in Scotland.

Rationale for occupational health models

OH delivery requires a multidisciplinary effort, with close co-operation between health and safety, occupational hygiene, ergonomics or other specialists, human resources, and legal advisers. Where the OH professionals are not an integral part of a multidisciplinary team, it will be necessary to liaise with these other disciplines. OH services, which do not have close operational links with other professionals, are more likely to undertake inappropriate health checks and health surveillance. Much OH provision is determined by the perceptions of the enterprise or

Table 17.1 Advantages and disadvantages of the different models

Model	Advantages	Disadvantages
Single OHP or OHN	Autonomy	Difficult to maintain clinical competence and establish clinical governance
OHP and OHN	Team work Appropriate use of resources	May do more health examinations than necessary Issues about adequacy of the risk assessment process
In-house OH service	Understanding of the organization's needs Knowledge of other members of the extended OH team	Can become institutionalized and inward looking; loss of independence (actual or perceived)
Group OH service: providing services to a number of enterprises	May have critical mass of resource and experience of different sectors More likely to have quality assurance processes if in a contracting situation with large commercial enterprises	May experience shareholder pressure for profit maximization, which can distort advice given to organizations May not be multidisciplinary, and have blind spots in provision
Multidisciplinary service	Potentially the best model, if well integrated and there is good teamwork Should be able to give the most appropriate advice to a client organization, i.e. advice not subject to the bias of a dominant professional group	Difficult for SMEs, micro-enterprises, and home workers to access such services unless provided within the public sector

employing organization. An organization that has financial problems is more likely to focus on the control of sickness absence, while a profitable organization (with low absence) may invest more in health improvement.

Current and future developments

Recent years have seen the decline of large within-company models and a growth of alternative models including contracted-in services. Many countries have strategies to address the lack of access to competent OH advice for many workers and employers in the SME sector (<250 employees). Across the world, OH services for this sector are very variable, and are generally inadequate. This has led to parallel developments in the countries of the UK. In Scotland the Healthy Working Lives service provides free Occupational health, safety and rehabilitation telephone advice to the employed and unemployed, access to a workplace visit and advice, and third-level access to OH advice.

One of the most highly developed models of OH provision is in Finland, which has a network of regional centres and high levels of coverage of the workforce.

Managing occupational health records 1: electronic record systems and security

Electronic records

Managing occupational health records 1: electronic record systems and security

Electronic records

Most occupational health services are now computerized. Their security is critical to the continued success of the OH service.

- Although IT security can be viewed in the narrow sense of hardware theft, protecting data is arguably more important
- Just as access to written OH records should be restricted, so data on an IT system must be protected. This is particularly important where the OH service uses an organization-wide IT system
- Medical information is deemed to be especially sensitive data by the Data Protection Act 1998, and particular care is required to protect it
- Staff should be trained on information security and how to report any security breaches
- Data security should be audited and any breaches or suspected breaches of security investigated
- Where management reports are e-mailed these should be encrypted (this is NHS policy) and sent in portable document format (pdf) to reduce the likelihood of the report being altered without the originator's permission.

Physical security

- Threats to the physical security of computer hardware may arise from theft, fire, flood, power surges, or accidental damage
- All IT hardware (monitors, printers, CPUs) should be security marked and kept on an asset register
- An uninterruptible power supply should be provided
- Building security should be at a level proportionate to local crime levels and the likely impact of loss of IT equipment on the OH service. This may include the provision of alarm systems, floodlighting, security patrols, etc.
- Particular care is needed when dealing with portable data storage devices such as data pens, detachable hard drives, lap tops and note books, or personal digital assistant (PDAs). Such devices are easily lost or stolen, and their contents should be protected using high quality encryption.

Software security

- Loss, corruption, theft, or unauthorized access to data should be guarded against
- Data should be backed up to a remote server on a daily basis, or saved on a detachable hard drive and stored in a fireproof safe. Small operations may be able to use CDs or other IT storage media to back up files. Ideally, these should be stored in a separate building
- Data back-ups should be checked for integrity, in case the back-up data is itself corrupt

- All data should be password protected and the passwords should be regularly updated
- Passwords should not be written down, nor should computer user names or passwords be shared
- All computers should be locked when not in use
- Computer users should log off any network application after use. This is especially important where the computer is shared with others
- Computer monitor privacy screen filters should be used to keep confidential data secure and prevent others viewing the screen's contents, e.g. clinic appointment lists
- Networked IT systems should have varying access levels, defined by operational need
- IT systems should provide an audit trail to identify unauthorized access, or attempts to access sensitive OH data. (Often the greatest threat to data security comes from within an organization)
- IT support staff, whether in-house or contracted to an OH department, should be asked to sign a confidentiality agreement
- Increasingly, smart cards (an identification card which carries an integrated computer circuit capable of holding personal data), are being employed to record health and safety data. Such cards require several layers of security to restrict access to data and to prevent unauthorized changes to existing electronic records
- Systems that allow remote working via the Internet should employon the highest possible security.

⚠ E-mail systems, where used for medical communications, should be secure and encrypted. Beware of similar e-mail addresses lest the wrong person receives the e-mail.

Computer viruses
- All IT systems should employ virus protection software to prevent computer viruses from compromising system operations
- Virus software must be kept up to date
- IT systems that connect to the Internet are especially vulnerable to infection with computer viruses, and this can lead to service loss for extended periods
- Unauthorized use or installation of pirated software may compromise IT security by introducing viruses, and should be forbidden.

IT policy
It is advisable for OH departments to have a written IT policy that covers the use of computer technology. This should cover the security issues outlined here as well as access to and use of stored data.

Managing occupational health records 2: security, transfer, and archiving of records

There are both legal and ethical issues around the security, transfer, and archiving of medical records. The General Medical Council (GMC), the Faculty of Occupational Medicine, the British Medical Association (BMA), and the Department of Health have all issued guidance on confidentiality. Concerns around confidentiality are a recurring issue in occupational medicine. OH professionals need to be aware of the many ways in which confidentiality may be compromised.

Security of occupational health records

- All contacts between an employee and an OH service should be recorded in the employee's OH record
- The medical records should be securely stored in a lockable cabinet or room or on a secure IT system
- Access to OH records should be restricted to OH staff
- All OH staff should sign a confidentiality agreement
- It is unethical to allow access to OH records to non-OH staff, such as personnel managers.

Transfer of occupational health records

- Companies may outsource OH services, change OH provider, or go out of business. Independent occupational physicians may retire or change jobs. In all these cases, OH records will need to be transferred to an individual or organization that is in a position to maintain them for the appropriate period (this may be 50yrs after the last entry in the records in some cases, e.g. ionizing radiation records)
- The Faculty of Occupational Medicine publication *Guidance on Ethics for Occupational Physicians* provides guidance on the transfer of OH records
- When it is proposed that OH records are to be transferred, employees should be informed and given the opportunity to request that their OH notes be archived, rather than transferred
- Where an organization closes, it may be appropriate to issue the OH records to the individual or (with their consent) their GP. In some situations, statutory records may be offered to the HSE for retention (again with the employee's consent).

Archiving

- Employees leave, are dismissed, or retire, and over time the number of inactive OH records held by an OH service will increase. Inactive files occupy valuable storage space. They can make it difficult for administration staff to locate current OH notes. As a result, all OH services need to have in place a standard operating procedure for archiving OH records
- Archives may be held on or off site, but it is important that archiving medical records does not compromise medical confidentiality

- Readily accessible records detailing the location of all archived notes should be maintained. The location of records should be tracked to avoid the loss or misfiling of records
- OH notes may need to be abstracted at a later date from an archive for a number of reasons, e.g. legal action, audit, or re-employment.

Relevant legislation and guidance

- GMC. *Confidentiality 2009: Disclosing information for insurance, employment and similar purposes.* Available at: ℰ http://www.gmc-uk. org/Confidentiality_disclosing_info_insurance_2009.pdf_27493823.pdf
- Faculty of Occupational Medicine (2006). *Guidance on Ethics for Occupational Physicians,* 6th edn. FOM, London.
- Revision to articles 3.37–3.40 of Guidance on Ethics for Occupational Physicians. Available at: ℰ http://www.fom.ac.uk/wp-content/ uploads/m_gmcconf_ethicsrev1.pdf
- British Medical Association. *Confidentiality and disclosure of health information toolkit.* Available at: ℰ http://bma.org.uk/practical-support-at-work/ethics/confidentiality-tool-kit
- Department of Health. (2003). *Confidentiality: NHS Code of Practice.* Available at: ℰ http://www.dh.gov.uk/en/Publicationsandstatistics/ Publications/PublicationsPolicyAndGuidance/DH_4069253

Quality and audit in occupational health practice 1: general principles

OH practice is naturally embedded within enterprises, or is supplied under contract. It faces scrutiny by purchasers, users, and enforcing authorities, who all wish to see evidence of compliance with standards. Standards can be derived from a number of sources, such as:

- The purchaser of services (e.g. contract specifications)
- The professional body (e.g. good OH practice guidelines)
- The statutory enforcing authority (e.g. standards for legal compliance).

Organizations strive constantly to improve the efficiency of their operation and also that of their suppliers of services. OH professionals must be able to show benefit, constantly seek to justify and improve what they do, and demonstrate the use of evidence-based best practice guidelines.

Quality

Definitions

- 'The degree and standard of excellence'
- 'Fitness for a purpose' (Juran).[1]

Customer-driven quality

This is a useful approach which ensures that the OH service meets the needs of its customers. It first requires that the customers are defined. There are many who could be considered as customers or stakeholders, and they all have different (real or perceived) needs:

- Service purchaser
- Patients or clients
- Legislative bodies
- Trade unions
- Other health care professionals
- Insurance companies
- Pension fund trustees.

The aim is to build a complex provider–client relationship, through which the needs of the many stakeholders can be addressed. This should not be an entirely reactive process. Many of the stakeholders and customers of OH services may be ignorant of the range of services available, and each will have a different perspective. The art of OH service practice is to meet the needs of the individual client (or patient), while at the same time taking into account the needs of the organization in which they work. To be successful, the OH professional must engage in a continuing educational dialogue with the various stakeholders of the service.

Quality improvement

Excellence in OH practice is not an endpoint, but is a continually moving target. Therefore, the pursuit of excellence requires continuous improvement. Juran suggested that up to 40% of all activity involved correcting

---

1 Joseph Juran—early proponent of benchmarking and quality costing.

iindividual or system failures. Quality principles provide a mechanism for continual improvement, which requires:
- Awareness of the need for improvement
- A willingness to improve
- A product or service
- Measurements.

Quality assurance

Quality assurance encompasses all the planned and systematic activities needed to demonstrate that the OH service is meeting all its defined standards and customer requirements. It includes processes:
- To eliminate faults
- Maintain consistent performance.

Audit

The systematic evaluation of the quality and effectiveness of OH service is a professional obligation. Audit is the process of observing the practice and comparing it against a defined standard. It may also be a high-level process used to undertake a needs assessment of an organization or review of an OH service.
- How many of your employees are sick?
- Who gets sick and why are they sick?
- How many accidents occur and what are the causes?
- Why do they retire?
- What do your people die from?
- What do you do?
- Do you have a mission statement?
- Do you have goals?
- Do you have specific objectives for this year?

Audit can be of the structure of an OH service, its processes, or its outcomes. An audit will compare practice against the standard as a means of establishing whether the standard is met or, if not, informing the need for change in either the standard or the practice—the audit cycle (see Fig. 17.1). Audit is an essential part of professional practice and is the tool that monitors and supports quality assurance and quality improvement.

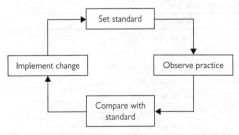

Fig. 17.1 The audit cycle.

Quality and audit in occupational health practice 2: systems and tools

Quality systems

A quality system requires that the OH service:
- Defines its processes
- Ensures that all staff know and understand these
- Ensures that the processes meet the needs of the customer
- Reviews standards and procedures regularly
- Improves continuously
- Audits all the above regularly.

Measurements

Measurements are important in OH practice. However, many organizations and individuals collect data of little relevance to health improvement, such as the numbers of people seen and other activity analysis. The data that any occupational health service or OH professional should strive to gather are given in Table 17.2. Outcomes are always more important than process measurements.

An effective OHS will be able to demonstrate positive change in some or all of the following:
- Attitudes, knowledge, or behaviour
- Health status or self-rated health
- Morbidity
- Mortality
- Occupational health process and practice
- Effects on work organizations

External quality standards

Internationally recognized quality systems have developed to support the assessment and maintenance of quality in industry. Many organizations routinely require that their suppliers of services operate a quality system, including external audit of their service.

Table 17.2 Data collection in OH

Outcome	Source
Morbidity	Sickness absence by location, occupation, function
Mortality	In service, pensioners
Occupational disease	Sickness absence by cause
Accidents and incidents	Reported accident statistics
Health	Health survey data
Stress	Employee Assistance Programme data
Litigation	Analysis of compensation claims

Examples of external standards can be:
- *Specific:* e.g. the UK Faculty of Occupational Medicine 'Safe Effective Quality of Occupational Health Services (SEQOHS)' and a German system for occupational physician practice
- *Generic:* industry standards, such as ISO 9000 and the European Foundation For Quality Management. These require that holders of their quality standard systematically apply all the principles described here.

Holders of a recognized quality standard will usually have some advantage with potential customers over their competitors who do not. However, possession of a quality standard will not necessarily ensure that the OH service is delivering the highest standards of occupational health and safety or clinical service—that still requires professional excellence and leadership.

National audit

A series of national audits of NHS occupational health services have been carried out by the Health and Work Development Unit of the Royal College of Physicians (see 📖 p. 355, Further information). This work is also relevant to other (non-NHS) providers. At present audit cycles are ongoing in two topics, screening for depression in employees who are on long term sickness absence, and the management of back pain.

Clinical governance

Clinical governance is defined as management's responsibility for clinical performance. This requires that managers of a service ensure that the highest standards of clinical performance are maintained by the consistent development and use of:
- Evidence-based guidelines (or consensus-based in the absence of evidence)
- Appropriate and ethical standard procedures
- Continuing professional development of clinical staff
- Peer review of clinical performance
- Monitoring of clinical outcomes.

Quality systems can encompass clinical governance processes. However, if the system does not apply to individual clinical performance, then separate procedures for ensuring clinical governance must be in place for the individual clinician or larger clinical team.

Further information

Royal College of Physicians. *Back pain management* audit. Available at: ℘ http://www.rcplondon. ac.uk/resources/back-pain-management-audit

Royal College of Physicians. *Depression screening audit.* Available at: ℘ http://www.rcplondon. ac.uk/resources/depression-screening-audit-2008

Royal College of Physicians. *Depression detection and management of staff on long term sickness audit.* Available at: ℘ http://www.rcplondon.ac.uk/resources/depression-detection-and-management-staff-long-term-sickness-audit

Guidelines in occupational health

Guidelines, governance, and quality

The development of clinical guidelines relevant to occupational health practice plays an important role in driving up clinical quality in the specialty. Guidelines form the link between scientific evidence (or professional consensus in the absence of clear evidence) and agreed standards for care. Clinical standards provide a framework for assuring:

- Consistency of practice across OH providers
- A baseline for continuous improvement in quality through repeated cycles of audit (see 🔲 p. 352, Quality and audit).

Guideline development methodology

A number of guideline methodologies have been used to develop guidelines in clinical medicine. These vary in complexity, but they have a common aim to use standardized tools to:

- Categorize evidence (peer reviewed papers, reviews or gray literature) in terms of quality
- Summarize the implications for practice.

▶ One of the main problems with the application of these methods in occupational health is the relative lack of evidence from experimental studies (randomized controlled trials being the gold standard). Much of the published research in OH is based on cross-sectional surveys and observational studies, so will score at the lower end of the quality rating scales within most of the agreed methodologies in Table 17.3. Nevertheless, a consistency of approach enables the reasonable justification of guidelines and the practice standards that are derived from them.

Table 17.3 Common methods for guideline development

Method	Web reference
Scottish Intercollegiate Guideline Network (SIGN)	ℛ http://www.sign.ac.uk/
National Clinical Guideline Centre (NCGC)	ℛ http://www.ncgc.ac.uk/Guidelines/Methodology/
Grading of Recommendations Assessment, Development and Evaluation (GRADE)	ℛ http://www.gradeworkinggroup.org/index.htm

Guideline development groups

The most important points to note when setting up a guideline development groups (GDG) are:

- Ensure all relevant stakeholders are included:
  - professional groups from OH practice (including a representative from a primary care background if relevant)
  - experts in the particular field (e.g. dermatology or microbiology)
  - users of a service (employers, employees or their representatives)

- patient representatives (patients who have personal experience of the condition in question)
- enforcing or regulatory agencies (HSE, Department of Health (DH)).
- Training will be required if GDG members will be appraising evidence
- Consider contracting out the systematic review and/or evidence appraisal to an experienced research unit
- A clear dissemination and implementation plan for any output is essential from early in the process
- The budget for a guideline should be split; 50% for development and 50% for dissemination and implementation.

Sources of occupational health guidance

The main sources of guidelines that are relevant for OH practice are outlined in Table 17.4.

Table 17.4 Main sources of guidelines that are relevant for OH practice

Source	Web reference
British Occupational Health Research Foundation (BOHRF)	http://www.bohrf.org.uk
Cochrane collaboration: Occupational Health and Safety Review Group	http://osh.cochrane.org/
Health and Work Development Unit (HWDU)	http://www.nhsplus.nhs.uk
National Institute for Health and Clinical Excellence (NICE)	http://www.nice.org.uk
NHS Plus	http://www.nhsplus.nhs.uk
Various other bodies including	
- Department of Health	http://www.dh.gov.uk
- NHS Employers	http://www.nhsemployers.org
- Health Protection Agency	http://www.hpa.org.uk
- Health and Safety Executive	http://www.hse.gov.uk

Further information

Although not specific for OH, the following are useful general evidence-based resources.

NHS (2011). *NHS Evidence*. Available at: http://www.evidence.nhs.uk/nhs-evidence-content

NICE (2012). NICE clinical pathways section. Available at: http://pathways.nice.org.uk/

- patient interviews with patients who have potential experience of the condition in question
- enhancing or developing a clear (HSE) step by step of Health Outcomes
- consulting with an opinion (NICE) methods, judge expert and evidence
  - OHA or implications out the systematic review and its evidence supporting to an appropriate research literature
- A clear classification and categorization plan for the output is reached from each step in the process
- The budget to a guideline should be with further development and budget requirements and implementation

Sources of occupational health guidance

The main sources of guidelines relating to the provision of practice are given in Table 17.3.

Table 17.3 Main sources of guidelines that are relevant for OH practice

Source	Main reference
British Occupational Health Research Foundation (BOHRF)	
Concawe	
Faculty of Occupational Medicine	
Health and Safety Executive (HSE)	
National Institute for Health and Care Excellence (NICE)	
SIGN	
World Health Organization (WHO)	
Cochrane	
NHS Plus	
Other	

Further information

Although much of the information that may be developed, the reproductivity over-researched from ref...

Ethics

Ethical principles in clinical occupational health practice

Role

The occupational physician is a registered medical practitioner (RMP) whose professional practice is concerned with the interaction between health and work. Their role is outlined on p. 386. Although general ethical principles (which would be appropriate for all doctors) apply in occupational medicine, special features of their role generate additional ethical issues for occupational physicians. These include:

- Having a largely preventive or rehabilitative role, rather than the traditional therapeutic role of the GP, or hospital specialist
- A need to maintain an objective and impartial position between various groups, including the employee (and his/her GP), the employer, and others (other employees, unions, local population).

Principles

The underlying ethical principles of medical practice (bioethics) for all RMPs, including occupational physicians are as follows:

- *Respect for autonomy:* competent adults may make decisions for themselves irrespective of the consequences to themselves
- Non-malfeasance: the doctor shall do no harm
- *Beneficence:* the doctor shall do good and act in the best interests of the patient
- *Justice:* how rights and responsibilities are equitably and fairly distributed (Distributive Justice).

In the UK and Europe respect for autonomy is the predominant principle. These ethical principles are further specified by ethical rules such as truthfulness, respect for privacy, fidelity, and confidentiality. These principles place active, relevant responsibilities on occupational physicians, which must be implemented even if not specifically required by law, rules or contract.

Rules

Occupational physicians are bound by 'the duties of a doctor' and *Good Medical Practice*, published by the GMC.[1] The Faculty of Occupational Medicine (FOM) has produced a specific version *Good Occupational Medical Practice*[2] that has been agreed with the GMC and comprehensively sets out professional practice. Occupational physicians are required, *inter alia*, to do the following:
Revalidate in accordance with the requirements of the GMC:

- Audit their work and demonstrate improvements in practice
- Evidence-based working must be at the heart of their activities
- Seek the views of their customers and clients and incorporate them

---

1 GMC. Regulating doctors, ensuring good medical practice. Available at: ℅ http://www.gmc-uk.org/index.asp

2. Faculty of Occupational Medicine (2010). *Good Occupational Medical Practice*. FOM, London.

- Have an effective complaints procedure in place
- Ensure appropriate arrangements for clinical governance in their work
- Support specialist training.

Ethical guidance

United Kingdom

- Faculty of Occupational Medicine (2006). *Guidance on Ethics for Occupational Physicians* (6th edn) FOM, London. ISBN 1860162800. It is recognized by the GMC as an authoritative source of guidance and is used by other occupational health professionals and lay people. 7th edition likely in 2012.
- British Medical Association (2003). *Medical Ethics Today*, 2nd edn. BMJ Books, London. Ethical guidance for all doctors is also published in the UK by the British Medical Association. 3rd edition likely to be published in February 2012.
- Nursing and Midwifery Council (2008). *Code of Professional Practice*. NMC, London. Available at: ℘ http://www.nmc-uk.org/Nurses-and-midwives/The-code/. Other health care professionals publish ethical guidance, such as the Nursing and Midwifery Council and the Royal College of Nursing.
- Royal College of Nursing (2005) *Confidentiality*. RCN, London. Available at: ℘ http://www.rcn.org.uk/publications/pdf/confidentiality.pdf
- Other non-health-care professionals, such as the Institute of Occupational Safety and Health, also produce ethical guidance.

International

- International Commission on Occupational Health (2000). *International Code of Ethics for Occupational Health Professionals*. ICOH, Singapore. The International Commission on Occupational Health (ICOH) publishes guidance that is recognized worldwide. The International Labour Office of the World Health Organization produces wide-ranging guidance for all those working in the field of health and safety.

Confidentiality, consent, and communication

General principles

The principles of communication in OH are different from normal doctor–patient relationship. Explain this to clients when first referred.

- The OH physician is impartial and aims to give objective advice to both employer and employee
- Personal information is kept confidential. Information is only disclosed if justified and then only with the employee's consent
- Any disclosure is the minimum required for the purpose, even if wider consent is available.

Legal requirements

In addition to the ethical requirement, confidentiality is ensured by:

- Data Protection Act 1998 (see ▢ p. 578, Data Protection Act 1998)
- Human Rights Act 1998
- Common law
- Access to Medical Reports Act 1988. This gives additional rights to individuals where an OH professional requests medical information from a doctor who has provided the individual with clinical care. This is covered more fully on ▢ p. 580, Access to Medical Reports Act 1988.

▶ Breaches of confidentiality may lead to action in the courts, by the GMC, or by the Information Commissioner.

Consent

In the setting of OH practice, consent may be required for any interaction with the client, including but limited to:

- Preventative or therapeutic interventions (e.g. immunizations)
- Assessment of risk to the employee or others (e.g. drug screening, assessment of immunity to infectious diseases)
- Health surveillance and biological monitoring
- Disclosure of confidential information held by the OH department
- Acquisition of confidential information by the OH department.

For consent to be ethically valid, it must be freely given by a competent individual who knows:

- What action is proposed (including the content of proposed disclosure of information)
- By whom
- To whom
- The benefits and adverse consequences of giving/withholding consent.

Consent may be:

- *Given explicitly:* either in writing or orally, and recorded in the contemporaneous medical record
- *Implied:* only used in obvious circumstances, such as a patient offering his/her arm for the taking of a previously explained blood specimen. Consent is freely given if no external pressure is put on the individual to agree or decline a particular course of action

- The fact that there are consequences to a particular decision does not render the consent ethically invalid
- The fact that an individual has to agree to an examination in order to gain a particular benefit (gain a pilot's license or obtain an ill-health retirement pension) does not invalidate the consent.

Consent is valid only for the purpose for which it was given. It may be withdrawn at any stage at which the change has practical effect (consent to disclosure cannot be withdrawn after disclosure has occurred).

Withholding consent

For assessment or treatment

If consent for risk assessment, health screening, or interventions is with-held, the consequences must be explained to the individual and recorded in the OH record. These will depend on the situation, but might include refusal to give health clearance for particular activities or jobs. The consequences of refusal to participate in screening programmes should be agreed in advance with employees' representatives.

Disclosing confidential information without consent

Rarely, confidential information may be disclosed without consent. Some examples include:

- Over-riding public interest (avoiding serious harm to third parties)
- Statutory requirement (terrorism, notifiable disease, GMC, road traffic accident, Driver and Vehicle Licensing Agency (DVLA))
- By order of a court.

However, occupational physicians who disclose information without consent may be required to justify their decisions. It is prudent to seek advice from senior colleagues, medical defence insurer, or lawyers before taking such action. Individuals must be informed about what information will be disclosed and to whom, and the possible consequences.

Communicating the output from OH assessments

It is essential that the individual is informed of the content of any reports that are generated by the OH department, and agree to their release. This applies even if the report does not contain sensitive or confidential medical information. A copy of the report should be offered to the individual, and their right of access to it should be explained clearly.

Further information

GMC guidance on confidentiality

GMC (2009). *Confidentiality: guidance for doctors*. Available at: ℘ http://www.gmc-uk.org/static/documents/content/Confidentiality_0910.pdf

GMC. Confidentiality: disclosing information for insurance, employment and similar purposes. Available at: ℘ http://www.gmc-uk.org/Confidentiality_disclosing_info_insurance_2009.pdf_27493823.pdfFaculty of Occupational Medicine (2006). *Guidance on Ethics for Occupational Physicians*, 6th edn. FOM, London.

Ethics in business and medico-legal work

Business ethics

Globalization has increased diversity in the workplace and companies increasingly operate their own ethical codes and values. Doctors should follow sound principles of business ethics where these do not conflict with their duties as a doctor.

- Occupational physicians remain as registered medical practitioners and are subject to the rules of the national medical regulator, the GMC in the UK; the lack of a therapeutic relationship in many activities does not absolve doctors working in business of their biomedical ethical responsibilities
- Occupational physicians have a duty to promote health and wellbeing in the workplace regardless of geography
- Commercial pressures can impact on occupational physicians, but do not justify breaches of ethical or legal rules
- Occupational physicians must not contract for work outside their own or their organization's competence
- Competitors must not be denigrated, and information gleaned by OH staff through their work should not be used for personal advantage
- Care must be taken that contracts or agreements for services do not contain unethical provisions such as a requirement to release confidential medical information to the employer
- When services are being transferred, the occupational health and safety of client organizations and their workforces must take primacy over commercial considerations.

Medico-legal work

Occupational physicians may be required to give evidence:

- As a factual witness, e.g. on some aspect of OH procedure or their personal input in a case. A factual witness does not give an opinion, just a statement of the facts or events as they occurred.
- As an Expert witness. An Expert witness gives an educated or expert opinion on a question e.g. the relationship between a workplace exposure and a particular health effect:
  - the expert witness is responsible to the court, not to the party who has funded the report.
  - independence and expert knowledge are paramount
  - never stray outside your area of expertise
  - expect to be challenged on your views; be prepared to produce evidence to justify your position.
- Legal report writing and giving evidence in court requires particular skills; ensure you have the appropriate training. The Expert witness Institute provides training programmes for doctors (🕮 http://www.ewi.org.uk).

Policies

Writing a policy

The purpose of any policy is to set out how an organization plans to conduct that aspect of its business in compliance with relevant legislation and current best practice. Behind the organizational policy may lie one or more operational procedures/protocols which document how the policy will be delivered. Well written, up to date, OH policies and procedures are one element of good clinical governance (see Fig. 19.1).

▶ To be effective, these policies must have support at the highest level of the organization.

A comprehensive policy sets out organizational intention, and explicit arrangements (who does what, and when) with respect to the management of any given organizational risk.

An effective policy should
- Define the purpose of the policy
- Define responsibilities from the top of the organization down the management tree
- Identify a director or senior manager responsible for that policy
- Describe the responsibilities of managers and supervisors
- Describe the responsibilities of employees
- Describe the responsibilities of other parties where relevant, e.g.
  - Occupational Health and Wellbeing service
  - Human Resources
  - Health and Safety Department
  - Training and Education Department
- Describe arrangements for:
  - monitoring and review of the policy
  - monitoring of the effectiveness of the policy
- Allocate appropriate resources
- Ensure the organization has access to competent advice
- Set a date for policy review.

Relevant legislation and guidance
- HSE (1997). *Successful health and safety management*, HSG65. HSE Books, Sudbury.
- TSO (2003). Chapter 37. In: *Health and safety at work, etc. Act 1974*. TSO, Norwich.
- HSE (2003). Management of Health and Safety at Work Regulations 1999. Approved Code of Practice and Guidance, 2nd edn, L21. HSE Books, Sudbury.

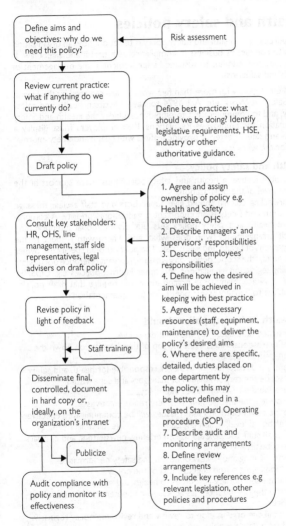

Fig. 19.1 Flow chart showing the key steps in drafting a policy.

Health and safety policies

The purpose of a health and safety policy is to set out how an organization plans to conduct its business in compliance with health and safety law. It expresses commitment to sustained improvement in the management of health and safety risk.

▶ All employers with more than five workers are required by the Health and Safety at Work etc. Act 1974 to have a written health and safety policy, and to communicate it to employees. Under the Health and Safety Information for Employees Regulations 1989 employers must display a health and safety poster or provide leaflets with health and safety information for the workers.

Health and safety policy

▶ To be effective, a health and safety policy must have support at the highest level of the organization.

The prevailing culture should give supervisors and staff a clear message that health and safety is an important organizational priority. A comprehensive health and safety policy sets out organizational intention, and explicit arrangements (who does what, and when) with respect to the management of health and safety risk. The policy should specify the owner of the policy, the scope, definitions/glossary, relevant reference documents including legislation, regulations and other internal policies e.g. COSHH, First Aid, Noise. Many large organizations will require that draft policies are subject to Equality assessment prior to implementation.

A health and safety policy should

- Be signed (and dated) by the chief executive
- Define responsibilities from the top of the organization down the management tree
- Identify a director/senior manager responsible for health and safety
- Describe the responsibilities of managers and supervisors
- Describe the responsibilities of employees
- Encourage the involvement of safety representatives
- Define how health and safety issues will be communicated effectively
  - at board level: health and safety on the agenda of all meetings
  - to all staff: toolbox talks/team briefing, newsletters, and circulars
- Describe arrangements for:
  - monitoring and review of health and safety performance
  - monitoring of the effectiveness of the policy
- Allocate appropriate resources to health and safety
- Ensure the organization has access to competent health and safety advice
- Commit the organization to review and revise the policy regularly, and set a date for policy review.

Principles of health and safety management: 'five steps'

The Health and Safety Executive describe five steps[1] to effective health and safety management.

1. Produce a health and safety policy

2. Develop a safety culture through control, competence, cooperation, and communication
- *Control:*
  - senior managers should lead by example
  - a senior manager should chair the health and safety committee
  - allocate and communicate health and safety responsibilities
  - company organizational chart
  - clear job descriptions
  - allocate appropriate resources (time, staff, finance)
  - identify especially hazardous tasks or jobs, and ensure that these workers receive appropriate additional training
  - monitor health and safety performance against agreed standards
- *Competence:*
  - recruit and train competent staff
  - provide or obtain specialist advice where required
- *Co-operation:*
  - work with safety representatives and trade unions
  - liaise with contractors to manage health and safety
  - consult with staff on health and safety issues
- *Communication:*
  - provide information, instruction, and training to staff, including short-term or agency workers
  - make health and safety a priority issue.

3. Planning and standard setting

4. Measure health and safety performance

5. Review and revise health and safety policy

Relevant legislation and guidance
- HSE (1997). *Successful health and safety management*, HSG65. HSE Books, Sudbury.
- TSO (2003). *Health and safety at work etc. Act 1974*, Chapter 37. TSO, Norwich.
- HSE (2003). Management of Health and Safety at Work Regulations 1999. Approved Code of Practice and Guidance, 2nd edn, L21. HSE Books, Sudbury.

Information from HSE
- HSE *Health and safety made simple: the basics for your business.* Available at: ℘ http://www.hse.gov.uk/simple-health-safety/write.htm
- HSE Do you have any information on how to compile a health and safety policy? Available at: ℘ http://www.hse.gov.uk/contact/faqs/policy.htm

Sickness absence policies

All employers should have a written policy, agreed between management and staff representatives, describing how the organization will manage absence attributed to sickness.

▶ Well-managed organizations record and monitor sickness absence and act on it at all levels—individual workers, departments, and work sites.

Purpose

To inform employees and managers about how the organization manages sickness absence.

Main requirements

The sickness absence policy should:
- Give a working definition of sickness absence
- Describe the arrangements for recording and analysing absence rates in the organization (see 🕮 p. 402, Sickness absence: general principles).
- Define the roles and responsibilities of senior managers, line manager, human resources (HR) advisers, occupational health service (OHS), and the employee in absence management
- Outline employees' rights to sick pay. Discretionary sick pay (not statutory sick pay (SSP)) may be withdrawn if the employer has information that the employee could do some work, but does not return to work despite appropriate adjustments (check employee's contract allows this)
- Enable the employer to seek a medical report with the employee's consent if there is no OH service
- Describe the practical arrangements to support 'return to work':
  - rehabilitation plans should be mutually agreed between employee and employer, including any temporary adjustments to duties or hours of work
  - pay arrangements during 'phasing-in' periods should be explicit
  - monitoring and review of rehabilitation programmes should be planned in advance
- Define training in sickness absence management for managers.

Managers' roles

Senior managers

Overall responsibility for absence management strategy, ensuring fair and consistent implementation.

Line managers

Day-to-day absence management is a fundamental part of a line manager's role. The line manager should:
- Monitor their team's attendance records, compare with absence levels in other teams/departments, and manage individual cases proactively
- Maintain contact with those employees on sickness absence and consider any work modifications/adjustments suggested by health professional in Fit Notes to hasten employee rehabilitation

- Hold a brief informal *return to work interview* with all employees following *any* sickness absence. This is a supportive fact-finding approach separate from any disciplinary process in poor attenders
- Refer to the OHS for medical input. Late referral to OH is associated with a poor prognosis for return to work. Therefore, early referral, within 4–6 weeks after absence begins, should be encouraged. Ideally a referral form or letter should include:
  - employee's details
  - job description
  - sickness absence record for last 12mths (causes and duration)
  - workplace adjustments/modifications already in place
  - specific queries to be addressed
  - confirmation that employee has given informed consent to referral.

Role of the human resources team

HR representatives have special expertise in managing absence. Their primary role is to advise managers on the correct and equitable implementation of absence policies and associated procedures. They play an important part in helping to resolve disputes or poor relationships bet-ween employee(s) and managers. HR representatives can be valuable in overcoming barriers to implementation of OH advice.

Role of the occupational health service

The OH professional aims to ensure that for all absence referrals:
- medical reasons for absence are assessed fully, whilst protecting the confidentiality of sensitive information
- both employer and employee receive impartial objective advice
- advice about adjustments to work are justifiable and appropriate.

Employees' responsibilities

Clarify employees' responsibilities in the event of sickness absence.
- When to inform the employer if they are ill
- Whom to inform—usually their line manager
- Requirement to maintain contact while off sick
- When to provide a self-certificate (SC2)
- When to provide a doctor's Statement of Fitness for Work.

Further information

HSE (2004). *Managing sickness absence and return to work. An employers' and managers' guide*, HSG249. HSE Books, Sudbury. Available at: ℘ http://www.cipd.co.uk/default.cipd. See absence management section.

Fit for work: the complete guide to managing sickness absence and rehabilitation. ISBN 1903461715.

National Institute for Health and Clinical Excellence. (2012). *Management of long-term sickness and incapacity for work*, PH19. NICE. Available at: ℘ http://guidance.nice.org.uk/PH19

Wellness/wellbeing policies

Purpose

Workplace wellbeing aims to take a holistic approach to wellness at work by preventing occupational illness and accidents while enhancing wellbeing in the workplace, but also addressing the physical and social factors that influence health such as:

- Poor nutrition
- Lack of exercise
- Work/home conflicts.

There are clear economic benefits for those employers achieving effective health promoting workplaces. These include reduced sickness absence rates, improved morale, and a better public image.

▶ The National Institute for Health and Clinical Excellence (NICE) has produced evidence-based guidance for employers including;
- Promoting physical activity in the workplace (PH 13)
- Workplace interventions to promote smoking cessation (PH5)
- Promoting mental wellbeing at work (PH22).

Workplace wellness/wellbeing

There are several aspects to a workplace wellness programme including physical, social and health initiatives.

A healthy physical environment

- Enhance the physical environment with better lighting, noise abatement, and action to reduce the risks of violence to staff
- *Develop a Travel Plan:*
  - encourage walking or cycling to encourage (provide bike lockers, shower facilities)
  - allow home working
  - encourage the use of stairs
  - promote walking to meetings nearby
- Organize lunch time walking groups, allow exercise groups to use rooms for yoga or aerobics, and offer discounted membership to gyms
- Participation in national or corporate challenges to increase physical activity among employees
- Workplace smoking controls including developing a Smoking policy

A healthy social environment

- Promote an open organizational culture
- Meet stress/mental health policy
- Employee assistance programme (EAP) or a staff counselling service
- Family friendly work policies e.g.
  - Home working
  - Flexi-time

• Staff 'climate' surveys to assess employee satisfaction

Health initiatives

• Health education for example on; safe drinking; time management; maintaining a healthy work-life balance
• Smoking cessation clinics
• Offering healthy eating options in the staff canteen and fruit as a snack
• Promote exercise/weight management
• Executive health checks.

Workplace wellbeing in the UK

The UK government's white paper *Choosing Health* has highlighted priority areas for lifestyle change in the interests of improving the public health. Key areas include healthy eating, stopping smoking, sensible alcohol drinking, and exercise. The importance of OH professionals in promoting healthy behaviours within the workplace is explicit in the document.

• The Healthy Workplace Initiative (HWI) is sponsored by the Department of Health and HSE and aims to promote workplace health in England and Wales.
• A similar initiative in Scotland is called Healthy Working Lives.

Main requirements

• To be successful a workplace wellness policy must involve all workers
• The policy must have the active support of senior managers
• The organizational culture should encourage employee participation
• The draft policy should be discussed and agreed by a working group of managers and staff before being circulated to staff for comment and feedback
• The final policy should commit the organization to integrating workplace wellbeing into its management systems
• The policy should affirm that all wellness initiatives are to be project managed and so require a needs analysis, priority setting, project implementation, continuous monitoring, and audit
• HR policies should reflect the wellbeing objective by embracing wellness issues, e.g. encouraging work–life balance
• The wellness policy should include the provision of a fully integrated occupational health and safety service.

Further information

🔊 European Network for Workplace Health Promotion (ENWHP) http://www.enwhp.org
Creating a Healthy Workplace. A Guide for Occupational Safety and Health Professionals and Employers. Faculty of Occupational Medicine and Faculty of Public Health Medicine, London, 2006.
NICE (2012). *Promoting physical activity in the workplace.* Available at: 🔊 http://www.nice.org.uk/PH13
NICE (2012). *Workplace interventions to promote smoking cessation.* Available at: 🔊 http://www.nice.org.uk/PH5
NICE (2012). *Promoting mental wellbeing at work.* Available at: 🔊 http://guidance.nice.org.uk/PH22
HSE Management Standards for work related stress. Available at: 🔊 http://www.hse.gov.uk/stress/

Immunization policies

Immunizations are commonly carried out by OH departments:
- To protect workers against vaccine preventable occupational infections
- To protect patients/colleagues (in health care setting) against infection
- For employees who are required to travel abroad.

Occupational health department policies

If immunization programmes are offered, a written immunization policy should be developed. As a minimum the policy should outline:
- The list of immunizations that are given
- The broad indications for immunization including staff groups who will normally be immunized and others according to a risk assessment
- Who will give immunizations, and arrangements for their training
- Arrangements for record keeping/advising worker of vaccination status
  - Arrangements for storage and disposal of vaccines
  - include arrangements for monitoring and recording of the cold chain, e.g. refrigerator temperatures
  - safeguards to protect expensive vaccines in the event of refrigerator power failure.
- Arrangements for recalls (e.g. for scheduled doses and boosters)
- Arrangements for reporting adverse events related to immunization
  - report to in-house adverse event monitoring system
  - report to Committee on Safety of Medicines (CSM) via 'yellow card' scheme (reports can be made electronically to Medicines and Healthcare Products Regulatory Agency (MHRA)).
- Arrangements for communication of fitness for work/necessary restrictions in light of outcome of immunization to the employer
- Arrangements for those who decline immunization or fail to attend
- Arrangements for monitoring including audit of immunization policy.

Vaccination procedures

These are usually outlined in a separate document or as an appendix to the main immunization policy. Checklists should include:
- Gaining and recording employees' consent
- Protocol for the safe administration of vaccines
- Recording immunizations in OH records, and communicating information to GPs (with employee's consent)
- Management of adverse events including anaphylaxis (see 🕮 p. 814, Management of anaphylaxis).

Patient group directions (PGDs)

OH nurses usually carry out immunizations under generic instruction from OH physicians. By law (Statutory Instrument 2000 No. 1917) vaccines that are given in this way must be the subject of written PGDs.

The legal definition of a PGD is:
a written instruction for the supply and/or administration of a licensed medicine (or medicines) in an identified clinical situation, signed by a doctor or dentist and a pharmacist.

- PGDs should be developed by:
  - a senior OH physician
  - a senior OH nurse
  - a senior pharmacist
  - the clinical governance lead
  - as a matter of good practice, local drugs and therapeutics committees and area prescribing committees should also be involved
- Each vaccine should have a separate PGD, which should include:
  - name of the body to which the PGD applies
  - dates of commencement and expiry of PGD
  - description of vaccine
  - class of registered health professionals who may administer vaccine
  - signature of a doctor and a pharmacist
  - signature by appropriate health organization
  - indications for vaccine
  - patients who should be excluded
  - description of circumstances when advice should be sought
  - dose, route, and schedule of administration
  - potential adverse reactions and actions to be taken
  - records to be kept for audit purposes.

Minimum training requirements

OH nurses who are giving immunizations must receive appropriate training. A set of national standards, defined by the Health Protection Agency, outline the basic training requirements including:

- Professional qualifications
- Specified training content, duration of baseline training and frequency of updates, post-training assessment
- Access to national immunization policies
- Inclusion of training in formal audit of immunization programmes
- Content of training for trainers.

Further information and guidance

Department of Health (2007). *Immunization against infectious disease—'The Green Book'.* Available at: ℘ http://www.dh.gov.uk/en/Publicationsandstatistics/Publications/PublicationsPolicyAndGuidance/DH_079917

Nursing and Midwifery Council (2008). *Standards for Medicines Management.* NMC, London. Available at: ℘ http://www.nmc-uk.org/Documents/Standards/nmcStandardsForMedicinesManagementBooklet.pdf

National Prescribing Centre: guidance and framework of competencies for the use of PGDs. 2009 ℘ http://www.npc.nhs.uk/non_medical/resources/patient_group_directions.pdf

Guidance and core curriculum for training on immunization delivery. ℘ http://www.hpa.org.uk/Publications/InfectiousDiseases/0506CoreCurriculumforImmunisationTraining/

Mental health policies

Purpose

To assist the organization in fulfilling its responsibilities to maintain the mental health and wellbeing of employees at work.

Development

Must have support from senior management, ideally at board level. Set up a steering group, chaired by a senior manager and include representatives from:

• Management
• Human resources
• Occupational health
• Safety
• Union(s) or other employee representatives.

Framework

Physical hazard model (see 📖 p. 134, Organizational psychosocial factors; 📖 p. 311, Stress 2: interventions/risk control).

A mental health policy should describe local arrangements for the prevention and management of mental ill health under the following headings.

Assessment of risk

• *Discussion between interested parties:*
  • satisfy HSE's requirement to consult
  • structured discussion around six key areas (HSE Management Standards)
  • give picture of current work situation
  • identify processes causing stress
  • facilitate practical recommendations, especially from employees
• Staff satisfaction surveys
• Sickness absence rates
• Employee turnover
• Business trends.

Prevention/risk reduction

Primary

• Supportive management culture
• Reporting outcome of risk assessment and resulting action plan to directors/board
• Effective leadership and management skills
• *Appropriate management systems:*
  • resource and project management
  • process management
  • interdependency and infrastructure management
• Change management
• Communication
• *HR-related policies and procedures:* appraisal and training; work–life balance; flexible working, including home working; bullying and harassment; violence at work; shift work; alcohol and drugs

- *Ergonomics:* job design, etc.

Secondary
- Mental Health First Aid or similar training
- Effective sickness absence policy
- Early referral of cases to OH; option of self-referral to OH
- Easy access to appropriate psychological treatment
- *General health promotion:*
  - regular exercise programme/relaxation regime
  - smoking cessation support
  - healthy eating/sensible alcohol consumption.

Tertiary
An effective rehabilitation policy has a joint approach towards individual case management through round-table discussions (see 📖 p. 311, Stress 2: interventions/risk control), where:
- *OH advise on:*
  - functional capacity
  - temporary or permanent nature of disability
  - types of reasonable adjustments
- *Management consider:*
  - business requirements
  - health and safety issues
  - training requirements
  - preparation of colleagues for return of employee's return to work
- HR co-ordinates programme.

Monitoring and auditing policy
- Trends in employee satisfaction
- Action plans for effecting appropriate interventions to address recognized difficulties
- Compliance with and effectiveness of the policy in managing employees' mental ill health.

Further information and guidance
HSE Work-related stress—together we can tackle it. Available at: ℅ http://www.hse.gov.uk/stress

Mental Health First Aid. Available at: ℅ http://mhfa.org.uk/en/

Substance abuse policies

Epidemiology of substance abuse

Alcohol and drug misuse is common in the UK (See Fig 19.2) with major societal costs.

Drug misuse is more common in younger people: 50% of 16–25-yr-olds have misused drugs and 15% currently do so. Cannabis accounts for 80% of illicit drug use. Each year there are ~100,000 offenders under the Misuse of Drugs Act 1971, 50,000 adults attend treatment and ~2000 suffer drug-related deaths. Statistics for alcohol abuse are much higher but are difficult to determine accurately.

Why have a policy?

Substance misuse has important implications for personal health, work performance (particularly if safety critical), protecting business probity and complying with customer requirements. A policy forms the framework for managing alcohol and drug misuse, ensuring clarity, consistency, and legal compliance (see Tables 19.1 and 19.2 📖 p. 758, Methods for alcohol and drug screening).

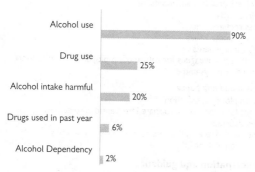

Alcohol use — 90%
Drug use — 25%
Alcohol intake harmful — 20%
Drugs used in past year — 6%
Alcohol Dependency — 2%

Fig 19.2 Population statistics show patterns of alcohol and drug use.

Table 19.1 The main substance abuse policy components

Purpose	Safe working arrangements, employee support
Roles and responsibilities	Management leadership, employee cooperation
Application	Applies to managers, employees, and contractors
Procedures	Communicated and understood by all
Discipline	Possible job termination for policy breach
Support	Managed as 'sickness' when worker seeks help
Testing	Defined testing reasons and Chain of Custody for quality assurance

Table 19.2 Legal obligations

Health & Safety at Work Act 1974	Employers have a duty to protect employees and others involved in their business. Employees have duty to cooperate in health and safety matters
Transport & Works Act 1974	Bans safety critical railway operations whilst under the influence of alcohol or drugs
Work in Compressed Air Regulations 1996	Prohibits working in compressed air whilst under the influence of alcohol or drugs
Road Traffic Act 1984	Employers must assure safe driving arrangements. Employees must not drive under the influence of alcohol or drugs
Misuse of Drugs Act 1971	Employers must not allow the use, possession, or production of any controlled substance, including cannabis on their premises

Policy components

A supportive approach should be taken, encouraging those with health problems to seek help. Principles should be aligned with the employer's values, the law, good employment, and medical practice.

Ethical considerations

These cover the right to personal privacy and the confidential management of sensitive personal information.
- International organizations need to respect legal and cultural differences between the countries in which they operate
- Observe reasonable standards of enquiry and respect privacy in searching personal belongings etc
- OH staff undertaking tests must avoid giving medical advice to individuals, to avoid confusing their testing and occupational health roles
- Disciplinary action following substance misuse testing should not involve OH staff: this would compromise employee relationships.

Roles and competencies

- Managers are responsible for the implementation of the policy
- Medical Review Officer (MRO) is a physician with specialist knowledge and training in specimen collection, chain of custody, analytical procedures, and alternative explanations for positive analytical results
- OH practitioners may advise on policy and test arrangements. They have a separate role in advising employers and managers in support and rehabilitation arrangements and assessing fitness for work.

Treatment and rehabilitation

Workers who volunteer a substance misuse problem may receive advice and support to seek treatment and rehabilitation. Subject to their co-operation, many organizations will maintain their employment.

Further information

Faculty of Occupational Medicine (2006). *Guidance on Alcohol and Drug Misuse in the Workplace.* FOM, London..

Travel policies 1: general travel policy

Employees who travel on company business should be assessed, screened, prepared, and cared for during and after their trip. Most business trips will be low risk, but the following factors ↑ risk.

- Travel to remote or underdeveloped areas
- Poor local infrastructure
- Restricted access to medical facilities
- Extreme climatic conditions
- Transportation challenges
- Individual's behaviours.

Travel policy

Implementing a corporate travel policy can mitigate risk. Such a policy should include the following headings:

Risk assessment

Risk assessment should include work activity; location; security situation; health care facilities; disease prevalence.

Insurance

- Comprehensive cover, appropriate to the individual and destination(s)
- Include insurance for emergency medical evacuation for remote areas
- Use insurers that provide remote access to health resource information, and identify and source medical assistance if required.

Security

- ▶ Awareness and understanding of local security issues are vital
- Include 24-h contact for emergency advice
- Give advice on personal behaviours that affect individual's risk
- ▶ Road traffic accidents are a common cause of morbidity and mortality due to poor vehicle maintenance; driving skills; and roads.

Immunizations: dependent on risk assessment

- Carefully define locations of country/region to be visited as there can be large differences between urban and rural disease vectors and risks
- Refer to regularly updated travel advice, on-line if possible (e.g. MASTA, Travax). Ascertain accurate immunization history
- Maintain documented mandated immunizations (e.g. yellow fever), to avoid entry denial or non-sterile local vaccination at borders.

Psychological stressors

Stressors include:
- Complex and long travel itineraries
- High expectations by the business
- Jet lag
- Cultural dysphoria
- Family separation.

Recognize the challenges and legitimize mitigating behaviours:
- Encourage adequate rest before meetings
- Consider Employee Assistance Programme for this high-risk group.

Personal guidance
- Ensure traveller is aware of potential health challenges that may be encountered
- Confirm traveller understands strategies to preserve health during trip
- Highlight potential ↑ risk behaviours during travel for business traveller
- Pay particular attention to alcohol, drug use, and sexual behaviours
- Give traveller resume of essential health tips as a simple guide.

Health screening
- Organizations may advise formal medical evaluation +/− additional tests (e.g. ECG, CXR) for frequent business travellers
- Quantify the potential impact of pre-existing health issues that may deteriorate during travel
- Define medication carried (also cold storage for drugs e.g. insulin)
- Consider the availability of health resources at the destination.

Malaria and insect borne diseases
- Malaria is a significant risk factor for travellers to endemic areas
- Chemoprophylaxis starts before trip to assess compliance issues
- *Promote ABCD:* Awareness; Bite prevention; Chemoprophylaxis; Diagnosis and treatment.

▶ Travellers perceive malaria risk as small and may not follow advice.

Circadian desynchrony (jet lag) (📖 p. 144, *Time zone changes*)
- Starts to have an effect after three time zones
- Resulting fatigue affects concentration and decision-making
- Allow time to acclimatize on arrival at destination in travel plans.

Travellers' deep vein thrombosis (DVT)
- Probably an effect of travel for >5h
- Risk factors include smoking, recent surgery (10 days), pregnancy, family history of DVT, malignancy, medication (oral contraceptive pill (OCP), hormone replacement therapy (HRT)).
- Advice on maintaining mobility and exercising during travel
- Discourage tranquillizing medication—may ↓ mobility during flights
- Encourage adequate hydration +/− compression stockings for journey.

Traveller's diarrhoea
The most common traveller's health problem. Avoid/mitigate by advice;
- Eating freshly cooked food
- Eating fruit that can be washed or peeled
- Drink safe potable water/ice; use boiled or reputable bottled water
- Consider self-treatment antibiotics (ciprofloxacin etc.) in travel kit.

Travel medical kits
- Content varies in relation to destination—from simple over-the-counter painkillers, insect repellents, and skin dressings to more comprehensive kits with stand-by antibiotics, anti-diarrhoeals, and malaria prophylaxis
- Instructions should be clear and comprehensive.

Post-trip precautions
- Early reporting of post-travel fever or illness
- ▶ Need to complete the full course of malaria prophylaxis, if prescribed
- EAP to be available for problems related to the stressors of travel.

Further information

MASTA. Available at: ℜ http://www.masta.org/
Travax. Available at: ℜ http://www.travax.scot.nhs.uk/
CDC. *Travelers health*. Available at: ℜ http://www.cdc.gov/travel/

Travel policies 2: expatriate policy

Definition of the expatriate worker

An employee who resides in another country for occupational purposes, but returns to their original country upon completion of the assignment.

Expatriate policies

Policies should include general travel advice (p. 382, Travel policy 1: general travel policies). However, prolonged residence requires extra considerations. Therefore, expatriate worker policies should also include the following sections.

Selection process
- Avoid pressing workers to accept postings i.e. for career progression
- Encourage spouse to be involved in decision-making, as family problems are a common reason for expatriate posting failure.

Pre-posting orientation
Family orientation visits are helpful before acceptance of posting. The employee and their family should consider lifestyle factors that will be affected by the move, including environmental, cultural and social changes, medical care, family adjustments, security, and schooling.

Fitness for duty
- Fitness for duty assessments should contain the following elements:
  - evaluation of current diagnosed medical conditions
  - evaluation of psychological suitability for overseas posting
  - physical capacity – if duties include physical fitness requirements.
- All family members should be examined at regular intervals, especially for locations with potential high risk health exposures.

Health resources at location
- Detailed evaluation of local and regional health care resources
- Include national, private, and if available, in-house health facilities
- Guidance on identified limitations of available health care
- Define how to assist expatriates identify/access routine health care
- Avoid single providers wherever possible as options allow choice.

Emergencies and medical evacuations (medivacs)
- Define emergency procedures to deal with illness or injury that may exceed the scope of local health care resources
- Include all management that need to authorize release of corporate resources or finance for management of the severely ill or injured.
- Identify in-country 'liaison physician' to assess and communicate the patient's condition to local management and/or corporate medical staff
- Understand evacuation alternatives and time delays for each option. In high-risk postings, consider a contract with air ambulance providers.

Medication supply
- Understand potential limitations in supply of prescribed drugs
- Encourage routine prescription-filling during scheduled home leaves
- Advise holding a minimum of 3mths supply of medication

- Where appropriate, communicate concerns related to counterfeit medicine supply in destination country or region
- Identify providers that will fill and ship personal prescriptions overseas.
- Some countries may require a formal doctor's prescription when carrying certain medications.

Medical insurance
- Insurance should cover expatriate to provide, as far as practicable, equivalent level of care to that in home country
- Include medical evacuation insurance where appropriate
- Ensure that excluded conditions are explicit, so that expatriates can mitigate potential gaps in care whilst on home leave
- Communicate processes for use of medical insurance and policy on reimbursement of any excess payments.

Other issues
Employee assistance programme (EAP)

▶ *Expatriates are at high risk for psychological difficulties; EAPs offer a valuable resource*
- Local EAP provider is preferable—home country resource as a default
- High-risk cases need 'red flag' to corporate OH department for follow-up.

Rotational assignments
- Complicated risk group because of swinging cultural exposures
- Often very extensive travel involved
- On-site behaviours may be negatively affected by poor perception of risk, including unrealistic beliefs about ready accessibility to home country health care.

Post-assignment
- Recognize the *reverse culture shock* of return to home country
- Consider medical screening (e.g. for tropical disease) in employees and families returning from high-risk postings
- Reiterate availability of the EAP service to returning expatriates.

In-patriates
Expatriates from another country who are on a temporary business related posting to the host country corporate office location:
- Need to understand scope of/access to, local health care provision
- Need to be appraised of cultural issues
- Recognize potential of employee importing illness not normally seen in host population, leading to difficulty/delay in diagnosis (e.g. malaria)
- EAP provision is essential for this high-risk group and families.

Violence management policies

Purpose

To assist the organization in protecting its staff from abuse, threats or violence. (See also 🕮 p. 136, Violence and aggression.) Policy documents should cover the following:

Arrangements for risk assessment and control

- Management responsibility for assessing the risk of violence in every workplace and for each job or group of jobs
- Examples of good practice in risk reduction can usefully be given in an appendix (see Table 19.3).

Promoting a culture where abuse is not permitted

Give a clear message that aggression towards staff is not appropriate, and offenders will be prosecuted i.e. a 'zero tolerance' approach.

Training for employees

All staff should be given basic information about violence and instructions for managing difficult behaviour including how to raise the alarm:

- Understand the mindset of the hostile or potentially violent person
- There may be a need to 'communicate' their grievance to someone
- Provide the hostile person with a verbal outlet
- Use 'active listening'
- Avoid confrontation
- Build trust with the hostile individual and provide help if needed
- Allow a total airing of the grievance without comment or judgment
- Preserve the individual's dignity, as fear of embarrassment will prevent hostile individuals from abandoning plans for violence
- Allow hostile people to suggest solutions for a win–win resolution.

Staff who are working in high-risk areas should have detailed training, including predicting and avoiding anger and aggression, defusion techniques, and using control and restraint as a last resort.

Management of staff who have been abused

- Debriefing by a manager to explore distress when staff are ready
- Information about routes to crisis organizations and helplines will allow employees to choose a source appropriate for their needs.
- Specialist counselling (including therapeutic techniques) may be needed if employees are severely traumatized.
- Affected individuals often need help and support to seek redress from attackers. Involvement of the police can be helpful.
- Where necessary, offer access to legal advice regarding civil claims or compensation from the Criminal Injuries Compensation Board.

Employees' responsibilities

- Employees must try, wherever possible, to defuse violent situations
- Report violent or aggressive incidents.

Table 19.3 Examples of practical risk management

Increased risk of violence	Risk control
Any jobs that involve public interface, especially if controlling or enforcing (e.g. traffic wardens)	Wide counters, barriers, security cameras, restricted access to work in areas for members of the public
Client group with risk factors for aggression: particularly, health care (ambulance workers, accident and emergency staff, mental health workers), custodial services (prison and probation officers)	Assessment of individual client's potential for violent behaviour should be a routine part of the care or service plan
Boredom, frustration, anxiety	Environmental factors: avoid long waits for services, provide comfortable waiting rooms, basic refreshments, children's play areas. Inform clients about delays and explain the reason
Control and restraint tend to escalate violence	Restraint techniques should be used only in extremes, as a last resort
Alcohol and drugs	Prohibit alcohol and drug use at high-risk events. Recognize intoxicated behaviours
Cash transactions	Avoid keeping large quantities of cash in work premises
Lone or night working	Avoid isolation. Have a means for lone workers to summon assistance. Pair-up staff for visits to high-risk clients. Ensure good lighting outside premises and in car parks

Arrangements for reporting incidents
The adverse event recording system must be clear to all employees.

Monitoring and review
- Regular monitoring of incidents, and link to review of risk assessments
- Staff surveys and exit interviews of staff who resign help to define the size and nature of the problem, and under-reporting of incidents.

Further information and guidance
Useful links (including some industry-specific guidance) are available via the HSE website. Available at: ℘ http://www.hse.gov.uk/violence/information.htm

The NHS Security Management Service gives sector-specific advice for health care. Available at: ℘ http://www.nhsbsa.nhs.uk/SecurityManagement.aspx

Special rules apply to the restraint or treatment of patients with acute mental illness. Further information is available in the Code of Practice, Mental Health Act 1983, revised 2008.

NICE, (2005). *Violence: the short-term management of disturbed/violent behaviour in psychiatric in-patient settings and emergency departments*, NICE clinical guideline 25. NICE, London.

Workplace smoking policies

Current practice

- Most employers have a policy on workplace smoking. However, UK research suggests that many organizations, especially small employers, may not have a written policy to support smoking controls
- Those workplaces to which the public has access (e.g. libraries, hospitals, shops) are more likely to have controls in place
- In some countries legislation has curtailed smoking in public places
- Under the Health and Safety at Work etc. Act 1974 employers have a duty to protect worker's health and this includes passive smoking
- Smoking is now banned in most indoor spaces, other than homes, including workplaces (e.g. vehicles) in the UK.

Purpose

- Concerns about employers' civil liabilities where non-smokers are exposed to environmental tobacco smoke (ETS) at work have encouraged some employers to develop and implement smoking controls
- There are many arguments against workplace smoking including breach of anti-smoking laws, annoyance to non-smokers, increased sickness absence among smokers, increased risk of fire, raised insurance costs, and inflated cleaning and redecorating costs
- One of the strongest arguments against workplace smoking is that passive smoking may have adverse effects on the health of some workers, especially pregnant workers, asthmatics, and COPD sufferers
- Smoking policy can aid corporate image.

Main requirements

- Set up a joint management–staff committee to discuss smoking controls and to develop a draft smoking policy
- A clear timetable for policy development, obtaining staff feedback, revising the policy, and implementing the final agreed policy should be made explicit at the outset of the process. The HSE recommend a minimum of 90 days for this process
- All employee groups should be represented, smokers and non-smokers alike. Union representatives, safety representatives, and members of the occupational health and safety team should be involved in the working group
- A draft policy should be drawn up, setting out the purpose of the smoking policy. Where restrictions on smoking are proposed, this may be a complete ban or a partial ban
- Where smoking is permitted, employees must smoke outside (this might affect evening/night shift workers' safety so this practice should be discouraged) Many NHS employers have banned smoking within hospital grounds
- Where smoking is permitted, this is usually only during scheduled tea or meal breaks. Alternatively, some employers allow smokers to work longer hours to make up for time lost due to smoking breaks

- The policy should define the responsibilities of supervisors to enforce the policy, and identify sanctions for those breaching the policy, e.g. disciplinary action
- The employer may wish to offer support for those who wish to stop smoking in the policy (as part of Wellbeing strategy) in addition to that available via NHS Direct/GP
- The draft policy should be distributed to all staff for discussion and feedback
- It is sensible to provide information to staff regarding the adverse effects of smoking and the hazard of passive smoking, using leaflets and posters
- To achieve optimum support for the policy it is important that the draft policy is well publicized using:
  - posters
  - staff e-mails/mailings
  - in-house magazine/newsletter
  - company intranet.

Staff feedback can be obtained in many ways including:
- Staff questionnaires
- Opinion survey
- Toolbox talks/staff briefings
- 'Town Hall' meetings.

Implementation
- Once the policy is agreed, further publicity is required to ensure that:
  - employees are aware of the new policy
  - know where smoking is banned
  - if smoking is permitted, staff know what restrictions are in place
- Some employers may opt to have a transitional period before full implementation of the workplace smoking policy
- The OH service may run a workplace smoking cessation programme in support of the policy. The employer may fund nicotine replacement therapy (NRT) for those employees wishing to stop smoking. NRT is now available on the NHS
- If smoking is to be permitted anywhere, then smoking and non-smoking areas should be designated, clearly signposted, and enforced.

Audit
Regular review of the effectiveness of the policy should be undertaken.

Further information
Action on Smoking and Health (ASH). Available at: ℘ http://www.ash.org.uk/
NICE (2012). *Brief interventions and referral for smoking cessation.* Available at: ℘ http://www.nice.org.uk/PHI001

Sickness absence, rehabilitation, and retirement

Improving health and wellbeing through work

Health and unemployment

There is good research evidence to suggest that unemployment is associated with poor health.

- Those who are out of work have an increased risk of:
  - mortality from coronary vascular disease, cancers, suicide, accidents, and violence
  - morbidity from depression, ischaemic heart disease
  - experiencing inequality in health and social opportunities
- In general, getting people back to work after illness or with disability is likely to benefit their long-term health
- Long-term absence from work due to sickness has a poor prognosis. The likelihood of returning to work is 20% after 6mths of absence.

Barriers to work and rehabilitation

- Cultural beliefs about the right of sick people to be excused from work, and failure to recognize that work is beneficial for most people
- Pressure on GPs from patients or relatives to certificate absence from work, and difficulty for GPs in declining to certificate
- Poor access to OH advice for many employees because of a shortage of OH professionals and other factors
- Employers' reluctance to arrange adjustments to work ('all or nothing' mentality), or poor understanding about positive effects for business
- Lack of practical support for rehabilitation.

Overcoming barriers to rehabilitation in the UK

The drive to improve return to work and rehabilitation has been helped by changes in legislation, primarily the Equality Act. However, cultural attitudes are slow to change. Pro-active and co-ordinated effort is required from political and social drivers and a range of stakeholders. A comprehensive description of solutions is beyond the scope of the handbook, but some broad approaches, current leads, and stakeholders are outlined here for reference.

Broad approaches

- Preventing ill health and injury in the workplace:
  - general measures to improve the public health
  - maximizing opportunities to support health promotion at work
  - managing specific risks to health and safety at work
- Encouraging all doctors to consider return to work as part of the clinical management plan, including introduction of the 'fit-note' (new Med 3 stating what work can be done by an employee, rather than automatically certificating off all work)
- Supporting employers to make adjustments to work
- Improving access to OH advice

- Improving the consistency and quality of OH advice (📖 p. 352, Quality and audit in occupational practice 1: general principles; 📖 p. 354, Quality and audit in occupational practice 2: systems and tools):
  - audit in OH practice
  - evidence-based guidelines on OH issues
  - accreditation for quality and governance
- Providing work rehabilitation schemes for those who are off work long term due to ill health, particularly using a case management approach
- Promoting good HR practice.

Government lead

The White Paper 'Choosing Health'[1] shows leadership in tackling the barriers to retaining, regaining, or accessing work. Work from a number of initiatives underpin this lead, including:

- *The Health, Work, and Well-being Unit:* established in 2005, and jointly sponsored by the Department for Work and Pensions (DWP), the Health and Safety Executive (HSE), the Department of Health (DH), the Scottish Government and the Welsh Assembly Government. The unit:
  - promotes the link between good work and health
  - collates and adds to the evidence base
  - drives change in this area
- The National Director for Health and Work has undertaken reviews, which outline relevant recommendations for improving health through work and for promoting early rehabilitation to work:
  - on the health of the working age population (2008, government response—Improving health and work—changing lives)
  - on sickness absence, jointly with the Director General of the British Chambers of Commerce (2011, government response awaited).

Other stakeholders

- OH professionals and service providers
- GPs and other health professionals, e.g. doctors in secondary care
- Faculty and Society of Occupational Medicine, Royal Colleges
- Employers and employers' organizations, e.g. Confederation of British Industry (CBI), UK manufacturers' organization (EEF), NHS Employers
- Employees and their representatives (e.g. trade unions), self-employed
- Human resources professionals
- Insurance companies
- Local authorities
- Voluntary sector organizations.

Table 20.1 lists the most important initiatives from the UK government and other stakeholders. It is not an exhaustive list.

---

1 Department of Health (2004). *Choosing health: making healthier choices easier*, Public Health White Paper. Department of Health, London.

Table 20.1 Supporting prevention, rehabilitation and healthy working in the UK

Driver	Strategy or initiative	Description	Web reference
National Director for Health and Work and Director General British Chambers of Commerce	Health and Work: an independent review of sickness absence	Review of the sickness absence system in Great Britain to help combat the costs and impact of sickness absence	http://www.dwp.gov.uk/policy/welfare-reform/sickness-absence-review
HSE	Health and Safety made simple 2011	Web-based guidance for employers on simplifying compliance with health and safety law	http://www.hse.gov.uk/simple-health-safety/
DWP	Good for Everyone. The next steps in the Government's plans for reform of the health and safety system in Britain 2011	Sets out a new start for health and safety regulation for businesses. Focus on deregulation for well-performing employers and making poorly performing employers bear the costs of inspection and rectification of non-compliance	http://www.dwp.gov.uk/docs/good-health-and-safety.pdf
Health, Work and Well-being Unit (DH, DWP, Scottish Govt, Welsh Assembly Govt)	Health, Work and wellbeing Baseline Indicators Report 2010	Sets out the available baseline data for the indicators of health and wellbeing at work described in Improving Health and Work: changing lives	http://www.dwp.gov.uk/docs/hwwb-baseline-indicators.pdf
HSE	The Health and Safety of Great Britain/Be part of the strategy 2009	Sets out the HSE Board's strategy for the health and safety system, recognizing the role of stakeholders in maintaining and improving health and safety standards	http://www.hse.gov.uk/strategy/strategy09.pdf

DH and DWP	Improving Health and Work: changing lives 2008	The Government's response to Working for a Healthier Tomorrow	http://www.dwp.gov.uk/docs/hwwb-improving-health-and-work-changing-lives.pdf
National Director for Health and Work	Working for a Healthier Tomorrow 2008	Report on the health of the working age population, presented to the Secretary of State for Health and the Secretary of State for Work and Pensions	http://www.dwp.gov.uk/docs/hwwb-working-for-a-healthier-tomorrow.pdf
DWP	Information for professionals and advisers	Various educational tools including desk-aids and web-based learning packages for doctors. Aimed at promoting good practice in relation to managing return to work after sickness or with disability	http://www.dwp.gov.uk/healthcare-professional/guidance/
DH	NHS Plus	A network of NHS OH departments that provide OH advice to SMEs	http://www.nhsplus.nhs.uk/
DH	NHS Health at Work Network	Network of NHS OH providers, working in partnership with NHS Plus and NHS Employers to promote collaborative working and exemplary provision of OH services to NHS staff	http://www.nhsplus.nhs.uk/providers/members.asp
HSE partnership	Workplace Health Connect	A free occupational health and safety advisory service for SMEs	http://www.workplacehealthconnect.co.uk/

Further information

DWP. *Health and well-being unit – resources*. Available at: ℘ http://www.dwp.gov.uk/health-work-and-well-being/resources/

Advice for employers and employees on returning to healthy work.

Healthy Working UK. *Fit note guide*. Available at: ℘ http://www.healthyworkinguk.co.uk/

Healthy working Wales. Available at: ℘ http://www.healthyworkingwales.com/splash_wales/en.html

Healthy working lives. Available at: ℘ http://www.healthyworkinglives.com/

Advising patients about work: an evidence-based approach for GPs and other health professionals. ℘ http://www.dwp.gov.uk/docs/hwwb-health-work-gp-leaflet.pdf

Sickness benefits

In the UK, state benefits are payable to those who cannot work due to illness. The process is summarized in Fig. 20.1.

Statutory Sick Pay (SSP) or equivalent[1]

- Payable by employer for spells of incapacity <28wks
- Certificated according to fitness for own occupation
  - <7 days, self-certificate SC1, SC2, or employers own form
  - >7 days, Med 3 (Statement of Fitness for Work) provided by GP or hospital doctor for out-patients or Med 10 provided by hospital doctor for hospital in-patients. Includes advice on rehabilitation.

State benefits[1]

Employment and Support Allowance (ESA)

- Entitlement depends on National Insurance (NI) contributions
- Those who have not paid sufficient NI, may qualify for income-based ESA depending on income and capital
- State benefits are subject to an assessment of work capability.

Work Capability Assessment (WCA)

- Eligible when SSP ended, self-employed or unemployed
- Assessment by a health professional +/− medical assessment
- Carried out during the first 13wks after application
  - assessment of limited capability for work—the focus is on what work activities the patient *can* carry out. The applicant has access to a personal adviser, training and condition management and is expected to move towards a return to work
  - assessment of limited capability for work-related activity—for the most severely affected, who are not expected to prepare for work
- GP no longer required to certificate if ESA awarded
- The WCA assesses:
  - the impact of health on daily life
  - the patient's view of the future from a health and work perspective
  - activities the patient enjoys or would like to develop to help them move into work
  - the support the patient feels they need to move into work
- Following WCA, support for those who are capable of work-related activities:
  - condition management programme
  - expert health advice
  - workshops on health topics, e.g. coping with pain, positive mood management, motivational support, preparing for work.

1 The newly published sickness absence review (21.11.11) proposes changes to the sickness absence and benefits system which will be subject to consideration and response by the UK government during 2012.

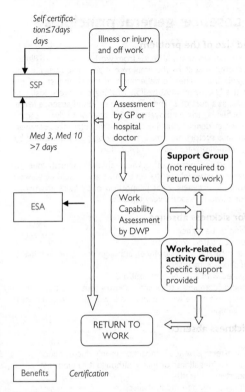

Fig 20.1 Summary of the process for assessing eligibility for benefits in relation to fitness for work[1]

Further information and guidance

For Occupational Health. Available at: ℛ http://www.dwp.gov.uk/docs/fitnote-occupational-health.pdf

For GPs. Available at: ℛ http://www.dwp.gov.uk/docs/esa-gp-leaflet.pdf; Also available at: ℛ http://www.dwp.gov.uk/docs/gp-benefit-guide.pdf; Also available at: ℛ http://www.dwp.gov.uk/docs/fitnote-gp-guide.pdf

Sickness absence: general principles

Definition and size of the problem

Sickness absence is defined as any absence from work attributed to illness or injury, and accepted as such by the employer. It gives rise to significant costs for all organizations. The Confederation of British Industry (CBI) estimate that in the UK, nearly 190 million working days were lost due to sickness in 2010, at a cost of £17bn.[1] That survey found absence levels of 8.1 days per public sector employee and 5.9 days per private sector employee. However, evidence from HSE suggests that differences between the public and private sectors are small, and may be partly explained by under-reporting in small private sector organizations.

💥 Estimates of the proportion of sickness absence actually due to non-medical reasons vary widely (~10% up to 30%) and should be viewed with great caution. Determining what proportion of sickness absence is not genuine is, for obvious reasons, very difficult.

Risk factors for sickness absence

Absence rates tend to be higher:
- Among women compared with men
- In older workers (total days of absence), although young workers have more spells of short-term absence
- In larger compared with smaller organizations
- In the public sector compared to private industry (but note that the public sector employs more women and older workers and comprises mostly large organizations).

Patterns of sickness absence

- *Short-term:*
  - frequent short-term absence is most commonly due to minor unrelated self-limiting illness or injury, although it can indicate chronic underlying ill health
  - however, it can mask non-medical absence
- *Long-term:* almost invariably due to significant medium- to long-term ill health
- Because of this general difference in the nature of short- and long-term absence, the broad approach to management also differs. See 📖 p. 404, Short-term sickness absence; 📖 p. 406, Long-term sickness absence).

Measurement of sickness absence

Simply counting hours or days lost as a proportion of total days worked by all staff (*crude absence rate*) may be misleading and does not show whether the main issue is short or long term absence.
- *Frequency rate:* shows the mean number of absences per worker as a percentage.

  (No. spells of absence in the period/No. employees) × 100

- *Lost time rate:* measures the mean number of working days lost as a percentage of total working days.

> [Total no. working days lost due to absence in a year/(Working days in year × total no. employees)] × 100

The lost time rate can be calculated across the company or for specific business units or by trade/profession, thus highlighting 'hotspots' of poor attendance. This calculation can also be made for lost hours rather than lost days—useful for employers with a large number of part-time staff.

Bradford score

$$S^2 \times D$$

Where S is the number of spells of absence and D is the number of days of absence in a given time period (e.g. rolling 52-wk interval).

The Bradford score is calculated for each worker individually. It highlights the disruption caused by repeated short-term absence by weighting the number of episodes (or spells) of absence. For example,

- Twelve 1-day absences: $12 \times 12 \times 12 = 1728$
- One 12-day absence: $1 \times 1 \times 12 = 12$
- Three 1-day absences: $3 \times 3 \times 3 = 27$
- One 3-day absence: $1 \times 1 \times 3 = 3$

The Bradford score may be used to set a threshold for case management so that consistency in approach between employees can be demonstrated. The threshold score can be based on the extreme of the distribution (upper 5–10% of all scores) rather than an absolute total score, avoiding the perception of a 'safe score' among employees. This measure tends to be used in organizations where most staff works shifts and short-term absence is more disruptive than long-term absence.

Further information

HSE (2005). *Survey of workplace absence sickness and (ill) health (SWASH)*. Available at: ℘ http://www.hse.gov.uk/sicknessabsence/

CBI absence survey 2011 ℘ http://www.cbi.org.uk/media/955604/2011.05-healthy_returns_-_absence_and_workplace_health_survey_2011.pdf

Short-term sickness absence

▶ Frequent short-term term absence is usually regarded as a management issue. The input from OH professionals generally has a different focus compared with long-term absence.

There is no accepted definition of short-term sickness absence—the National Institute for Health and Clinical Excellence (NICE) define it as any absence of less than 28 days and recurrent short-term absence as more than one episode of short–term absence, each episode lasting less than 28 days.

Factors that affect short-term absence

Medical
- Self-limiting illness
- *Poor control of chronic medical conditions:*
  - inadequate treatment
  - poor self-management
  - side-effects of treatment
- *Substance misuse:*
  - alcohol misuse
  - drug misuse
- Epidemics.

Organizational
- Sick pay
- Personnel policies
- *Poor working conditions:*
  - long or unsociable hours
  - boring or unpleasant work
  - poor training or supervision
  - shift work
- *Interpersonal difficulties in the workplace:*
  - between manager or colleagues
  - ⚠ suspect bullying if absences mirror the supervisor's shifts
- Poor labour relations
- Change, e.g. redundancies.

Psychosocial and cultural
- Retirement age
- Local unemployment
- *Domestic factors:*
  - childcare
  - elderly relatives
  - sick or disabled relatives
  - intimate partner violence—the British Crime Survey found that 20% of employed female victims and 6% of employed male victims took time off work and 2% of both sexes lost their job as a result
- *Poor work motivation:*
  - young people
  - temporary workers

- *Social and cultural factors:*
  - sporting events
  - appointments with hairdressers, tradesmen, etc.
  - holidays
  - cultural, e.g. a widespread belief that employees are entitled to a level of sick leave, to be used as additional holiday.

Role of occupational health

When an employee with repeated short-term absence is referred, the main purpose is to ensure that medical issues are properly taken into account by the employer in managing the absence pattern. The role of OH is to identify medical reasons why the employee's absence pattern might deviate from the average for the organization.

- In the absence of medical factors, the OH practitioner should give a clear message that no underlying chronic or recurrent illness explains the excess absence. This is the case when absences are a collection of minor self-limiting illness that are no more likely to occur in the referred employee than in any other. It can be helpful to add that there is no medical intervention that would have an important impact on the pattern of absence
- If an underlying health problem makes the employee more susceptible to short-term absence, the OH practitioner should communicate the susceptibility (but not necessarily the diagnosis) clearly. It is helpful to comment on the likely future pattern of absence (taking into account any medical intervention), and how much excess absence might reasonably be expected
- In the case of recurrent short-term sickness absence due to a single medical condition then the same approach as NICE recommends for the management of long-term sickness absence (NICE PH19) is appropriate. (See 📖 p. 406, Long-term sickness absence).

Interacting psychosocial factors

- The division between medical and psychosocial is rather more blurred than implied by the checklist here. Factors such as difficulties at home and work often impact on wellbeing even if they do not cause a well-defined 'illness'
- The OH adviser should facilitate the raising of any workplace issues that might be influencing absence, so that these can be addressed
- It can also be helpful to highlight any major domestic problems so that the manager and HR can at least take these into account, offering support or adaptations where this is appropriate. However, this must be done sensitively, and with the employee's consent.

Further information

NICE (2009). *Management of long-term sickness absence and incapacity for work*, PH19. Available at: 🔗 http://www.nice.org.uk/PH19

Long-term sickness absence

Absences >28 days are usually due to significant illness/injury. OH input aims to enable rehabilitation where possible: ill-health retirement is a last resort. The most common causes of long-term absence are:
- Mental illness (stress, anxiety/depression)
- Musculoskeletal disorders (MSDs) (low back pain, osteoarthritis).

NICE guidance on sickness absence management (PH19)

NICE guidance on sickness absence management advises early contact with absent employees, ideally at 2–6wks absence, and suggests a tiered response.

Initial enquiries

Employers should task someone impartial to make initial enquiries to:
- Identify reasons for sickness and barriers to returning to work
- Discuss return to work options and agree any action needed
- If necessary appoint a case worker to contact the worker, agree management plan and co-ordinate interventions

Detailed assessment

If needed, arrange assessment by a relevant specialist—may include:
- Specialist advice on diagnosis and treatment
- Use of a screening tool
- A combined interview and work assessment
- Develop a return-to-work plan, and if needed, interventions.

Level of interventions (if needed)

In addition to usual treatment consider:
- 'Light' interventions for workers likely to return to work
- 'Intensive' interventions for those unlikely to return to work (e.g. CBT or physiotherapy).

Occupational health assessment

Process frequent and active case management, clinical assessment +/– discussion with manager or HR +/– workplace visit.

Purpose

- Establish the nature of the underlying medical condition
- In a minority of cases it is useful to obtain a report from the GP, hospital doctor, or other specialist (physiotherapist or psychologist)
- *Facilitate optimal medical management:*
  - some employers provide treatment or fund private health care
  - careful communication with the GP essential, as is written consent from employee. If medical intervention is arranged, inform GP
- Carry out a functional assessment. This is crucial to the OH management of long-term absence, as it informs rehabilitation (see Box 20.1)
- Identify precipitating or exacerbating factors at work
- Explore and address psychosocial factors (see Box 20.2), Facilitation of self-directed goal-setting and use of positively influencing consultation skills (e.g. motivational interviewing) by the OH team can be helpful.

Output

Written report to management +/− human resources detailing:

- Prognosis for work including likely duration of absence and likelihood of recurrent absence in the future
- Need for adjustments to work, where relevant:
  - to facilitate rehabilitation. Agree a rehabilitation programme with employer/employee. It is sometimes helpful to share the rehabilitation plan with the GP (with the employee's consent)
  - to reduce the risk of recurrence
- Outline the plan for review (clinical +/− workplace)
- Do not disclose medical details to the employer, except where:
  - required by law (e.g. RIDDOR), but obtain employee's consent
  - disclosure (with consent) to facilitate the employer's/co-workers' understanding of impact of condition, e.g. if an insulin-dependent diabetic is at high risk of hypoglycaemic attacks, informed intervention by colleagues is important
  - the minimum necessary information should be disclosed. The worker must know what will be disclosed and to whom
- Advise manager if the Equality Act is likely to apply. Only an employment tribunal can decide if the definition of disability is actually fulfilled

Identify and try to resolve disparity between sources of medical advice. In the event of unresolved disparity, the employer can take their occupational physician's advice if their expertise is the most appropriate.

Box 20.1 Functional assessment

Record symptoms (severity and duration), but the emphasis should be on *functional capacity*. A useful checklist includes:

- *Generic capabilities:* duration of sitting, standing, walking, reading/concentrating. Ability to bend, lift/carry, reach up. 'Down time': time spent in bed during the day
- *Day-to-day activities:* washing/dressing, cooking, housework, gardening, driving, shopping, computer use, sport and social activity
- *Work activities:* enquiry tailored to specific job tasks.

⚠ This is not intended to be a complete list.

Box 20.2 Psychosocial factors

Successful return to work dependent on employee's motivation/beliefs about health/work—belief is that they will never again be fit for work means they are unlikely to return to work, irrespective of medical condition. Useful to assess such beliefs at an early stage.

Further information

NICE (2009). *Management of long-term sickness absence and incapacity for work*, PH19. Available at: ℘ http://www.nice.org.uk/PH19

Evidence-based recovery times

Increasingly, evidence-based guideline material is being used to promote consistency of medical advice in the assessment of fitness for work. Table 20.2 is based on average recovery times for common surgical procedures. It is not intended to be an exhaustive list, or to be used inflexibly. However, it does provide a 'rule of thumb' to be adjusted according to the clinical and job details of individual cases.

Further information and guidance

Royal College of Surgeons. (2012). *Get well soon: helping you make a speedy recovery after your surgery.* Available at: ℜ http://www.rcseng.ac.uk/patient_information/get-well-soon

Royal College of Obstetricians and Gynaecologists.(2012). *Return to fitness: recovering well.* Available at: ℜ http://www.rcog.org.uk/recovering-well/

Table 20.2 List of expected time off work for uncomplicated procedures

Operation	Minimum expected (wks)	Maximum expected if no complications (wks)
Angiography/angioplasty	<1	4
Appendectomy	1	3
Arthroscopy	<1	<1
Cataract surgery	2	4
Cholecystectomy	2	5
Colposcopy +/– cautery	<1	<1
CABG or valve surgery	4	8
Cystoscopy	<1	<1
D&C, ERPC, or TOP	<1	<1
Femoro-popliteal grafts	4	12
Haemorrhoid banding	<1	<1
Haemorrhoidectomy	3	6
Hysterectomy	3	7
Inguinal or femoral hernia	1	3
Laparoscopy +/– sterilization	<1	<1
Laparotomy	6	12
Mastectomy	2	6
Pacemaker insertion	<1	<1
Pilonidal sinus**	<1	<1
Retinal detachment	<1	Avoid heavy work, lifelong
Total hip or knee replacement	12	26
TURP	3	6
Vasectomy	<1	<1

Key: CABG, coronary artery bypass graft; D&C, dilatation and curettage; ERPC, evacuation of retained products of conception; TOP, termination of pregnancy; TURP, trans-urethral resection of prostate.

Taken from table 8.2 (p. 199), Chantal Simon et al (2005). *Oxford Handbook of General Practice* 2e, with kind permission of Oxford University Press.

** If time off for dressings is allowed.

Rehabilitation and disability services

A range of facilitative services are available for disabled people who are trying to maintain or regain employment:

- These are provided by a variety of organizations including charitable trusts and government-funded departments
- These resources can be accessed by employees themselves, but OH departments can usefully signpost routes of contact
- The services include provision of financial support for employers of disabled people, and provision of sheltered employment opportunities for those who are out of work because of disability.

Jobcentre plus

This government agency is part of the DWP. It aims to support people of working age, who are on state benefits, in overcoming barriers to gainful employment. Further information is available at ℗ http://www.dwp.gov.uk/jobcentreplus/ ℗ http://www.direct.gov.uk/en/Employment/Jobseekers/ContactJobcentrePlus/DG_186347

Access to work scheme (AtW):

Advice and grants towards additional employment costs. For new employees, the grant is up to 100% of the approved costs. For existing employees, the grant is up to 100% of the approved costs up to £10 000 depending on the size of the organization. Larger employers are expected to share a proportion of the costs. ℗ http://www.direct.gov.uk/en/DisabledPeople/Employmentsupport/WorkSchemesAndProgrammes/DG_4000347

The range of services includes the following:

- Support at interview
- Special equipment, e.g. induction loops for hearing impaired individuals
- Adaptations to premises (e.g. improving wheelchair access)
- Help with travel costs if disabled employees cannot use public transport.

Work Choice: special advice and support for disabled people to find or stay in work and whose needs cannot be met by other Jobcentre plus services.

Residential training: for disabled adults.

Adaptations for disabled drivers

A network of independent regional mobility centres in the UK, offering advice and assessment for drivers with medical problems. ℗ http://www.mobility-centres.org.uk/

Information technology (IT) and disability

Ability Net is a charitable organization that provides free information and advice, individual assessment of technology needs, the supply of assistive technology with free support, a programme of awareness education, and consultancy for employers on system and workstation adaptations and web accessibility. ℗ http://www.abilitynet.org.uk/

Disability in education/ universities

Under the Equality Act 2010, universities and other educational establishments are required to make adjustments for disabled students. Many universities have well-defined resources for supporting disabled students, and these are often a source of useful information. ℘ http://www.cam.ac.uk/cambuniv/disability/university/trainingdb/

Charities and organizations that support disabled people in work

- The Shaw Trust. Available at: ℘ http://www.shaw-trust.org.uk/
- Remploy. Available at: ℘ http://www.remploy.co.uk/
- Scope. Available at: ℘ http://www.scope.org.uk/

Ill-health retirement

Ill-health retirement (IHR) is not a decision to take lightly. However, if an individual will never again be fit for his/her designated post, no suitable alternative employment is available, and he/she fulfils pension scheme criteria, further delay in recommending ill-health retirement is undesirable and unethical. Factors to consider in assessing whether an individual is eligible include the following.

Medical factors

- *Diagnosis*: seek medical reports and/or interview and examine the applicant in person. Seek consent for up-to-date medical reports from the individual's doctors:
  - a GP's report is helpful in giving an overview of an employee's health including psychosocial factors
  - a specialist can best address issues around prognosis and treatment options
  - in cases of doubt, an independent medical report for occupational purposes may be helpful, and some Pensions Boards require independent reports as a matter of routine
- *Duration of illness*: a reasonable period should have elapsed to allow for appropriate treatment to be instituted and its effect assessed. As a general guide, it should be possible to make a decision after 6–9mths of incapacity
- *Treatment*: has a range of treatment options been explored? This does not mean all available treatments, but several options should be explored before concluding that a condition is permanent
- *Permanence*: usually interpreted as meaning that the illness will persist until the normal retirement age. Some schemes require that the condition should be permanent before IHR will be approved. Others apply the less stringent criterion that the condition is expected to persist for the 'foreseeable future'. However, 'foreseeable future' can be difficult to define, and discussion with the other doctors advising within a particular pension scheme is desirable in order to maintain consistency. Permanence is easier to demonstrate in those close to normal retirement age
- *Comorbidity*: where an individual has several conditions, these may make the difference between the employee coping with his/her designated post and being unfit
- *Ageing*: an employee with a fixed deficit (e.g. polio) may find that, although the condition itself has not changed, he/she is no longer able to cope with work owing to age-related loss of physiological reserve. However, be absolutely sure that you can demonstrate a clear deterioration in a function that is a recognized feature of the disease
- *Sickness absence*: a pattern of increasing sickness absence (frequency, duration) may indicate that an employee is no longer able to offer regular effective service. In that case, IHR may be appropriate if the condition is permanent. An individual applying for IHR is, by definition, unfit for work and should be on sick leave

- *Reasonable adjustments*: (see 📖 p. 410, Rehabilitation and disability services). IHR is a last resort, only after adjustments and redeployment have been carefully considered
- *Limited life expectancy*: terminally ill employees may have their application fast-tracked by the pension scheme. Depending on scheme rules, it may be financially advantageous to some employees to remain in employment until death (death in service) rather than seek IHR. Some schemes offer an enhanced lump sum and commuted pension if an individual, usually without dependents, has limited life expectancy.

Non-medical factors

- *Organizational pressures*: requests to retire on health grounds may increase at times of reorganization or downsizing for one of two reasons:
  - IHR may be financially more attractive than redundancy to some long-serving staff
  - some staff may genuinely be unfit, but have been 'carried' by colleagues. Restructuring may reveal such problems
- *Operational pressures*: managers may try to remove incompetent staff by persuading them to retire on health grounds; this pressure should be resisted
- *Financial pressures*: once occupational sick pay has ceased, both employer and employee may be keen to seek IHR rapidly. Financial pressures are not in themselves a reason to advise IHR.

Pension scheme membership

- Retirement is distinguished from termination of employment on medical grounds by the payment of a 'pension'
- It is not usually a requirement of employment that a worker be a member of a company pension scheme or indeed any scheme.

▶ Do not assume that an employee is a pension scheme member: check.

Scheme rules

- *Pension scheme rules*: these vary and it is imperative to be aware of the relevant scheme's rules before offering an opinion
- *Length of service*: many schemes will not award a pension to members with short service (<2yrs); instead contributions are refunded
- *Approved doctors*: some schemes will only accept a recommendation for IHR from a qualified occupational physician. Others restrict this role to doctors on an approved list, e.g. an organization's chief medical adviser
- *Added years*: some schemes offer 'added years' of reckonable service where a member is retired on health grounds. This increases the value of the final pension, but can have unintended consequences where employees select the financially optimum time for ill health retirement
- *Higher/lower tier*: some schemes have two tiers—retirees unfit for their job, but fit for other work (*lower tier* retiral) receive a smaller pension than those permanently unfit for all employment (*higher tier*).

Chapter 21

Principles of risk assessment and risk management

Introduction and terminology

Need and context

Decisions in OH often entail a choice between two or more options, the comparative merits of which are not immediately obvious. The decision may be for an individual (e.g. whether to ground a pilot because of a health problem), for the whole of a workforce (e.g. whether to immunize HCWs against smallpox), or at a societal level (e.g. whether to permit the use of a pesticide). Risk management is the process by which decisions of this sort are made, following an assessment of the risks and benefits associated with each option. Depending on the nature of the decision, the process of risk assessment and management may be more or less formalized.

Terminology

In the context of risk management, several terms have a more precise meaning than when they are used in everyday language.

Hazard

A hazard is a potential adverse effect of an agent or circumstance. For example, mesothelioma is a hazard of asbestos, and physical trauma from a fall is a hazard of working at heights. A hazard may be serious (e.g. death) or relatively trivial (e.g. transient irritation of the upper airways).

Risk

Risk is the probability that a hazard will be realized, given the nature and extent of a person's exposure to an agent or circumstance. For example, the risk of mesothelioma from asbestos depends on the type of fibre and the amount that it is inhaled. There is no risk of mesothelioma from the handling of intact asbestos products if no fibres are inhaled.

A risk in an individual corresponds to an excess rate of the adverse outcome in a population of exposed people. Thus populations of asbestos workers have an elevated rate of mesothelioma.

Uncertainty

Often there is uncertainty about the existence of a hazard (e.g. does radiofrequency radiation from mobile phones carry a hazard of brain cancer), or about the levels of risk associated with exposures to a hazardous agent or circumstance (e.g. how much the risk of leukaemia is increased by low levels of exposure to benzene). In managing risks, it is important to take account of uncertainties in the assessment of hazards and associated risks.

Conceptual model

A number of similar models are used in OH practice to summarize and guide the process of assessing and managing risks in the workplace and the environment. One example is given in Fig. 21.1.

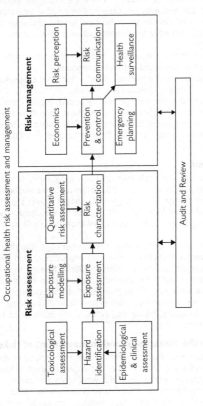

Fig. 21.1 Health and safety management. S. Sadhra and K.G. Rampal. Occupational Health: Risk assessment and Management. Copyright (1999). By permission of Blackwell Publishing.

General principles

Risk assessment

Assessing the risks and benefits from a possible course of action requires evaluation of relevant scientific evidence. There are four main elements to this. Typically, these elements are described in relation to potential adverse effects, but beneficial effects can be considered analogously.

- *Hazard identification:* what are the potential adverse effects of the agent or circumstance?
- *Hazard characterization:* how does the probability of these hazards vary according to the nature and extent of exposure?
- *Exposure assessment:* what are the nature and extent of the exposures that will occur if the course of action is followed?
- *Estimation of risk:* what is the likely probability of each hazard if the course of action is followed? For each risk estimate there should be an evaluation of the associated scientific uncertainty (might the true risk be much larger or smaller than the figure estimated, and if so, how likely is this?).

Risk management

Risk management entails the application of value judgements to decide between possible courses of action, given the estimated risks and benefits associated with each option. Value judgements should reflect the interests of all people who could be materially affected by the decision, with greatest weight being given to the interests of those who will be most affected.

Who makes the decision will depend on the number of people affected. If the important risks and benefits involve only one person, then ideally that individual should decide which option to follow. If more than one person will be affected and their interests conflict, then the decision may require societal input (e.g. through an elected government or the judiciary). For example, governments set exposure limits on hazardous substances in the workplace, taking into account the interests of both workers and employers.

Frameworks for the assessment and management of risks

Where complex, but similar risk management decisions must be made on a regular basis (e.g. in the regulation of toxic chemicals in the workplace), a generic framework may be established within which risks are assessed and managed. This has the advantage of transparency (it is easier for affected parties to understand the basis on which decisions are made) and promotes internal consistency of decisions. For example, the framework for regulation of pesticides in the EU specifies standard requirements for scientific data and the approaches that should be used to determine whether potential risks will be acceptable.

The precautionary principle

As defined in 1992, the precautionary principle stated that 'where there are threats of serious or irreversible damage, lack of full scientific certainty shall not be used as a reason for postponing cost-effective measures to prevent environmental degradation'. It has since been extended to encompass hazards to health as well as to the environment. Essentially, it is an affirmation that decisions in risk management should take appropriate account of scientific uncertainty.

Sources of scientific evidence and uncertainty

Sources of scientific evidence on hazard and risk

Information about hazard and risk may come from various sources:

- *Extrapolation from accepted scientific theory:* for example, in assessing the health risks from static magnetic fields, account is taken of the relevant principles of biophysics
- *Experiments* in vitro: e.g. tests for mutagenicity in bacteria
- *Toxicological experiments in live animals:* these can be more informative, but are relatively expensive and must be justifiable in relation to the impact on animal welfare
- *Studies investigating risk in humans:* these may be experimental (e.g. randomized controlled trials (RCTs)) or observational (e.g. cohort and case-control studies). They have the advantage of avoiding the uncertainties of extrapolation between species, but are limited by the practical and ethical constraints on research in humans. Moreover, they can only be conducted after human exposure to a potentially hazardous agent has occurred
- *Studies to assess patterns of exposure that may result from a risk management decision:* depending on the nature of the exposure, these may use methods of occupational hygiene, ergonomics, microbiology, psychology, or other scientific disciplines.

Reasons for scientific uncertainty

Scientific uncertainty in the assessment of risks may occur for various reasons.

- Doubts about the validity of accepted scientific theory and of its extrapolation to the exposure of interest
- Possible differences in susceptibility to a hazard between humans and the animal species in which toxicology has been investigated, sometimes taken into account by application of an 'assessment factor' ('safety factor')
- Possible differences between individuals in susceptibility to a hazard (e.g. because of differences in genetic constitution, sex, age, coincident disease, and medication, or aspects of lifestyle and environment). Again, an assessment factor may be used to allow for this
- Deficiencies in the design or execution of studies
- Statistical uncertainties when results are based on finite samples of observations that may be unrepresentative by chance. Confidence intervals can be used to help gauge the potential for error of this type.

Risk communication and perception

Risk communication

Good communication of risk is important for two main reasons:

- People who take decisions in risk management ('risk managers') need to understand the likely risks and benefits of each possible course of action. This information must be conveyed to them by the scientists who have assessed the risks and benefits
- Where decisions in risk management are made at a societal level, the people affected need to understand the basis on which decisions are made, and to have an opportunity for informed contribution to the decision-making (e.g. through consultation processes or lobbying of politicians).

▶ Conveying a clear assessment of risk is not easy, especially when the target audience is not scientifically trained. Language should be tailored to the audience, and it may help to draw analogies with other risks that are more familiar (e.g. how risk compares with that of a road traffic accident or from living with a smoker).

⚠ It is best to avoid referring to a situation as 'safe', since nothing in life can ever be guaranteed as totally free of risk. The term 'at risk' is also unhelpful without some indication of the level of risk implied.

Perceptions of risk

The value judgements that are applied in risk management will depend on people's perceptions of hazards, risks, and uncertainties. A number of factors influence perceptions.

- *The nature of the hazard:* this encompasses not only the gravity of the hazard (e.g. is it life-threatening?), but also its nature (e.g. cancer may generate more fear than heart disease even though the risk of fatality is similar).
- The risk of the hazard being realized.
- *The timeframe within which the risk will apply:* is it transient (e.g. the risk of acute injury from undertaking a dangerous activity), prolonged (e.g. the risk of cancer from ionizing radiation), or delayed (e.g. the risk of cancer from taking up smoking)?
- *Whether the risk is offset by an obvious personal benefit:* e.g. there is more public concern about risks from mobile phone masts than from mobile phones themselves, although the latter give higher exposures to radiofrequency radiation.
- Whether the risk is voluntary or imposed.
- *The familiarity of the risk:* risks that are well understood (e.g. of road traffic accidents) are less threatening.
- *Risk experience:* e.g. someone who has lost a relative to cancer is likely to be more worried about contracting the disease themselves than someone who has had no personal experience of it.

Health surveillance

Health surveillance: general principles

General principles

- Health surveillance should only be introduced where the risk assessment indicates that it is required (Regulation 6, Management of Health and Safety at Work Regulations 1999) or it meets the criteria listed in the associated Approved Code of Practice:
  - an identifiable disease or adverse effect is associated with the work activity
  - appropriate methods are available to identify such ill effects
  - it is reasonably likely that the adverse effect will occur given the prevailing work conditions
  - health surveillance will offer additional protection to the workforce's health
- Health surveillance should be supported by a health surveillance policy agreed between management and the employees or their representatives
- The health surveillance policy should document the roles and responsibilities of the line manager, employee, OH service, and HR department
- The health surveillance policy should clearly state how results are to be handled and records stored
- Where an employee's continued fitness for work may be affected by the outcome of health surveillance, an agreed policy on redeployment should be in place
- Informed consent to participate in the health surveillance programme should be sought from each employee at the outset
- The consequences of refusal to participate in health surveillance where this is legally required for work with an agent/process should be made explicit.

Frequency of health surveillance

- An initial assessment of fitness is required prior to exposure commencing. This provides a baseline against which subsequent changes can be compared. In addition, it identifies those workers with pre-existing deficits not attributable to that employment
- Thereafter, the risk assessment dictates the frequency of workers' health surveillance unless published guidance stipulates a greater frequency of checks.

Quality assurance

- All staff involved in health surveillance should be appropriately trained and understand the purpose of the surveillance programme
- Equipment used for health surveillance should be well maintained, regularly calibrated, and fit for purpose
- Any samples taken for health surveillance, e.g. biological monitoring should be analysed in a laboratory that participates in a recognized quality assurance programme
- Any abnormal results should be checked and repeated before further action is taken.

Results

The results of health surveillance should be fed back to the worker and a decision made on his/her continuing fitness for work. If a predetermined action level is exceeded, the employer should investigate the reasons for this and review the efficacy of control measures.

Grouped, anonymized, results of health surveillance should be fed back to staff and the health and safety committee. No personally identifiable data should be disclosed except to the individual employee unless consent has been given for such release.

The health surveillance programme should be regularly audited and any adverse trends investigated and acted on.

Health records

- An entry documenting the individual's fitness status (fit/fit with restrictions/unfit) for work with the relevant agent should be made in the worker's health record and be sent to their employer
- The medical surveillance records should be retained by the OH health service for 40yrs.

Relevant legislation

HSE (2000). *Management of Health and Safety at Work Regulations 1999*, Approved Code of Practice and Guidance, 2nd edn, L21. HSE Books, Sudbury.

HSE (2005). *The Control of Substances Hazardous to Health Regulations 2002* (as amended), Approved Code of Practice and Guidance, L5. HSE Books, Sudbury.

Faculty of Occupational Medicine (2006). *Guidance on Ethics for Occupational Physicians*, 6th edn. FOM, London.

Skin surveillance

Skin surveillance is appropriate where there is a recognized risk of occupational skin disease as defined in COSHH 2002, Regulation 11. This decision may be based on previous experience, Manufacturer's Safety Data Sheets (MSDS), or industry advice. Following the introduction of new agents suspected of causing skin problems, skin surveillance may be instituted.

✇ Value of skin surveillance is contested by some occupational physicians. A recent NHS Plus systematic review failed to find any published evidence regarding skin surveillance for occupational hand dermatitis.

Frequency

Frequency of skin inspection depends on the agents in use. Monthly skin inspection is usual.

Methods

- Annual hand dermatitis screening questionnaire to identify those workers who need to be seen by an OH professional for assessment.

⚠ Such questionnaires should be validated against direct skin inspection in that workforce: some questionnaire validation studies have shown disappointing agreement levels with direct skin inspection.

- Regular skin inspection of 'at-risk' staff by an OH nurse or a responsible person. Those deemed 'at-risk' may be based on:
  - occupational exposure, e.g. hairdressers
  - occupational exposure and a history of hand dermatitis
- Vinyl chloride workers must be subject to skin surveillance under the supervision of an HSE appointed doctor or employment medical adviser (EMA)
- *Patent fuel manufacture from pitch:* workers are subject to skin surveillance under the supervision of an HSE appointed doctor or EMA.

Results

- Individuals with skin problems should be referred to a medical practitioner for further assessment
- A health record should be kept as required by COSHH
- Further tests may include:
  - patch testing
  - skin-prick testing for urticaria
  - blood tests for IgE and RAST
  - skin biopsy (skin cancer).

Relevant legislation and guidance

HSE (1998). *Medical Aspects of Occupational Skin Disease*, guidance note MS24, 2nd edn. HSE Books, Sudbury. Available at: ℘ http://www.hse.gov.uk/pubns/ms24.pdf

Respiratory health surveillance

Respiratory health surveillance is required under COSHH, Regulation 11, for employees who are exposed to known respiratory sensitizers (asthmagens). The purpose is to identify cases of occupational asthma (OA) as early as possible. A list of asthmagens for which surveillance is likely to be required is given in 📖 p. 198, Occupational asthma and rhinitis.

Methods

Screening methods

- Questionnaire (baseline and follow-up) based on a symptoms checklist. Enquiry covers exposure in the proposed job, previous history of exposure to asthmagens, asthma, or work-related respiratory symptoms, and any changes to exposure or symptoms, during follow-up (see Box 22.1)
- *Spirometry:* forced expiratory volume in 1s (FEV_1) and FVC
- *Education:* an important part of screening is to inform employees about the nature and level of the risk to their health, and to counsel them about early reporting of symptoms. Explanation should be given about the possibility of late symptoms.

Format and frequency

This depends on the level, duration, and frequency of exposure (and therefore the risk of sensitization). Two levels of health surveillance are defined in HSE guidance (MS25, see 📖 p. 429, Further information and guidance).

- *Low level:* where there is only suggestive evidence of a hazard, or a low likelihood of exposure:
  - baseline questionnaire and spirometry
  - annual follow-up questionnaire
- *High level:* where there is strong evidence of a hazard and it is not possible to exclude a risk of sensitization:
  - baseline questionnaire and spirometry
  - follow-up of newly exposed employees is by questionnaire (+ spirometry if the risk of sensitization is significant) after 6wks and 12wks, respectively; the interval can fall to annually thereafter in the absence of positive findings.

Responsible person

Questionnaires may be administered by a responsible person (usually a line manager) who has been trained appropriately by an OH doctor or nurse. Positive questionnaire responses must be referred to a competent OH professional for further investigation.

Investigation and management of potential cases

This is usually carried out by an occupational physician.

- *Investigation aims to distinguish the following:*
  - work-related from non-work-related disease—usually possible from a detailed history and lung function, but may need further investigation by serial PEFR testing (see 📖 p. 762, Serial peak flow testing)

Box 22.1 Example questions for baseline questionnaire*

1. Do you believe that your chest has suffered as a result of previous employment?
2. Have you ever left a job because of your chest?
3. Do you have or have you ever had (do not include isolated colds, sore throats, or flu):
   a) Recurring soreness or watering of your eyes?
   b) Recurring blocked or running nose?
   c) Bouts of coughing?
   d) Chest tightness?
   e) Wheezing?
   f) Breathlessness?
   g) Any persistent of history of chest problems?

Example questions for follow-up questionnaire*

Since you last answered our questionnaire
1. Has your job changed?
2. Have you had any of the following symptoms? (list 3, a to g)

* Adapted from HSE sample questionnaire (see web reference in Further information and guidance).

- true immunological sensitization (OA) from non-specific irritation of pre-existing reversible airways disease—it is often impossible to distinguish these on history or PEFR testing alone. Exposure to a known sensitizing agent might give rise to a presumptive diagnosis of OA. However, the gold standard investigation is specific broncho-provocation challenge testing (see ☐ p. 198, Occupational asthma and rhinitis)
- *Management of OA:* confirmed cases should be restricted from exposure, or exposure controlled to the level where symptoms are not detectable. Frequent follow-up should occur if exposure continues.

Other surveillance
- Employers should monitor trends in sickness absence to detect any excess absence that might be due to allergic respiratory disease
- Useful information can be gained from exit interviews: employees with OA and rhinitis often select themselves out of work with the allergen.

Further information and guidance

HSE (1998). Health surveillance for occupational asthma. In: *Medical Aspects of Occupational Asthma*, MS25. HSE Books, Sudbury. Available at: ℅ http://www.hse.gov.uk/asthma/employers. htm#health

Sample baseline and follow-up questionnaires. Available at: ℅ http://www.hse.gov.uk/asthma/samplequest2.pdf; also available at: ℅ http://www.hse.gov.uk/asthma/samplequest3.pdf

BOHRF asthma review. Available at: ℅ http://www.bohrf.org.uk/downloads/OA_Guide-1.pdf

Classification of hearing loss

Screening for hearing loss is required under the Control of Noise at Work Regulations 2005 (📖 p. 548, Control of Noise at Work Regulations 2005). The method of screening is by audiometry (📖 p. 764, Screening audiometry).

Purpose of hearing loss classification

There are a number of hearing loss classification systems developed for the purposes of:
- Determining compensation in civil litigation
- Determining disability benefits
- Monitoring hearing in audiometric surveillance programmes.

One method of classifying occupational hearing loss which is employed in the UK is that published in Appendix 5 of the HSE publication *Controlling Noise at Work 2005*.

▶ Whether or not such a classification scheme is employed all audiograms should be reviewed by a competent health professional.

Method of classification using revised HSE scheme

- The results of audiometry are summed across 1, 2, 3, 4, and 6kHz frequencies in each ear separately
- Audiograms are classified using the information in Table 22.1
- Table 22.2 is used to determine whether the hearing loss exceeds the warning or referral levels for that age band
- Where the sum for either ear is greater than or equal to the warning level for the worker's age and gender, he/she is graded category 2 (mild hearing impairment)
- Where the sum for either ear is greater than or equal to the referral level for the worker's age and gender, he/she is graded category 3 (poor hearing). Such individuals should be referred to a doctor
- Where the previous test took place within 3yrs and ↑ in hearing threshold of 30dB or greater is found (as the sum of 3, 4, and 6kHz), the worker is graded category 4 (rapid hearing loss) and should be referred to an occupational physician or GP
- To assess unilateral hearing loss, take the sum of the hearing level at 1, 2, 3, and 4kHz for both ears. If the difference between the ears is >40dB, notify the worker and refer for medical advice
- Where referral is indicated, an occupational physician should review the worker and consider the need for further assessment by an ear, nose, and throat (ENT) surgeon.

Actions following audiometry

- Offer all workers advice on the use of hearing protection and the health effects of noise
- Workers in category 2 should be notified of the presence, and implications of any hearing loss and the advice recorded in the OH notes
- Give workers a copy of their audiogram
- Workers in category 4 may need audiometry more frequently.

Table 22.1 The HSE categorization scheme

Category	Calculation	Action
1 *Acceptable hearing ability* Hearing within normal limits	Sum of hearing levels at 1, 2, 3, 4, and 6kHz	None
2 *Mild hearing impairment* Hearing within 20th percentile, i.e. hearing level normally experienced by 1 person in 5. May indicate developing NIHL	Sum of hearing levels at 1, 2, 3, 4, and 6kHz. Compare value with figure given for appropriate age band and gender in Table 22.2	Warning
3 *Poor hearing* Hearing within 5th percentile, i.e. hearing level normally experienced by 1 person in 20. Suggests significant NIHL	Sum of hearing levels at 1, 2, 3, 4, and 6kHz. Compare value with figure given for appropriate age band and gender in Table 22.2	Referral
4 *Rapid hearing loss* Reduction in hearing loss of 30dB or more within 3yrs or less. Such a change could be caused by noise exposure or disease	Sum of hearing levels at 3, 4, and 6kHz	Referral

© Crown copyright, material is reproduced with the permission of the controller of HMSO and Queen's Printer for Scotland.

Table 22.2 Classification of audiograms into warning and referral levels

Age	Sum of hearing levels 1, 2, 3, 4, and 6kHz			
	Males		Females	
	Warning level	Referral level	Warning level	Referral level
18–24	51	95	46	78
25–29	67	113	55	91
30–34	82	132	63	105
35–39	100	154	71	119
40–44	121	183	80	134
45–49	142	211	93	153
50–54	165	240	111	176
55–59	190	269	131	204
60–64	217	296	157	235
65	235	311	175	255

© Crown copyright, material is reproduced with the permission of the controller of HMSO and Queen's Printer for Scotland.

Relevant guidance/legislation

HSE (2005). *Controlling noise at work*, Guidance on the Control of Noise at Work Regulations 2005, L108. HSE Books, Sudbury. Available at: ℘ http://www.hse.gov.uk/pubns/indg362.pdf

Patterns of hearing loss

The audiogram varies with the age of the individual, the degree of noise exposure, and any co-existing auditory conditions.

Normal audiogram

Fig. 22.1 shows a normal audiogram of a young person with a hearing threshold of approximately 0dBHL. In older workers the hearing threshold will be lower than this, although in most normal individuals it will remain above 20dBHL.

Noise-induced hearing loss

- Typically, noise-induced hearing loss will produce a notch lying between 3 and 6KHz with recovery (see Fig. 22.2). This dip is usually most prominent at 4KHz
- In older workers with co-existing presbyacusis (age-related hearing loss) the audiogram may not show recovery at higher frequencies
- Firearms use can lead to hearing loss. Initially this loss may be unilateral, but with continued exposure the hearing loss will affect both ears although asymmetry may be evident.

Otosclerosis

- This conductive hearing loss (Fig. 22.3) is due to an autosomal dominant disorder that causes progressive conductive deafness due to a localized disorder of bone metabolism
- Family history may be positive
- In women this disease may first present during or following pregnancy
- Typically, the audiogram shows hearing loss more marked at low frequencies than at high frequencies
- Carhart's notch may be observed with a dip at 2kHz.

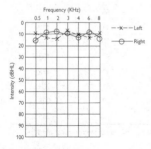

Fig. 22.1 Normal audiogram: X left; O right.

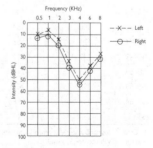

Fig. 22.2 Noise-induced hearing loss: X left; O right.

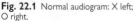

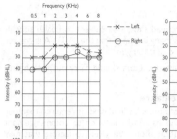

Fig. 22.3 Otosclerosis: X left; O right.

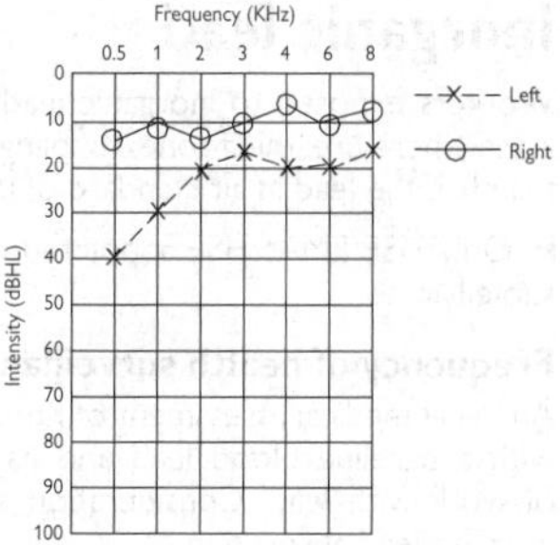

Fig. 22.4 Ménière's disease: X left; O right.

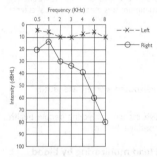

Fig. 22.5 Acoustic neuroma: X left; O right.

Ménière's disease
This condition (Fig. 22.4) produces a low-tone hearing loss often accompanied by tinnitus.

Acoustic neuroma
- A schwannoma of the vestibulocochlear nerve. It presents with unilateral hearing loss (Fig. 22.5), tinnitus, and sometimes vertigo
- Workers with unilateral hearing loss and associated tinnitus should be referred for ENT investigations to exclude an acoustic neuroma: the diagnostic yield of such investigations is, however, low.

Inorganic lead

Workers exposed to inorganic lead should be subject to health surveillance where breathing zone sampling indicates that the 8h TWA is greater than half the lead in air standard of 0.15mg/m^3.

▶ Only HSE EMAs/HSE appointed doctors should carry out such health surveillance.

Frequency of health surveillance

An initial medical assessment of fitness for lead work is required together with a baseline blood lead and haemoglobin prior to commencement of work with lead. Consideration should be given to factors that may increase lead absorption:
- Nail biting
- Smoking
- Poor personal hygiene.

Thereafter, the work activity and/or blood lead level dictates the frequency of workers' health surveillance. As a minimum this means an annual clinical review, including:
- Physical examination
- Review of medical records
- Review of blood lead levels
- Other relevant tests
  - haemoglobin
  - zinc protoporphyrin (levels in unexposed workers are usually <2µg/g haemoglobin).

However, for women of reproductive capacity or young people health surveillance should take place at 3-monthly intervals.

Maximum intervals for blood lead monitoring by blood lead levels

Blood lead	Maximum interval for surveillance
<30µg/dL	12mths
≥30–<40µg/dL	6mths
≥40–<60µg/dL	3mths
≥60µg/dL	At doctor's discretion, but not >3mths

Samples

A 5-mL blood sample should be collected in an EDTA tube. The timing of sampling is not critical. A laboratory participating in the joint HSE/UK NEQAS programme should carry out atomic absorption spectroscopy to determine blood lead levels.

Results

- Results of blood lead monitoring should be fed back to worker and a decision made on their continuing fitness for work with inorganic lead
- If an action level is exceeded the employer should investigate the reasons for this and review the efficacy of control measures. Aim is to prevent the worker's blood lead level reaching the suspension level
- Where the relevant suspension level is reached, the appointed doctor must decide whether to certify that the employee is no longer fit to work with lead.

The Control of Lead at Work Regulations 2002 indicates the following action and suspension levels (Box 22.2).

Box 22.2 Actions required for given blood lead level

	Action level	Suspension level
Adult (not of reproductive capacity)	50µg/dL	60µg/dL
Young person	40µg/dL	50µg/dL
Woman of reproductive capacity*	25µg/dL	30µg/dL

*A woman of reproductive capacity is a woman medically and physically capable of conceiving. This includes any woman on hormonal contraceptives.

- Background blood lead levels in the general population are usually <10µg/dL
- ▶ Pregnant workers should be suspended from work involving significant exposure to lead
- ▶▶ Where a worker's blood lead level reaches the suspension level, the blood lead should be re-checked as a matter of urgency.

Health records

An entry documenting the individual's fitness for work with inorganic lead should be made in his/her health record and be sent to his/her employer. The medical surveillance records should be retained for 40yrs.

Relevant legislation

- HSE (2002). *Control of Lead at Work Regulations 2002*, Approved Code of Practice and Guidance, L132. HSE Books, Sudbury. ℅ http://www. hse.gov.uk/pubns/priced/l132.pdf
- HSE (2000). *Management of Health and Safety at Work Regulations 1999*, Approved Code of Practice and Guidance, 2nd edn, L21. HSE Books, Sudbury.

Organic lead

Workers exposed to lead alkyls (e.g. tetraethyl lead, tetramethyl lead) should be subject to health surveillance where breathing zone sampling indicates that the 8h TWA is greater than half the lead in air standard of 0.10mg/m^3 or there is a risk of dermal absorption of lead alkyls. Most exposure to organolead occurs in the manufacture or use of lead alkyls employed as anti-knock agents in leaded petrol.

▶ Only HSE EMAs/HSE appointed doctors should carry out such health surveillance.

Frequency of health surveillance

An initial medical assessment of fitness for lead work is required together with baseline urinary lead prior to work with lead commencing. Those with a recent history of psychiatric illness should not work with organic leads to avoid confusion between organic lead poisoning and a relapse of pre-existing mental illness. Consideration should be given to factors that may increase lead absorption:
- Nail biting
- Smoking
- Poor personal hygiene.

Thereafter, the work activity and/or urine lead level dictates the frequency of workers' health surveillance. As a minimum this means an annual clinical review, including:
- Physical examination
- Review of medical records
- Review of urinary lead
- Annual blood lead.

Samples

A 25-mL urine sample should be collected at the end of the shift at the end of the working week. Analysis is by atomic absorption spectrophotometry to determine urinary lead levels.

Results

The results of lead monitoring should be fed back to the worker and a decision made on his/her continuing fitness for work with organic lead. Where the relevant suspension level is reached and is confirmed by repeat testing, the appointed doctor will certify that the employee is no longer fit to work with organic lead. The Lead at Work Regulations 2002 indicate the following suspension levels (Box 22.3).
- ▶ Pregnant workers should be suspended from work involving significant exposure to lead
- ▶▶ Where a worker's urinary lead level reaches the suspension level, the urinary lead should be re-checked as a matter of urgency.

Health records

An entry documenting the individual's fitness for work with organic lead should be made in his/her health record and be sent to his/her employer. The medical surveillance records should be retained for 40yrs.

Box 22.3 Suspension levels for urinary lead

	Suspension level
Adult (not of reproductive capacity)	110µg Pb/g creatinine
Young person (aged 16 or 17)	110µg Pb/g creatinine
Woman of reproductive capacity*	25µg Pb/g creatinine

* A woman of reproductive capacity is a woman medically and physically capable of conceiving. This includes any woman taking hormonal contraceptives.

Relevant legislation

- HSE (2002). *Control of Lead at Work Regulations 2002*, Approved Code of Practice and Guidance, L132. HSE Books, Sudbury. available at: ℘ http://www.hse.gov.uk/pubns/priced/l132.pdf
- HSE (2000). *Management of Health and Safety at Work Regulations 1999*, Approved Code of Practice and Guidance, 2nd edn, L21. HSE Books, Sudbury.

Surveillance for hand–arm vibration syndrome

The health surveillance requirements for HAVS are described in the Control of Vibration at Work Regulations 2005.

Main requirements

Health surveillance should be provided for vibration-exposed employees who:
- Are likely to be regularly exposed above the exposure action value of 2.5m/s^2 A(8)
- Are likely to be exposed occasionally above the exposure action value and where the risk assessment identifies that the frequency and severity of exposure may pose a risk to health
- Have a diagnosis of HAVS (even when exposed below the exposure action value).

Process and methods

The HSE recommends a tiered approach to health surveillance for HAVS. Further information and example questionnaires are available through the HSE website (℅ http://www.hse.gov.uk/vibration/hav).
- *Tier 1—initial baseline assessment:* a short questionnaire to be used for people moving into a job involving exposure to vibration. Questionnaire responses determine whether the individual is referred for health assessment (tier 3)
- *Tier 2—annual (screening) questionnaire:* a short questionnaire to be used annually for individuals exposed to vibration, to determine whether they need to be referred to tier 3
- *Tier 3—assessment by qualified person:* this involves a HAVS health assessment by a qualified person, e.g. an OH nurse. A clinical questionnaire asks about relevant symptoms, and limited clinical examination is recommended. If the assessment shows that the individual has HAVS, he/she should be referred to tier 4
- *Tier 4—formal diagnosis:* at this stage a formal diagnosis is made by a doctor qualified in OH. The reported history of symptoms is considered to be the most useful diagnostic information. Information from tiers 1–4 is also used to make decisions on fitness for work
- *Tier 5—standardized tests (optional):* this stage is optional and involves referral for certain specialized tests for individuals who have signs and symptoms of HAVS.

Tests include:
- *Vascular tests:*
  - finger rewarming after cold provocation (CPT)
  - finger systolic blood pressure test (FSBP)
- *Sensorineural:*
  - vibrotactile perception threshold (VPT)
  - thermal (temperature) perception threshold (TPT).

Symptoms related to carpal tunnel syndrome may need to be investigated by nerve conduction tests (see 📖 p. 294, Compression neuropathies).

- Specialist training is required to carry out clinical assessments for HAVS. The Faculty of Occupational Medicine (UK) has developed a syllabus for approved training in health surveillance for HAVS
- As part of the health surveillance programme a record-keeping system is needed for results of reports of symptoms and medical examinations.

Related legislation

Occupational cases of HAVS and carpal tunnel syndrome are reportable to HSE by the employer under RIDDOR 1995.

Further information

HSE (2005). *Hand arm vibration: the Control of Vibration at Work Regulations 2005*. HSE Books, Sudbury.

HSE. *Health Surveillance—guidance for occupational health professionals*. Available at: ℘ http://www.hse.gov.uk/vibration/hav

Section 4

Fitness for work

Generic fitness for work issues and specific disorders

General principles of fitness for work assessments

Purpose

The purpose of undertaking fitness for work assessments is to try to achieve the best possible job–person fit. Knowledge of workplace hazards and job demands should inform the assessment. The objective should be to be inclusive and, where practicable, to make reasonable adjustments to accommodate those with disabilities. Such assessments may be carried out pre-placement, prior to promotion or job transfer, or following sickness absence or work-related injury. Other reasons for carrying out a fitness for work assessment include:

- *Legislative compliance:* for example, medical assessments under the Control of Asbestos Regulations 2012, Diving at Work Regulations 1997
- *Infection control:*
  - food industry (product safety)
  - health services (patient safety)
- *Baseline data for health surveillance:* e.g. audiometry, spirometry.

Routine periodic medicals, unless subject to rigorous assessment, may generate activity but fail to achieve any useful purpose. Employers may be under the mistaken impression that a 'rigorous' medical will reduce or eliminate sickness absence.

▶ The rationale for the fitness assessment should be clear to all parties, as should the procedures to be followed where an individual is deemed unfit following assessment.

Key information

- Knowledge of workplace hazards and task demands
- Special requirements, e.g. emergency response duties, working in isolation, driving
- Current job description
- The assessor should be familiar with the workplace, or should specifically visit the workplace to ensure appropriate knowledge of the job. This is especially important where the post makes unusual demands of employees
- Any legislative fitness standards should be observed
- Company or industry sector guidance, where available, is helpful in identifying relative and absolute medical contraindications to work.

Reports to employer

- The employer should be informed in writing of the individual's fitness for his/her designated post
- Any restrictions on fitness should be clearly stated
- Identify any adjustments the employer may wish to consider under the Equality Act 2010

- No information regarding underlying medical conditions should be disclosed except with the employee's consent and where disclosure is necessary for health and safety reasons or for the employer to comply with legislation.

Record keeping

- Clear legible contemporaneous notes should be kept (see 📖 p. 748, Recording an occupational health consultation)
- Entries in the employee's OH record should be signed and dated
- Health questionnaires and records of any medical assessment should be filed in the employee's medical record
- All OH files should be securely stored in the OH department. It is illegal and unethical for sensitive health records to be stored where others may have access to them (see 📖 p. 350, Managing occupational health records 2: security, transfer and the archiving of records 📖 p. 362, Confidentiality, consent, and communication, 📖 p. 578, Data Protection Act 1998).

Relevant legislation and guidance

- Faculty of Occupational Medicine (2012). *Fitness for work*, 5th edn. Oxford University Press, Oxford.
- Equality Act 2010.
- Faculty of Occupational Medicine (2012). *Guidance on ethics for occupational physicians*, 7th edn. Faculty of Occupational Medicine, London.

Occupational history

Purpose
- Identify occupational risk factors for disease
- Understand job demands
- Advise on fitness for work
- Inform efforts at rehabilitation or redeployment

▶ It is not sufficient to ask 'What is your job?' although even that may be overlooked by some doctors. Job names vary and may mislead. It is much more useful to know what an employee actually does at work, or has done in his/her previous main job. This should be followed by enquiry about the main workplace hazards, the likely intensity and route of any exposures, and any control measures in place (including personal protective equipment).

⚠ Ask about concurrent jobs (paid or unpaid) as otherwise these may not be declared. This includes second jobs, evening or weekend work, participation in family businesses, such as farms or shops, and moonlighting, i.e. work not declared for tax purposes.

Some jobs place workers at high risk of certain occupational diseases. For example, spray painters are at risk of occupational asthma (due to isocyanates in 'two-pack' paints). Such a work history should prompt the physician to consider whether the patient may have that disease.

> ## Key questions
> - What do you do at your work?
> - Do you have another job?
> - Does anyone else at work have this problem?
> - Does it get better away from work?
>
> *and sometimes:*
> - Have you ever worked with …?
> - What are your hobbies?

Diseases of long latency
Some diseases, such as bladder cancer or pneumoconiosis have a long latent interval between exposure and presentation. To establish an occupational cause in that situation requires a lifetime occupational history. Sometimes, it is more efficient to ask if the patient has ever worked with the suspected agent, e.g. for mesothelioma ask about asbestos exposure.

Hobbies
Pastimes can lead to significant non-occupational exposures especially in those whose hobby occupies many hours per week. Prolonged exposure may be compounded by a lack of health and safety knowledge and inadequate control measures. As a result hobbies may cause occupational-type illness.

Pre-placement assessment

Purpose

The purpose of a pre-placement health assessment is to establish a prospective employee's fitness for employment, including his/her ability to offer regular effective attendance. Consider relevant previous and current health problems and significant workplace risks.

Process (see Fig. 23.1)

⚠ Prospective employees should be advised *not* to submit their resignation to their current employer until their fitness is confirmed (including results of drug screen where relevant).

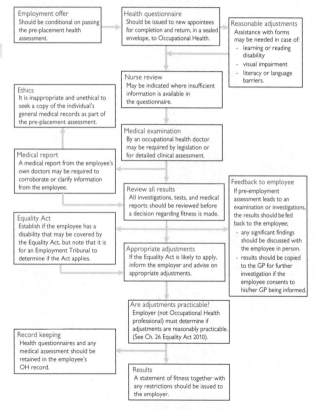

Employment offer
Should be conditional on passing the pre-placement health assessment.

Health questionnaire
Should be issued to new appointees for completion and return, in a sealed envelope, to Occupational Health.

Reasonable adjustments
Assistance with forms may be needed in case of:
- learning or reading disability
- visual impairment
- literacy or language barriers.

Nurse review
May be indicated where insufficient information is available in the questionnaire.

Ethics
It is inappropriate and unethical to seek a copy of the individual's general medical records as part of the pre-placement assessment.

Medical examination
By an occupational health doctor may be required by legislation or for detailed clinical assessment.

Medical report
A medical report from the employee's own doctors may be required to corroborate or clarify information from the employee.

Review all results
All investigations, tests, and medical reports should be reviewed before a decision regarding fitness is made.

Feedback to employee
If pre-employment assessment leads to an examination or investigations, the results should be fed back to the employee;
- any significant findings should be discussed with the employee in person.
- results should be copied to the GP for further investigation if the employee consents to his/her GP being informed.

Equality Act
Establish if the employee has a disability that may be covered by the Equality Act, but note that it is for an Employment Tribunal to determine if the Act applies.

Appropriate adjustments
If the Equality Act is likely to apply, inform the employer and advise on appropriate adjustments.

Are adjustments practicable?
Employer (not Occupational Health professional) must determine if adjustments are reasonably practicable. (See Ch. 26 Equality Act 2010.)

Record keeping
Health questionnaires and any medical assessment should be retained in the employee's OH record.

Results
A statement of fitness together with any restrictions should be issued to the employer.

Fig. 23.1 Flow chart showing the process for pre-placement assessment.

PRE-PLACEMENT ASSESSMENT **449**

- The Equality Act 2010 requires that only the successful applicant should be offered a pre-placement assessment. It is crucial that assessment is undertaken *after* selection or outcome should not be known to employer at the time of selection. Thus, the term pre-placement is often used, rather than the previously common term 'pre-employment assessment'.

▶ Where there is high turnover (e.g. service industries) a rapid access scheme (same-day clinical assessment, where indicated, by rapid screening questionnaires) reduces costs, while managing the associated risk.

Key information
- Current job description, including special job requirements
- Knowledge of workplace risks and task demands
- Sickness absence record for last 2yrs
- Any legislative fitness standards
- Industry sector guidance, where available.

Clinical investigations
Depending on the post, these may include tests listed in Table 23.1.

Legislation and guidance
- Faculty of Occupational Medicine (2007). *Fitness for Work*, 4th edn. Oxford, Oxford University Press.
- Equality Act 2010. Available at: ✍ http://www.legislation.gov.uk/ukpga/2010/15/contents
- *Guidance on Ethics for Occupational Physicians* (6th edn). Faculty of Occupational Medicine, London, 2006.

Table 23.1 Clinical investigations*

Test	Example
Spirometry	Animal house technicians
CXR	Commercial divers
Audiometry	Call centre workers, pipe fitters
Visual acuity and visual fields	Occupational drivers
Colour vision	Seafarers, electricians
Exercise test	Firefighters
Full blood count	Divers, lead workers
Immunity to infectious diseases (rubella, varicella, hepatitis B)	Health care workers (📖 p. 494, Fitness for exposure prone procedures 1; 📖 p. 496, Fitness for exposure prone procedures 2)
Drug screening	Safety critical jobs

* This list is not exhaustive.

Psychosocial factors and fitness for work

Psychosocial factors have been recognized increasingly over the past 10yrs as having an important impact on work capacity and the risk of work-related ill health.

The factors listed here increase the risk of occurrence or recurrence of psychological morbidity and musculoskeletal disorders. However, they should also be taken into consideration when advising about fitness for work, likelihood of absence, and adjustments required, thus facilitating rehabilitation and reducing risk.

Personal psychosocial factors

- *Personality type:* type A personality, and perfectionist and obsessional traits
- *Pre-existing psychiatric morbidity:*
  - depression and anxiety
  - psychotic disorders
- Health beliefs
- Somatizing tendency
- Conflicting family responsibilities
- Poor work–life balance.

Workplace psychosocial factors

These factors and their control are covered in detail on 🕮 p.134, Organizational psychosocial factors. However, the most important are:
- Job demands
- Excessive or insufficient workload
- *Control over work:*
  - lack of control over the volume or rate of work, or achievement of targets
  - low decision latitude
- *Monotonous or repetitive work:* intellectual demands mismatched with the individual's ability or professional background
- Low job satisfaction
- Low perceived value by service users or colleagues
- *Poor relationships with others:*
  - managers
  - colleagues
  - customers
- Bullying and harassment.

Control of psychosocial hazards at work

- Organizational psychosocial hazards (see 🕮 p. 134, Organizational psychosocial factors)
- Violence and aggression (see 🕮 p. 136, Violence and aggression), Violence policies (see 🕮 p. 388, Violence management policies)
- Low back pain (see 🕮 p. 254, Low back pain), WRULDs (see 🕮 pp. 254, 258) Work-related upper limb disorders 2)
- Stress (see 🕮 p. 311, Stress 2: interventions/risk controls)
- Depression and fitness for work (see 🕮 p. 458, Depression).

Ageing and fitness for work

Epidemiology and workforce demographics

- The demographics of populations are changing. The proportion of the UK population who are in the 50–64-yr age group is increasing.
- Changes in UK pension arrangements are likely to increase retirement age, with more individuals working beyond the age of 65yrs.
- It is predicted that within the next 25yrs, 30% of the workforce in Europe will be >50yrs old.

Physiological changes with age

There is some evidence that certain physiological and cognitive parameters change with ↑ age.

Physical

↓ Cardiovascular capacity (measured by VO_2 max)

↓ Musculoskeletal capacity.

↓ *Heat tolerance:* unclear whether this is simply a function of age, or whether it reflects a higher incidence of cardiovascular disease

↑ Sleep disturbance.

△ There is wide individual variation in the baseline level and rate of decline of physiological parameters. A physically fit 50-yr-old can have a greater physical capacity than an unfit 20-yr-old.

Cognitive

↓ Precision

↓ Speed of perception and cognitive processing

↑ Control of language

↑ Ability to process complex information in difficult situations.

Overall function in ageing workers

▶ There is good evidence that job performance does *not* weaken markedly with age; indeed, it can improve.

'Workability' is a concept that assumes that overall performance derives from a portfolio of skills and attributes. The relative contribution of various attributes changes with age; overall performance is preserved. Motivation, loyalty, and experience all generally improve with age, and these factors tend to compensate for physiological decline. If better use is made of enhanced attributes in older workers (e.g. using their experience to train and mentor others), their work potential is maximized.

Sickness absence

Long-term absence is more common in older employees as a group because of the higher incidence of serious or degenerative diseases. However, short-term absence is lower in this group because of a combination of factors including lack of immediate dependents (e.g. time off to look after children) and higher levels of motivation.

△ As with overall function, there is a wide individual variation in absence-taking, and generalization is unwise in decision-making about individuals.

Risks for older workers

The following factors are associated with ↓ work ability and ↑ risk of ill health, and it is particularly important to be aware of them in older workers:

- Role conflict
- Fear of error
- Poor control over work
- Lack of professional development
- Lack of feedback and appreciation
- High speed of decision-making.

Interventions to manage an ageing workforce

There is little direct evidence of benefit from the scientific literature because of a lack of intervention studies. However, these adjustments are based on enhancing 'workability' as described here.

- *Careful management of change:*
  - tailored re-training for new technology
  - flexible career development initiatives for older workers.
- Train supervisors to be aware of age management
- *Apply age ergonomics:*
  - special attention to ergonomics solutions for manual handling tasks and avoiding *extremely* heavy physical work
  - adaptations to man–machine interfaces for long-sightedness (clear controls, large visual displays) and slower reaction times
  - avoiding *extremely* hot working environments
- Health promotion and facilitation of exercise programmes to promote general physical fitness. This is clearly a matter of personal choice for employees, but the effect of physical fitness on overall work capacity with increasing age is often not appreciated
- Adopt a generally positive approach and supportive culture for older employees; value their experienced input.

Relevant legislation

The Equality Act 2010 (📖 p. 562, Equality Act 2010, 📖 p. 572, Age discrimination) puts an onus on employers not to discriminate in employment on the grounds of age. Because of the wide variation in fitness in older people, it will be necessary to carry out a careful individual assessment of capacity, and make adjustments where these are practicable.

Obesity

Definition 'A disorder in which excess fat has accumulated to an extent that health may be adversely affected'. (Royal College of Physicians)

Epidemiology

According to the World Health Organization (WHO) there is an epidemic of obesity. In the UK obesity (body mass index > 30kg/m^2) affects
- 22% of ♂ population
- 24% of ♀ population.

Risk factors

Predisposing factors for obesity include:
- Age (obesity rises with age)
- Gender (females>males)
- Social class (risk increases with lower social class)
- Genetic
- Marital status (married>single).

It can be precipitated by:
- Smoking cessation (e.g. by substituting food for cigarettes)
- Physical inactivity (e.g. due to ill health, work and family pressures)
- Increased dietary calorie intake (e.g. holidays, psychological distress)
- Rarely, sympatho-adrenal or other endocrine disorders
- Drugs e.g. anti epileptics, anti-psychotics, anti-depressants, and insulin.

Classification

WHO classifies weight as in Table 23.2).

▶▶Waist circumference is important because abdominal fat deposition dictates risk of medical complications. Risk is increased with increasing waist circumference:
- Europeans/Caucasians: men > 102 cm, women > 88cm
- South Asians: men >90 cm, women > 80 cm.

Table 23.2 WHO classification of weight

	BMI (Caucasians) Kg/m^2	BMI (South Asians) Kg/m^2
Overweight	25.0–29.9	>23.0
Obese (class 1)	30.0–34.9	>25.0
Obese (class 2)	35.0–39.9	
Obese (class 3) (morbid obesity)	>40	

Clinical features

Obesity is important because is associated with an increased risk of:
- Type 2 diabetes

- Cardiovascular disease (hypertension, angina, myocardial infarction, cerebrovascular accidents)
- Respiratory complications, e.g. sleep apnoea
- Cancers, e.g. of breast, colon, uterus, kidney, and oesophagus.
- Other conditions, e.g. gout, varicose veins, gallstones, fatty liver, menorrhagia.

Sickness absence
Obesity is a predictor of:
- Short-term sickness absence in men and women
- Long-term sickness absence in men and women.

Overweight is a predictor of:
- Short-term absence on men
- Long-term absence on women.

Obesity can accelerate physical disorders (e.g. osteoarthritis of the knees). In terms of work limitations, the effects of obesity are estimated to be the equivalent of the worker being 20yrs older.

Other potential occupational issues
- Increased travel costs due to the need to use two seats (air, rail travel)
- Impaired fit of personal protective equipment, e.g. face masks, clothing
- Costs of adapted furniture
- Special arrangements for evacuation during emergencies
- Inability to mount an emergency response.

Prevention
The workplace is an important opportunity for the prevention of overweight and obesity. See 📖 p. 368, Health and safety policies.

Clinical management
- Dietary advice
- Physical activity management

National Institute for Health and Clinical Excellence (NICE) (SIGN in Scotland) have produced guidelines on the use of drugs and surgery.
- *Orlistat, lipase inhibitor:* improves weight loss if taken with a low fat diet
- *Surgical interventions:*
  - laparoscopic banding (least invasive)
  - gastric bypass (effective weight loss, but significant complications).

Compensation/legal aspects
Obesity is recognized as a clinical condition and appears in ICD-10. It is associated with frequent reports of disability both in mobility and activities of daily living, and may be covered by the Equalities Act 2010. Any adjustments/adaptations should be consistent with the medical advice on the importance of physical activity.

Further information
Nerys W (2008). *Managing obesity in the workplace.* Radcliffe Publishing Oxford.

Cognitive impairment and fitness for work

Causes of cognitive impairment

- Dementia
- Pseudo-dementia in those with severe depression
- Space-occupying lesions, e.g. subdural haematoma
- Brain injury
- Alcohol or substance misuse
- Hypothyroidism
- Vitamin B_{12} or folate deficiency
- Vasculitis.

Epidemiology

- Alzheimer's disease (AD) and vascular dementia are the most common forms of dementia
- There are ~17,000 dementia sufferers under age 65 in the UK
- 5% of people over the age of 65yrs have dementia, rising to 20% over the age of 80yrs
- Evidence that work is a risk factor for AD is conflicting. Some evidence that blue-collar work ↑ risk, but this may be confounded by premorbid ability and/or socio-economic status
- Exposures to organic solvents, lead, mercury, aluminium, or pesticides have all been implicated, but the evidence is inconclusive.

Symptoms and practical problems at work

- *Impairment of:*
  - memory
  - reasoning
  - personality
  - communication (word finding difficulties)
- Workers may be referred to the OH service owing to concerns regarding their memory, decision-making, time-keeping, communication, interpersonal relationships, attendance, or overall performance
- Initial signs and symptoms of cognitive impairment are subtle and may go unrecognized, or be misdiagnosed as stress or depression
- Poor insight can make management challenging.

Clinical assessment and diagnosis

History

It is helpful if managers give specific examples of workplace difficulties as this may alert the assessing physician to the possibility of cognitive impairment. If suspected then explore the following;

- The employee's perceptions of their difficulties
- Family history of dementia
- *Past medical history:* history of head injury, brain tumour, etc.
- Drug/alcohol history
- Educational history

- Occupational history (exposure to occupational neurotoxins).
- ⚠ *Consider treatable causes of dementia:*
  - pseudo-dementia in those with severe depression
  - space-occupying lesions
  - alcohol misuse
  - hypothyroidism
  - vitamin B_{12} or folate deficiency
  - vasculitis.

Investigation

- If cognitive difficulties are suspected then tests to screen for cognitive impairment such as the Addenbrooke's Cognitive Examination – Revised (ACE-R) or the widely used, but less sensitive Mini-Mental State Examination (MMSE)[1] may be helpful. An MMSE score of <29–30 in a person of working age is unusual (anxiety may compromise performance). An MMSE score <24 indicates significant cognitive difficulties
- Referral to a psychologist for formal cognitive assessment.

Prognosis

- Prognosis depends on cause and the outcome of treatment
- The prognosis of dementia is one of declining cognitive function, and employment cannot usually be sustained in the medium term
- *Workplace adjustments:*
  - highly structured/routine work
  - regular supportive supervision
  - predictable workload.
- *Factors that reduce the feasibility of remaining at work:*
  - highly variable work pattern
  - high decision latitude
  - multi-tasking
  - time pressures
  - cognitively demanding work
  - behavioural problems.
- Caution should be exercised in assessing workers in safety critical posts or key decision-makers.

Medical management

- Identify reasonably practicable workplace adjustments
- If, despite adjustments, the worker is unable to cope with his/her current post, he/she may be eligible for ill-health retirement (if the condition is progressive and untreatable).

Relevant legislation

The Equality Act 2010.

---

1 Folstein MF, Folstein SE, McHugh PR (1975). 'Mini-mental State': a practical method for grading the cognitive state of patients for the clinician. *Psychiatry Res*, **12**, 189–98.

Depression

Types The most common type of depression is unipolar depression; bipolar disorder (manic depression) affects around 1%.

Prevalence

- *Major depressive episode:* males – 1.9%. females – 2.8%
- *Mixed anxiety and depression:* males – 6.9%, females – 11.0%
- *Lifetime risk of depression:* 10–12% in men, 20–26% in women.

Causation

Predisposing factors

- Genetic (> ×2 increased risk if first degree relative affected)
- Adverse childhood experiences
- Previous history of depression
- Underlying physical illness.

Precipitating factors

- Major adverse life events
- Physical illness, e.g. onset, worsening of symptoms
- Drug therapy, e.g. corticosteroids
- Work-related difficulties, especially bullying.

Perpetuating factors

- Lack of confiding relationship with partner
- Misuse of alcohol or drugs
- Combination of work and domestic problems
- Isolation and lack of adequate support.

Diagnostic assessment

- *Classification:*
  - DSM-IV (APA) – 'Major depressive disorder'
  - ICD10 (WHO) – 'Depressive episode'/'Recurrent depressive disorder'
  - both sets of criteria require impairment of social, *occupational* or other important areas of functioning.

Clinical treatment

- *Psychological:*
  - CBT – linking thoughts, feeling and behaviours to challenge negative patterns of thinking
- *Pharmacological:*
  - SSRIs most commonly used, e.g fluoxetine, sertraline, citalopram
  - Other drugs include, e.g. mirtazapine, venlafaxine, agomelatine
  - Maintain treatment for at least 6mths from point of maximum recovery (2yrs if recurrent depression)
- Relapse rate of major depression: 60% in 5yrs if untreated.

Occupational health input

Facilitate early referral for psychiatric assessment/psychological treatment.

Fitness for work

- *Performance:*
  - poor motivation
  - reduced concentration and poor decision-making
  - lack of confidence
  - impaired communication, withdrawal and/or irritability
  - lack of energy
  - antidepressant medication.
- *Sickness absence:*
  - significant impairment of performance
  - non-compliance with medication
  - side effects of medication
  - premature reduction of dose.

Fitness to attend disciplinary hearing

- Legal fitness to plead criteria relate mainly to capacity. Main question is whether the employee understands the allegations and their significance—can they take part in the decision making process?
- Useful guide to cognitive ability is the employee's own correspondence with the employer
- Understandable that employee is likely to feel anxious and preoccupied, and to eat and sleep badly around the time of any hearing but postponement of the hearing can only protract and intensify this natural reaction
- Speedy resolution helps to prevent chronicity and secondary morbidity, and can help both parties move on
- Location of the hearing is important; the workplace might be too aversive and a meeting in the employee's home would be intrusive. Therefore a neutral location, e.g. hotel suite, might be more acceptable.

Time off work

See 📖 p. 308, Stress 1 recognition and assessment; 📖 p. 311, Stress 2: interventions/risk control.

Rehabilitation and reasonable adjustments at work

- 'Round-table' discussions can be helpful:
  - shared problem-solving approach
  - OH, HR, employee, manager +/– treating psychiatrist/psychologist
  - realistic goal setting, job definition, and work routine
  - agreed hours and days of work, and how these change over time
  - manager's involvement
  - preparation of work colleagues for employee's return.

Further information

Workplace intervention for people with common mental health problems: Evidence review and recommendations. British Occupational Health Research Foundation, available at: 🔗 http://www.bohrf.org.uk/downloads/cmh_rev.pdf

Chronic fatigue syndrome/myalgic encephalomyelitis

There is a broad range of disability among patients with CFS. Some at the mild end of the spectrum manage to work normally, while others will need protracted adjustments to work.

- Intervention studies have shown that ~30–60% of chronic fatigue syndrome/myalgic encephalomyelitis (CFS/ME) patients do not return to work after treatment. Between 25 and 42% of CFS/ME patients are on disability benefits
- Work status is an important predictor of recovery. CFS/ME patients who are out of work have a poor overall prognosis compared with those who manage to maintain some employment (even after adjustment for severity)
- Low likelihood of a good treatment outcome in CFS/ME predicted by:
  - severe symptoms
  - psychiatric co-morbidity
  - long duration of symptoms.

The prediction of return to work might be assumed for practical purposes to reflect these factors, although, because few studies look at work outcomes, there is little direct evidence on this question.

Medical management of CFS/ME

The approach to clinical management follows a bio-psychosocial model. It is recognized that outcome is greatly influenced by psychosocial factors including illness beliefs, personal experience, personality, and coping skills. Treatment includes:

- A multidisciplinary approach to rehabilitation, including the input of physicians, pain specialists, psychologists, dieticians, physiotherapists, and sometimes alternative therapists
- Medical control of symptoms (e.g. treating pain and sleep disturbance)
- Management of comorbid conditions (e.g. depression)
- Of the specific treatment modalities, CBT and graded exercise therapy (GET) have been shown to be effective for CFS/ME, although GET is not popular among patients
- Employers or insurance companies will sometimes fund or facilitate treatment by multidisciplinary clinical teams. This is particularly helpful in view of the scarcity of NHS resources in this area.

Adjustments to work in CFS/ME

It may be difficult for an employer to implement or sustain prolonged adjustments to work. Therefore, it is important that there is close liaison between treating physicians and allied specialists, OH advisers, managers, and HR advisers in supporting a return to work. In CFS/ME it is best if a work rehabilitation can be coordinated as part of an overall graded activity programme.

- A protracted phasing up of working hours with a low baseline (e.g. 2–3h, 2–3 days/week) and very gradual increase may be necessary. It may take many months (or even more than a year in some cases) to reach premorbid working hours

- If a long commute to work exacerbates fatigue, home working or a change of work site should be considered. Alternatively, working hours can be tailored to avoid peak traffic times
- Frequent rest breaks should be built in to the work schedule
- Reduction in heavy physical work or repetitive work is sometimes appropriate
- Permanently reduced hours of work may be required for those unable to return to their previous contracted hours.

💣 Tolerance of a higher level of sickness absence by the employer might be reasonably expected if there are frequent exacerbations of symptoms.

Overlap with other conditions

There is considerable overlap between CFS/ME and a number of other conditions for which the precise pathology and aetiology are unknown, including fibromyalgia and irritable bowel syndrome. For example, 20–70% of patients with fibromyalgia meet the diagnostic definition for CFS/ME, and 35–70% of patients with CFS/ME could also be defined as having fibromyalgia.

Relevant legislation

The Equality Act 2010 would apply to individuals with CFS/ME and employers would be expected to make reasonable adjustments to work.

Further information and guidance

NHS Plus/Department of Health (2006). *Occupational aspects of the management of chronic fatigue syndrome: a National Guideline*, related leaflets for employers and employees. Available at: 🔗 http://www.nhsplus.nhs.uk/providers/clinicaleffectiveness-guidelines.asp

Diabetes mellitus

Terminology and diagnostic criteria

- Type 1 usually develops in childhood and adolescence.
- Type 2 predominantly occurs in adults and accounts for 90% of cases.

WHO criteria for diagnosis

Depends on symptoms of diabetes (polydypsia, polyuria and weight loss) plus:

- a random venous plasma glucose › 11.1mmol/L *or*
- a fasting plasma glucose concentration ›7.0mmol/L (whole blood ›6.1mmol/L) *or*
- plasma glucose concentration ›11.1mmol/L 2h after 75g anhydrous glucose in an oral glucose tolerance test.

If asymptomatic the diagnosis requires at least one additional glucose test result on another day.

General occupational health considerations

Fitness to work should be based on an individual risk assessment taking into account the nature of the work, the health status of the worker and how well their diabetes is controlled. A report from the individual's specialist or GP may be useful. Employers must make reasonable adjustments to employee's duties as required by the Equality Act 2010.

From an occupational aspect, the most important clinical complications of diabetes are:

- *Hypoglycaemia:* premonitory warning signs include hunger, sweating and dizziness, but these may be reduced or absent. Risk factors for hypoglycaemia are:
  - treatment with insulin or sulphonylureas
  - poor compliance with medication or diet
  - excessive exercise
  - alcohol
  - renal failure
  - intensification of treatment.
- *Impaired visual acuity:* proliferative retinopathy, maculopathy and pan-retinal laser photocoagulation may bring individuals below DVLA standards for Group 1 driving
- *Neuropathy:* this may lead to a reduction in fine motor skills, reduced positional awareness and postural hypotension. Sensory loss leads to an increased risk of accidental damage to peripheral tissues.

Sickness absence

Studies of sickness absence in employees with diabetes show increases in absence rates (estimates between 50–100% increase compared with non-diabetics). However, the better controlled the diabetes, the less likely the person is to take sick leave.

Shiftwork

In theory, timing of insulin and meals can be difficult with rotating shifts. However, modern insulin treatments have made shift work less problematic than previously and most diabetics cope well.

Safety critical jobs

In the UK, people on insulin are barred from some jobs e.g. airline pilot, the Armed Forces. The jobs for which there is a blanket ban are frequently reviewed and the latest list is available from Diabetes UK. Since October 2011, insulin-treated diabetics have been able to apply for a group 2 driving license, subject to strict DVLA qualifying criteria.

A careful risk assessment needs to be done to assess the suitability of people with insulin-treated diabetes for employment where there may be a risk of injury or harm to the individual or the public, for example firefighting. Suitability for such employment should be assessed annually by an occupational health professional in consultation with a diabetes specialist; and should be based on the following criteria:

- Be physically and mentally fit in accordance with non-diabetic standards
- Be under regular (at least annual) specialist review and their diabetic control must be stable
- Be well motivated and be able to self-monitor their glucose levels at least bd
- Have full awareness of hypoglycaemic symptoms
- Be able to demonstrate an understanding of the risks of hypoglycaemia.

Further information and guidance

DVLA. *At a glance guide to the current medical standards of fitness to drive.* Available at: ℜ http://www.dft.gov.uk/dvla/medical/ataglance.aspx

Diabetes, UK. *Meet our new Peer Support Network.* Available at: ℜ http://www.diabetes.org.uk/

Epilepsy

Defined by the International League Against Epilepsy (ILEA) as two or more epileptic seizures unprovoked by any immediate identifiable cause.

Epidemiology

Depends on definition, but the most commonly quoted statistics are:
- Prevalence 5–10 per 1000 population
- Incidence 50 (range 40–70) first fits per 100,000 population/yr.

Clinical classification of seizures

Partial seizures
- Simple partial seizures (no loss of consciousness)
- *Complex partial seizures:*
  - with impairment of consciousness at onset
  - simple partial onset followed by impairment of consciousness
  - partial seizures evolving to generalized tonic–clonic (GTC) seizures.

Generalized seizures
Convulsive or non-convulsive with bilateral discharges involving subcortical structures:
- Absence
- Myoclonic
- Clonic
- Tonic
- Tonic–clonic
- Atonic.

Unclassified epileptic seizures
Usually used when an adequate description is not available.

Treatment and prognosis

Treatment
Treatment is with anticonvulsants. Chronic stable treatment rarely affects performance significantly. Acute drug over-dosage can cause serious impairment, but is rapidly reversible.

Prognosis
The risk of further seizures depends on the clinical situation:
- *First seizure (see Fig. 23.2):*
  - 67% have a second seizure within 12mths
  - if seizure-free for 6mths, 30% have a further seizure within 12mths
- *Established epilepsy (more than one seizure):*
  - most patients who achieve remission (seizure-free for 5yrs) do so within the first 2yrs; >95% remain seizure-free for 10yrs
  - approximately 20–30% will have further seizures despite treatment
  - the risk of further seizures ↑ with ↑ duration of poor control and ↑ frequency, combination of partial and tonic–clonic seizures, structural cerebral lesions, and impairment of cerebral function.

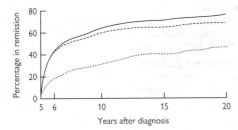

Fig. 23.2 Actuarial percentage recurrences after first seizure and after 6, 12, and 18mths without seizures (From Hart YM, Sander JW, Johnson AL, Shorvon SD (1990). National General Practice Study of Epilepsy. *Lancet*, **8726**, 1271–4. Reproduced by kind permission of Elsevier.)

Fitness for work
General issues
Advice about fitness for work should consider the risk to the individual and to others (e.g. passengers). ⚠ Never base risk assessment on the label of epilepsy, but on individual clinical and job details.

Specific issues
- *High-risk activities:* restrict those with epilepsy from:
  - lone working
  - working at heights
  - swimming or working unprotected near water
  - working with dangerous or unguarded machinery, or fire
  - carrying out or assisting at surgical procedures
  - sole care of dependent (e.g. ventilated or unconscious) patients
  - sole manual handling of patients, e.g. carrying infants
  - usually excluded: aircrew, armed forces, police, firefighters
- *Driving:* see DVLA guidance, but in general:
  - *group 1* – restrict until seizure-free for 1yr (+/– treatment), unless seizures only occur during sleep, and the last seizure was >3yrs ago
  - *group 2* – restrict until seizure-free *off* treatment for 10yrs (5yrs if seizure due to substance abuse and abuse is controlled)
  - advise not to drive during and 6mths after treatment withdrawal
  - provoked seizures (e.g. eclampsia) will be advised on an individual case basis by the DVLA
- Jobs that are associated with sleep disturbance or fatigue (e.g. shift work) are not contraindicated, but can exacerbate epilepsy
- Visual display equipment is associated with an extremely low risk of seizure provocation, and it is usually inappropriate to restrict.

Disclosure
Individuals are often reluctant to disclose a diagnosis of epilepsy; 50% do not declare it at pre-employment assessment. It can be useful to inform the line manager, but only with the individual's consent.

Adjustments to work

Diagnosis of epilepsy likely to qualify under Disability Discrimination Act 1995/2005. Where practical, employer must provide adjustments/redeployment as indicated by a risk assessment.

Further information and guidance

DVLA. *At a glance guide to the current medical standards of fitness to drive.* Available at: ℅ http://www.dft.gov.uk/dvla/medical/ataglance.aspx

Alcohol misuse and fitness for work

- An increasing use of alcohol (especially among women) means that more workers are likely to present with alcohol misuse or alcoholism
- People who are alcohol dependent may not accept that a problem exists, making management challenging
- Initial signs and symptoms of alcohol misuse may go unrecognized or be 'overlooked' by well-intentioned colleagues.

Guidelines on sensible drinking limits

	Men	Women
Daily consumption	3–4U	2–3U
Weekly consumption		
Safe drinking	21U	14U
Hazardous	22–50U	15–35U
Harmful	>50U	>35U

- ▶ Binge drinking is defined as consuming, in one episode, 8–10U for men and 6–8U for women
- A unit of alcohol is 10mL, by volume, of pure alcohol.

Epidemiology

- 22% of UK men drink more than 21U/wk
- 6% of UK men drink more than 50U/wk
- 22% of UK women drink more than 14U/wk
- 6% of UK women drink more than 36U/wk
- Alcohol-related deaths doubled from 4023 in 1992 to 8664 in 2009
- 17% of deaths on UK roads in 2009 were alcohol related
- 5% of road casualties in 2009 involved someone driving 'over the limit'.

'Soft' signs of substance misuse

- Variable work performance
- ↑ Accidents
- ↑ Errors
- ↑ Complaints
- ↑ Absenteeism, especially around weekends and holidays
- Poor time-keeping.

Clinical assessment and diagnosis

Workers may be referred to the OH service because of ↑ sickness absence, ↓ performance, work attendance while intoxicated, or alcohol consumption at work. Not all will have alcoholism.

It is helpful when referring an employee to the OH service if the manager gives examples of workplace difficulties. This may alert the occupational physician to the possibility of alcohol misuse. If suspected, then explore the following:

- The employee's perceptions of their difficulties
- Medical history, focusing on illnesses associated with alcohol misuse:
  - dyspepsia
  - jaundice
  - cirrhosis
  - cardiac arrhythmia
  - peripheral neuropathy
  - hypertension
- Alcohol history
- Family history of alcohol misuse
- Accidents or assaults
- Money problems due to alcohol misuse
- Legal problems, e.g. drink driving convictions
- Clinical examination, seeking the stigmata of alcoholism
- Use the Alcohol Use Disorders Identification Test (AUDIT) to establish severity of misuse
- If cognitive difficulties are suspected, arrange a cognitive assessment.

Prognosis

- The prognosis for a worker with alcoholism is guarded.
- Some problem drinkers aim for 'controlled drinking'. In practice, this is rarely achieved and may indicate a failure to acknowledge the problem.
- Special caution should be exercised in assessing workers in safety critical posts, such as vocational drivers, or key decision-makers.
  - See also 📖 p. 472, Fitness to drive 1; 📖 p. 474, Fitness to drive 2
  - See also 📖 p. 504, Fitness for safety critical work.

Alcohol testing

Where supported by an alcohol policy, pre-employment, with cause, or random breath or blood alcohol testing may be undertaken.

Medical management

- Identify a treatment provider, usually via the GP
- In-patient care for assisted alcohol withdrawal is not usually required, but may be required in those;
  - consuming >30U/day
  - with significant co-morbidities
  - history of seizures or delirium tremens
- Agree a contract with the worker for regular follow-up including, where obtainable, regular reports from treatment agency
- A sustained period of abstinence is required before any return to work
- Once at work, monitor time-keeping, performance, and absences
- Prolonged OH service follow-up (up to 12mths) may be appropriate.

Relevant guidance and legislation

- The Equality Act 2010
- Faculty of Occupational Medicine (2006). *Guidance on alcohol and drug misuse in the workplace.* FOM, London.

Further information and guidance
- NICE (2012). *Alcohol dependence and harmful alcohol use*. NICE Clinical Guidance CG115. Available at: ℛ http://www.nice.org.uk/CG115
- See also ⊞ p. 378, Substance abuse policies.

Fitness for specific work

Fitness to drive 1

The DVLA is responsible for licensing drivers in the UK.
- Group 1 drivers are licensed to drive cars and motorbikes
- Group 2 drivers are licensed to drive buses and lorries
  (passenger-carrying vehicle (PCV) and large goods vehicle (LGV)
  licenses).

Ultimately, it is for the DVLA's medical advisers to determine an individual's fitness to drive. However, if driving is a special requirement of a job, employers may make their own assessment of fitness.

Driving for employment purposes

Decisions about fitness for vocational driving may be challenged under the Equality Act. Therefore OH professionals should carry out a risk assessment, and be prepared to justify their advice. Examples where Group 2 standards may be applied are as follows:
- Driving in hazardous areas such as quarries or construction sites
- Driving emergency response vehicles (ambulances, police cars, fire engines):
  - the NHS employing authority determines whether Group 2 standards shall apply to their ambulance drivers
  - ◆ *Note* that insulin-dependent diabetics have been advised by the Medical Advisory Panel on Diabetes and Driving not to drive emergency vehicles. However, this is an extremely contentious issue, and the situation may be subject to change
- Carrying passengers (see 📖 p. 474, Fitness to drive 2).
  ◆ The Medical Commission on Accident Prevention (now discontinued) recommended that Group 2 fitness standards be applied to taxi drivers, by their local authority, prior to licensing. More than half of local authorities follow this advice
- Driving large vehicles (see 📖 p. 474, Fitness to drive 2).

General principles

- It is the duty of the license holder to notify the DVLA of any medical condition, or change to a medical condition, which may affect his/her fitness to drive
- Drivers need not notify the DVLA if their medical condition is not expected to last >3mths, but they should be guided by medical advice and refrain from driving if advised to do so
- Any person suffering from a medical condition that is likely to cause sudden incapacity should not drive
- Any person who is unable to control his/her vehicle safely should not drive.

Assessment frequency

- A Group 1 license is valid until age 70, and thereafter is renewable every 3yrs
- License applications must be accompanied by a self-declaration of fitness.

Specific medical conditions

The DVLA publishes extensive guidance on fitness to drive in respect of a range of important medical conditions (see 📖 p. 473, Legislation and guidance).

Ethical issues

- Where an employee is medically unfit to drive, the OH doctor should confirm that the employee understands that his/her condition may impair his/her fitness to drive
- The doctor should advise the employee verbally, and in writing, of his/her legal duty to notify the DVLA if he/she is medically unfit to drive. This advice should be recorded in the medical records
- If an employee who is medically unfit to drive refuses to notify the DVLA, then the doctor should offer to arrange a second medical opinion on the understanding that the employee does not drive pending reassessment
- The GMC advises that a doctor should make every reasonable effort to persuade an individual who is unfit to drive not to do so
- If an individual continues to drive despite the advice, then the DVLA medical adviser should be informed in confidence (having first advised the employee in writing of the intention to do so).

⚠ Always check current GMC guidance before notifying the DVLA in this situation.

Adjustments to driving work

- An OH professional should advise reasonable adjustments to the job (including adaptations to vehicles) if this would enable an employee, whose ability to drive is impaired by a medical condition, to work
- Such adjustments would be a matter of good practice for all employees. However, the employer has a legal obligation if the Equality Act applies
- Disabled drivers and their advisers can access expert advice and driving assessment through the forum of mobility centers. ℘ http://www.mobility-centres.org.uk

Legislation/guidance

- At a Glance Guide to the Current Medical Standards of Fitness to Drive—A Guide for Medical Practitioners, February 2011. Available online (and updated every 6mths) at: ℘ http://www.dft.gov.uk/dvla/medical/ataglance.aspx
- General Medical Council Guidance for Doctors. Confidentiality: Protecting and Providing Information FAQs #17. Available at: ℘ http://www.gmc-uk.org/index.asp
- *Medical Aspects of Fitness to Drive*. Medical Commission on Accident Prevention, London, 1995.

Fitness to drive 2

LGV/PCV drivers

The DVLA sets the fitness standards for UK drivers, including drivers of LGVs or PCVs with more than eight seats.

General principles

The fitness standards for HGV or PCV drivers (Group 2 drivers) are more stringent than these for Group 1 drivers. The reasons for this are the higher annual mileages driven by occupational drivers and the potentially greater consequences of an accident involving an HGV or PCV.

Assessment frequency

A Group 2 license is usually issued at age 21, and is valid until age 45 unless medical fitness changes. Thereafter, it is subject to review every 5yrs, or shorter periods depending on medical conditions until age 65. After age 65 licenses are renewable annually.

Specific issues

- It is the duty of the license holder to notify the DVLA of any medical condition that may affect his/her fitness to drive
- Any person suffering from a medical condition likely to cause sudden incapacity should not drive
- Any person unable to control his/her vehicle safely should not drive
- A medical practitioner must prepare a medical report using Form D4.

Medical assessment

- Height
- Weight
- Smoking history
- Alcohol consumption
- Current medication
- Corrected visual acuity >6/9 in the better eye and >6/12 in the other eye with uncorrected visual acuity being >3/60 in each eye
- Visual fields intact
- Medical history
  - epilepsy
  - other neurological conditions
  - diabetes
  - psychiatric illness
  - cardiovascular disease
  - blood pressure
  - musculoskeletal disease sufficient to interfere with vehicle control.

The final decision regarding fitness for Group 2 driving lies with the DVLA's medical adviser and not the examining doctor.

Forklift truck operators

Task demands

Operation of a forklift truck, whether in a factory, on a farm, or on a building site, can be associated with the following hazards:

- Proximity to other vehicles and people

- Noisy environments
- Relatively confined spaces
- Frequent reversing and manoeuvring.

General principles

- There are no regulations governing fitness to operate forklifts on private ground. HSE has published useful guidance (see 📖 p. 475, Legislation and guidance)
- If the forklift is to be operated on the public highway, the operator must meet current DVLA standards on fitness to drive
- Operators should be 17 or over. Construction workers must be age 18. Agricultural workers should be over school-leaving age
- The fitness required is only that sufficient for the task to be carried out safely and efficiently. Individuals with a disability should be assessed bearing in mind good employment practices and disability legislation.

Fitness requirements

Include good eyesight, adequate hearing, and reasonable head/neck mobility. The ability to look over the shoulder is important; no condition that predisposes to sudden loss of consciousness.

Assessment frequency

- Assess at pre-employment
- Assess at 5-yearly intervals from age 40
- Over age 65 review annually
- An operator with a medical condition should be reviewed more frequently if this is indicated.

Specific issues

- Visual acuity should be 6/12 (corrected) with adequate visual fields
- Hearing should be sufficient to understand instructions and warnings
- Alcohol/drug addiction renders a worker unfit to operate a lift truck
- Careful assessment is necessary where there is a history of psychosis
- Poorly controlled angina or conditions predisposing to loss of consciousness (arrhythmias, transient ischaemic attack (TIAs)) are a bar to work with lift trucks
- Epilepsy is acceptable where the criteria for a car license are met
- Diabetes is permitted subject to good glycaemic control. Loss of awareness of hypoglycaemia will probably render the diabetic unfit
- Musculoskeletal problems should not significantly impair the driver's ability to look up, sideways, or over the shoulder.

Legislation and guidance

- A guide to vehicle licensing requirements including definitions of license categories and vehicles is given at: ℘ http://direct.gov.uk/
- HSE (2000). *Safety in Working with Lift Trucks*, HS(G)6. HSE, London. Available at: ℘ http://www.hse.gov.uk/pubns/priced/hsg6.pdf

Fitness for professional diving

Purpose

To establish whether a worker is fit to undertake diving at work and to identify, at an early stage, diving-related illnesses such as dysbaric osteonecrosis. Difficulties may arise when individuals undertake diving activity for hire or reward and do so out with (and in breach of) regulations (see ⬛ p. 544, Diving at Work Regulations 1997).

General principles

- Statutory medical assessments can only be carried out by an HSE approved medical examiner of divers. The examiner has to satisfy the HSE that they have the required knowledge of diving medicine to carry out this work. Usually, this knowledge is acquired by attending a 5-day diving medicine course
- The initial medical assessment involves the prospective diver completing a medical questionnaire, which is then validated by his/her GP. The approved medical examiner then reviews this and advises whether the individual has a medical condition that would disqualify him/her from diving without a full assessment
- Prior to commencing diver training the prospective diver should undergo a full diving medical examination. The results of this are recorded on form MA2 which includes the certificate of fitness to dive. The white copy of MA2 is given to the diver and the pink lower copy should be retained by the medical examiner for 7yrs
- Where a diver is found unfit to dive, he/she has the right to appeal this decision to HSE within 28 days.

Assessment frequency

- The medical certificate is valid for any period stipulated by the examining doctor up to a maximum of 12mths
  - Where a diver is medically unfit for work for >14 days *or* suffers a neurological, cardiorespiratory, or ear disorder, his/her fitness to dive must be reassessed by an approved examiner.

Specific issues

- Female divers should not dive when pregnant
- CXR and long-bone views are only required where clinically indicated
- The British Thoracic Society has issued guidelines on respiratory aspects of fitness for diving
- Extensive guidance on diving fitness standards is provided in the HSE publication MA1 which is available on the HSE website. The underlying principle is that the diver should not be at increased risk of a diving accident because of an existing medical condition.

Investigations required at diving medical

Initial examination	Annual review
Exercise testing (step test)	Exercise testing (step test)
Resting ECG	Resting ECG (5-yearly from age 40)
Urinalysis	Urinalysis
Spirometry	Spirometry
Audiometry	
Full blood count	

Relevant legislation and guidance

- Diving at Work Regulations 1997
- HSE *The Medical Examination and Assessment of Divers*, MA1. HSE Books, London. Available at: ℜ http://www.hse.gov.uk/diving/ma1.pdf
- British Thoracic Society (2003). Guidelines on respiratory aspects of fitness for diving. *Thorax*, **58**, 3–13.

Fitness for work in food handlers

Definition of a food handler

A food handler manufactures, prepares, or transports food, and may come into direct contact with the food or with machines handling unwrapped food. This definition includes engineers, cleaners, and those visiting the premises. The definition also includes those preparing or serving food in canteens and shops.

Health screening

Fitness for work is assessed by health screening. The screening process aims to exclude individuals with medical conditions that may pose a risk of microbiological or general contamination of food products. The assessment should also identify conditions that may be caused or exacerbated by work, or jeopardize employee safety. Therefore, it should identify the following:

- Those suffering from, or carriers of, infectious disease which can be transmitted to the product, e.g. Norovirus infection of the GI tract
- Those suffering from conditions, such as an infected wound or skin condition, which can transmit pathogens
- Those suffering from conditions (e.g. respiratory/musculoskeletal) which may be exacerbated by work or make work unsafe (allergies/blackouts).

Screening process

A questionnaire is completed before starting work, by visitors, or existing employees returning from absence from work. Examples of questions are shown in the box opposite. Those with no positive answers can start work; those with a positive response must be assessed by a competent OH professional. Questionnaires are confidential and must be handled as sensitive information under the Data Protection Act.

▶ By law all food handlers must receive training in food hygiene.

Legislation and guidance

- NHS Plus, Royal College of Physicians, Faculty of Occupational Medicine (2008). *Infected food handlers: occupational aspects of management. A national guideline.* RCP, London. Available at: ℘ http://www.nhsplus.nhs.uk/providers/clinicaleffectiveness-guidelines-evidence based.asp
- Food Handlers: Fitness to Work. Food Standards Agency. ℘ http://www.food.gov.uk/multimedia/pdfs/publication/fitnesstoworkguide09v2.pdf

Fitness for air passenger travel 1: the physics and physiology of air travel

Many employees are required to fly as part of their job. This can cover a large spectrum from frequent to infrequent flying, and short to long-haul flight. The main issues to consider when advising about air travel are summarized here.

Relative hypoxia

- Most passenger aircraft are pressurized to between 4000 and 8000 feet at their cruising altitude. This 20–30% reduction in air pressure results in a reduction of the partial pressure of oxygen inspired
- Due to the sigmoid nature of the oxyhaemoglobin dissociation curve, this only results in about a 10% fall in oxyhaemoglobin saturation in healthy people (Fig. 24.1)
- However, those with significant lung disease and a degree of hypoxia will operate on the steeper section of the curve (Fig. 24.1). They are at risk of significant desaturation. The risk varies between patients, particularly depending on hypoxic drive
- As a rough guide, in-flight oxygen is likely to be needed if the individual's oxygen saturation (SaO_2) at sea level is less than 90%.

Pressure change

The reduction in ambient pressure also results in an increase in volume of any gas trapped in a body cavity:

PV = constant (Boyle's law).

Gas expansion in an aircraft cabin can be of the order of 20–40%. This is demonstrated by the need to 'clear the (middle) ears' when ascending or descending. Other closed and semi-closed cavities will be similarly affected.

⚠ In ascending to altitude, passengers are effectively decompressing in a similar way to an ascending diver. Therefore, travellers who have been on diving holidays should carefully plan their last days of diving to reduce the risk of decompression illness during their flight home.

Low humidity

The air conditioning of cabin air results in low humidity and can lead to a modest drying of mucous membranes. There is no evidence that even the longest flight would contribute to passengers becoming dehydrated.

Seated immobility

- Air travel leads to long periods of sitting with limited posture changes. Flights longer than 4h are considered a risk factor for developing DVT
- Travellers with pre-existing risk factors (e.g. recent surgery, known clotting disorders, malignancy, etc.) should seek medical advice. Preventative strategies range from leg exercises/stockings to medication (e.g. aspirin, heparin).

Noise and motion

Noise (engine noise, cabin ventilation systems, and airflow over the external surfaces) is not a hazard to hearing, but may be a factor in travel fatigue. Studies have shown that 0.5% of passengers have vomited and 8.4% experience nausea in flight, especially in turbulence.

Stress

New environments, time pressures, and delays can increase stress in vulnerable people. Fear of flying is common and can normally be dismissed, but desensitization is available for the few who are severely affected.

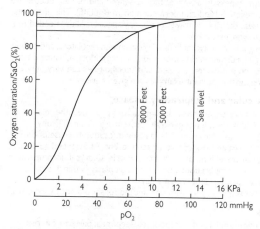

Fig. 24.1. Effect of cabin pressure on oxygen saturation in a healthy passenger. Those with cardiovascular and respiratory disease where SaO_2 is below 90% may operate on the steeper part of the curve with significant desaturation at altitude.

Fitness for air passenger travel 2: specific medical conditions

Medical conditions that need assessment prior to flight can be divided:
- Stable chronic (e.g. chronic obstructive pulmonary disease)
- Chronic with recent change (myocardial infarction and angina)
- Acute (e.g. illness, injury, surgery).

The physiological challenges of air travel outlined on the previous page need to be taken into account in the assessment of fitness to fly.

Most large airlines have medical advisers who advise on fitness to fly. Usually, a few weeks in advance, the passenger and his/her doctor are asked to complete a Medical Information Form (MEDIF). This allows the airline to assess the risks of travel and/or any special facilities needed (e.g. stretcher, oxygen, escort).

Extensive guidance is available from government, regulators, and airlines (see 🕮 p. 483, Further information and guidance). Most guidance is pragmatic and often not evidence based, and specific rules can vary between carriers. The most important examples are given here.

Cardiovascular and respiratory disease
- Broadly, if a passenger can walk 50m without dyspnoea, the relative hypoxia at altitude will not generally present significant difficulty
- Recent cardiovascular event should result in caution because of the relative hypoxia and risk of further acute event. As a general guide, do not allow air travel if myocardial infarct within 10 days if uncomplicated (3–4wks with complications), coronary angioplasty within 3–5 days, cerebrovascular accident within 3 days
- *Pneumothorax:* passengers with pneumothorax should not fly for 6wks.

Diabetes
- Crossing time zones and disruption of sleep/meal patterns can risk destabilizing control
- Diabetic passengers should be advised to stay on home time for medication until arrival
- Modern (basal bolus) regimes make problems less likely with good education, and medication should be carried in hand baggage because of low temperatures in the aircraft hold. Sharps (e.g. needles) must be declared for security reasons.

Pregnancy
Most carriers will allow travel up to the 36th week for single pregnancies and the 32nd week for multiple pregnancies.

Infectious disease
- It is an international health regulation that individuals should not fly during the infectious phase of a contagious disease
- The main risk is the proximity of others (rather than spread via the cabin air, which is filtered) and acute worsening of the condition.

Other

- *Recent surgery:* advise against flying within 10 days, because of risk of trapped gas (eye, abdomen) and DVT
- *ENT conditions:* those affecting Eustachian tube patency can cause tympanic membrane rupture
- *Anaemia:* risk of severe hypoxia if haemoglobin is <7.5g/dL
- *Psychiatric:* patients with acute psychotic illness require an escort and available sedation
- *Fractures:* restrict flying for 24–48h.

On-board facilities for dealing with medical emergencies

All cabin staff are trained in first aid, including defibrillation when automatic external defibrillators (AEDs) are carried. Aircraft are required to carry extensive first aid and medical packs, which include drugs to treat the commonly occurring ailments. Many airlines also subscribe to air-to-ground medical services which can advise crew and medical attendants.

Further information and guidance

Federal Aviation Administration. *Passenger health and safety guidance.* Available at: ℘ http://www.faa.gov/passengers/fly_safe/health/

British Thoracic Society Guidelines (2011). *Air travel guidelines.* Available at: ℘ http://www.brit-thoracic.org.uk/guidelines/air-travel-guideline.aspx

British Lung Foundation leaflet on flying with a lung condition. ℘ http://www.lunguk.org/you-and-your-lungs/living-with-a-lung-condition/air-travel

Fitness for work in professional pilots: commercial pilots/aircrew

Regulation/standards

- The international standards for the medical fitness of aircrew are maintained and updated by the International Civil Aviation Organization (ICAO)
- In the UK, the European Aviation Safety Agency (EASA) currently define standards for airworthiness, operations, and licensing compliant with the ICAO standards. A number of private or sport flying regulations remain under UK Civil Aviation Authority (CAA) oversight
- These regulatory provisions cannot cover every aeromedical situation. Therefore, to facilitate flexibility, 'accredited medical conclusion' (a decision by one or more medical experts), operational limitations, and relevant pilot skill and experience can be taken into account if the licensing authority believes that this would not jeopardize flight safety. However, this flexibility standard has resulted in different national regulators around the world applying different standards.

Medical assessment of pilots

Process

- Aircrew are medically examined annually under the age of 40yrs, and 6-monthly thereafter if undertaking single pilot operations
- A health declaration is completed and a physical examination performed. Clinical tests focus on visual performance and ECG and audiogram when required
- Any pilot not meeting the standard is referred to the regulatory authority, who defines what further investigation/evidence is required
- A medical certificate to fly may be temporarily or permanently suspended at any time if there is a risk to flight safety.

Principles

Fitness for aircrew is based on two broad principles: the physical and mental capability to fly/operate the aircraft, and the risk of an acute incapacitating event whilst flying (which could lead to a fatal accident).

Functional capability

- *Visual acuity:* good vision is required for long distance (to taxi, take off, and land the aircraft under visual conditions), intermediate (reading and operating cockpit instruments), and near distance (reading maps/ flight plans, etc.)
- *Colour vision:* acceptable colour discrimination is required to identify signal lights from air traffic control, and other aircraft, vehicles, buildings, etc.
- *Visual field:* a normal visual field is required to maintain an adequate look-out to identify and avoid other aircraft
- Good hearing is required for communicating with and understanding instructions from air traffic control and other members of the flight crew, sometimes on a noisy flight deck

- Physical operation of aircraft controls and switches, and ability to assist passengers in the event of emergency
- *Psychological stability*: cognitive functions are important in dealing with complex aircraft and air traffic environments. Also, a proportion of accidents worldwide have been attributed to untreated depressive illness, alcohol and substance misuse, and the suicidal intent of one or more of the crew.

Incapacitation risk

- Over the last two decades in the UK and elsewhere, and latterly within the European member states, an annual medical incapacitation risk limit of 1% has been applied in two-pilot public transport operations. This is known as the '1% rule', and assumes a target all-cause fatal accident rate for large public transport aircraft of 1 per 10^7 flying hours, not more than 10% of which should be due to one system failure (e.g. pilot failure), and not more than 10% of system failures should be due to a subsystem failure (e.g. medical incapacitation)
- This gives a target fatal accident rate due to aircrew medical incapacitation of 1 accident per 10^9h. This is almost unachievable in single-pilot operations
- The times during which the aircraft is closest to the ground (i.e. take-off and initial climb, and approach and landing) are the accident-critical phases. At the time the 1% rule was formulated, it was considered that in-flight incapacitation of one of the pilots would result in a fatal accident in about one in 1000 such events. Therefore in order to achieve the target medical cause fatal accident rate of one accident per 10^9h, neither pilot should have a risk of medical incapacitation greater than one in 10^6h, i.e. approximately 1% in 1yr. Note that the maximum DVLA Group 2 (LGV) driving risk is 2%.
- ☞ However, since its development there have been important changes to airline operations. Flights have become longer and aircraft more automated, so a higher risk might be tolerable whilst maintaining flight safety. Some States accept risks of 2% per annum, although this has not been accepted universally.

Cabin crew

Cabin crew fitness is currently not formally regulated in the UK, and there is no published work supporting health standards in relation to safety. New EASA standards for cabin crew are to be introduced based on an initial medical examination followed by periodic reassessment. Clinical examination/investigation is only required if an abnormality or condition is disclosed/discovered. Most airlines rely on a focused health enquiry by questionnaire, which relates to international travel health and providing regular and efficient service. This minimizes operational difficulties due to recurrent sickness absence.

Further information

ICAO. Available at: ☞ http://www.icao.int/Pages/default.aspxpilots/aircrew

Fitness for military service

Recruits

Principles of screening

- Recruits to the armed forces must undergo intensive training, which is physically arduous and mentally taxing. They need to be of robust constitution, free from disease and injury. Given the investment placed in individuals in military training, those who are likely to be lost from training on medical grounds need to be screened out
- On completion of training, personnel may operate in locations remote from medical care, and in situations where illness or injury of one individual may have profound and immediate effects on units
- Opportunities for flexibility of employment are very limited, and to remain in the military most individuals will need to be fit for unrestricted active service (i.e. at sea or on operations)
- This isolation means that medical follow-up of existing conditions can be impossible, and medication may not be available
- An initial engagement in the military can be for many years, and so any chronic effects from past conditions or injuries must be considered
- These all mitigate towards setting a high initial standard of fitness for the military. This standard needs to be generic since many different centres are providing recruitment medicals. The minimum standards apply across all three services, but certain branches of the military, notably aircrew and divers, have higher requirements (see 📖 p. 487).

Screening process

- In the UK, initial medicals will normally be carried out by uniformed or civilian medical officers on contract to MOD, and where appropriate a full history will also be obtained from the recruit's GP. Specialist referral may be necessary
- Candidate is assessed using a grading system PULHHEEMS and compared with a pre-determined profile for his/her chosen specialization
- If successful, following the medical examination, the candidate will be required to complete a fitness assessment.

In service

- Many countries maintain a separate military health system. In the UK this is limited to responsibilities for primary care (including occupational health, community mental health, and rehabilitation) and operational medical care. Secondary care is the responsibility of the NHS, although some cases may be fast tracked to obtain an early return to service
- Decisions on fitness for work are the prerogative of service medical officers and MOD civilian medical practitioners. NHS GPs may only treat military personnel as temporary residents, and can only certify them as unfit to travel rather than unfit to work
- A detailed system of Medical Employability Standards (MESs) describing capability in each environment has now been introduced

- Where individuals fall below standards in the long term (normally >12mths), they will be required to appear before a medical board to assess functional capacity. The relevant service personnel departments will subsequently decide if they can continue to serve under specified restrictions. If long-term employment is not available, they will be medically retired.

Specific medical conditions affecting fitness for entry to UK Armed Services

- Personnel with a history of anxiety do not do well in the armed forces, and so equal weight must be given to mental fitness. Repeated self-harm, mood disorders, and ongoing medication will normally be a bar to entry
- Chronic medical conditions such as asthma, epilepsy, eczema, and migraine are usually incompatible with service
- Orthopaedic conditions or injuries, particularly affecting the lower limbs, are likely to prejudice new entry training
- There are specific eyesight requirements for individual branches and services, as well as an overall minimum generic standard. If in doubt, a proper opthalmological evaluation is essential
- Conditions requiring regular medication, specific diets, and allergies will normally be unacceptable for service because of operational constraints affecting supply, catering, etc.
- Many conditions, such as cardiological murmurs, will require formal specialist evaluation
- Further information is available from Armed Forces Careers Offices.

Military pilots

In the UK and many countries, civilian aviation authorities have no jurisdiction over aircraft on the military register. Furthermore, the high medical standards set for commercial aircrew in order to ensure flight and passenger safety are not always enough to satisfy the demands of military flying. Therefore, a separate system of standards and regulatory systems is required. These are additional to the considerations that apply to any military recruit outlined here.

Standards

- In view of joint operations with other air forces, some joint standardization is also necessary
- These standards will be reflected in a system of medical grading which should only be applied by those specifically trained and familiar with the requirement
- There may be an additional requirement imposed for aptitude testing, and cognitive testing may form part of a separate non-medical assessment. May include ability to tolerate high G forces where appropriate.

Medical standards for military pilots

The following are relevant in the assessment of medical standards for military pilots:

• Flight safety	• Risk of incapacitation
• Aviation environment	• Hypoxia, hypobaria, acceleration, extremes of temperature, noise, vibration
• Mission accomplishment	• Ability to complete task
• Operational efficiency	• Ability to perform task repeatedly
• Cost effectiveness	• Is outcome worth investment
• Escape and evasion	• Ability to survive if shot down
• Nuclear biological chemical	• Ability to operate warfare environment
• War role	

Relevant legislation

The Armed Services are currently exempt from the disability provisions of The Equality Act 2010.

Fitness for work in health care

Definition

HCWs are those whose work involves medical management of patients, and wider aspects of their health and social care. Health care work is one of the most common occupations in the UK, including almost 2 million employees in the public (NHS) and private sectors.

Three groups of HCW have been defined for practical purposes:

- *Clinical and other staff:* including those in primary care and students, who have regular clinical contact with patients. This includes doctors, dentists, nurses; paramedical professionals such as occupational therapists, physiotherapists, radiographers; ambulance workers
- *Laboratory and other staff* (including mortuary staff): who have direct contact with potentially infectious clinical specimens and may additionally be exposed to pathogens in the laboratory. This includes those in academic (or commercial research) laboratories who handle clinical specimens. They do not normally have direct contact with patients
- *Non-clinical ancillary staff:* who may have social contact with patients, but not usually of a prolonged or close nature. This group includes receptionists, ward clerks, administrative staff working in hospitals and primary care, and maintenance staff such as engineers, gardeners, cleaners, etc.

Specific hazards and occupational disorders in health care

- Infection (see ◻ p. 103, Biological hazards and ◻ p. 149, Occupational infections, for individual hazards and diseases)
- Violence (see ◻ p. 136, Violence and aggression)
- *Musculoskeletal disorders:* low back (see ◻ p. 254, Low back pain) and neck/shoulder pain)
- Stress (see ◻ p. 308, Stress 1: recognition and assessment; ◻ p. 311, Stress 2: interventions/risk controls)
- Latex allergy (see ◻ p. 202, Latex allergy)
- Dermatitis (see ◻ p. 242, Dermatitis 1; ◻ p. 244, Dermatitis 2)
- Radiation (see ◻ p. 18, Ionizing radiation 2: principles of radiation protection)
- Cytotoxic drugs.

Fitness assessment

Health care work covers a very wide range of duties. HCWs often change role, and robust arrangements should be made to identify internal job changes, with reassessment of fitness where appropriate. Standard health clearance[1] for new HCW includes checks for tuberculosis disease/immunity, HBV immunization with post-immunization testing of immunity, and the offer of HIV and HCV tests.

Immunity from vaccine-preventable infections is advisable (Table 24.1)

---

1 Department of Health. (2007). Health clearance for tuberculosis, hepatitis B, hepatitis C and HIV: new healthcare workers'. DH, London.

Table 24.1 Immunization requirements for HCWs

Recommended routine assessment of immunity and immunization	Clinical (1)	Laboratory (2)	Non-clinical (3)
History of routine childhood immunization: diphtheria, polio, tetanus (DPT); mumps, measles, rubella (MMR); tuberculosis (BCG) or positive measles, rubella antibodies, and Mantoux test if no satisfactory history of immunity and immunization of non-immune	+	+ For polio, only boost those handling faecal specimens; diphtheria special arrangements to boost those handling organisms	DPT and MMR BCG not routinely recommended
History of infection with varicella (chicken pox) or positive varicella antibodies if history unsatisfactory and immunization of non-immune	+	+	+
History of immunization against hepatitis B and immunization, followed by check of serology in non-immune	+	+	+ If exposed to blood or body fluids
History of immunization against hepatitis A and typhoid and immunization of non-immune		Only if handling specific organisms	Only if exposed to sewage, e.g. drainage engineers
Influenza: offer of annual immunization	+	Only if handling organisms	
Cholera, meningococcus ACW 135Y, smallpox, tick-borne encephalitis, yellow fever, rabies, Japanese encephalitis, anthrax		Only if handling specific organisms	

Detailed guidance: Department of health. Chapter 12. In: *Immunization against infectious disease.* Available at: ℅ http://www.dh.gov.uk/health/category/publications/reports-publications/

Special fitness requirements
- Fitness for exposure prone procedures (see 🕮 p. 494, Fitness for exposure prone procedures 1; 🕮 p. 496, Fitness for exposure prone procedures 2)
- Fitness to work with children and vulnerable patients (see 🕮 p. 498, Fitness to work with children).

Transfer of information about fitness for work

Transfer of OH records or conclusions about fitness for work (including immunization status) should only be done with the employee's consent. Smart cards (transferable electronic record) are increasingly used for some staff groups, e.g. junior doctors and medical students.

Specialist skills for professionals who care for HCWs

It is recognized that OH and other health professionals who provide care and support to healthcare practitioners need particular skills, including the management of alcohol and substance abuse. The Faculty of Occupational Medicine and Royal College of Psychiatrists have published guidance on competencies for OH Physicians and psychiatrists, respectively.

Fitness for exposure prone procedures 1

Definition of EPPs

EPPs are health care procedures where there is a risk that injury to the HCW may result in the exposure of the patient's open tissues to the blood of the worker (bleed-back). Procedures include those where the worker's gloved hands may be in contact with sharp instruments, needle tips and sharp tissues (spicules of bone or teeth) inside a patient's open body cavity, wound, or confined anatomical space where the hands or fingertips may not be completely visible at all times.

Categorization of EPPs

EPPs are classified according to the likelihood that infection would be transmitted from an infected HCW to the patient.

Category 1

Procedures where the hands and fingertips of the worker are usually visible and outside of the body most of the time and the possibility of injury to the worker's gloved hands from sharp instruments and/or tissues is slight. This means that the risk of the HCW bleeding into the patient's open tissues should be remote.

Category 2

Procedures where the fingertips may not be visible at all times but injury to the worker's gloved hands from sharp instruments and/or tissues is unlikely. If injury occurs it is likely to be noticed and acted upon quickly to avoid the HCW's blood contaminating the patient's open tissues.

Category 3

Procedures where the fingertips are out of sight for a significant part of the procedure, or during certain stages, and in which there is a distinct risk of injury to the worker's gloved hands from sharp instruments and/or tissues. In such circumstances it is possible that exposure of the patient's open tissues to the HCW's blood may go unnoticed or would not be noticed immediately.

Transmission from infected HCW to patients following EPPs

- HBV transmission from HbeAg positive HCW is well documented. Several transmissions from HbeAg negative HCW prompted the use of HBV viral load testing in determining fitness for EPPs
- HCV—5 reported incidents of transmission to 15 patients in the UK, and at least 4 other incidents worldwide
- HIV—3 reported incidents with 8 possible transmissions worldwide. None in the UK despite 28 notification exercises in 7,000 patients up to the year 2003. The risk of transmission to patients is very low.

Duties of health care workers

HCWs who carry out EPPs and believe they have been exposed to BBV have a duty to seek professional advice on whether they should be tested. HCWs who know they are infected *must* seek and follow confidential occupational health and expert medical advice.

Duties of employers

Employers in the health care sector must

- Ensure that staff are aware of the guidance on BBV and EPPs
- Make every effort to arrange occupational adjustments, re-training, or (as a last resort) ill health retirement for infected employees
- Promote a climate which encourages confidential disclosure
- Arrange for HCW to have access to a Consultant Occupational Physician.

Table 24.2 Summary of testing protocol to assess fitness for EPPs

Initial screening (minimum documentation of fitness for EPPs)	Periodic annual screening
All HCW undertaking EPPs HBsAg −ve or HBsAg +ve, *but* HBeAg −ve *and* HBV DNA<10³ copies /mL	Annual HBsAg if non-responder to vaccine (persistent anti-HBs <10 IU/L) and not naturally immune (anti-HBc −ve) Annual HBV DNA (must remain below 10³ geq/mL)
New HCW Anti-HCV −ve or Anti-HCV +ve AND HCV RNA −ve *and* Anti-HIV −ve	

Routine assessment of fitness for EPPs

Laboratory tests (summary in Table 24.2)

- In new HCW:[1]
  - HBsAg (and, if negative, HBeAg with viral load testing (HBV DNA) in those who are HBeAg +ve)
  - *and* HCV antibody (and, if +ve, HCV RNA)
  - *and* HIV antibody.
- Must be carried out on an identified validated sample (IVS), i.e.:
  - blood sample taken in an occupational health department
  - photographic proof of identity provided
  - sample not delivered to laboratory by HCW
- Must be carried out in an accredited laboratory. Only two specific laboratories are designated by DH for HBV DNA testing (see HSC 2000/020 under Further reading and guidance (📖 p. 496, Exposure prone procedures 2).

---

1 *New* HCW are defined as those who are new to the NHS, those who are starting a post or training involving EPPs for the first time, and those who are returning to the NHS and many have been exposed to BBV while they were away. All locum and agency recruited HCW performing EPPs should be treated as *new* HCW.

Fitness for exposure prone procedures 2

Restrictions from work involving EPPs

Box 24.1 summarizes the current UK guidance on initial restriction of the practice of HCWs who are infected with blood-borne viruses, and the specific circumstances under which HCWs can be allowed to return to EPPs following appropriate treatment.

> **Box 24.1 UK guidance on initial restriction of the practice of HCWs who are infected with blood-borne viruses**
>
> *Restrict from work involving EPPs*
> HCW with the following serological markers of infection:
> - Hepatitis B e antigen (HBeAg) +ve
> - Hepatitis B surface antigen (HBsAg) +ve, but HBeAg –ve *unless* viral load (HBV DNA) <10^3geq/mL
> - Hepatitis C antibody (anti-HCV) +ve *AND* HCV RNA +ve
> - HIV antibody +ve ($\triangle$ this guidance is subject to current public consultation—see following bullet points).
>
> *Fitness for EPPs following treatment for BBV infection*
> HBV and HCV infected HCW can recommence EPPs under specified circumstances following successful antiviral treatment.
> - If HBV DNA levels are <10^3 copies/mL *during continuous* antiviral treatment or 12mths *after* treatment ceases
>   - during treatment, monitoring HBV DNA at 3-monthly intervals by a designated hepatologist is mandatory
>   - and they must cease EPPs immediately if treatment stops
>   - sharps injuries to an infected HCW during EPP must be reported, and the patient offered counselling and post-exposure treatment with HB immune globulin, according to a risk assessment
>   - an infected HCW must cease EPPs if HBV DNA rises >10^3geq/mL either during or after treatment
> - If HCV RNA is negative 6mths *after* cessation of therapy. A further check on HCV RNA should be carried out 6mths later. HCV infected HCW may not carry out EPPs *during* treatment
> - Currently HIV infected HCW who are on antiviral treatment cannot resume EPPs.
> $\triangle$ However, a public consultation is in progress regarding a change in policy to allow EPPs if viral load remains consistently <200 copies/mL on combination antiretroviral treatment subject to explicitly defined 3-monthly monitoring and follow-up by a consultant occupational physician and HIV specialist.

Patient notification exercises

- Notification of patients who are known to have been exposed to a risk of infection from an infected HCW is necessary:
  - to inform the patient about the nature and magnitude of risk
  - to enable treatment and prevention of onward transmission; and

- to inform existing estimates of the risks of nosocomial transmission
- Newly identified cases of infected HCW who have carried out EPPs should be discussed with the local Director of Public Health (DPH), who will decide on the need to notify patients
- In the presence of an index case of transmission from the HCW to a patient, a patient notification exercises will be required in the case of:
  - HBV
  - HCV
  - HIV
- In the absence of proven transmission:
  - HBV or HCV—there is no automatic requirement for a patient notification exercise, but anonymized case-specific advice must be sought from UKAP (see 📖 p. 497, Specific advisory bodies)
  - HIV—in the absence of known transmission, notification will be confined to patients who have undergone Category 3 EPPs by the infected HCW.[1]

Specific advisory bodies

Advice about restrictions to work and the need for notification exercises for new cases of BBV-infected HCW is available from the UK Advisory Panel for health care workers infected with blood-borne viruses (UKAP).

Further legislation and guidance

Department of Health (2007). *Health clearance for tuberculosis, hepatitis B, hepatitis C and HIV: new healthcare workers.* Available at: 🔗 http://www.dh.gov.uk/en/Publicationsandstatistics/Publications/PublicationsPolicyandGuidance/DH_073132

Department of Health (2005). *HIV infected health care workers: guidance on management and patient notification.* Available at: 🔗 http://www.dh.gov.uk/assetRoot/04/11/64/16/04116416.pdf

Department of Health (1993). *Protecting health care workers and patients from hepatitis B,* HSG(93)40. Available at: 🔗 http://www.dh.gov.uk/assetRoot/04/07/93/06/04079306.pdf

Department of Health (1996). *Protecting health care workers and patients from hepatitis B,* Addendum to HSG(93)40. Available at: 🔗 http://www.dh.gov.uk/assetRoot/04/08/06/26/04080626.pdf

Department of Health (2000). *Hepatitis B infected health care workers,* guidance on implementation of Health Service Circular 2000/020. Available at: 🔗 http://www.dh.gov.uk/assetRoot/04/05/75/38/04057538.pdf

Department of Health (2007). Hepatitis B infected healthcare workers and antiviral therapy. Available at: 🔗 http://www.dh.gov.uk/en/Publicationsandstatistics/Publications/PublicationsPolicyAndGuidance/DH_073164

Department of Health (2002). Hepatitis C infected health care workers. Available at: 🔗 http://www.dh.gov.uk/en/Publicationsandstatistics/Publications/PublicationsPolicyAndGuidance/DH_4010554

UK Advisory Panel for health care workers infected with blood-borne viruses. Available at: 🔗 http://www.hpa.org.uk/Topics/InfectiousDiseases/InfectionsAZ/BloodborneVirusesAndOccupationalExposure/UKAP/

---

1 Department of health (2005). *HIV infected health care workers,* guidance on management and patient notification. DH, London.

Fitness to work with children

General considerations

Considerable psychological and emotional demands are placed on people who work with children. Some jobs involve the worker acting in *loco parentis*, or supervision of potentially hazardous sports, such as swimming. Workers need to be able to relate to children and be able to maintain control without loss of temper or physical violence.

Hazards associated with working with children

- Voice trauma
- Communicable diseases
- Ergonomic (bending, manual handling, sitting on small chairs)
- Physical or verbal assault from children or parents.

Criminal record

Individuals whose work will involve contact with children should have their records checked by the Criminal Records Bureau. This will undertake a level of disclosure appropriate to the post applied for ℗ http://www.homeoffice.gov.uk/agencies-public-bodies/crb/

Statutory requirements

The Education (Health Standards) (England) Regulations 2003 state that employers and training providers must ensure that a person has the health and physical fitness to teach. If it appears to an employer that a teacher may no longer have the health or physical capacity to carry out a relevant activity, the employer must follow the procedures under the 2003 regulations.

Occupational health assessment

The decision on fitness should be made following an individual risk assessment based on

- The nature of the work
- The age group of the children
- The health status of the worker.

General factors

- Ability to undertake the duties of the post (adjusted if necessary), without constituting a health or safety risk to the children
- Ability to communicate effectively with children, parents and colleagues
- Ability to deal with an emergency situation and administration of first aid
- Any adverse effect the job may have on the individual's health
- Individuals whose responsibility includes driving children should meet the DVLA driving standards
- A history of pedophilia or voyeurism (e.g. child pornography websites) precludes working with children.

💣 Any decision to find an individual unfit should be made only if the individual has been fully investigated by their GP or specialist and has been given appropriate treatment. Such decisions are often difficult and may be contentious; therefore discussion with a more experienced colleague may be helpful.

The following specific conditions would need careful consideration in consultation with a specialist:

- *Specific psychiatric conditions:*
- Schizophrenia
  - poorly controlled bipolar affective disorder
  - persistent or recurrent severe depression resistant to treatment
  - anxiety disorder with uncontrolled panic attacks
  - eating disorders associated with self-injury
  - Fabricated or Induced Illness (FII) (previously known as Munchausen's syndrome and Munchausen's syndrome by proxy)
  - profound personality disorder
  - drug or alcohol dependency
- Individuals with epilepsy (see 📖 p. 464, Epilepsy), or impairment of vision or hearing must have a full risk assessment
- Individuals with active tuberculosis should not work with children until they are non-infectious.

Protection of employees

- Consider testing female staff of childbearing age for rubella antibodies and offer immunization well in advance of pregnancy if non-immune
- Consider Hepatitis B vaccine if working with children with learning difficulties or behavioural problems, due to the risk of biting or scratching.

Legislation and guidance

- The Equality Act 2010
- The Education (Health Standards) (England) Regulations 2003
- Fitness to Teach. Occupational health guidelines for the training and employment of teachers. Department of Education and Employment.

Fitness for work in confined spaces (or with respirators)

Task demands

Confined spaces can be found in many workplaces. Hazards in confined spaces include:
- Difficult access/egress
- A non-respirable atmosphere
- Low oxygen levels
- Toxic gas
- An explosive atmosphere.

One means of controlling some of these risks is a full-face respirator or, in some circumstances, an escape set.

General principles

- The worker should not be suffering from a medical condition that would be aggravated by wearing a respirator
- Any illness should not pose an unacceptable risk to the health or safety of the individual or other workers. Examples of conditions which may cause problems include:
  - cardiac disease
  - chronic obstructive pulmonary disease (COPD)
  - musculoskeletal problems
- A doctor should carry out a pre-placement medical assessment focusing on fitness to use a respirator
- Test lung function using spirometry to identify individuals with impaired lung function as this might compromise their ability to tolerate a respirator or to escape in an emergency
- Getting the prospective worker to use the relevant respirator is a useful exercise to see if he/she has any difficulties.

Assessment frequency

- Every 2yrs for workers over age 18
- Following illness or injury if it is believed the operator may be unfit.

Specific issues

- *Vision should be adequate:* 6/6 corrected vision in the better eye without visual field deficit
- *Asthma:* some asthmatics cannot tolerate a respirator
- *Claustrophobia:* is a contraindication to work in confined spaces.
- *Respirator fit:* should be tested[1] ideally by a Fit2Fit accredited fit tester. Factors that influence respirator fit:
  - facial deformity, e.g. retrognathia
  - beard
  - other PPE.

---

1 HSE *Fit testing of respiratory protective equipment face pieces,* HSE operational circular OC282/28. Available at: ℜ http://www.hse.gov.uk/foi/internalops/fod/oc/200–299/282_28.pdf

Legislation and guidance

- *Confined Spaces Regulations 1997. Approved Code of Practice, Regulations and Guidance.* L101, HSE Books, Norwich, 1997. ISBN 071761405.
- Cox R, Edwards F, Palmer K (eds) (2007). *Fitness for Work: The Medical Aspects* (4th edn). Oxford University Press, Oxford.
- British Safety Industry Federation Fit2Fit RPE fit testers accreditation scheme ℘ http://www.fit2fit.org/

Fitness for seafaring

Task demands

- Seafaring is a diverse occupation that encompasses those operating in near-coastal waters and those sailing in distant waters. The latter group may be at sea for many weeks in remote locations far from medical assistance
- Broadly speaking, there are three categories of crew:
  - deck crew (cargo handling, watch keeping)
  - engineers and radio operators
  - support staff (caterers, stewards, etc.)
- Fitness standards and task demands vary by occupation, but in any event crew must be fit to undertake emergency response procedures (e.g. abandon ship, firefighting)
- MSN1765 (M) provides guidance on task demands and the rationale for fitness standards for specific conditions.

General principles

- The seafarer should not be suffering from a medical condition that would be aggravated by being at sea
- Any illness should not pose an unacceptable risk to the health or safety of the individual, other crew, or the vessel
- A doctor approved by the Maritime and Coastguard Agency (MCA) carries out seafarer medical assessments
- The doctor assesses the individual's fitness against occupational demands and the medical and eyesight standards
- Following assessment the doctor issues a medical fitness certificate (form ENG1) for category 1 or 2. An ENG3 form Notice of Failure/ Restriction is issued for categories 3 or 4
- If the ENG3 form runs for longer than 3/12 the seafarer may appeal against the examining doctor's decision.

Assessment frequency

- Every 2yr for seafarers over age 18
- Annually for seafarers aged less than 18yrs old
- Where, as a result of illness or injury, it is believed that the seafarer may no longer be fit.

Fitness categories

- *Category 1:* Fit for sea service, with no restrictions
- *Category 2:* Fit for sea service but *with restrictions* (e.g. near-coastal waters only)
- *Category 3:* Temporarily unfit for sea service
- *Category 4:* Permanently unfit for sea service

Specific issues

- *Vision:* deck crew should have 6/6 corrected vision in the better eye and 6/12 vision in the other eye without visual field deficits

- *Colour vision:* deck crew must have normal colour vision assessed using Ishihara test plates to undertake watch keeping. Where an individual fails this test, he/she may be tested using the Holmes Wright B Lantern at an MCA office.

Legislation and guidance

Merchant Shipping (Medical Examination) Regulations 2002: Seafarer Medical Examination System and Medical and Eyesight Standards. Maritime and Coastguard Agency, Merchant Shipping Notice MSN 1765 (M).

Fitness for safety critical work

Definition

Safety critical work is any task that (in the event of failure) may lead to an accident, or otherwise compromise the safety of:

- People (employees, clients or service users, the public)
- Plant or premises
- The environment.

Safety critical work

- Regular vehicle driving, particularly passenger vehicles, e.g. train drivers, pilots
- Work at heights
- Work in confined spaces
- Work with, or near, electrical or mechanical equipment, including those in customer's houses
- Managing safety critical control systems, e.g. plant control rooms, air traffic controllers, nuclear industry
- Working on railway premises or infrastructure; this includes drivers, guards, and signalmen
- Work on construction sites, e.g. banks men, tower crane operators.

Task demands and fitness standards

Safety critical jobs depend on the employee being competent to undertake the required task, and being fit to do so.

- Fitness standards for safety critical work vary by industry. Some are statutory and others advisory (see ⬚ p. 474, Fitness to drive 2; ⬚ p. 476, Fitness for professional diving; ⬚ p. 484, Fitness for work in professional pilots)
- Doctors who advise about fitness for safety critical work must have special knowledge of both task demands and statutory or industry fitness standards.

General principles

- A useful rule of thumb is 'Would this person be able to drive an LGV/PCV under DVLA rules?'
- A disease or disability may affect fitness for safety critical posts where the condition is a fixed disability (e.g. loss of a limb) or a progressive condition that may compromise fitness in the future, such as multiple sclerosis
- Pharmacological treatment of a condition may compromise fitness for safety critical posts, e.g. by leading to increased drowsiness (these effects may be temporary)
- Broadly speaking, conditions that may compromise fitness for safety critical posts are those that:
  - lead to sudden incapacity/altered consciousness (e.g. epilepsy, diabetes)
  - affect mobility (e.g. rheumatoid arthritis)
  - affect balance (e.g. Ménière's disease)
  - affect cognition (e.g. dementia, brain damage)

- affect risk perception (e.g. mental handicap)
- affect behaviour (e.g. psychosis, personality disorder, substance misuse)
- affect communication (e.g. deafness, visual impairment, speech problems, abnormal colour vision)
- Review of the job description, task analysis, a workplace visit, and discussion with experienced supervisors will assist in determining the demands of a safety critical post
- When assessing an individual's fitness for a safety critical post it may be difficult to obtain sufficient information to make an informed decision based solely on a health questionnaire. In such cases a consultation for a detailed medical history and examination will be necessary
- Useful additional information regarding the medical condition may be obtained from the individual's GP or specialist, especially when dealing with an employee suffering from a rare condition
- In cases of doubt, discussion with a senior OH physician may be helpful
- In some cases a supervised workplace assessment may be necessary to establish an individual's fitness for the task.

Specific issues

Health and safety reasons may genuinely preclude an individual with a disability from undertaking a safety critical task. However, before concluding an employee is unfit, an employer should consider whether any reasonable workplace adjustments would allow the employee to undertake safety critical work. The employer should carefully document their reasoning in case it is subsequently challenged at an employment tribunal under the Equality Act 2010.

Assessment frequency

This will vary by industry sector. Generally, annual review is the minimum assessment interval, but longer intervals may be stipulated where dealing with young fit workers without pre-existing disease. Where an employee suffers from a progressive medical condition, more frequent review of fitness by the physician may be indicated.

Legislation and guidance

Guidance on Alcohol and Drug Misuse in the Workplace. Faculty of Occupational Medicine, London, 2006. ISBN 1860162819.

Occupational health law

UK health and safety legislation

Health and safety regulation in the UK

Background

Health and safety legislation in the UK developed in a piecemeal fashion from the early nineteenth century onwards. This had the unfortunate consequence of some sectors being heavily regulated by many separate pieces of legislation, while others were effectively unregulated.

In 1970, the Robens Commission was set up to review the UK's workplace health and safety laws. Their report led to:

- The Health and Safety at Work, etc., Act of 1974 (HSW)
- The establishment of the Health and Safety Executive (HSE).

Health and Safety Executive

- Exists to protect the health and safety of workers (including the self-employed) and the public from hazards arising from work
- Governing board of up to 12 persons, appointed by the Secretary of State for Work and Pensions in consultation with key stakeholders:
  - employers' organizations
  - employee organizations – trade unions
  - local authorities
- Proposes health and safety legislation and associated guidance to government ministers
- Responsible for enforcement of health and safety legislation in conjunction with local authorities
- Undertakes reactive and planned inspection of workplaces
- Funds research into health and safety issues in support of regulation.

HSE strategy 2011

Good for Everyone. The next steps in the Government's plans for reform of the health and safety system in Britain. 2011.

See ℘ http://www.dwp.gov.uk/docs/good-health-and-safety.pdf

This document sets out a new plan for health and safety regulation in the UK, with a deregulatory agenda that aims to reduce the burden of bureaucracy for businesses. The key features are:

- Reducing the number of HSE inspections, but
- focusing inspections on high risk industries
- shifting away from scrutiny of low risk organizations
- Taking strong action against employers who breach seriously health and safety law, and making them responsible for the costs of inspections and rectification of the breach
- Developing a register of competent Health and Safety Consultants, and clamping down on a perceived plethora of health and safety advisers who are not competent
- Simplifying health and safety legislation and providing simple summary advice to low risk businesses

A review of health and safety regulation.

Local authorities
- Statutory responsibility for health and safety inspection and enforcement in:
  - shops
  - offices
  - leisure
  - residential homes
  - hotels and restaurants
  - distribution (wholesale and retail) including petrol stations
- Links with HSE through the Health and Safety Executive/Local Authorities Enforcement Liaison Committee (HELA) to ensure conformity of approach by Local Authorities across the UK (see 📖 p. 512, Health and safety inspectors).

Relevant legislation
- Legislation.gov.uk (2003). *Health and Safety at Work etc. Act 1974*, Chapter 37. TSO, Norwich. Available at: ᔥ http://www.legislation.gov.uk/ukpga/1974/37
- The Legislative Reform (Health and Safety Executive) Order 2008. Available at: ᔥ http://www.legislation.gov.uk/uksi/2008/960/contents/made

Further information
The health and safety system in Great Britain ᔥ http://www.hse.gov.uk/pubns/ohsingb.pdf

Health and safety inspectors

Enforcement of workplace health and safety law in the UK is the responsibility of HSE inspectors and their equivalents in local authority environmental health departments.

HSE inspectors

HSE inspectors are normally graduates, from a range of industry backgrounds. On appointment, they receive extensive additional training in health and safety and the relevant law. Currently, inspectors are organized into several directorates.

- Field Operations Directorate (FOD) is the largest grouping of inspectors, and covers a number of sectors excluding railways (the rail industry is the responsibility of the Office of the Rail Regulator): the regional offices also house the occupational physicians and nurses who work with FOD
- Office for Nuclear Regulation: an agency of the HSE: regulates the nuclear industry
- Hazardous Installations Directorate covers health and safety in the following sectors:
  - petrochemical industry
  - explosives industry
  - mines
  - diving
  - sites where genetically modified organisms or biological agents are handled
  - transport of hazardous agents.

Role of HSE inspectors

The role of HSE inspectors includes:
- *Inspection of workplaces:* this may lead to:
  - advice to the employer
  - improvement notice
  - prohibition notice
  - prosecution
- Accident investigation
- Liaison with local authorities
- Advice to the public
- Information gathering.

Local authority inspectors

Local authority inspectors are generally environmental health officers (EHOs). Some inspectors, in larger authorities, specialize in a specific area such as health and safety. In contrast, EHOs in smaller authorities may also be responsible for dealing with food hygiene, noise pollution, and other statutory duties placed on local authorities.

Powers of inspectors

- Statutory right of entry to work places (without notice)
- Right to interview staff and supervisors

- Right to take samples and photographs
- Right to seize dangerous equipment
- *Enforcement:* inspectors can take enforcement action against employers, the self-employed, or employees where the prevailing standards of health and safety management are unacceptable. They can issue either an improvement notice or a prohibition notice. In serious cases they may also pursue a prosecution through the criminal courts.

Improvement notice

This notice requires an organization to address a named health and safety breach within a specified period. An employer may appeal to an employment tribunal against an improvement notice. In this case, the notice is suspended pending the decision of the tribunal.

Prohibition notice

Issued by an inspector where there is thought to be a risk of illness or injury. Work must stop until the breach is addressed. Generally, a prohibition notice takes immediate effect unless stopping a process immediately will be dangerous. In that situation a prohibition notice will be delayed until the process is complete. No suspension occurs if an appeal against a prohibition notice is made to an employment tribunal.

Relevant legislation

HM Govt. (2003). *Health and Safety at Work, etc., Act 1974*, Chapter 37. TSO, Norwich. Available at: http://www.legislation.gov.uk/ukpga/1974/37

Regulations, approved codes of practice, and guidance

The Health and Safety at Work etc. Act 1974 laid down the framework for subsequent health and safety legislation in the UK. The Act has been supplemented by various regulations that relate to particular topics (e.g. manual handling at work). Regulations set out general principles, and are supported by more detailed codes of practice.

Regulations

The Secretary of State, on the recommendation of the Health and Safety Executive, makes new regulations under the umbrella of the Health and Safety at Work etc. Act 1974. Increasingly, new regulations are brought forward in response to EC directives. Any proposed new regulation under the Health and Safety at Work etc. Act 1974 must be laid before parliament for a period of 21 days. Thereafter, it becomes law, provided that no objections are raised during this period.

Approved codes of practice

Approved Codes of Practice (ACOPs) have a special status within the UK regulatory framework. The Health and Safety Executive approve ACOPs after agreement by the relevant Secretary of State. Failure to comply with an ACOP can be held to be evidence of a breach of the Health and Safety at Work etc. Act 1974, or a breach of the specific regulations to which the ACOP relates.

In principle, an employer can choose not to follow an ACOP. However, in the event of challenge by an inspector, defendants must demonstrate that they have complied with regulations in an equivalent manner to that recommended by the ACOP.

- In practice, it is easier for employers to comply with an ACOP than to justify their own approach
- As an ACOP can be readily updated, this allows health and safety standards to be kept up to date.

Guidance

The Health and Safety Executive regularly issue guidance on health and safety matters, and on the implementation of health and safety regulations. Unlike ACOPs, employers are not compelled to follow guidance notes. However, compliance with regulations must still be achieved.

Relevant legislation

HM Govt. (2003). *Health and Safety at Work, etc., Act 1974*, Chapter 37. TSO, Norwich. Available at: http://www.legislation.gov.uk/ukpga/1974/37

Safety committees and safety representatives

The Safety Representatives and Safety Committees Regulations 1977 cover the prescribed functions of union-appointed safety representatives.

Representatives of employee safety are the equivalent of union-appointed 'safety reps' in non-unionized workplaces. Their more limited role is defined in the Health and Safety (Consultation with Employees) Regulations 1996,

Separate regulations, the Offshore Installations (Safety Representatives and Safety Committees) Regulations 1989, apply to workers on offshore installations.

Safety representatives

- Represent employees' interests on matters of workplace health and safety
- Are immune from prosecution for their actions as safety reps
- Must be given paid time off work to act as safety reps, and to attend training relevant to their role and responsibilities. If an employer fails to give paid time off, the safety rep. can complain to an industrial tribunal.

Representatives of employee safety

Although the role of representatives of employee safety is more limited than that of safety reps, it is open to the employer to give them a wider remit. Their role, as defined in legislation, is:

- To represent workers' interests to the employer
- To approach the employer about workplace hazards/dangerous occurrences
- To approach the employer about issues affecting the workers they represent.

Purpose

- Under the Health and Safety at Work etc. Act 1974, employers are required to consult with safety representatives to ensure health and safety at work
- Workplaces with safety committees have lower accident rates than workplaces where managers only are responsible for health and safety.

Main requirements of the Safety Representatives and Safety Committees Regulations 1977

A union may appoint a person to represent its members at a work site.

Role of the safety representative

- To investigate complaints on health and safety or workplace welfare issues
- To represent employees in meetings with the employer about health and safety issues
- To undertake workplace inspections (Regulation 5), usually at 3-monthly intervals

- To investigate workplace accidents and dangerous occurrences (Regulation 6)
- To raise health and safety or welfare issues with the employer
- To consult with HSE/LA inspectors regarding workplace health and safety
- To attend safety committee meetings as a safety representative.

Role of employers
- Discuss with safety reps any changes that may affect health and safety
- Communicate to safety reps the results of any risk assessments
- Discuss emergency and worksite evacuation plans with safety reps
- Provide any health and safety information to safety reps that is necessary for them to fulfill their role (excludes individual health data)
- If requested by two safety representatives, an employer must set up a safety committee within 3mths.

Legislation and guidance
- HM Govt. (1977). *Safety Representatives and Safety Committees Regulations 1977*. Available at: ✍ http://www.legislation.gov.uk/uksi/1977/500/contents/made
- HM Govt. (1996). *Health and Safety (Consultation with Employees) Regulations 1996*. Available at: ✍ http://www.legislation.gov.uk/uksi/1996/1513/contents/made
- Consulting workers on health and safety. Safety Representatives and Safety Committees Regulations 1977 (as amended) and Health and Safety (Consultation with Employees) Regulations 1996 (as amended) Approved Code of Practice and Guidance 2008 L146 HSE.

Health and Safety at Work etc. Act 1974

Purpose

The purpose of this Act is to secure the health, safety, and welfare of workers, and others affected by work activities. It is termed an enabling act, as it empowers the Secretary of State to create regulations under the Act. The HSC and HSE were set up as result of this act, and merged in 2008 as the HSE (see 📖 p. 510, Health and safety regulation in the UK).

Application

The Act applies to all workers except those employed as domestic servants.

Definitions

'So far as is reasonably practicable' is a key phrase in UK health and safety legislation, which requires an employer to assess the risk posed by a hazard against the costs of addressing it: the greater the risk, the greater the effort that should be employed to address it. If prosecuted, the burden of proof lies with the employer to demonstrate that it was not reasonable to do more to control a risk.

⚠ Limited financial resources are not a justification for failing to do all that is 'reasonably practicable'.

Main provisions

- *Section 2:*
  - places a *duty on employers* (including self-employed) to ensure, so far as is reasonably practicable, the health, safety, and welfare of workers
  - the provision and maintenance of safe plant and procedures (systems of work)
  - requires that employers maintain a written health and safety policy
  - provides for the election of workers' safety representatives and, if requested, for the creation of a safety committee
- *Section 3:* creates a general duty of care on employers (and the self-employed) towards those who are not in their employ, but who may be affected by their work activities
- *Section 4:* places a *duty on those who control premises* to ensure:
  - they are maintained
  - they do not pose a health and safety risk to people (other than employees) who may work there
- *Section 5:* places a general *duty on those who control premises* to prevent and control harmful/offensive releases into the environment
- *Section 6:* a *duty on manufacturers, importers, and suppliers* to:
  - ensure, so far as is reasonably practicable, that any work equipment or agents for use at work do not pose a risk to health and safety
  - arrange appropriate testing, unless information is already available

- provide information to ensure that the equipment or substance is used safely, and for its intended purpose
- *Section 7:* places a general *duty on workers* with regard to ensuring the health and safety of themselves and others:
  - this section places a duty on employees to co-operate with employers to comply with health and safety legislation
- *Section 8:* requires that no person shall interfere with any measures provided to protect health, safety, and welfare
- *Section 9:* employers are forbidden from charging workers for anything done in respect of the Health and Safety at Work, etc. Act (e.g. health and safety training or provision of PPE).

Relevant legislation

HM Govt. (1974). *Health and Safety at Work, etc., Act 1974*, Chapter 37. Available at: ✍ http://www.legislation.gov.uk/ukpga/1974/37

Management of Health and Safety at Work Regulations 1999

Purpose

The Management of Health and Safety at Work Regulations are generally referred to as the 'Management Regulations'. They provide an overarching framework for the management of health and safety at work. More specific regulations give additional detail regarding the assessment and control of key hazards. Generally, compliance with these more specific regulations will fulfill the requirements of the Management Regulations.

Exemptions

- These regulations do not apply to:
  - the captain and crew of sea-going vessels, except where the ship is in harbour, e.g. for ship repair
  - domestic staff in private homes.

Main requirements

- Every employer is required to undertake a suitable and sufficient risk assessment of the risks to the health and safety of staff and others (Reg. 3)
- Regulation 3 places a similar duty on the self-employed
- Where a number of different employers share premises, they must co-operate to produce an overall risk assessment (Reg. 11)
- Organizations with more than five employees should record risk assessment findings
- Regulation 4 covers the application of preventative measures. The principles of prevention are:
  - avoid risks
  - evaluate unavoidable risks
  - control risks at source
  - fit the workplace to the human
  - update work practices as technology improves
  - substitute with less hazardous agents/processes
  - have a comprehensive workplace health and safety policy
  - measures that protect everyone should be preferred over those that protect the individual
  - provide information, instruction, and training (Reg. 13)
- Employers and the self-employed must have in place effective health and safety arrangements (Reg. 5). This covers:
  - planning
  - organization
  - control
  - monitoring
  - review
- Employers must provide health surveillance, where appropriate (Reg. 6). This mirrors the requirements of other regulations including COSHH (see 📖 p. 532, Control of Substances Hazardous to Health

Regulations 2002 and 📖 p. 538, Control of Lead at Work Regulations 2002
- Employers must have competent assistance to manage health and safety (Reg. 7)
- Employers must have procedures to deal with dangerous situations (Reg. 8)
- Links must be established with the emergency services for situations such as fire, bomb threats, or other dangerous occurrences (Reg. 9)
- Employers must provide information to staff regarding the results of any risk assessment, control measures in place, and emergency procedures (Reg. 10)
- Where a child below minimum school-leaving age is employed, special attention must be paid to health and safety risks (Reg. 19). There is a duty to communicate the results of the risk assessment to the child's parents (see 📖 p. 522, Young people at work)
- Employees must co-operate with health and safety measures
- Special measures are required to control any risk that may affect the health of a new or expectant mother, or her baby (see 📖 p. 524, New and expectant mothers).

Legislation and guidance
HSE (2000). *Management of Health and Safety at Work Regulations 1999, Approved Code of Practice and Guidance*, 2nd edn, L21. HSE Books, Sudbury. Available at: ℅ http://www.legislation.gov.uk/uksi/1999/3242/contents/

Young people at work

Purpose

The Management of Health and Safety at Work Regulations 1999 contains measures intended to protect the health and safety of young people at work.

Application

Young people are recognized as being at particular risk in the workplace by virtue of their lack of work experience, in some cases compounded by psychological or physical immaturity. The guidance associated with the regulations gives a number of examples where the young worker may be at special risk. The risks of some work activities are deemed unacceptable, and young people are prohibited from such work (e.g. lead glazing). The regulations do not apply to short-term employment in domestic service or to non-harmful work in a family business.

Definitions

- A *young worker* is someone aged less than 18yrs of age
- The *minimum school leaving age* (MSLA) is age 16 or just before.
- A *child* is someone below the minimum school leaving age.

Main requirements

- Employers should, when undertaking a risk assessment, pay particular attention to vulnerable groups of workers including young people
- Employers must carry out the assessment before the young person starts work
- Where a risk assessment identifies a process or agent that may affect the health of the young worker, the employer should inform the employee and explain how they intend to protect health
- When dealing with children under school-leaving age, the employer must communicate the risk assessment findings and control measures to their parents
- Where, despite controls, significant risks remain, a young person under MSLA cannot be employed to do that work.

Legislation and guidance

- Management of Health and Safety at Work Regulations 1999. ℘ http://www.legislation.gov.uk/uksi/1999/3242/contents/made
- HSE *Young People at Work. A Guide for Employers.* HS(G)165, HSE Books, Sudbury. ISBN 0717618897.

New and expectant mothers

Purpose

The Management of Health and Safety at Work Regulations 1999 contains measures intended to protect the health and safety of pregnant workers and their unborn children, and also breast-feeding mothers and their children.

Application

The guidance to the regulations gives a number of examples where occupational exposures may be harmful to the worker or her child. These include work with lead, mercury, diving, underground mining, hyperbaric work, ionizing radiation, biological agents, carcinogens, and mutagens.

Definitions

- A *new or expectant mother* is a woman who is pregnant, has given birth in the preceding 6mths (delivered a living child or suffered a stillbirth after 24wks pregnancy), or is breast-feeding
- Note that there is no limit on the duration of breast-feeding. It is for the nursing mother to determine for how long she wishes to breast-feed. The employer must then apply the regulations to protect her and her child's health.

Main requirements

- Employers should, when undertaking a risk assessment, pay particular attention to vulnerable groups of workers including pregnant workers and breast-feeding mothers
- Where a risk assessment identifies a process or agent that may affect the health of this group of workers, the employer should inform all female employees of child-bearing age and explain how they intend to protect workers' health
- If the risk assessment indicates that, despite appropriate controls, a significant risk to health remains, the employer has to take other measures to protect the worker's health:
  - first, consider adjusting the work conditions or working hours
  - if this is not possible, the employer should offer suitable alternative work
  - if this is not possible give paid leave
- The risks to health during pregnancy may change and so employers must regularly review their risk assessment
- Employers must provide suitable facilities for pregnant workers and breast-feeding mothers to rest
- There is currently no requirement for employers to provide a suitable place for breast-feeding women to express or store breastmilk. However, enlightened employers will wish to make suitable provision. Toilets would not be deemed suitable for this purpose.

Legislation and guidance

- HSE (1999). *New and expectant mothers*. Management of Health and Safety at Work Regulations 1999. Available at: ℘ http://www.hse.gov.uk/pubns/indg373hp.pdf
- HSE (2002). *New and expectant mothers at work. a guide for employers*, HSG122, HSE Books, Sudbury.

Workplace (Health, Safety and Welfare) Regulations 1992

Purpose

These regulations expand on the duties placed on employers by the Health and Safety at Work, etc., Act 1974. While the welfare requirements may seem detailed, they are largely based on common sense.

Application

All workplaces are covered with the exception of transport (Reg. 13 applies to planes, trains, and road vehicles if stationary in a workplace), mines and quarries, oil rigs, or building sites (Reg. 3). Work on farms or forests away from main buildings, and temporary work sites such as carnivals, have more limited requirements covering provision for sanitation, washing, and drinking water 'so far as is reasonably practicable'.

Definitions

- *Workplace* means any place of work including shops, offices, factories, schools, and hospitals. The definition includes private roadways, corridors, and temporary workplaces (excluding building sites)
- *Domestic premises*: a private dwelling where the regulations do not apply.

Main requirements

- The employer must maintain the workplace:
  - keep it clean (Reg. 5)
  - and well ventilated (Reg. 6)
  - and dispose of waste (Reg. 9)
- Any indoor workplace should have a reasonable temperature (usually no lower than 16°C, but 13°C if work is physically demanding) (Reg. 7). No maximum temperature is given; instead the regulations refer to 'reasonably comfortable' temperatures
  - this does not apply where it conflicts with food safety or is impractical e.g. vehicle loading bays
  - thermometers should be provided
  - measures to prevent excessive solar gain should be taken
  - heating systems should be maintained so they do not produce noxious fumes, e.g. carbon monoxide
  - where temperatures cannot be maintained at comfortable levels, task rotation should be employed
- Every workplace shall have suitable lighting, including emergency lighting if necessary (Reg. 8)
- Room dimensions must be sufficient for health, safety, and welfare purposes (Reg. 10). This does not apply to sales kiosks or parking attendants' cabins where space is limited. The minimum space per person is $11m^3$ (maximum ceiling height for calculation is 3m)
- Seating should be fit for the task and the person doing the task (Reg. 11)
- Floors, paths, and roadways should be well maintained (Reg. 12)

- Guard rails, fences, or covers must be provided where there is a risk of falls from height or into a tank or pit (Reg. 13)
- Windows and transparent doors, gates, and walls must be made of safety materials, e.g. polycarbonate, annealed glass or safety glass (Reg. 14)
- *Windows:*
  - should be capable of being opened and cleaned safely (Reg. 16)
  - should not pose a hazard once open (Reg. 15)
- Workplaces should be organized so that pedestrians and vehicles can move around the site safely (Reg. 17), ideally by separating people and vehicles
- Doors and gates must be suitably constructed and operate safely (Reg. 18)
- Escalators and moving walkways must operate safely and have an emergency stop button (Reg. 19)
- Provide suitable and sufficient toilets and washing facilities (Regs 20 and 21)
- Potable water should be readily available (Reg. 22)
- *Provide facilities for:*
  - changing clothes (Reg. 24)
  - storage for work clothing and the worker's own clothing (Reg. 23)
- Provide suitable canteen and rest areas (Reg. 25). Facilities for making a hot drink should be available. Pregnant workers or nursing mothers should be provided with somewhere to rest and, if necessary, to lie down.

Legislation and guidance
- Workplace (Health, Safety and Welfare) Regulations 1992.
  ℘ http://www.legislation.gov.uk/uksi/1992/3004/contents/made
- HSE (1996). *Workplace (Health, Safety and Welfare) Regulations 1992. Approved Code of Practice and Guidance.* L24, HSE Books, Sudbury.

Health and Safety (Display Screen Equipment) Regulations 1992

Purpose

The Health and Safety (Display Screen Equipment) Regulations 1992, as amended by the Health and Safety (Miscellaneous Amendments) Regulations 2002, implement an EC directive on minimum health and safety standards for display screen equipment (DSE) and its use.

Application

Display screen equipment includes:
- Computer monitors (also termed visual display units (VDUs))
- Microfiche readers
- Laptop or notebook computers (depends on usage).

It excludes:
- DSE equipment intended for short-duration public use, e.g. bank automated teller machine (ATMs)
- Laptops/notebooks used for short periods
- DSE on board a means of transport
- Calculators
- Cash registers
- Medical/scientific instruments used for short periods, e.g. heart monitors.

The regulations cover DSE users and do not apply to infrequent users of visual display units or to the general public.

Definitions

Who is a DSE user?

Someone who fulfils most of the following:
- Depends on DSE to do their job
- Has no discretion as to use
- Uses DSE for >1h
- Uses DSE daily.

Main requirements

- Risk assessment (Reg. 2) (see 🕮 p. 780, Carry out a display screen equipment assessment). This may involve a generic assessment for a group of workers doing similar tasks, and a user questionnaire completed by each user
- Workstation minimum requirements (Reg. 3) cover the workstation including hardware, software, working environment, and the user interface. Specific requirements are described in Annex A of the Guidance on Regulations:
  - Equipment
  - Environment

- Tasks and software should be designed using good ergonomic practice with an effective equipment–user interface, and software should be fit for purpose
  - Work schedules (Reg. 4)—there is no specific guidance on break timing and frequency. In general, short frequent breaks away from the workstation are preferable. Users should have some discretion as to how they manage their work
- *Vision and vision testing (Reg. 5):* users may request an eye and eyesight test at the employer's expense. An optometrist or a registered medial practitioner must carry out the test. Some employers offer vision screening prior to sight testing. The user is not obliged to accept such screening and may proceed directly to sight testing
- Employers must pay for spectacles, where these are required solely for DSE use ('special' corrective appliances):
  - the employer is only required to provide corrective appliances that are fit for purpose and not designer spectacle frames
  - an employer may specify which professional undertakes sight tests and dispenses spectacles
- *Information, instruction and training (Regs 6 and 7):* users should receive health and safety training regarding DSE workstations and their safe use.

Legislation and guidance

- Work with display screen equipment. Health and Safety (Display Screen Equipment) Regulations 1992 as amended by the Health and Safety (Miscellaneous Amendments) Regulations 2002. Guidance on Regulations L26 (2 edn). Available at: ℘ http://www.legislation.gov.uk/uksi/1992/2792/contents/made; also available at: ℘ http://www.hse.gov.uk/pubns/indg36.pdf
- Guidance on Eye Examinations for VDU Users: Association of Optometrists. Available at: ℘ http://www.aop.org.uk/uploads/uploaded_files/guidance_on_Eye_Examinations_for_vdu_users.pdf
- E03: Examining patients who work with visual display screen equipment College of Optometrists Guidelines for Professional Conduct, 2011. Available at: ℘ http://www.college-optometrists.org/en/utilities/document-summary.cfm/docid/570D3F84–5B24–4DBF-B7145510CBBC5B15

Provision and Use of Work Equipment Regulations 1998

Purpose

The aim of the regulations is to ensure that the use of work equipment does not affect worker's health and safety.

Application

The regulations apply to all work sites covered by the Health and Safety at Work etc. Act 1974. It covers the provision and use of all work equipment including lifting equipment, although additional regulations govern lifting operations and lifting equipment (LOLER 1998). PUWER applies to employers, the self-employed, and persons controlling equipment such as plant hirers (Reg. 3). Domestic work in a private house is excluded from the regulations.

Definitions

- Work equipment means any tools, machinery, appliances, apparatus, or installations (e.g. a production line) provided for use at work (Reg. 2). This is true even if the employee provides the tools, as occurs in garages
- The definition excludes privately owned cars, but does include vehicles not in private ownership when they are off public roads, e.g. within a factory.

Main requirements

- The regulations cover the management of the provision and use of work equipment. They also deal with features of the equipment itself, such as the provision of emergency stop buttons, guards, and safety markings
- Employers must ensure that equipment is suitable for its intended use (Reg. 4), and that it is only used for those activities for which it is intended
- High-risk equipment must be regularly inspected (Reg. 6) and maintained (Reg. 5) by competent persons. Records should be kept of maintenance to high-risk equipment such as fairground rides
- Information, instruction, and training must be provided to equipment users (Regs 8 and 9). Special attention should be paid to the training of young people
- Any equipment should conform to European Community requirements and be CE marked[1]
- Equipment should have suitable guards on dangerous parts (Reg. 11)
- Measures to protect workers and others from objects falling or being ejected from equipment. Controls should protect against equipment failure, fire, explosion, overheating, or discharge of substances from equipment (Reg.12)

---

1 CE Marking indicates that a product conforms to EU product safety rules.

- Workers must be protected from very hot or cold parts of a machine or articles produced by the machine (Reg. 13)
- Equipment should have appropriate controls, including emergency stop controls (Regs 14–16)
- Any controls should be clearly visible and located in safe areas, and there should be a safe system of operation
- Audible or visible warnings should be in place, where employees may be at risk if the machine starts unexpectedly while they are in a danger area, e.g. inside a paper-making machine (Reg. 17)
- Control systems should 'fail to safe' in the event of malfunction (Reg. 18)
- Any power source should be capable of being isolated for maintenance, or where operating conditions are unsafe. This may require interlocks and isolating devices to be fitted (Reg. 19)
- Equipment should be stable and secure, e.g. ladders should be properly footed
- Adequate lighting must be provided where equipment is operated. This may require additional lighting, especially during construction or maintenance
- Equipment should be designed such that maintenance operations do not place workers at risk (Reg. 22)
- Any work equipment must be clearly marked with any necessary health and safety warnings. Any warnings (reversing alarms, 'power on' lights etc.) must be clear and unambiguous (Regs. 23 and 24)
- Additional rules cover the use of mobile equipment, in particular its movement (Regs 25–30):
  - the use of roll-over protection (rather than a cab) on mobile equipment such as forklift trucks will often require the use of restraining devices
  - mobile equipment should be designed so that it is safe to move, and does not place the operator or others at risk
  - drive shafts or power take-offs (PTOs) should be guarded, and have a slip-clutch to prevent catastrophic equipment failure if the shaft seizes.

Legislation and guidance

- HSE (1998). *Provision and Use of Work Equipment Regulations 1998. Approved Code of Practice and Guidance*, L22. HSE Books, Sudbury, Available at: ℜ http://www.opsi.gov.uk/si/si1998/19982306.htm
- HSE (1998). *Lifting Operations and Lifting Equipment Regulations 1998. Approved Code of Practice and Guidance*, L113. HSE Books, Sudbury. Available at: ℜ http://www.opsi.gov.uk/si/si1998/19982307.htm

Control of Substances Hazardous to Health Regulations 2002

Purpose
The regulations are intended to protect workers from risks posed by chemical hazards in the workplace. The Regulations and ACOP specify how chemical hazards should be assessed, controlled, and monitored (including health surveillance).

Application
These regulations apply to employers and the self-employed. They cover most hazardous substances excluding the following, for which specific regulations apply:
- Asbestos
- Lead
- Radio-active agents
- Substances being used in medical treatment
- Substances hazardous because of flammable/explosive properties.

Definitions
- *Substance*: a natural or artificial substance whether a solid, liquid, gas, dust, fibre, mist, smoke, or vapour. This term includes micro-organisms. It encompasses individual agents and mixtures which are impurities, intermediates, by-products, wastes, or final products
- *Workplace*: any place where work is being carried out, including domestic premises and the public highway
- *'So far as is reasonably practicable'*: financial factors may be taken into account when determining whether risk controls are reasonably practicable. Note that the level of risk outweighs the financial resources of the organization in determining practicability. The greater the health risk, the greater the expectation of effort and expense
- Biological agents are categorized under COSHH as follows:
  - *Group 1*—unlikely to cause human illness
  - *Group 2*—can cause human disease. Usually effective treatment or prophylaxis is available
  - *Group 3*—can cause severe human illness and may be a serious hazard to employee's health
  - *Group 4*—causes severe human disease. Usually no effective treatment is available for such agents.

Main requirements
- The duties placed on employers under COSHH also apply to the self-employed (Reg. 3), except for the duty to undertake workplace monitoring and health surveillance
- The use of substances listed in Schedule 2 are either restricted or prohibited, as they are deemed too hazardous to health (Reg. 4)
- Employers are required to carry out a risk assessment before exposing employees to a hazardous substance (Reg. 6). If an organization has more than five employees, this risk assessment must be recorded

- Employers must prevent or control exposure to hazardous substances (Reg. 7). This includes substitution of a less hazardous agent, reformulation of an agent (e.g. using a paste instead of a powder), process re-engineering, industrial hygiene controls, and administrative control measures. Appendix 1 of COSHH guidance provides further information on the control of carcinogens and mutagens. Schedule 3 lists additional provisions for biological agents
- Employers must ensure that employees use control measures provided, and employees have a duty to do so (Reg. 8). If an employee finds a defect in a control measure, he/she must inform the employer
- Control measures must be maintained, examined, and tested regularly (Reg. 9). Suitable records of such tests must be retained for at least 5yrs. All control measures should be regularly inspected. For most processes (except those in Schedule 4), regular inspection means weekly visual checks, and examination and testing every 14mths
- Where a risk assessment indicates that workplace monitoring is needed to confirm the effectiveness of control measures, an employer must comply (Reg. 10). Processes and agents listed in Schedule 5 must have specified workplace monitoring. Suitable records of employee monitoring should be maintained for 40yrs
- Health surveillance (Reg. 11) (see Chapter 22 Health surveillance: general principles) is required where the worker is exposed to an agent or process listed in Schedule 6 or exposure to a hazardous substance is such that:
  - an identifiable disease is related to exposure
  - there is a reasonable likelihood of the illness occurring
  - valid methods exist to detect the disease
- Health records must be kept for 40yrs after the last entry. A health record (which should not include confidential clinical information) is distinct from medical records of health surveillance maintained by health professionals
- Information, instruction, and training should be provided for employees who may be exposed to hazardous substances (Reg. 12)
- Regulation 13 requires employers to make plans to deal with emergencies such as spills, fires, or leaks. These requirements may overlap with other regulations relating to major accident hazards (📖 p. 590, Control of Major Accident Hazards Regulations 1999).

Legislation and guidance
- Control of Substances Hazardous to Health Regulations 2002 (as amended). Approved Code of Practice and guidance, 5th edn, L5. HSE Books, Sudbury. 🔗 http://www.legislation.gov.uk/uksi/2002/2677/contents/made
- HSE (2005). *Workplace exposure limits: containing the list of workplace exposure limits for use with the Control of Substances Hazardous to Health Regulations 2002* (as amended), EH40. HSE Books, Sudbury.
- COSHH. Available at: 🔗 www.coshh-essentials.org.uk

Reporting of Injuries, Diseases, and Dangerous Occurrences Regulations 1995

Purpose

To ensure that injuries, accidents, and dangerous incidents arising from work are reported to the relevant enforcing authority (HSE or local authority). They provide a single set of reporting rules applicable to all work. A 2° benefit is that RIDDOR provides information on trends for workplace accidents and some occupational illnesses. In reality, significant under-reporting across all sectors compromises the system.

Application

- Regulations apply to Great Britain including the offshore oil industry.
- Separate regulations apply to Northern Ireland
- Incidents arising directly from medical treatment are excluded.

Definitions

- *Enforcing authority:* either HSE or the local authority
- *Over-7-day injury:* a worker is unfit for his/her normal work for 7 days excluding the day of the incident
- *Responsible person:* the employer, the person in control of the workplace, or the individual, if self-employed
- *Accident:* defined as 'an act of non-consensual violence done to a person at work' and excludes injuries to professional sportsmen in the normal course of play.

Main requirements

Reportable incidents, diseases, and dangerous occurrences

All incidents can be reported online to HSE, but a telephone service remains for reporting fatal and major injuries only. The following must be reported by the responsible person to the enforcing authority:

- Death due to an accident
- *Major injury:*
  - any fracture, other than to fingers, thumbs, or toes
  - any amputation
  - dislocation of the shoulder, hip, knee, or spine
  - loss of sight (temporary or permanent)
  - a chemical or metal burn to the eye or any penetrating eye injury
  - any injury due to an electric shock or burn leading to unconsciousness or requiring resuscitation or admittance to hospital for >24h
  - any injury leading to hypothermia, heat illness, or unconsciousness
  - any injury requiring resuscitation
  - any injury needing hospital admission for >24h
  - loss of consciousness due to asphyxia or exposure to a harmful agent
  - absorption of any agent causing acute illness requiring medical treatment or loss of consciousness

- acute illness requiring medical treatment due to exposure to a
  biological agent, its toxin, or infected material; this covers needlestick injuries where the exposure is to blood or body fluids infected
  with agents such as hepatitis B, C or HIV
- From April 2012 over-7-day injuries (excluding day of incident) must
  be reported within fifteen days. A record (e.g. accident book) of
  over-3-day injuries must still be maintained despite the move from
  reporting of over-3-day injuries to over-7-day injuries
- *Notifiable diseases:* an employer must notify the relevant authority
  using Form F2508A where one of their workers develops a prescribed
  occupational disease (see 📖 Appendix 3). This applies where the
  employer is notified in writing by a doctor that the employee has a
  disease listed in Schedule 3, Part 1, of the regulations and the worker
  is involved in the relevant work listed in column 2 of that list (Reg. 5)
- Any dangerous occurrence listed in Schedule 2 of the regulations. This
  covers incidents such as the collapse of a crane, failure of a pressure
  vessel, or a fire or explosion leading to plant shutdown for >24h.

Other provisions

- Death or major injury is reportable whether the affected individual is
  an employee or a member of the public
- There is no duty on anyone to report to the HSE the death of a
  self-employed person who dies on his or her own premises
- Injuries sustained in 'hazing' (initiation ceremonies) would be
  reportable if the new worker was forced to take part in such an event
- Injuries to members of the public, where they are taken to hospital,
  are reportable even where no treatment is administered (Reg. 3)
- Regulation 4 requires that, where a worker (but not a member of the
  public) dies as a result of an accident within 12mths, the responsible
  person must inform the enforcing authority
- Gas Safe registered gas fitters[1] are required to report dangerous gas
  fittings or installations to HSE
- Gas suppliers must notify HSE when they learn of an incident involving
  gas they supply which causes injury or death (Reg. 6)
- Regulation 7 places a duty on the responsible person to keep a record
  of any report for 3yrs after the incident
- Where an employer was unaware of an incident, they can use this
  as a defence if subsequently prosecuted for failing to report it. The
  employer would have to demonstrate they had taken reasonable steps
  to have such incidents reported.

Legislation and guidance

- Reporting of Injuries, Diseases and Dangerous Occurrences
  Regulations 1995. Available at: ℘ http://www.legislation.gov.uk/
  uksi/1995/3163/contents/made
- RIDDOR reporting online. Available at: ℘ http://www.hse.gov.uk/
  riddor/report.htm

---

1 Gas Safe Register.

First Aid at Work Regulations 1981

Purpose

To describe the first aid provision that employers must make in workplaces.

Application

Apply to all employers in the UK, except where other regulations apply (Reg. 7) in offshore oil, diving and merchant shipping. The armed forces are exempt.

Definitions

First aid means the provision of immediately necessary care to ill or injured people and, where necessary, calling an ambulance. It does not include the administration of drugs to treat an illness (e.g. paracetamol for headache).

Main requirements

- Employers must assess likely first aid needs (Reg. 3) having considered:
  - workplace risks such as machinery, chemicals
  - high-risk areas, e.g. laboratories
  - staff numbers
  - shift work and out-of-hours work
  - accident history
  - location of workplace, e.g. remote forests
  - lone workers
  - trainees on work experience
  - needs of any disabled or young persons employed
  - workers who travel
  - general public[1]
  - multiple buildings on a single site, e.g. universities
  - arrangements for workers on shared sites, e.g. construction sites
  - availability of first-aiders due to holidays, sickness
  - staff with language/reading difficulties
- The minimum first aid provision is:
  - a first aid container stocked with the recommended contents
  - an appointed person to take charge of first aid arrangements
  - information for workers on first aid provision (Reg. 4).

▶ The self-employed must undertake a risk assessment and make suitable first aid provision (Reg. 5).

- Employers must provide suitable and sufficient first aid materials in an easily identifiable first aid container. First aid kits may be issued to lone workers, those in remote locations, or those who travel at work.
- *First aid rooms:*
  - should be provided if the risk assessment identifies a need
  - should have a couch, desk, chair, phone, sink with hot/cold water, soap and paper towels, adequate heating and lighting

---

1 Employers are not required to make first aid provision for the public but many in the retail and hospitality industries will wish to do so.

- should be clearly identified, with a notice identifying first aiders, their locations, and how to contact them
  - should be easily accessible, clean, and ready for use
- *First aiders:*
  - select on aptitude; should hold a valid first aid certificate
  - first aid certificates are valid for 3yrs
  - the number of first aiders is determined by the risk assessment
- *Record keeping:* an accident book should be maintained to record incidents including the date, time, and location of any incident, the name and job of the injured/ill person, details of the injury or illness, what first aid was administered, disposal of the casualty (e.g. return to work, sent to hospital), and the name and signature of the first aider.

Other regulations and guidance

The Offshore Installations and Pipeline Works (First-Aid) Regulations 1989 address the provision of first aid on offshore oil installations. The NHS does not provide medical cover to oil platforms and so operators must make their own arrangements for nursing cover onboard (rig medics) and for land-based medical support (topside medical cover). The oil industry has produced guidance on suitable first aid and medical equipment on offshore platforms.

The Diving at Work Regulations 1997 require the diving contractor to provide first aid during a diving project (see 📖 p. 544, Diving at Work Regulations 1997).

Legislation/guidance

- The Health and Safety (First-Aid) Regulations 1981. Available at: ℅ http://www.legislation.gov.uk/uksi/1981/917/contents/made
- HSE (1997). *The Health and Safety (First-Aid) Regulations 1981. Approved Code of Practice*, L74. HSE Books, Sudbury.
- The Offshore Installations and Pipeline Works (First-Aid) Regulations 1989. Available at: ℅ http://www.legislation.gov.uk/uksi/1989/1671/contents/made
- HSE (2000). *Offshore Installations and Pipeline Works (First-Aid) Regulations 1989. Approved Code of Practice and Guidance*. L123, HSE Books, Sudbury.
- *First Aid and Medical Equipment on Offshore Installations*, Issue 1, HS 013, 2000. Oil & Gas UK.

Control of Lead at Work Regulations 2002

Purpose
Lead regulations were first introduced in the early twentieth century in an effort to protect workers' health. Historically, lead toxicity was an important occupational disease in the UK. It still causes much morbidity in developing countries. (Lead as a hazard is covered in 📖 p. 70, Lead).

Application
CLAW applies to all work that exposes workers to lead in any form in which it may be absorbed by:
- Inhalation
- Dermal absorption
- Ingestion.

Definitions
- 'Lead exposure is significant' means that one of the following applies:
  - exposure exceeds half the occupational exposure limit for lead
  - there is a substantial risk of ingesting lead
  - skin contact with dermally absorbed lead may occur (lead alkyls, lead napthenate)
- Where exposure is significant, all regulations apply, and in particular the need for hygiene surveys and health surveillance
- 'Woman of reproductive capacity' is a woman medically capable of conceiving.

Main requirements
Risk assessment (Reg. 5)
- The employer must assess the risks to workers and others, who may be affected by lead, record their findings, retain the record for 5yrs, and review the assessment as necessary
- This complements the duty placed on employers by the Management of Health and Safety at Work Regulations to undertake suitable and sufficient risk assessments using competent personnel.

Prevention and control (Reg. 6)
Employers must prevent or control exposure to lead, *so far as is reasonably practicable*, without resort to personal protective equipment. In other words, respiratory protective equipment (RPE) should be the last, not the first, means of control. The hierarchical principles of occupational hygiene apply (see 📖 p. 636, Control hierarchy: source, transmission, and the individual):
- *Substitution:*
  - lead-free compounds
  - low solubility lead compounds
  - use pastes, emulsions or liquid formulations
- *Engineering controls:*
  - enclose work processes

- low-temperature processes < 500°C to ↓ lead fume
- local exhaust ventilation (LEV)
- wet processes
- design plant for easy cleaning
- *Administrative controls:*
  - maintenance and testing of controls
  - provide suitable washing facilities
  - ensure washing facilities are used at breaks/meals
  - provide 'clean' canteen/rest facilities (Reg. 7)
  - enforce 'clean' and 'dirty' areas
  - ban smoking, drinking, eating in lead-contaminated areas (Reg. 7)
  - identify areas where smoking, eating, or drinking is/is not permitted
- *PPE:*
  - suitable protective clothing; impermeable coveralls/gloves are required for work with organolead
  - RPE
  - provide suitable storage for PPE.

Maintenance and testing of control measures (Reg. 8)
LEV maintenance:
- LEV should be visually inspected once a week and fully tested every 14mths
- All control measures must be maintained
- Keep records of maintenance and testing.

Hygiene surveys (Reg. 9)
Breathing zone sampling should be carried out every 3mths. The exception is where work practices are unchanged and on the two previous consecutive occasions the lead in air concentration was <0.10mg/m^3. In that case testing every 12mths is permitted.

Medical surveillance
Special rules apply for young persons (aged 16 or 17) and women of reproductive capacity. These are covered in 📖 p. 423, Health Surveillance: general principles; 📖 p. 434, Inorganic lead; 📖 p. 436, Organic lead.

Information, instruction, and training (Reg. 11)
Training and communication should include:
- Risks to health of lead exposure
- Control measures and precautions
- Results of lead in air monitoring
- Grouped anonymized health surveillance results; communicating this information is very important as it allows the employer and employees to confirm that controls are adequate.

Legislation
HSE (2002). *Control of Lead at Work Regulations 2002*, 3rd edn. *Approved Code of Practice and Guidance*, 3rd edn, L132, HSE Books, Sudbury. http://www.legislation.gov.uk/uksi/2002/2676/contents/made

Control of Asbestos Regulations 2012

Purpose
To protect workers and the public from exposure to asbestos.

Application
The Control of Asbestos Regulations (CAR) 2012 replaces the Control of Asbestos Regulations 2006 and cover most work with asbestos in the UK. Most of the requirements of the 2006 regulations are unchanged but the 2012 Regulations introduces a third category of work; notifiable non-licensed work (NNLW) in addition to the existing categories of licensed work and non-licensed work with asbestos.

- Notifiable non-licensed work requires;
  - Notification to HSE before work commences
  - Medical examinations every 3 years
  - Health records
  - Compliance with risk assessment
  - Control of exposure
  - Training.

Definitions
- The *control limit* for asbestos is 0.1 fibre/cm^3 over any 4 hour period
- Exposure must not exceed 0.6 fibres/cm^3 in any 10 minute period

Main requirements
- Asbestos work is licensable where it is not sporadic and low intensity (SALI) or the risk assessment shows the *control limit* will be exceeded or work on asbestos coating, or work on asbestos insulation board or insulation where the risk assessment shows work is not SALI; the *control limit* will be exceeded; work is not short duration (short duration means all work is less than 2 hours/no-one will work > 1 hour)
- Non-licensed work is not notifiable where exposure is SALI and less than the control limit and involves;
  - short, non-continuous maintenance where only non-friable materials are handled
  - removal without deterioration of non-degraded materials in which the asbestos fibres are firmly linked in a matrix.
- No asbestos work is of low intensity if exposure is > 0.6 fibres/cm^3 over 10 minutes
- Employers must manage asbestos in non-domestic premises
- Assess, by survey, whether buildings contain asbestos
- Assess the risk from any asbestos so identified.

There are two levels of survey:
- Management survey: this is the standard survey to identify any material that might contain asbestos and assess its condition. Such a survey may employ a mix of;
  - sampling to identify asbestos and
  - the presumption that material contains asbestos, and is managed as such.

- *Refurbishment and demolition survey*: suspect materials are sampled and analysed with a view to asbestos removal. The condition of the asbestos is not generally assessed. This approach is employed where demolition or major rebuilding is planned.
- Before commencing work that might lead to exposure to asbestos; the employer must:
  - identify the presence and type of asbestos
  - assess risks, identify control measures, and record findings.
  - draw up a site-specific plan of how the work is to be done (method statement)
  - notify HSE of the planned work.
- Any employer undertaking asbestos work (this covers work with asbestos, ancillary work or supervision), except where exempt under Reg. 3(2) must have an HSE asbestos licence.
- Employers must give employees information, instruction, and training, and maintain training records.
- Where possible, exposure to asbestos should be prevented or, if not feasible, reduced to as low a level as practicable.
- Control measures must be used and maintained. Employees must report defects in controls.
- Employers must make arrangements to deal with emergencies arising during asbestos work and with unplanned releases of asbestos.
- Employers must prevent or reduce the spread of asbestos by using enclosures, restricting access, using decontamination procedures (preliminary and final), and waste removal.
- Good housekeeping with clear procedures for cleaning
- Before re-occupation the site must be certified clear.
- Areas where exposure may exceed the action level must be signed as a designated asbestos area. If exposure may exceed the control limit, the area must be signed as a respirator zone.
- Those undertaking air sampling or laboratory analysis must be accredited to ISO 17025 by UKAS.
- *Medical surveillance* by an HSE appointed doctor including respiratory questionnaire, respiratory examination, and spirometry is required before licensable work begins and every 2 years thereafter (see MS31). Employers must retain the health record for 40 years.
- *Medical examinations* are required for notifiable non-licensed work every three years and must include a chest examination and be carried out by a registered medical practitioner.
- Asbestos waste must be disposed of in suitable labelled containers, and transported in an enclosed vehicle to a licensed disposal site.

Legislation and guidance

- The Control of Asbestos Regulations 2012
- http://www.legislation.gov.uk/uksi/2012/632/contents/made
- Guidance for appointed doctors
- http://www.hse.gov.uk/pubns/ms31.pdf

Ionizing Radiation Regulations 1999

Purpose
The Ionizing Radiation Regulations (IRR) provides the framework for the management of hazards arising from ionizing radiation (naturally occurring or man-made) in the workplace. The objective is to reduce, so far as is reasonably practicable, occupational exposure to radiation.

Application
These regulations apply in the UK and cover three areas of work:
- Practice, which means work involving the production, use, storage or transport of radioactive substances, or operation of electrical equipment that emits ionizing radiation
- Work where the concentration of radon gas exceeds 400Bq/m³ over a 24-h period, e.g. mines
- Work with naturally occurring radionuclides where employees are likely to receive >1mSv in a year, e.g. naturally occurring radioactive material (NORM) deposited in pipework in the oil industry
- The regulations apply to both employers and the self-employed.

Main requirements
- Employers who wish to use radiation in their practice must seek authorization from HSE, unless they comply fully with the conditions stated in one of HSE's generic authorizations (Reg. 7)
- Radiation employers must undertake a risk assessment prior to commencing work with radiation (Reg. 8) and record their findings
- Employers must take all steps required to reduce radiation exposure.
- The employer may employ dose constraints[1] when assessing the risk to carers of patients, when the patient is receiving radiopharmaceuticals.

Risk controls
- Any personal protective equipment provided must be fit for purpose, and comply with the Personal Protective Equipment Regulations 1992
- Any personal protective equipment or engineering controls should be maintained and examined regularly (Reg. 10)
- The employer must prepare local rules for radiation use (Reg. 17)
- The employer must designate controlled areas where the external dose rate exceeds 7.5μSv/h over a working day or employees are likely to receive >6mSv in 1yr
- Monitoring of designated areas is required to assess likely radiation exposures
- Employers are required to account for all sources held by them.

Competent advice and training
Radiation employers must:
- Consult with a recognized radiation protection adviser for advice on compliance with the IRR regulations

---

1 Dose constraint: the upper limit of exposure likely to be received by a non-professional carer when supporting a relative or friend receiving medical treatment with a radiopharmaceutical.

- Provide information, instruction, and training to all relevant staff (Reg. 14).

Monitoring and classification of workers
Dose limits are as follows;
- 20mSv for workers >18yrs
- 6mSv for workers aged 16–18yrs
- 1mSv for members of the public
- For women of reproductive capacity radiation exposure to the abdomen must not exceed 13mSv in any 3-mth period
- Employees shall be designated as 'classified' workers under the IRR (Reg. 20) if personal exposure is likely to be >6mSv, or three-tenths of any other exposure limit
- An approved dosimetry service (ADS) must be appointed by the employer to undertake exposure monitoring of employees
- An employer must investigate when personal annual exposure to radiation exceeds 15mSv. The results of such investigations should be retained for 2yrs.

Medical assessments
- Must be undertaken by a doctor appointed by the HSE who is known as an 'Appointed doctor'
- Prospective classified workers must be examined prior to commencing work with radiation (Reg. 24). Caution should be exercised when assessing:
  - skin problems which might increase the dose received when exposed to unsealed sources
  - mental health problems that might affect safety behaviour
  - fitness to wear PPE.
- Periodic reviews (usually annual) involve review of dosimetry results and sickness absence records. Medical examination may be required at the doctor's discretion
- Health records must be kept for 50yrs after the last entry.

Accidents and over-exposures
- Where a radiation accident occurs, the ADS should be contacted and arrangements made to determine employees' radiation exposure as soon as possible
- Where an over-exposure occurs the employer must investigate the circumstances, having notified the affected individual and HSE of the suspected over-exposure.

Legislation and guidance
Ionizing Radiation Regulations 1999. Approved Code of Practice and Guidance. L121, HSE Books, Sudbury. ISBN 9780717617463. Available at: http://www.legislation.gov.uk/uksi/1999/3232/contents/made

Diving at Work Regulations 1997

⚠ Assessment of fitness to dive at work is the remit of an HSE Approved medical examiner of divers (AMED). Where such an assessment is required, the diver should be referred to such a doctor.

Purpose

To regulate diving operations at work.

Application

The Diving at Work Regulations apply to all diving at work, but different codes of practice apply to the five industry sectors and give sector-specific information on the management of health and safety in diving operations.

The ACOPs cover:

- Commercial diving inland/inshore
- Commercial diving offshore
- Media diving
- Scientific and archaeological diving
- Recreational diving projects.

▶ Hyperbaric treatment at a hospital is excluded from the regulations.

Definitions

- *Diver:* a person who dives at work
- *Diving operation:* that portion of a diving project which can be safely supervised by one diving supervisor
- *Diving project:* the overall job, which may be a single dive or series of dives
- *Diving contractor:* each diving project can have only one diving contractor (Reg. 5), usually the divers' employer. Most of the duties under these regulations fall on the diving contractor.

Main requirements

- The ACOP relevant to a diving project is usually obvious. However, any diving project using a closed diving bell or saturation diving automatically falls under the commercial diving projects offshore ACOP, irrespective of dive location
- The dive contractor must ensure that the diving project is safely run, and that risk assessments are undertaken
- A project plan must be prepared for each diving project (Reg. 6)
- All staff involved in a diving operation must be competent
- A diving supervisor must be appointed in writing
- All equipment and plant must be suitable and well maintained (Reg. 6)
- Only one diving supervisor can supervise a diving operation at a time (Reg. 9), and there must be well-documented handovers between supervisors
- All divers must possess:
  - an HSE approved qualification to dive (Reg. 12)
  - a valid medical certificate of fitness to dive issued by an AMED.

Legislation and guidance

- Diving at Work Regulations (SI 1997 No2776). Stationery Office, Norwich. Available at: http://www.legislation.gov.uk/uksi/1997/2776/contents/made
- HSE (1998). *Commercial Diving Projects Inland/Inshore*, Approved Code of Practice, L104. HSE Books, Sudbury.
- HSE *Commercial Diving Projects Offshore*, Approved Code of Practice, L103. HSE Books, Sudbury.
- HSE *Media Diving Projects*, Approved Code of Practice, L106. HSE Books, Sudbury.
- HSE *Scientific and Archaeological Diving Projects*, Approved Code of Practice, L107. HSE Books, Sudbury.
- HSE *Recreational Diving Projects*, Approved Code of Practice, L105. HSE Books, Sudbury.
- HSE further information and list of Approved Medical Examiner of Divers. Available at: http://www.hse.gov.uk/diving/index.htm

Work in Compressed Air Regulations 1996

Purpose
These regulations govern the conduct of construction works in compressed air.

Application
Applies to all construction work under pressures >0.15bar, except where the Diving Operations at Work Regulations apply.

Definitions
Dysbaric illness
- *Barotrauma:* usually affects sinuses, ears or lungs
- Dysbaric osteonecrosis (see Table 25.1)
- Decompression illness.

Table 25.1 Radiological surveys to detect dysbaric osteonecrosis

Pressure	X-rays	Frequency
<1.0bar	Not required	None
>1.0bar	AP of both shoulders and hips including proximal third of shafts together with AP and lateral views of distal two thirds of both femurs and proximal third of both tibia including knees	Within 3mths of commencement Annually while work continues and 1yr after exposure ceases
>2.0bar	As above	> than annual

Main requirements
- The compressed air contractor must have a safe system of work in compressed air (Reg. 7)
- The contractor must appoint competent personnel as the:
  - person in charge
  - compressor attendant
  - lock attendant
- For work at >1bar the contractor must appoint a medical lock attendant
- The contractor must notify in writing 14 days before and on suspension/completion of compressed air work (Reg. 6):
  - HSE
  - local hospital casualty department
  - emergency services (fire, ambulance)
  - local hyperbaric facilities
- The contractor must provide suitable equipment, fit for use at pressure.

Medical adviser and examinations

- A contract medical adviser (Reg. 9) shall be appointed. This person may also be the HSE appointed doctor
- The contract medical adviser's role includes:
  - planning for compressed air work including health surveillance (Reg. 10)
  - treatment of dysbarism
  - record keeping (retain for 40yrs)
  - occupational medical advice
- No-one can work in compressed air unless passed fit by the appointed doctor (Reg. 16)
- Medical surveillance requires:
  - full medical examination of fitness for work at pressure at entry
  - review every 3mths (<1.0bar) or every month (>1.0bar)
  - full medical assessment every 12mths
- medical assessment following illness >3 days
- medical assessment after any dysbaric illness
- The content of the full medical examination and review are described in Appendix 7 of the regulations. The initial assessment includes detailed history and examination, spirometry, and audiometry
- For work at pressures >1.0bar, an exercise step-test, initial CXR, and full blood count are also required
- The employer shall maintain a health and exposure record for 40yrs, including employee's and employer's details, appointed doctor's details, health surveillance results, exposure record, and training record.

Treatment

- The contractor must provide treatment facilities for dysbaric illness (Reg. 12)
- Provision for emergencies, including fires, must be made
- Decompression from >1.0bar normally employs the Blackpool tables. Rates of decompression illness associated with these tables exist and can be used to benchmark decompression illness rates on a project
- All workers must be provided with a badge to alert others to their work in compressed air should they be incapacitated owing to dysbarism.

Training

Employees and other workers must receive information, instruction, and training (Reg. 15) as to safe operating procedures, hazards of compressed air work, and health surveillance.

Legislation and guidance

- The Work in Compressed Air Regulations 1996. Available at: ℘ http://www.legislation.gov.uk/uksi/1996/1656/contents/made
- Construction (Design and Management) Regulations 2007. Available at: ℘ http://www.legislation.gov.uk/uksi/2007/320/contents/made
- Reporting of Injuries, Disease and Dangerous Occurrences Regulations 1995. Available at: ℘ http://www.legislation.gov.uk/uksi/1995/3163/contents/made

Control of Noise at Work Regulations 2005

Purpose
The aim of the regulations is to ensure that workers are protected from the risks to health caused by noise. The noise regulations implement the EU directive 2003/10/EC on the minimum health and safety requirements regarding the exposure of workers to the risks arising from physical agents (noise).

Application
- The regulations apply to employers, the self-employed, and trainees
- The regulations do not apply to the master and crew of a merchant ship during normal shipboard activities
- Members of the public are not covered where they are exposed to noise through their own activities (e.g. DIY) or where they have made a conscious decision to enter a noisy place (e.g. a nightclub).

Definitions
- *For daily or weekly exposure:*
  - lower exposure action value is 80dB(A)
  - upper exposure action value is 85dB(A)
  - exposure limit value is 87dB(A).
- *For peak sound pressure:*
  - lower exposure action value is 135dB(C)
  - upper exposure action value is 137dB(C)
  - exposure limit value is 140dB(C).

Main requirements
- Employers must undertake a 'suitable and sufficient' risk assessment (Reg. 5) of the risks of noise exposure and identify control measures
- Employers must ensure that the risk from noise exposure is either eliminated at source or, where this is not possible, reduce exposure to as low a level as is reasonably practicable (Reg. 6)
- Where employees are likely to be exposed at, or above, the lower exposure action value, the employer must provide hearing protectors on request
- Any area where employees are likely to be exposed at, or above, the upper exposure action value must be signed as a hearing protection zone and, where possible, demarcated
- Where the upper exposure action value is likely to be exceeded, the employer must eliminate exposure at source or reduce exposure to a level as low as is reasonably practicable, (excludes hearing protection)
- Workers must not be exposed to noise above an exposure limit value.
- Where an exposure limit value is exceeded, after allowing for any noise attenuation afforded by hearing protectors, the employer must take immediate action to reduce exposure. This may include stopping the work

- Hearing protectors must be provided in a hearing protection zone (Reg. 7)
- Employers must enforce the use of hearing protectors where they are required (Reg. 8)
- Any noise control equipment must be used and maintained (Reg. 8).
- Employees have a duty to use personal hearing protectors provided in compliance with Reg. 7 and other noise control measures provided
- Employees should report promptly, any defects in noise control measures, including hearing protectors, to their employer
- Where the risk assessment indicates a risk to workers' health because of noise exposure, suitable health surveillance must be provided (Reg. 9)
- Appendix 5 of the guidance gives detailed information on audiometric testing and Part 6 of the guidance gives more information on health surveillance for noise-induced hearing loss
- Where, following health surveillance, hearing damage due to noise is found the employer shall ensure that:
  - a suitably qualified person notifies the employee
  - the noise risk assessment is reviewed
  - the employer considers redeploying the worker to a non-exposed job
- Employees must cooperate with health surveillance and attend appointments
- The employer must pay the employee when attending health surveillance and meet any associated costs (Reg. 9)
- Where employees are likely to be exposed above the lower action value, the employer must provide suitable information, instruction, and training (Reg. 10). This should cover the risks of noise exposure, the results of any risk assessment, and the measures in place to control noise
- Employees should be advised of the availability of hearing protectors and how to obtain them
- Workers should be told how to detect and report hearing damage
- Employees should be given an explanation of the reasons for health surveillance and informed of the grouped results of any health surveillance.

Legislation and guidance

- HSE (2005). *Controlling Noise at Work*, The Control of Noise at Work Regulations 2005. Guidance on regulations, L108. HSE Books, Sudbury.
- The Control of Noise at Work Regulations 2005. Available at: ℰ http://www.legislation.gov.uk/uksi/2005/1643/contents/made
- See also 📖 p. 4, Noise 1: legal requirements, and risk assessment; 📖 p. 6, Noise 2: instrumentation and determination of LEP,d; 📖 p. 302, Noise induced hearing loss; 📖 p. 430, Classification of hearing loss; 📖 p. 432, Patterns of hearing loss; 📖 p. 764, Screening audiometry; 📖 p. 778, Carry out a noise assessment.

Control of Vibration at Work Regulations 2005

Purpose

To protect against risks to both health and safety from hand-transmitted vibration. This includes risk of hand–arm vibration syndrome (HAVS) and carpal tunnel syndrome in exposed workers and situations where vibration may affect the ability to handle controls safely.

Application

- Duties apply to both employers and self-employed persons
- The specific regulation dealing with compliance with exposure limits will not apply to agricultural and forestry until 2014 for work equipment provided to employees before July 2007
- The regulations do not apply to the master or crew of a merchant ship during normal shipboard activities.

Definitions

- Hand-transmitted vibration is the vibration which enters the body through the hands, e.g. tools used in construction, agriculture, and mining
- *Daily personal exposure or A(8):* average vibration over a working day of 8h
- Daily exposure limit value (ELV) is 5m/s^2 A(8)
- Daily exposure action value (EAV) is 2.5m/s^2 A(8).

Main requirements

Part 1 of the guidance on regulations deals with the legal duties of employers:

- The ELV is the maximum amount of vibration to which an employee may be exposed in any single day. The EAV is the daily exposure to vibration above which action needs to be taken to reduce exposure (Reg. 4)
- An employer who carries out work which is liable to expose employees to risk of vibration is required to assess the risk to the health and safety of employees and identify measures needed to prevent or adequately control exposure (Reg. 5)
- The risk assessment should take into consideration the following:
  - the type of vibration, and its magnitude, and duration
  - the effect of vibration on employees whose health is at particular risk from exposure to vibration
  - information from manufacturers of equipment used
  - work conditions, e.g. temperature
  - information from health surveillance
- Significant findings of the assessment should be recorded together with measures taken to minimize risks
- Action must be taken to eliminate risks from vibration exposure completely wherever it is reasonably practicable to do so (Reg. 6).

Hence there is a need to consider alternative processes, choice of work equipment, and/or better working methods
- Health surveillance (Reg. 7) to be provided for:
  - employees likely to be exposed above the EAV *or*
  - where the risk assessment indicates individuals may be at risk, e.g. those more sensitive to vibration
- A health record must be kept for each employee who undergoes health surveillance. This should contain information on the outcome of the health surveillance and the individual's fitness to continue to work with vibration exposure
- Where as a result of health surveillance an employee is found to have a disease from exposure to vibration, the employer must ensure that a qualified person informs the employee. The employer should also review the risk assessment and the health of other employees
- Employers should ensure that employees understand the level of risk they may be exposed to, how it is caused, possible health effects, safe work practices, and how to detect and report signs of injury (Reg. 8)
- Parts 2–5 of the guide to the regulations provide practical information for employers on carrying out risk assessment, estimating exposure, controlling risks, and arranging health surveillance, and the duties of machinery manufacturers and suppliers. Part 6 provides technical guidance on exposure measurement and Part 7 provides guidance on health surveillance.

Legislation and guidance
- HSE *Hand–arm vibration*, The Control of Vibration at Work Regulations 2005. Guidance on Regulations, L140, HSE Books, Sudbury
- HSE *The Control of Vibration at Work Regulations 2005*. Available at: ℘ http://www.legislation.gov.uk/uksi/2005/1093/contents/made
- HSE *Control the risks from hand–arm vibration*, INDG175 (rev2), HSE free leaflet. Available at: ℘ http://www.hse.gov.uk/pubns/indg175.pdf
- HSE *Hand–arm vibration: advice for employees*, INDG296 (rev1), HSE free pocket card. Available at: ℘ http://www.hse.gov.uk/pubns/indg296.pdf
- See also ▯ p. 10, Vibration 2: hand-transmitted vibration, ▯ p. 438, Surveillance for hand–arm vibration syndrome; and ▯ p. 768, Clinical assessment of hand–arm vibration syndrome.

Food Hygiene Regulations 2006

Purpose

The Food Hygiene (England) Regulations 2006 were introduced to ensure food hygiene regulations in England met EU directives. Similar regulations apply in Wales, Northern Ireland and Scotland. They apply to anyone who owns, manages or works in a food business. They cover primary producers, large manufacturers and restaurants, as well as small mobile catering vans or fast food outlets.

Main provisions

In summary the regulations require:
- Food businesses to register all premises with the local authority. New premises must be registered 28 days before food production begins
- Meat, egg, fish or dairy producers must have their premises approved by the local authority
- Food safety management should be *based* on the principles of Hazard Analysis and Critical Control Points (HACCP)
- Food premises to be clean and well maintained
- Food premises to have adequate handwashing and toilet facilities
- Raw materials to be free from contamination
- Water used to be of drinking quality
- Measures to avoid contamination during transport
- Food handlers to be trained in hygiene procedures and to report conditions such as diarrhoea or vomiting to their manager
- Foods that need temperature control must be hot at or above 63°C, or cold at or below 8°C.

HACCP

In order to manage the potential risks to food in a complex business, a management system is required. HACCP is an internationally recognized system used to identify hazards and control risks along the production line.

The business must:
- Identify hazards such as contamination with bacteria or foreign bodies (e.g. glass)
- Look for critical points where the contamination can take place
- Implement control measures at these points
- Check that control methods work
- Put in place procedures to review these points regularly
- In a small business the system will be simpler, but will (for example) involve regular checks of refrigerator temperatures.

Further information and guidance

HM Govt (2006). Food Hygiene (England) Regulations 2006. Available at: ℜ http://www.legislation.gov.uk/uksi/2006/14/contents/made

Food Standards Agency. Hygiene legislation. Available at: ℜ http://www.food.gov.uk/foodindustry/regulation/hygleg/hygleginfo/foodhygknow/

See also ▢ p. 478, Fitness for work in food handlers.

Registration, evaluation, authorization, and restriction of chemicals

Purpose
REACH is a single, unified framework for the regulation of chemical substances throughout the EU. Its purpose is to:
- Provide a high level of protection for human health and the environment
- Improve the competitiveness of the EU chemical industry
- Promote the development of test methods other than animal testing.

Application
- REACH was launched in 2007 and applies to manufacturers or importers (M/I) that supply chemical substances to the EU market in quantities greater than one ton per year. A substance cannot be manufactured or imported into the EU without prior registration. Registration is due to be completed in 2018
- REACH applies to chemical substances, mixtures and (with qualifications) substances released from preparations or articles. However, REACH assessment is conducted only in relation to a single substance regardless of potential co-exposure to other substances whether added intentionally or occurring as waste products
- The European Chemicals Agency (ECHA) is responsible for the implementation of REACH. In the UK, the Competent Authority is the HSE and enforcement is through the REACH Enforcement Regulations, 2008.

Definitions
Key definitions of relevance to occupational health in REACH are:
- *Chemical safety assessment (CSA):* determination of risk presented by a substance
- *Chemical safety report (CSR):* documentation of the CSA
- *Derived no-effect level (DNEL):* level of exposure below which no adverse effects are expected to occur
- *Exposure scenario:* set of conditions defining the use of a substance through its life cycle
- *Risk characterization:* estimation of the incidence and severity of adverse effects due to actual or predicted exposure
- *Substance of very high concern (SVHC):* substances that are carcinogenic, mutagenic, persistent bioaccumulative and toxic (PBT), very persistent and very bioaccumulative (vPvB) or otherwise SVHC assessed on a case-by-case basis
- *Technical Dossier:* description of intrinsic properties, classification and guidance on safe use of a substance.

Main requirements

Registration

Remaining timelines for registration:
- 100–1000tons/yr, 31 May 2013
- 1–100tons/yr, 31 May 2018.

Main M/I and related responsibilities

- Submission of a technical dossier (> 1ton/yr) and CSA (>10tons/yr). CSA is to include calculation of the DNEL
- If a substance is 'dangerous' (under REACH Article 10a), PBT or vPvB, CSA is also to include exposure scenarios, exposure assessment and risk characterization. These are to incorporate the effect of existing or planned Risk Management Measures (RMM)
- M/I is to convey information on the safe use and necessary RMM to downstream users (DU). DU have a responsibility to apply the necessary RMM
- CSA to be documented in the CSR
- M/I may pool data through a substance information exchange forum (SIEF) and apply for joint registration though a lead registrant.

Evaluation

ECHA and member states' (MS) competent authorities are responsible for the examination of dossiers for completeness, testing proposals in relation to health effects and substance evaluation i.e. need for further information.

Authorization

Specific conditions may apply to authorization of SVHC with consideration of the following; the suitability of alternative substances or technologies, a study of the feasibility of substitution, socio-economic analysis to assess overall risk/benefit and the effectiveness of existing RMM.

Restriction

Provision for a limitation on use or complete prohibition of substances that present an unacceptable risk at a community-wide level.

Further information

ECHA issues guidance on the application of REACH which is available at: ℘ http://guidance.echa. europa.eu

Employment law

Employment law

This is, of necessity, an abridged account of detailed and complex legislation. The interested reader is referred to more detailed texts.

Employment law

- Employment law in the UK is a mixture of civil law, concerned with compensation, and criminal law, concerned with punishment. Some employment law is in the form of case law, and some in the form of statute law, setting standards for the behaviour of employers in terms of equality, data protection, and health and safety at work (see Table 26.1)
- The courts of law, in deciding cases brought before them, create precedents which may be applied in future similar disputes. Decisions of higher courts, like the Supreme Court and Court of Appeal, are binding on lower courts. Much of the civil law is made by the judges in this way, without recourse to Parliament. We call this judge-made law the common law
- Statutes are Acts of Parliament; that is the House of Commons, the House of Lords, and the Queen. The Scottish Parliament and the Welsh Assembly have limited powers to create legislation for Scotland and Wales. Statute law takes precedence over case law, but the courts in interpreting the meaning of statutes also create precedents
- Statutory instruments, or statutory regulations, are delegated legislation made by a government minister by virtue of the authority given to him/her in a statute. They do not need to be debated in Parliament, unless an MP questions them. Delegated legislation is used to provide detailed provisions which Parliament has insufficient time to create. The statute lays down the principle, which is then expanded in regulations.

Employment tribunals

- Employment tribunals are specialist employment courts which deal with unfair dismissal, redundancy payments, and laws against discrimination at work
- They sit in several large towns and are composed of a legally qualified judge who sometimes sits with two lay members, one representing employers and the other employees
- They can award money compensation and make recommendations, but have no power to force an employer to reinstate an employee
- The law that the employment tribunals administer is laid down in a number of statutes and regulations, which have been interpreted by the courts.

Enforcement of civil law

- The enforcement of the civil law is not a matter for the HSE, the local authorities, or the police. A civil action is brought by the person claiming a remedy: the claimant
- In England and Wales actions for damages for personal injury must be brought in the County Court or the High Court

- In Scotland actions for damages for personal injury are brought in the Sheriff Court or the Court of Session
- Appeals against a refusal of social security benefits must be taken to a first tier tribunal
- Complaints that an employer has unfairly dismissed an employee, or unlawfully discriminated against him/her because of a protected characteristic under the Equality Act 2010 must be taken to an employment tribunal.

Table 26.1 The main differences between civil law and criminal law

	Civil law	Criminal law
Main purpose	Compensation	Punishment
Source of law	Statute or case (common) law	Statute law
Prosecuting authority	None—civil action by claimant	Crown Prosecution Service[a]
		Procurator Fiscal[b]
		HSE
		Local authority
Insurance	Employers' Liability Insurance	None

[a]England and Wales
[b]Scotland

Compensation

State benefits

- A system of no-fault compensation for occupational injuries and diseases, originally named Workmen's Compensation, now the Industrial Injuries Benefits Scheme, has existed in the UK since 1897
- Financed through taxation; administered by the State (now the DWP)
- The scheme covers all employed earners, but not the self-employed
- A disablement pension is payable to a person who has:
  - suffered a personal injury caused by accident arising out of and in the course of employment, *or*
  - contracted a prescribed disease, i.e. one designated by the Secretary of State as a special risk for a particular occupation
- The Industrial Injuries Advisory Council (IIAC) advises the Secretary of State regarding the diseases that should be considered for prescription under the scheme, and generally on its operation
- Prescription will be recommended when epidemiological evidence shows that a particular job is associated with a doubling of risk of the disease (compared with a member of the general public)
- A list of prescribed diseases is found in the Social Security (Prescribed Diseases) Regulations 1985 (see ▱ Appendix 2: list of prescribed diseases). Regularly updated by statutory instrument. Prescribed diseases are divided into:
  - conditions due to physical agents, e.g. tenosynovitis for manual labour or frequent repetitive movements of the hand or wrist
  - conditions due to biological agents (e.g. anthrax for work involving contact with animal products or residues)
  - conditions due to chemical agents (e.g. lead poisoning for work involving exposure to lead), *and*
  - miscellaneous conditions (e.g. asthma for work involving exposure to any of a long list of agents including isocyanates).

Claims for industrial injuries disablement benefit (IIDB)

- Claims must be made to the DWP, where assessment is made by a civil servant aided by medical evidence from the DWP's doctors. Appeal to a tribunal consisting of a legally qualified judge and two doctors
- A tax-free pension is payable to those who qualify for benefit only where the disability is assessed as at least 14% (except noise-induced hearing loss (>20%) and pneumoconiosis, byssinosis, or diffuse mesothelioma (no level))
- Lump sum payments and death benefits have been abolished
- A reduced earnings allowance to compensate for incapability to follow the regular occupation is payable to those injured by an accident or the onset of a prescribed disease before 1 October 1990
- Those who are 100% disabled and need constant care are also entitled to a constant attendance allowance or an exceptionally severe disablement allowance.

Civil compensation

- Compensation can be obtained through a civil action in tort. A tort (from the Latin for twisted) is a civil wrong, which gives rise to an action for damages. The equivalent in Scotland is a delict. In almost all cases liability is based on fault
- A successful claimant must deduct from the damages awarded all social security benefits received over 5yrs, to reimburse the DWP
- Legal aid is now available in only a few cases. Most claimants finance their actions through a conditional fee agreement with the lawyer, under which the lawyer is paid only if successful
- An action must normally be brought within 3yrs of the damage. Therefore it is important to advise an individual when an occupational disease is diagnosed, and to make a written record of this advice in the medical records. Where the claimant is unaware of the damage (as where an illness has a long latency period), he/she has 3yrs from the date he/she discovers the illness or ought reasonably to have discovered it
- In the field of industrial injury or disease the claimant usually alleges negligence by the employer
- Negligence is defined as a failure to take reasonable care to prevent foreseeable harm
- Employees often also sue their employer for breach of statutory duty
- Most of the statutory regulations, like the COSHH Regulations 2002 and the Manual Handling at Work Regulations 1992, give rise to a civil action for breach of statutory duty, as well as the possibility of a criminal prosecution
- Since the numbers of prosecutions brought by the enforcing authorities are relatively few, a civil action is a more likely sanction for breach of health and safety laws
- The Health and Safety at Work Act 1974 does not give rise to a civil action. It lays down a framework for the criminal law of health and safety at work. The common law of negligence already provides a civil action for damages for negligence
- Damages are awarded for loss of earnings, and also for pain and suffering and loss of amenity
- The employer is vicariously liable for the wrongdoing of its employees in the course of employment
- The Employers' Liability (Compulsory Insurance) Act 1969 imposes an obligation on employers to take out insurance against a claim by an employee for an industrial injury.

Relevant legislation

- Social Security (Industrial Injuries)(Prescribed Diseases) Regulations 1985, as amended
- Social Security Act 1998.

Further information

Kloss D (2005). *Occupational Health Law*, 5th edn, Chapter 7. Wiley-Blackwell, Oxford.
DWP. Available at: ◌ http://www.dwp.gov.uk for information about welfare benefits.

Equality Act 2010

The protected characteristics

- This Act, most of which came into force in England and Wales and Scotland on 1 October 2010, repeals previous legislation dealing with discrimination, including:
  - the Sex Discrimination Act 1975
  - the Race Relations Act 1976
  - the Disability Discrimination Act 1995 *and*
  - the Employment Equality (Age) Regulations 2006
- The law is based on EU directives. It covers discrimination in employment, education, transport, and the provision of goods, facilities, and services. It brings together all the anti-discrimination legislation into one comprehensive statute
- The Equality and Human Rights Commission oversees and polices the Act
- The employment provisions are enforced through employment tribunals
- A claim of unlawful discrimination must be commenced in an employment tribunal within 3mths of the act complained of or, where there are a series of complaints, within 3mths of the last incident
- The Equality Act does not apply to Northern Ireland where the old legislation is, for the time being, still in force.

Characteristics protected by the Act

The following are characteristics protected by the Act:

- Age
- Disability
- Gender reassignment
- Marriage and civil partnership
- Pregnancy and maternity
- Race
- Religion or belief
- Sex
- Sexual orientation.

Disability discrimination 1: the definition of disability

A disabled person is one with a physical or mental impairment that has a substantial and long-term adverse effect on his/her ability to carry out normal day-to-day activities. These activities may be carried out in employment or outside employment, but must be activities common to many jobs, such as reading, writing, walking, and climbing stairs, not those special to a particular job, such as assembling a watch or playing a violin in an orchestra.

- Physical impairment includes sensory impairments such as those affecting sight or hearing
- Mental impairment includes learning difficulties and any mental disorder. Since 2005 it is unnecessary to show that a mental illness is clinically well recognized
- A substantial adverse effect is one that is more than minor or trivial
- Long term means having lasted for 12mths or more, likely to last for 12mths or more, or terminal
- The Equality Act removes the need to prove impairment of one of a list of capacities, for example mobility, manual dexterity or memory. It is now ultimately for the employment tribunal to decide what is a normal day-to-day activity
- Pain and fatigue must be taken into account, and the fact that disabled people develop coping mechanisms to avoid tasks they find difficult
- Where a condition would be disabling if not controlled by drugs (e.g. epilepsy, diabetes) or assisted by prosthesis or other aid (e.g. hearing aid, counselling), it counts as a disability under the Act. Only exception to this is defective eyesight assisted by spectacles or contact lenses
- A severe disfigurement is treated as a disability (unless self-inflicted), even though it does not interfere with normal day to day activities
- Cancer, HIV, and multiple sclerosis are disabilities from diagnosis
- Other progressive conditions, e.g. muscular dystrophy, are disabilities from when the impairment has some effect on the ability to carry out normal day-to-day activities, even though not yet substantial
- Recurrent disabling conditions, e.g. rheumatoid arthritis, are disabilities despite periods of remission if a substantial adverse effect is likely to recur
- Where a person has suffered from a substantial and long-term disabling condition in the past and has now recovered, he/she will be protected by the Act if discriminated against because of the past disability. This is particularly important to those who have had a mental illness
- The Equality Act 2010 (Disability) Regulations 2011 provide that a person is disabled if certified as blind, severely sight impaired, sight impaired or partially sighted by a consultant ophthalmologist
- These regulations also provide that certain conditions are to be treated as not amounting to impairments, i.e.
  - a tendency to set fires
  - a tendency to steal

- • a tendency to physical or sexual abuse of other persons
  - • exhibitionism, *and*
  - • voyeurism
- Seasonal allergic rhinitis is to be treated as not amounting to an impairment unless it aggravates the effect of another condition
- Addiction to alcohol, nicotine or any other substance is to be treated as not amounting to an impairment unless originally the result of administration of medically prescribed drugs or other medical treatment
- Where addiction causes a disabling medical condition, e.g. alcoholism and liver cirrhosis, the consequent impairment is a potential disability under the Act.

Occupational health reports

- A medical report on a worker should not state definitively that he/she is disabled, since that is a legal question for an employment tribunal. However, it is acceptable for a doctor to state that in his/her opinion it is likely or unlikely that the worker qualifies as disabled, without making a definite ruling
- If it is appropriate, a report should set out whether there is an impairment, the effect on normal day-to-day activities, and how long it is likely to last
- It may also recommend adjustments to the working environment or working practices that could enable to worker to do the job, despite the disability. The latter is good employment practice even when there is doubt about whether the worker is disabled, and this is supported by the Equality and Human Rights Commission's Code of Practice on Employment 2011
- In order to be legally defensible, occupational health reports must be written by a suitably qualified expert, based on evidence, and must be logical and reasoned. Suitable expertise would include being an accredited specialist in occupational medicine.[1]

Further information

Guidance on Matters to be Taken into Account in Determining Questions Relating to the Definition of Disability (2011).

Kloss D (2010). *Occupational Health Law*, 5th edn, Chapter 9. Wiley-Blackwell, Oxford.

---

[1] Jones v Post Office [2001] EWCA Civ 558, [2001] IRLR 384, Court of Appeal.

Disability discrimination 2: employers' duties

The disability provisions of the Equality Act apply to all employers, except for the armed forces. They apply to job applicants, employees, self-employed, contract workers, and office-holders, but not to volunteers. A complaint of unlawful disability discrimination must be made to an employment tribunal within 3mths (of the act or the last incident).

Direct discrimination

- This is treating someone less favourably because of the fact of the disability—a 'blanket ban', e.g. 'job is not open to those with epilepsy'
- Direct discrimination is unlawful and cannot be justified. Each job applicant or employee must be treated as an individual
- Direct discrimination against a non-disabled person because of association with a disabled person is unlawful, e.g. mother of a disabled child rejected because of fear she will take time off to care for her child.

Pre-employment screening

- Employers must not normally ask health questions, including questions about sickness absence, before offering a job applicant work
- However, an offer of work can be made conditional on satisfactory health clearance and health questions can then be asked
- The employer is allowed to ask an applicant, before offering work:
  - if s/he needs adjustments to the selection process, e.g. an interview
  - questions about functions intrinsic to the job, e.g. eyesight
- Health questionnaires should be drafted, processed, and interpreted by health professionals and stored as confidential medical records. Nothing in the pre-employment health questionnaire should be disclosed to the manager without the consent of the worker, or a court order. Such information should only be disclosed to managers in as far as this is necessary for them to undertake their management responsibilities.

Disability-related discrimination

- This is treating someone unfavourably because of something that arises in consequence of his/her disability, e.g. rejecting a wheelchair user for a job as a firefighter. This discrimination is justifiable if the employer can prove it is a proportionate means of achieving a legitimate aim
- Employers should consider reasonable adjustments before rejecting someone for a disability-related reason, e.g. dismissal for unacceptable sickness absence without considering adjustments to the attendance management procedure may be discrimination. However, employers are not obliged to continue to employ a disabled employee whose attendance has been seriously unsatisfactory for a long period.

- An employer may be able to justify discrimination on health and safety grounds, but only if it is proportionate to the risk. Decisions must be based on a risk assessment and reasonable adjustments must be made
- Employers must not exclude a disabled person if there is no explicit statutory prohibition and no clear evidence that the risk to the disabled person is substantially greater than to the non-disabled employee, or employment would create a significant hazard to others.

The duty to make reasonable adjustments

- There is a duty to consider adjustments to the working environment and practices, and the provision of auxiliary aids (including services)
- There is a duty to consider adjustments to recruitment
- The duty only arises when the employer either knows or ought to know of the disability
- The employer only has to do what is reasonable. Reasonableness depends on practicability and cost. The extent of an employer's resources, the nature of its activities, and the size of the undertaking are relevant. Financial assistance through the Access to Work scheme, or sponsorship by a charity or local authority, must also be explored
- The employer must not seek payment from a disabled employee for the costs of complying with the duty of reasonable adjustment
- Examples are given in the Code of Practice on Employment 2011:
  - making adjustments to premises
  - providing information in accessible formats
  - allocating some of the disabled person's duties to another worker
  - transferring the disabled person to fill an existing vacancy
  - altering hours of work or training
  - assigning to a different place of work or training, or home working
  - allowing the disabled person to be absent during working or training hours for rehabilitation, assessment, or treatment
  - providing training/mentoring for disabled person or other worker
  - acquiring or modifying equipment
  - modifying procedures for testing or assessment
  - providing a reader or interpreter
  - providing supervision or other support
  - allowing a disabled worker to take a period of disability leave
  - participating in supported employment schemes, such as Workstep (see 📖 p. 410, Rehabilitation and disability services)
  - employing a support worker to assist a disabled worker
  - modifying disciplinary or grievance procedures
  - adjusting redundancy selection criteria
  - modifying performance-related pay arrangements
- Reasonable adjustments include moving a disabled employee to a higher grade job (if s/he has the necessary qualifications), or to a lower-paid job (if that is all that is available within his/her competence)

- In general, a disabled employee is not entitled to a longer period of sick pay than the non-disabled. However, the Court of Appeal has held that, where an employer is at fault in not making a reasonable adjustment, they must pay full pay throughout a resulting period of absence
- Disability-related leave, e.g. to attend physiotherapy or counselling, is not sick leave and should be recorded separately
- Failure to make adjustments deemed reasonable by an Employment tribunal (EmT) cannot be justified.

Relevant legislation and further information

- Equality Act 2010 (Disability) Regulations 2010.
- Equality and Human Rights Commission (2011). CoP on Employment.
- Kloss D (2010). *Occupational Health Law*, 5th edn, Chapter 9. Wiley-Blackwell, Oxford.

Sex discrimination

It is unlawful to treat a person of one sex less favourably than someone of the opposite sex because of their gender. Stereotypical assumptions should not be made about women being weaker and more vulnerable than men. Each person should be treated as an individual.

Indirect discrimination

- Indirect discrimination is treating a member of one sex unfavourably because of a provision, criterion or practice which puts members of one sex at a disadvantage, e.g. a requirement to work shifts or to work away from home
- Indirect discrimination can be justified if the employer has used a proportionate means of achieving a legitimate aim, e.g. the needs of his/her business require these methods of working.

Sexual harassment

Sexual harassment is a form of sex discrimination. It is unwanted conduct either of a sexual nature or on the grounds of sex that has the purpose or effect of violating the employee's dignity, or creating an intimidating, hostile, degrading, humiliating, or offensive environment. If not done with that intention it is to be regarded as having such an effect only if it should reasonably be considered as doing so.

Pregnancy discrimination

- The Equality Act 2010 provides that it is unlawful to treat a woman unfavourably in the protected period because she is pregnant or because of illness suffered by her as a result of it or because she takes statutory maternity leave
- The protected period begins when the pregnancy begins and ends at the end of her statutory maternity leave or, if earlier, when she returns to work after the pregnancy. If she does not have the right to maternity leave it ends 2wks after the end of the pregnancy
- After the end of the protected period, the employer is entitled to treat any sickness absence of the woman in the same way as he would treat that of a man, even though it may be pregnancy or maternity related
- Nothing shall render unlawful any act done in relation to a woman if it is necessary to protect women as regards pregnancy or maternity, e.g. work with lead or ionizing radiations, or work on a ship or aircraft
- Pregnant employees are entitled to reasonable time off work with pay to attend antenatal care recommended by a doctor, midwife, or health visitor (Employment Rights Act 1996)
- Where a job is hazardous for a pregnant employee or one who has recently given birth, the employer must not dismiss her. Either a suitable alternative must be found or she must be sent home on full pay
- If a doctor or midwife has certified that night work is hazardous, the employer must either offer her suitable day work or suspend her on full pay

- Under the Management Regulations 1999 an employer must carry out a risk assessment of the specific risks posed to the health and safety of pregnant women or new mothers when employing any woman of childbearing potential. Further risk assessment should be performed when a female employee informs the employer she is pregnant, and update as necessary. Failure to do so is unlawful sex discrimination
- The main hazards are:
  - physical agents (e.g. shocks, vibrations, handling of loads, noise, non-ionizing radiation, extremes of heat and cold)
  - chemical agents (e.g. mercury, lead, antimitotic drugs, CO)
  - biological agents (e.g. listeria, rubella, chickenpox, toxoplasma, cytomegalovirus, hepatitis B, and HIV)
  - working conditions (e.g. mining)
- If the woman informs her employer after her return to work that she is breastfeeding, a risk assessment should be done
- Employers have a duty to provide suitable workplace rest facilities for women at work who are breastfeeding
- There is no statutory right for workers to take time off to breastfeed, but an employer who unreasonably refuses to allow a woman to express milk or to adjust her working conditions to allow her to continue to breastfeed may be liable for unlawful sex discrimination
- A woman must not be at work within 2wks of giving birth
  - from 1 April 2007 she has the right to up to 52wks maternity leave
  - statutory maternity pay is payable for up to 39wks.

Gender reassignment

- Discrimination against a person who is proposing to undergo, is undergoing, or has undergone a process (or part of a process) for the purpose of reassigning sex by changing physiological attributes, or who is living as a member of the opposite sex without undergoing medical treatment, is unlawful under the Equality Act 2010
- Absence from work to undergo gender reassignment must be treated in the same way as absence due to sickness or injury, and the employer must not treat a transsexual's absence less favourably than that of other workers if it is unreasonable to do so, e.g. the transsexual asks to take a day's holiday to attend counselling and the employer refuses without good reason
- There is an exception where the job involves the holder of the job being liable to be called upon to perform intimate physical searches pursuant to statutory powers. However, under the Gender Recognition Act 2004 a person who has successfully undergone gender reassignment can register his/her acquired gender and thereafter is entitled to be regarded for all purposes as possessing that gender.

Relevant legislation

- Equality Act 2010
- Workplace (Health, Safety and Welfare) Regulations 1992
- Management of Health and Safety at Work Regulations 1999
- Employment Rights Act 1996
- Gender Recognition Act 2004.

Age discrimination

- Discrimination against employees because of their age is unlawful under the Equality Act 2010 unless the employer can justify it as a proportionate means of achieving a legitimate aim. This applies to both direct and indirect discrimination, and to both young and old
- Employers are permitted to ask for training and experience where it can be shown that this is a genuine requirement for the job, and to refuse to give training where the employer will be unlikely to work for long enough to justify the expenditure on training
- In 2011 the employers' right to force employees to retire at 65 was repealed. Employers now have to justify forcing an employee to retire at any age. However, the Supreme Court decided in 2012 that a policy that specifies a compulsory age of retirement can be defended if it is reasonably necessary to assist workforce planning, or to preserve the dignity of older workers
- There is no age limit for unfair dismissal and redundancy rights
- Case law from the European Court of Justice has held that assumptions based on statistical averages showing that older workers are likely to be less physically and intellectually competent than younger workers can justify the imposition of age restrictions on recruitment and retirement
- Employers are justified in imposing fitness testing on older workers, where fitness is a necessary job requirement.

Young workers

- Employers are under a special duty to protect young workers
- No person under 13 may lawfully be employed in any capacity and from 13–16-yrs-old only outside school hours and not for more than 2h a day, except for approved work experience for children in their last year of school
- The employer must conduct a risk assessment of a young person under 18yrs old before he/she starts work and has a duty to take into account inexperience, lack of awareness of risk, and immaturity
- Young persons must not be employed on work which is:
  - beyond their physical or psychological capacity
  - involves harmful exposure to agents which are toxic
  - carcinogenic, cause heritable genetic damage or harm to the unborn child, or in any other way chronically affect human health
  - involves harmful exposure to radiation
  - involves a risk of accidents which it may reasonably be assumed cannot be recognized or avoided by young person's owing to their insufficient attention to safety or lack of experience or training
  - or presents a risk from extreme cold or heat, noise, or vibration.

Relevant legislation

- Equality Act 2010
- Management of Health and Safety at Work Regulations 1999.

Working Time Regulations 1998

Working Time Regulations 1998

These provisions are very complex, and only a general account is given, with only a few of the many amendments being considered in this section. Issues around working time inevitably link in with shift working and related health issues.

Main provisions and definitions

- The regulations impose a limit on working hours, including overtime, of an average of 48h for each 7 days, taken over a period of 17wks, but there are many exceptions. Doctors in training were included from 1 August 2004. They were restricted to 58h until 31 July 2007, and 56h until 31 July 2009. The 48h limit now applies
- Working hours include hours when the worker is on call on his/her employer's premises, but not when he/she is on call at home. They do not include travel to and from work unless the worker's job involves travel, e.g. a travelling salesman
- Employers are permitted to ask workers to opt out by agreement in writing. Workers must not be penalized for refusing to do so
- Employers must keep records, and are subject to inspection by the HSE
- There is a general duty in the Health and Safety at Work Act to prevent risks to health and safety. This applies to overlong working hours
- Young workers (under 18yrs old) are prohibited from working more than 8h a day or 40h a week
- The regulations extend to self-employed workers as well as employees.

Night workers

- There are special provisions relating to night workers, defined as working at least 3h of daily working time between 23.00 and 06.00 hours
- An employer shall ensure that no night worker, whose work involves special hazards or heavy physical or mental strain, works for more than 8h in any 24h period during which the night worker performs night work.

Night workers' health assessments

- Every adult worker assigned to night work must have the opportunity of a free health assessment before he/she takes up the assignment, and at regular intervals as appropriate. This should be done through a screening questionnaire, compiled with guidance from a qualified health professional. (See 📖 p. 756, Night worker health assessment). Where a potential problem is disclosed, referral to a health professional is advised
- Where a doctor has advised an employer that a worker is suffering from health problems that the practitioner considers to be connected with night work, the employer should, where possible, transfer the worker to suitable day work.

Rest periods and holidays

- Adult workers must be given a rest period of at least 24h every week and a rest break of at least 20min after 6h. They must have a rest period of at least 11h in each 24h period
- There are special provisions for workers under 18yrs old:
  - they must have a rest period of at least 48h a week and a rest break of at least 30min after 4.5h
  - they are entitled to a rest period of at least 12h in each 24h period
  - young workers should not normally be employed to work at night, but in exceptional cases they may be assigned to night work, e.g. work in hospitals
  - young workers assigned to night work must have the opportunity of a free assessment of their health and capacities before they take up the assignment
- Workers are entitled to a minimum of 28 days a year paid holiday, which includes bank holidays. Part-time workers are entitled to paid holidays *pro rata*
- Employees who are absent on sick leave continue to accrue rights to paid holidays which can be taken after they return to work
- The holiday provisions are enforced through the employment tribunals.

Relevant legislation

Working Time Regulations (1998) (as amended).

Further information

Department of Trade and Industry (2003). *Your Guide to the Working Time Regulations (VRN 00/1068)*. Department of Trade and Industry, London. Available at: ℘ http://www.dti.gov.uk/employment/employment-legislation/employment-guidance/page28978.html

HSE (2006). *Managing shift work*, HSG 256. HSE Books, Sudbury.

Legislation related to occupational health records

Data Protection Act 1998

Purpose

The Data Protection Act 1998 came into force in 2001 and governs the collection, holding, use or release of data on individuals as required by EC Directive 95/46/EC. It sets out principles of good data handling ('the eight principles') and confers several rights on individuals. This Act replaces the Data Protection Act 1984 and the Access to Health Records Act 1990, although the latter still applies to access to the medical records of dead people.

⚠ An organization found in breach of the Act may face a substantial fine.

Application

The Act applies to individuals and organizations (data controllers) based in the UK or processing data in the UK. The Act covers all health records including X-rays, video, and audiotapes.

Definitions

- *Data controller*: the person who determines the purpose and manner of data processing
- *Data* is information which is:
  - processed by computer
  - recorded to be processed by a computer
  - held in a 'relevant filing system'
  - part of an accessible record
- *Data subject*: the person to whom the data relates
- *Personal data* relates to a living individual who may be identified from that data alone, or in combination with other data, held by the data controller
- *Sensitive personal data* includes:
  - an individual's race or ethnicity
  - political beliefs
  - religious or other beliefs
  - trade union membership
  - health
  - sex life
  - crimes or alleged crimes
  - criminal convictions
- *Caldicott guardian:* a senior health or social services professional responsible for controlling the management, use, and disclosure of health or social services data sets. A system set up following the report by the Caldicott Committee to the Department of Health in 1997 on the use and transfer of patient identifiable information for purposes other than patient care, research or statutory notification.

Main requirements

- Data processors must register with the Information Commissioner's Office and pay a small fee. Failure to register is a criminal offence

- The Data Protection Act confers a right of access to health records irrespective of when the health record was created:
  Subject access request should be made in writing (or by email).
  ▶ It is important to confirm the identity of the person making the request, especially where the records requested are old. Where a third party, e.g. a solicitor, makes the request you must satisfy yourself that they have the subject's permission to do so
  - All requests should be acknowledged, logged and tracked to completion. This permits subsequent audit
  - Access may be denied where information in the health record may cause serious harm to the physical or mental health of the applicant or any other person. A medical practitioner must make this decision and should carefully document their reasoning
  - Access may be denied where disclosure would release information regarding or provided by a third party who had not consented to disclosure
  - Fees may be charged by the data controller to reflect the actual costs incurred to produce copies of health records up to a maximum of £10 for computer records and £50 for paper records
  - Alternatively, the individual may inspect their records at no cost
  - Access to health records should be provided within 40 days.

The eight principles of good practice
- Data processors must comply with 'the eight principles of good practice' such that:
  - data are fairly processed
  - processing is for limited purposes
  - data are adequate, relevant, and not excessive
  - data are accurate and up to date
  - data are retained only for as long as necessary
  - data processing is in line with subjects' rights
  - data are secure
  - data are not transferred out with the European Economic Area except to a country with adequate data protection laws*.

* Privacy laws in the USA differ from the EU, and so the US–European Union Safe Harbor Framework was set up. US companies that self-certify to the US EU Safe Harbor Framework demonstrate that their organization provides 'adequate' privacy protection, as defined by the Directive, so allowing data transfers from EU countries to that US company.

Legislation and guidance
- Website of the Information Commissioner. ℘ http://www.ico.gov.uk/
- The Employment Practices Code 2005
- Data Protection Act 1998
- Confidentiality: NHS Code of Practice, Department of Health, 2003.
- Website of Business USA detailing the Safe Harbor framework. Available at: ℘ http://export.gov/safeharbor/

Access to Medical Reports Act 1988

Purpose
This Act gives a person a right of access to medical reports regarding themselves prepared by a medical practitioner, who has provided care to them, for the purposes of employment or insurance.

Application in occupational health
The Act applies to any person or organization that wishes to obtain a medical report on an individual for employment or insurance purposes.

Reports requested by an OH professional
The Act clearly applies when an Occupational Health professional requests a report from an employee's doctor.

Reports produced by an OH professional
✍ Some have argued that this legislation does not apply to reports produced by OH professionals as they do not provide care. However, there may be situations where they do provide care and the Act does apply: see the Faculty of Occupational Medicine's Guidance on Ethics for examples. In addition:
- It is good practice to discuss with an employee the contents of any medical report to an employer. Failure to do so can undermine the doctor–patient relationship
- The individual can request access to a medical report under the Data Protection Act
- The GMC has produced guidance for doctors stating that a patient must have the right of access to any reports written about them for insurance or employment purposes, including receiving a copy (if they wish) before the report is released:
  - the GMC do not explicitly allow a 21-day period for the patient to have access to the report before it is sent
  - although the GMC guidance does not strictly apply to OH nurses, it is good practice for them to follow these principles.

Definitions
- *Applicant:* the person requesting a medical report
- *Medical report:* a report regarding the physical or mental health of an individual prepared by a medical practitioner responsible (now or in the past) for the clinical care of that individual.

Main requirements
- An employer wishing to obtain a medical report on an employee or prospective employee can only do so with his/her consent. (This should be in writing and a copy of the signed consent provided to the medical practitioner.)
- The employee must be informed of his/her rights under the Act and most employers will provide this information in writing. The employee's rights are:
  - to withhold consent for the report

- to have access to the report before consenting to its submission to the employer
- to make a written request to the medical practitioner for amendment of any part of a report which he/she considers wrong or misleading
- to have access to the report up to 6 months after submission.

- Where an employee wishes to see the medical report the applicant must advise him/her that they have requested the report so that the individual can contact the medical practitioner to see the report within 21 days
- Having seen the report, the employee may decide to withhold consent for the report to be provided to the applicant
- If an individual indicates that he/she wants to see the report but then fails to contact the doctor within 21 days to see it, the doctor can submit the report to the applicant
- If an individual believes a report is wrong or misleading and the medical practitioner does not agree to amend the report, the individual may request that a statement of his/her views be attached to the report before he/she consents to release the report. Alternatively, the employee may decide to withhold consent to release the report
- A doctor can withhold access to any part of a report he/she believes may cause serious harm to the individual's health. The doctor should inform the individual of his/her decision to deny access. In practice it is rare to withhold access to part of a report
- A medical practitioner can withhold access to any part of a report where it would reveal the identity of a third party who had provided information about the individual unless that third party consents or is a health care worker and the information was imparted as part of his/her job
- The individual has a right of access to a medical report for a period of 6mths, and so the medical practitioner must retain a copy for 6mths after the report is provided.

Legislation and guidance

- Access to Medical Reports Act 1988
- Faculty of Occupational Medicine (2006). *Guidance on Ethics for Occupational Physicians*, 6th edn. FOM, London.
- BMA (2009). *Access to medical reports – guidance from the BMA Medical Ethics Department*. Available at: ℘ http://www.bma.org.uk/ethics/ health_records/accessmedreports.jsp
- GMC (2009). *GMC supplementary guidance. Confidentiality: disclosing information for insurance, employment and similar purposes*. available at: ℘ http://www.gmc-uk.org/static/documents/content/Confidentiality_ disclosing_info_insurance_2009.pdf

Freedom of Information Act 2000

The Freedom of Information Act 2000 provided for public access to information held by, or on behalf of, publicly funded bodies in England, Wales, and Northern Ireland. Similar legislation applies in Scotland: the Freedom of Information (Scotland) Act 2002. These pieces of legislation were intended to create a culture of openness among public bodies. The Freedom of Information Act 2000 created the Information Commissioner's Office (ICO) whose role is to enforce the Act. The Act was subsequently updated by the Environmental Information Regulations 2004 (EIR). In Scotland the Scottish Information Commissioner fulfils the ICO's role.

Definitions
- *Public authorities* include:
  - central government
  - local authorities
  - police
  - prison service
  - health authorities
  - NHS GPs, dentists, opticians, and pharmacists
  - educational establishments.

Main requirements
- All public bodies must produce a publication scheme (approved by the Information Commissioner) stating what information they routinely make available (e.g. annual reports, committee minutes) and how to obtain it
- An information request may be made verbally, in writing, or by email.
- Public bodies must respond promptly to such information requests and in any event within 20 days
- There are 23 exemptions from disclosure in the Act. Some are absolute while others are qualified exemptions:
  - information covered by an absolute exemption includes personal information
  - information covered by a qualified exemption may only be withheld where the public interest is best served by withholding it. The presumption is that disclosure is preferred
- Where a public body refuses to release information application may be made to the Information Commissioner to review the decision. Where the ICO disagrees with the decision not to release information, the public body can be required to release the information
- Where an individual or a public body disputes the ICO's decision, an appeal can be made to the Information Tribunal
- Failure to comply with a decision of the Information Tribunal may be held to be contempt of court.

Legislation and guidance
- HMSO (2000). *Freedom of Information Act 2000*, Chapter 36. Stationery Office, London.

- HMSO (2002). *Freedom of Information (Scotland) Act 2002*, asp 13. Stationery Office, London.
- HMSO (2004). *The Environmental Information Regulations 2004*. Stationery Office, London.
- Information Commissioner's Office. ✍ http://www.ico.gov.uk/
- Scottish Information Commissioner ✍ http://www.itspublicknowledge. info/

Environmental legislation

Environmental Protection Act 1990

The Environmental Protection Act 1990 aimed to improve control of pollution arising from industrial processes by integrating pollution control (IPC). It represents the most recent in a series of laws that began with the Alkali Acts in the Nineteenth century. This legislation covers air, water, and soil pollution, and also covers the release of genetically modified organisms. The Act gave the Secretary of State power to prescribe substances subject to controls on their release into the environment. The Act was subsequently updated by the Environment Act 1995, which created the Environment Agency (England and Wales) (see 📖 p. 588, The Environment Agency) and its equivalent Scottish body, the Scottish Environment Protection Agency.

Definitions
- *Pollution:* of the environment means release into air, water, or land of any substance capable of causing harm to living organisms, e.g. humans
- *Release:* includes emissions into the air, discharge of substances into water, and the disposal, deposit, or keeping of substances in or on land
- *Waste:* includes any scrap material, effluent, or unwanted substance
- *Controlled waste:* means household, industrial, or commercial waste
- *Special waste:* is controlled waste that is so dangerous to keep, treat, or dispose of, that special provision is required for dealing with it.

Main requirements
- No-one may carry out a prescribed process unless authorized by the enforcing authority (Regulation 6)
- When carrying out a prescribed process, the operator should employ the best available techniques, not entailing excessive cost ('Batneec') to prevent the release of prescribed substances, to minimize any release or to render harmless any substance released (Regulation 7)
- If a prescribed process has not been carried out for >12mths, the enforcing authority may revoke the authorization (Regulation 12)
- If a prescribed process is carried out in breach of its authorization, an enforcement notice can be served
- If there is an imminent risk of serious pollution, a prohibition notice may be served
- An appeal against an enforcement or prohibition notice may be made to the Secretary of State
- The enforcing authorities are required to maintain a register of prescribed processes available for inspection by the public (Regulation 20)
- Any organization that carries on a prescribed process without authorization, fails to notify a transfer of undertaking involving a prescribed process, or fails to comply with a prohibition or enforcement notice is liable on conviction to a fine not exceeding £20 000, or if convicted on indictment to a fine and/or imprisonment for up to 2yrs
- Disposal of controlled waste is prohibited (Regulation 33) except in accordance with a Waste Management License. This excludes storage of household waste in domestic premises

- Transport by road of controlled waste, except in accordance with the controls imposed by a Waste Management License, is an offence
- Regulation 34 creates a duty of care for any person or organization producing, carrying, keeping, or disposing of controlled waste, to prevent the escape of waste from his control, and on transfer of the waste to ensure the transfer is only made to an authorized person
- A written description of the waste must be provided to the Waste Collection Authority or a holder of a Waste Management license
- Where controlled waste is deposited on land in breach of the regulations, the enforcing authority may require the occupier to remove the waste. Where the occupier did not deposit the waste, the authority may remove the waste from the land.

Legislation and guidance
- Environmental Protection Act 1990, Chapter 43. Stationery Office, London.
- Environment Act 1995, Chapter 25. Stationery Office, London.

The Environment Agency

Background

- The Environment Agency (EA) and the Scottish Environmental Protection Agency (SEPA) were created by the Environment Act 1995 and came into being in 1996
- The Environment Agency is a non-departmental public body of the Department of Environment, Food and Rural Affairs (DEFRA) and an Assembly Sponsored Public Body of the National Assembly for Wales
- The Agency exists to protect the environment of England and Wales. It covers all of England and Wales including the land, rivers, and coastal waters
- SEPA has a similar role in Scotland to the Environment Agency south of the border.

Both agencies work with the HSE in the licensing of major industrial sites under the Control of Major Accident Hazards Regulations 1999 (COMAH) (see 📖 p. 530).

Structure of the environment agency

- Supervised by a board of 12 members:
    - Eleven members are appointed by the Secretary for Environment, Food and Rural Affairs
    - one member is appointed by the National Assembly for Wales
- Managed by a Chief Executive and six directors
- Employs ~12 000 staff
- Operates through six regional offices in England and one in Wales (Environment Agency Wales) and 21 area offices.

Role of the Environment Agency

The Environment Agency is a regulatory body which has a wide remit covering issues such as the following:

- Water resources and water quality
- Flood prevention and management
- Leisure and recreation
- Navigation
- Fisheries
- Soil quality and land contamination
- Air quality and air pollution
- Waste transport and disposal
- Radioactive substances
- Pollution prevention and control (PPC), which involves the enforcement of environmental regulations in a range of industries:
    - agriculture
    - chemical
    - food and drink
    - power stations, fuel stores, etc.
    - metals
    - minerals, e.g. cement works
    - nuclear waste

- radioactive substance users
- pulp and paper
- wood
- waste management
- textiles and tanneries.

Relevant legislation

Environment Act 1995, Chapter 25. Stationery Office, London. Available at: ℘ http://www.opsi.gov.uk/acts/acts1995/Ukpga_19950025_En_1.htm

Control of Major Accident Hazards Regulations 1999

Purpose

COMAH implements the European Commission's Seveso II directive on the control of installations that may pose a major accident hazard. The aims of the regulations are:

- To identify sites where a major accident may occur
- To put in place control measures to prevent such an accident
- To mitigate the impact of an accident should it occur.

Application

The COMAH regulations apply to any lower tier or top tier site as defined in the regulations.

Definitions

- *Competent authority*. Because of the overlap between workplace health and safety and environmental protection, the competent authority for the COMAH regulations comprises:
  - HSE and the Environmental Protection Agency (EPA) in England and Wales
  - HSE and SEPA in Scotland
- *Major accident:* means an uncontrolled event at a site covered by the COMAH regulations that leads to serious danger to people or the environment, and involves an agent defined in the regulations.

Main requirements

- Operators shall take all measures needed to prevent accidents (Regulation 4), and to limit the harm caused by any accident that may occur, by reducing risk to a level as low as is reasonably practicable (ALARP)
- All operators must produce a major accident prevention policy (MAPP) and keep it up to date (Regulation 5)
- Operators of new or planned installations must notify the competent authority as soon as possible, to allow planning of assessments
- Operators of existing installations must notify the competent authority if a significant change is anticipated, such as an increase in dangerous substances on site, a change to processes, or closure of the site
- Where an installation is a top-tier site, its operator must prepare a safety report (Regulation 7) demonstrating that all necessary measures to prevent an accident have been taken
- The safety report must be revised:
  - every 5yrs (Regulation 8)
  - when there is a change in the safety management system
  - when new knowledge dictates that a review is needed.

Legislation and guidance
HSE *A Guide to the Control of Major Accident Hazards Regulations 1999.*
HSE Books, Sudbury.

Environmental impact assessment

European Council Directive 97/11/EC on the assessment of the effects of certain public and private projects on the environment came into force in 1999. It extended the range of development projects for which Environmental impact assessment (EIA) was required under Council Directive No. 85/337/EEC. A range of planning regulations has since implemented the amended directive in the UK, and The Town and Country Planning (EIA) Regulations 2010 and its Scottish equivalent are expected to come in to force in 2011.

Purpose

- To ensure that the planning authority, when giving consent for a project, is aware of any likely environmental impacts of the development
- EIA is a procedure for systematically assessing the environmental impacts of land use change (development), including ↑ noise, ↑ pollution, ↑ traffic, etc. It is a multidisciplinary activity that requires a range of expertise, as each project raises different issues
- EIA may indicate the ways in which a project can be modified to ↓ or eliminate adverse impacts, ideally by designing out the nuisance at source.

Application

- Planners may require developers to prepare an EIA prior to giving *development consent*. It is the developer who then commissions and pays for the EIA
- All schedule 1 projects must have an EIA carried out. Schedule 1 includes major hazards such as oil refineries and nuclear power stations, as well as motorways, waste incineration plants, and large quarries
- Schedule 2 projects are only required to have an EIA if the project is likely to cause significant environmental impact.[1]

Definitions

- EIA, when applied to the environmental impact of government or other public policy, is termed *strategic environmental assessment* (SEA)
- *Development consent*: the decision of the competent planning authority to allow the development to proceed
- The *competent authority* is the public body giving the primary consent for a particular project
- *Economic impact assessment* (cost-benefit analysis) forms part of an EIA in some circumstances
- *Health impact assessment* (HIA): the requirements for this component of an EIA in the UK vary depending on the specific development, but broadly cover two areas:

- social effects of a development (e.g. ↑ access to amenities from a new bridge). These can be beneficial or deleterious, and will embrace quality of life as well as more direct outcomes
- adverse effects of the development (e.g. ↑ hospital admissions due to ↑ factory emissions).

Main requirements

- EIA can be:
  - prospective for a new development
  - retrospective for an existing situation
- In some cases, prospective assessments should include a monitoring component to quantify the *actual impact*, and compare that with the *estimate of impact* made in the EIA.

Quantification of impacts

Should be attempted wherever possible. Use established effects size coefficients, as has been done for air pollution, applying these to the specific population at risk.

⚠ Bear in mind the dangers of applying health data gathered from one population to a different population.

Relevant guidance and legislation

This is not an exhaustive list of the regulations relating to EIA.

- Town and Country Planning (Environmental Impact Assessment) (England and Wales) Regulations 1999
- The Environmental Impact Assessment (Scotland) Regulations 1999
- Planning (Environmental Impact Assessment) Regulations (Northern Ireland) 1999.

---

1 See Town and Country Planning (Environmental Impact Assessment) (England and Wales) Regulations 1999 for a full list of schedule 1 and 2 projects.

Human requirements

Relevant guidance and legislation

Occupational hygiene

Occupational hygiene overview

Role and function of occupational hygienists

Introduction

Occupational hygienists have a role in identification, evaluation, and management of work-related hazards, as part of an OH team.

Definition of occupational hygiene

The BOHS defines occupational hygiene as 'The applied science concerned with the identification, measurement, appraisal of risk and control to acceptable standards of physical, chemical, and biological factors arising in or from the workplace, which may affect the health or wellbeing of those at work, or in the community'. The Faculty of Occupational Hygiene (FOH) within BOHS develops and maintains the professional standards of occupational hygienists.

Scope and functions

- *Hazard identification:*
  - anticipate and recognize health hazards that may result from operational processes, work tasks/method, equipment, tools and the work environment
  - identify the location and nature of hazards and number exposed
  - understand the possible routes of entry of hazardous agents into the human body, and the potential health effects of such agents
- *Exposure evaluation:*
  - evaluate work processes and methods of work so as to understand exposure pathways and factors affecting the level of exposure
  - design suitable sampling strategies
  - assess workers' exposure to hazards, including exposure measurement (personal or static) and interpretation of data
- *Management/control of hazards:*
  - evaluate effectiveness of administrative, organizational and engineering controls used to minimize exposure to hazards
  - advise on risk control strategies, including prioritization and ranking of risks
  - advise on the selection of risk management measures
  - understand the legal framework for occupational hygiene practice
  - educate, train, inform, and advise persons at all levels in all aspects of hazard and risk communication
  - record findings and review
- *Environmental risk management:* recognize agents and factors that may have environmental impact; understand the need to integrate occupational hygiene practice with environmental protection.

Code of ethics Codes of ethics for certified occupational hygienists exist in the USA and UK, relating to the responsibility of professional occupational hygienists to employers and clients. BOHS code of ethics available at: ℜ www.bohs.org

Classification of occupational hazards

Hazards in the working environment can be divided into five main categories (Table 29.1). These may produce an immediate or delayed response dictated largely by their inherent characteristics and the intensity and frequency of exposure.

Table 29.1 Types of occupational hazard

Hazard category	Examples
Chemical	Solids (dusts), liquids, fibres, gases, vapours, fumes, mists, and smoke
Physical	Noise, vibration, ionizing and non-ionizing radiation, extremes of temperature, humidity, pressure, electricity, illumination, and visibility
Biological	Viruses, bacteria, fungi, protozoa, nematodes
Ergonomics and mechanical	Loading/lifting, repetitive action, posture, traps, impact, contact, entanglement, ejection
Psychosocial and organizational	Individual characteristics, work demand and conditions, work environment, organization

Use of occupational hygiene exposure data

Exposure monitoring may be conducted for the following reasons:
- To identify hazards
- To demonstrate compliance with occupational exposure limits (OEL)
- As part of health risk assessments/investigations
- When conducting epidemiological studies
- When designing and selecting appropriate control measures
- When assessing the effectiveness of control measures
- To identify individuals for inclusion in health surveillance programmes
- Litigation and insurance purposes.

Hazard identification
- Information sources/techniques include inventories of materials and material safety data sheets, understanding processes and work environments, and observing actual work practices
- This may not enable the identification of all hazards, particularly those generated from non-routine activities or as a result of chemical processing, e.g. thermal degradation.
- Exposure monitoring can provide useful information on the location and spread of contaminants in the workplace.

Monitoring compliance
- The most common reason for sampling is to determine whether the exposure of an individual or group of individuals exceeds an OEL
- In the case of hazardous substances, monitoring is necessary in the following circumstances as defined in the COSHH Regulations 2002 (amended):
  - when failure or deterioration of the control measures could result in a serious health effect because of the toxicity of the contaminant, or the extent of potential exposure, or both
  - when measurements are necessary to ensure that WELs are not exceeded, and always in the case of the substance or process specified in schedule 5 of COSHH
  - as an additional check on the effectiveness of the control measures provided
  - when any changes occur in the conditions affecting employees' exposure, which could mean that adequate control is no longer being maintained.

Standard setting
Occupational exposure data are used to draw and understand dose–response relationships when deriving OELs for different hazards. Dose–response data are used to determine the no adverse effect level (NOAEL). The measured exposure level for the hazard is compared with its derived NOAEL to determine whether it presents a risk to health for defined workplace scenarios (see 📖 Chapter 33).

Epidemiological study

Ideally, occupational epidemiological studies should include exposure estimates of all employees to essentially all contaminants over all of the time period of the study. Data on the degree of exposure will help the epidemiologist to identify a dose–response relationship, which can aid the confirmation of a causal relationship between an agent and a disease. Various surrogates for exposure have also been used, such as job title, which is crude and can lead to misclassification of employees and exposure categories. Retrospective exposure assessment can be impaired by recall bias, and by poor quality or missing data. Prospective exposure assessments may be hindered by data which is not representative of the whole study population.

Monitoring the effectiveness of controls

Control measures such as engineering need to be assessed for their continued effectiveness. This can be achieved by comparing the performance of the control measure against its design specification e.g. for ventilation systems (velocities, pressure and flow rates) or by monitoring changes in exposure level for the pollutant that the system is designed to control / minimize (see 📖 Chapter 32).

Informing the process of litigation

Exposure data may be used in medico-legal cases. The relevance and reliability of the measured data may have an impact for both the plaintiff and the defendant.

Epidemiological study

Monitoring the effectiveness of control

Informing the process of litigation

Monitoring exposure

Sample types for workplace pollutants

Measurement of exposure in occupational hygiene normally involves collecting a sample from the breathing zone using personal sampling equipment. However, in some cases air-sampling techniques alone may not provide a reliable indicator of exposure, e.g. where there is potential for skin absorption or ingestion, or where RPE is used to control exposure (see 📖 p. 652, Selecting respiratory equipment).

Monitoring techniques

Monitoring techniques for airborne pollutants can be divided into several categories.

- *Instantaneous monitoring (direct reading):* refers to the collection of samples, usually for a relatively short period. Instantaneous monitors may be used to detect explosive concentrations of solvents, oxygen deficiency, or physical hazards such as noise and light levels. The instrument may be linked to an alarm device or data downloaded to a computer to examine the exposure profile with time (see Fig. 30.1)
- *Integrated monitoring:* provides a single TWA concentration over a defined sampling period, i.e. averaging peaks and troughs, e.g. when sampling personal exposure to organic solvents using charcoal adsorbent tubes
- *Personal sampling:* involves the placement of a monitoring device within the individual's 'breathing zone' (approximately 20–30cm from the nose/mouth) to sample the microenvironment from which the person breathes
- *Static (area or fixed) samples:* can be taken to check the effectiveness of process controls, to identify emission sources, to determine background concentrations in the work environment (mapping), and in some cases as a surrogate for personal sampling
- *Active and passive monitoring:* active monitoring techniques involve use of a sampling pump to pull airborne pollutant through a sampling device, while the passive technique relies on molecular diffusion, e.g. diffusion badges
- *Bulk samples:* large volume of air, liquids, or settled particulates collected e.g. for qualitative analysis to determine the nature/composition of pollutant.

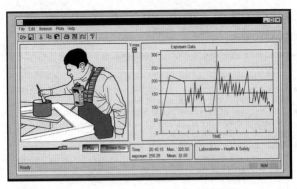

Fig 30.1 Video exposure monitoring. Combining a direct reading monitor with a video to examine the relationship between work practices and exposure.

Selection of sampling and analysis methods

- Decisions on the selection of control measures frequently depend on measured exposure levels. Therefore, it is essential that measurements are made using appropriate sampling and analytical methods
- The inherent limitations of the sampling and analysis methods used for data collection must be understood fully
- The objectives of the occupational hygiene survey and its design will help to define the acceptable accuracy, precision, and limit of detection for the pollutant(s) of interest
- Where available, standard methods of sampling and analysis should always be used. In the UK, sampling and analysis methods for a wide range of substances are detailed in the HSE MDHS series which are available on line at: ℘ http://www.hse.gov.uk/pubns/mdhs
- The International Standard Organization (ISO), the European Committee for Standardization (CEN), and various national bodies, e.g. the US National Institute for Occupational Safety and Health (NIOSH), also publish methods for the measurement of workplace contaminants
- In the absence of a recommended reference sampling method, the following factors should be considered when selecting an appropriate method:
  - nature of the pollutants (gases, vapours, mists, fibres, particles, etc.) to be collected and the stability of the sampling medium
  - compatibility of the sampling medium with the subsequent analytical technique, e.g. GC, AAS, XRD
  - capacity and collection efficiency of the sampling medium
  - intrinsic safety of the sampling equipment, its ease of use, and portability for personal sampling.

Analytical definition of terms

- *Specificity:*[1] the ability of the assay to measure one particular substance in the presence of another substance in the sample
- *Sensitivity:*[1] smallest amount of substance in a sample that can be accurately measured by an assay
- *Accuracy*: difference between the measurements and the true or correct value for the quantity measured
- *Precision*: closeness of agreement between the results obtained by applying the method several times under prescribed conditions. Precision can be expressed by the standard deviation
- *Limit of detection (LOD)*: the smallest amount of a substance that can be reliably measured by the instrument which is distinguishable from the background.

---

1 ▶▶ The definitions of sensitivity and specificity are those used in occupational hygiene practice and differ from those used in epidemiological surveys.

Minimum sampling volume

When sampling it is important to ensure that a sufficient quantity of sample is collected to enable the analyst (laboratory) to determine the amount of contaminant accurately. The minimum sampling volume (time) can be calculated from the following equation:

Min. sampling vol. (m³) = (10 × LOD for analytical technique (mg)/OEL (mg/m³))

Sampling and analysis errors and corrections

When comparing measured exposure data with relevant OELs it is important to consider the following:

• Instrumental and analytical errors
• Potential for contamination of sampling device
• Sampling efficiency of collecting devices and desorption efficiency of solid adsorbents
• Ensure that the measurements and OELs are expressed at standard temperature and pressure. For example, as the exposure limits are based on a temperature of 20°C and a pressure of 760mmHg, the concentrations of any measured pollutant not measured at these values should be corrected as follows:

$$C_{corr} = C (760/P) (T / 293)$$

Where C_{corr} is the corrected concentration, P (mmHg) is the actual pressure of air samples, and T (K) is the absolute temperature of air sampled.

Quality assurance (laboratory analysis)

When sending samples to analytical laboratories for analysis (after a exposure survey), e.g. analysis of sorbent tubes for solvents include:

• 'Field blanks' for analysis. 'Field blanks' are samples taken to the worksite and treated and handled in the same way as other samples with the exception that no air is drawn through the sampling media
• Samples that are 'spiked' with a known amount of the substance(s) sampled in the workplace. -

For information on practical methods for sampling hazards (chemical, physical, and biological agents) in the workplace, see Further reading.

Further reading

Cherrie J, Howie R, Semple S (2010). *Monitoring for health hazards at work*, 4th edn. Wiley-Blackwell, Oxford.

Workplace exposure survey types

Three stages

The design of the monitoring programme will be strongly influenced by the aim of the survey. The HSE has produced an outline for monitoring exposure, which includes three stages (initial appraisal, basic survey, and detailed survey). These are summarized here. The structured approach is summarized in Fig. 30.2.

Initial appraisal

This step helps to establish the need for, and the extent of, monitoring. Information is required on the following factors:

- The substance to which individuals are exposed
- The hazardous and physical properties of the substance
- The airborne form of the substance
- The process or operations where exposure is likely to occur
- The number, type, and position of sources from which the substance is released
- The groups of employees who are most likely to be exposed
- The pattern and duration of exposure, including exposure routes (inhalation, dermal, ingestion)
- Actual work practices
- The means by which the release of the substance is controlled
- Whether personal protective equipment is used and its effectiveness
- The OELs for the substances involved.

Basic survey

This step involves identifying and monitoring exposure of employees who are likely to be at significant risk. Individuals at risk and processes of concern are identified using information collated in the initial appraisal, including situations when employees complain.

The exposure is estimated using either semi-quantitative or validated laboratory-based sampling and analysis methods. The survey also includes an indication of the efficiency of process and engineering controls.

Detailed survey

This is conducted when:

- The extent and pattern of exposure cannot be confidently assessed by a basic survey
- Exposure is highly variable between employees doing similar tasks
- Carcinogenic substances (R45) or respiratory sensitizers (R42) are involved
- The initial appraisal and basic survey suggests that:
  - TWA personal exposure may be very close to the OEL
  - costs of additional control measures cannot be justified without the evidence of the extent of exposure variability
  - specific non-routine tasks are undertaken which require further investigation.

Prioritization of sampling needs

Having determined the need and reasons for sampling, it may be necessary to make an *a priori* prioritization of contaminants and/or processes to be assessed. The following factors should be considered when prioritizing sampling

- Number of individuals potentially exposed to the substance
- Toxicity of the substance(s)—acute and chronic effects
- Quantities (substance) used over some arbitrary reference period
- Pattern and estimate of exposure levels
- Existence of, and confidence in, control measures used to minimize exposure
- Reported symptoms
- Findings from previous risk assessments.

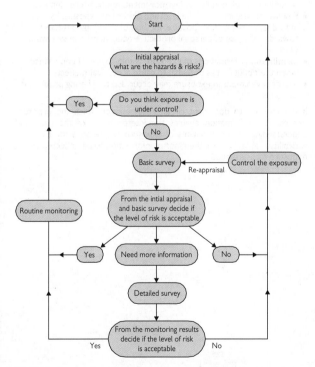

Fig. 30.2 Structured approach for assessing exposure to substances hazardous to health (from HSE (1997). *Monitoring strategies for toxic substances*, HSG173. HSE Books, Sudbury. © Crown copyright, reproduced with the permission of the Controller of HMSO.

Exposure variability

Exposure to hazards (e.g. chemicals, noise, vibration.) in the workplace can vary both within and between individuals, days, shifts, etc. In order to obtain representative exposure data for risk assessment these variables need to be understood and considered carefully in the design of occupational hygiene sampling surveys.

- Factors which influence the release and airborne concentrations of substances include:
  - physical and chemical properties of the substance
  - number of sources
  - rate, speed, and duration of release from each source
  - variation in the process, job, and tasks carried out
  - dispersion and mixing of agent in the workplace
  - ambient work conditions (air movement, temperature, humidity)
- Employees may influence the level and pattern of exposure by their individual work practice (posture, method of work) and attitudes towards risks (use of personal protective equipment) and systems of work
- Identification of variations of exposure within-days is of importance when the pollutant has potential to cause acute health effects
- Seasonal variations in exposure may occur due to differing production demands.

It is important to document circumstances under which the exposure occurs. This information enables the interpretation of the data, and understanding the determinants of exposure and reasons for exposure variability. Table 30.1 lists the types of information to be collected during exposure measurement.

Table 30.1 Information to be collected during exposure measurement

Category	Information
Strategy	Reason for collecting measurements
	Worst case or randomly chosen worker
	Task-specific or full-shift based
	Duration of sample
	Sampling and analytical method
Location	Type of industry
	Department
	Number of employees in the department
Worker	Personal identification code
	Gender, age
	Worker behaviour (e.g. tasks performed)
	Personal protective equipment used
	Machines and tools used
	Pace of work
	Degree of training
	Mobile or stationary work
Process	Level of automation
	Continuous or intermittent
	Control or exposure-reducing measures
Environment	Indoors or outdoors
	Temperature, atmospheric pressure, relative humidity
	Weather conditions (for outdoor work)
	Local and/or general ventilation
	Room volume (e.g. confined space <$50m^3$)
	Day or night shift
Agents	Likely source (e.g. composition of raw materials)
	Physical characteristics (e.g. particles, vapours, mists, fibres, etc.)

Based on: Kromhout H (2002). Design of measurement strategies for workplace exposures. *Occup Environ Med*, **59**, 286, 349–54.

Designing exposure monitoring programmes

Occupational exposure monitoring programmes should address the following questions:
- Whose exposure should be measured?
- Where to collect the sample?
- When to measure?
- How long to sample?
- Number of samples?
- How often?
- How to interpret the data?

When evaluating these questions, consider the following points:
- For compliance purposes, sampling can be carried out on a group basis where groups of employees are performing identical or similar tasks and are exposed to similar risks to health, i.e. homogenous groups. HSE (1989) states that if an individual's exposure is less than half or more than twice the group mean, he/she should be reassigned to another group
- For the assessment of human health risks personal sampling is preferred, as this is most likely to reflect the individual's exposure. In fact, for all, but a few substances (e.g. cotton dust, vinyl chloride monomer, and subtilisins (proteolytic enzymes)) the assigned OELs are specific to personal exposure
- When locating personal samplers consideration must be given to source(s) of exposure, work tasks, and individual work practices. Studies have shown up to twofold differences in dust level for samples placed equidistant from the nose/mouth on each lapel
- Start-up procedures at the beginning of the shift and end-of-shift procedures such as clean-down as well as unplanned events (chemical spillage) can make an important contribution to daily exposures
- When sampling exposure to demonstrate compliance with OELs, the duration over which the sample should be taken is dictated by the reference period of the OEL. In the UK, OELs are expressed over two reference periods, i.e. 15min and 8h. Fig. 30.3 shows different sampling strategies for obtaining 8h TWA concentrations
- Given the variability of occupational exposure data (see 🕮 p. 610), one or two samples taken on one day may be insufficient to reach reliable exposure estimates. The sample size requirements can be related to closeness of measured mean personal exposure levels to OEL for the contaminant of interest (Table 30.2)
- The decision on the frequency of monitoring should be based on factors such as reliability of controls, closeness of exposure levels with limits (Table 30.3), changes in work practices, work equipment, work environment, and reported symptoms
- Exposure data is usually log normally distributed and can be expressed as a range, arithmetic mean, geometric mean and geometric standard deviation or as a log probability plot to estimate percentiles points.

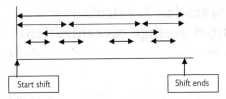

Start shift

Shift ends

Fig. 30.3 Four different strategies for estimating the 8-h TWA concentration. Each offers different advantages and limitations. The arrowheads indicate the number of samples taken over the shift and their duration.

Table 30.2 Sample size requirements for testing mean exposure from log normal distribution of 8-h TWAs (95% significance and 90% power)

| Mean/OEL | Sample size n | | | | |
	SD = 1.5	SD = 2.0	SD = 2.5	SD = 3.0	SD = 3.5
0.1	2	6	13	21	30
0.25	3	10	19	30	43
05	7	21	41	67	96
0.75	2	82	164	266	384
1.25	25	82	164	266	384
1.50	7	21	41	67	96
2.00	2	6	11	17	24
3.00	1	2	3	5	6

SD, Geometric standard deviation.

Table 30.3 Minimum frequency of regular monitoring

Shifts to be sampled (per 10 employees)	Exposure/occupational exposure
1/month	1–2
1/quarter	0.5–1 or 2–4
1/annum	0.1–0.5 or 4–20
None	<0.1 or >20

Data interpretation 1: calculating time-weighted average concentrations

Air-borne concentrations of substances are calculated using the following equation;

$$C = M/V$$

where C is the concentration (mg/m^3), M is the mass of substance (mg) and V the volume of air sampled (m^3).

Calculating 8-h time-weighted average

If exposure is measured by collecting a number of samples over an 8h period, then the 8h time-weighted average (TWA) is calculated by multiplying each exposure concentration by the corresponding exposure duration.

$$8h\ TWA = (C_1 \times T_1 + C_2 \times T_2 .... CnTn)/8$$

where C (mg/m^3) is the concentration and T the time (h).

Example

A machinist in a wood workshop works an eight hour shift. A personal sample was taken using an IOM sampling head connected to a sampling pump for 2h. The sampling pump was calibrated at a flow rate of 2.0L/min. The difference (gain) in the weight of the sampling filter before and after sampling was 5mg.

Personal sampling was conducted for two further periods on the same day, i.e. 2h and 4h which produced TWA concentrations of 6.0 and 2.0mg/m^3, respectively.

Question

(a) What is the 2-h TWA personal dust concentration for the first sampling period?
(b) What is the 8-h TWA?

Calculation

(a) 2h TWA =
   Mass(mg)/Vol. (m^3)
   5.0mg/0.24m^3
   21.0mg/m^3
(b) 8h TWA = $(21.0 \times 2.0) + (6 \times 2) + (2.0 \times 4.0) = 8.0$mg/m^3

Period of work >8h: adjustment of OEL

- The use of unusual work schedules is now fairly common. Consequently, workers will not experience occupational exposure over the traditional 8h per shift, 5 days a week, which is that used in setting OELs
- A work shift longer than 8h will result in additional exposure and also a shorter period of recovery before the next insult. This may not be a problem with substances with very short half-lives. However, the body burden for substances with half-lives approaching or exceeding 16h (the period of recovery for an 8h working day) may rise over the week/shift period

- A number of sophisticated models utilizing pharmacokinetics have been put forward to adjust for exposures greater than the reference period of 8h. Unfortunately, they require a great deal of substance-specific information, which is very rarely available. A more simplistic equation is given here which can be used to adjust the 8h OEL:

  OEL multiplication factor = $8/H [(24 - H)/16]$

where H is the number of hours worked.

▶▶Note that the formula does not apply to continuous 24h exposure, work periods of <7–8h/day or 35h/wk, or concentration-dependent acute toxicants.

Data interpretation 2: exposure to chemical mixtures

Occupational exposure seldom involves exposure to a single substance. Exposure to mixtures is of concern in both measuring exposure and estimating their biological significance. Potential adverse effects may be greater than, less than, or equal to the sum of the effects of the individual components of the mixture.

Evaluating exposure to mixtures

- The majority of the substances encountered in occupational settings are assigned an individual WEL. Some WELs relate to substances commonly encountered as complex mixtures, e.g. welding, rubber, and solder fumes
- When individuals are exposed to mixtures, the first step is to ensure adequate control of each individual substance. It may then be necessary to assess whether further control is needed so as to counteract any increased risk due to presence of other substances in the mixture. Interaction should be considered in the following order:
  - synergistic effect—occurs when the combined effect of the two agents is greater than the effect of each agent given alone. Antagonistic effects occur when the combined effect of two agents is less than the sum of the effects of each agent given separately
  - additive effect—is an example of a non-interaction, i.e. the combined effect of two agents is equal to the sum of the two effects of each agent given alone
  - independent effects—i.e. the other components do not add, enhance, or diminish the effect of the most active component, e.g. where each component acts on a different organ in the body and the magnitude of each effect is not influenced by the other effects
- When there is reason to believe that the effects of constituents are additive, and where the WELs are based on the same health effects, the mixed exposure should be assessed using the formula.

$$C_1/L_1 + C_2/L_2 + C_3/L_3 + \ldots < 1.0$$

where C_1, C_2, etc. are the airborne TWA concentrations and L_1, L_2, etc., are the corresponding WELs.

Dermal exposure

Workers may be exposed to hazardous substances by inhalation, ingestion, and contact with the skin or eyes. Exposure by the dermal route may result in local (skin irritation, ulceration) as well systemic effects (neurotoxicity, hepatotoxicity).

- Dermal exposure occurs in a number of jobs, examples include:
  - agricultural workers (pesticide sprayers)
  - painters (solvents)
  - hairdressers (dyes)
  - engineers (metalworking fluids)
  - construction workers (cements, solvents, resins)
  - cleaners (solvents, skin irritants)
- Chemicals diffuse through the stratum corneum because of the concentration gradient between the skin contamination layer (SCL) (mixture of sweat, sebum, and other material on the skin) and the tissue around the peripheral blood supply
- Most gases/vapours are not taken up by the skin in significant quantities as the concentration gradient is too low
- The mass (surrogate for concentration) of a substance absorbed through the skin depends on the following properties of the substances, which are used to predict the permeability coefficient of the substance (Kp):
  - solubility in oils and water
  - chemical structure
  - and molecular weight
- Dermal exposure assessment should include information on the following:
  - substance type
  - intensity (concentration or mass of substance on skin) of exposure
  - duration and frequency of exposure
- High molecular weight liquids (>500Dal) with an octanol–water partition coefficient <−1 or >4 are unlikely to permeate skin
- Occlusion of the exposure site by clothing or personal protective equipment may ↑ absorption through the skin.

Skin notation 'Sk'

Many national authorities publish occupational exposure limits and assign a 'skin notation' to substances when they judge that dermal exposure may make a significant contribution to total exposure. List of chemicals (more than 100) assigned 'skin notation' can be found in the HSE guide note EH40.

Examples of Hazard Statements relevant to dermal exposure include H312 (harmful in contact with skin), H314 (causes severe skin burns), H315 (cause skin irritation), H317 (may cause an allergic skin reaction). See 📖 Appendix 1 for health hazard statements.

Conceptual model of dermal exposure

- Dermal exposure can be conceptualized according to a number of compartments and transfer routes (Fig. 30.4)
- Key transfer routes depend on the particular work situation, e.g. someone handling pesticide in a container may have direct splashes onto the SCL and the outer clothing contaminant layer from the source, together with direct contact of these layers with surfaces contaminated by pesticides
- Use of this conceptual model can help in the analysis of the main routes and compartments for different workplace exposure scenarios.

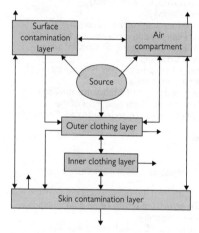

Fig. 30.4 Conceptual model of dermal exposure.

Dermal: exposure measurement and estimating uptake

Assessing the contribution of skin exposure to systemic uptake

Several methods are used to measure dermal exposure:
- Intercepting contaminants before they land on the SCL or clothing
- Removal of contaminants from the SCL after exposure
- *In situ* methods, e.g. use of fluorescent tracer compounds.

Qualitative assessment of dermal exposure

To investigate skin exposure, collect good descriptive information:
- Record contact with contaminated surfaces (number of contacts, area of SCL in contact, duration of each contact)
- Evidence of splash (liquids) or powder (solids) on surfaces
- Large particles/droplets that may impact on worker or work surfaces
- Type of clothing worn (note visible contamination), glove type, whether gloves are worn continuously, reuse of gloves.

▶ Videos are useful in analysing worker behaviour and dermal exposure.

Interception methods

Patch sampling
- Widely used to sample low-volatility liquids, e.g. pesticides
- Patches are attached to workers' clothing or the skin
- Patches attached outside clothing are said to assess potential exposure
- Samples inside clothing are said to assess actual dermal exposure
- Patches are analyzed to assess contaminant mass (and total body contaminant mass by multiplying the area of the body part by contaminant mass on the patch and summing overall).

Suit sampling
- An alternative interception sampler is the cotton 'suit sampler'
- Suit analysis gives a direct estimate of whole-body contaminant mass landing on the SCL and/or clothing.

Skin stripping
- Skin stripping is a removal technique which can assess contaminant, e.g. acrylate, jet fuel, metal, that has started to permeate skin
- Adhesive tapes are used to remove ('strip') sequential layers of stratum corneum and any contaminant residues present in the skin.

Removal techniques
- Hand washing
- Rinsing
- Skin wiping.

In situ methods
- Fluorescent tracer methods are highly specialized research tools
- Small amounts of a fluorescent agent are added to the contaminant source

- After work the skin is imaged with UV light using a video camera linked to a computer system to estimate tracer mass and hence contaminant mass.

Biological monitoring and dermal exposure

- Biological monitoring provides indirect assessment of dermal exposure, but without exposure information it is of limited value
- Biological monitoring is often limited by availability of suitable method to measure the substance (parent compound or its metabolite) in the body
- Biological monitoring provides an assessment of PPE efficacy where data are available for workers with and without protective clothing.

Surface monitoring

- Surface contamination and transfer to skin play an important part in many dermal exposure situations (see Fig. 30.4)
- Surface contamination monitoring provides a measure of workplace contamination and its probable contribution to dermal exposure
- Surface wipe sampling is extensively used, but has high variability
- Techniques are similar to those described for skin removal techniques.

Estimating dermal uptake

The dermal uptake (mass) of a chemical can be estimated from the following equation:

$$U_{sk} = K_p \times C_{sk} \times A \times t$$

where K_p is the permeability coefficient (cm/h), C_{sk} is the concentration of the substance on the skin (mg/cm^3); A is the area of skin exposed; t the duration of exposure (hours).

For a defined exposure scenario the relative uptake of a substance by both the dermal and inhalation route can be compared, i.e. contributions to total boy burden. The inhalation uptake (U_{inh}) can be estimated from the following equation:

$$U_{inh} = C_{air} \times B \times t$$

where C_{air} is the air concentration (mg/m^3); B the breathing rate (m3/h); t the exposure time (h).

Further information

Cherrie J, Howie R, Semple S (2010). Dermal and ingestion exposure measurement In: *Monitoring for health hazards at work*, 4th edn. Wiley-Blackwell, Oxford.

Biological monitoring

Biological monitoring and biological effect monitoring

Definitions

Biological monitoring

The measurement and assessment of hazardous substances or their metabolites in tissue, secretions, excreta, expired air, or any combination of these in exposed workers. Examples of blood and urine biological monitoring (BM) are shown in Table 31.1.

Biological effect monitoring

The measurement and assessment of a biological effect (early consequences of exposure) in exposed workers, caused by absorption of chemicals.

BM provides an indication of a workplace agent causing some detectable biochemical alteration. Unlike BM, biological effect monitoring BEM is not a surrogate of absorbed dose, but provides evidence of exposure. Examples of BEM include measuring the following biochemical responses:

- Cholinesterase activity following an acute exposure to organophosphorus pesticides
- Urinary β_2-microglobulin proteins following exposure to cadmium
- Free erythrocyte protoporphyrin (FEP) in blood or δ-aminolaevulinic acid (ALA-D) in urine for workers exposed to inorganic lead.

Biological monitoring

- Unlike air monitoring (external exposure) BM integrates exposure received from all routes
- BM can be a useful complementary technique to air monitoring, particularly when exposure via the dermal route is significant. Examples of chemicals which have the potential to penetrate skin include those assigned the 'Sk' notation
- BM data can give useful information on the effectiveness of industrial hygiene controls, e.g. personal respiratory protective equipment as well as individual work practice
- BM sampling methods may be invasive and it may be difficult to distinguish between exposure at and away from work.

Table 31.1 Biological (blood and urine) samples and analytes

Biological sample	Example of parent compound	Examples of metabolite
Urine	**Metals:** mercury, lead (organic), cadmium, chromium, cobalt, vanadium **Organic solvents:** methyl ethyl ketone (MEK), acetone, phenol, pentachlorophenol, 4,4'-methylene bis-2-choroaniline (MbOCA)	**Aromatic compounds:** phenylmercapturic acid (for benzene), hippuric acid (for toluene), methyl hippuric acids (for xylene), mandelic acid (for styrene and ethyl benzene), 1-hydroxypyrene (for PAHs) **Chlorinated solvents:** trichloroacetic acid (for trichloroethylene, perchloroethylene, 1,1,1 trichloroethane) **Other organic compounds:** e.g. dialkylphosphates (for organophosphorous pesticides), 2,5-hexanedione (for n-hexane)
Blood	**Metals:** inorganic lead, mercury, cadmium, cobalt *Organic solvents:* aromatic compounds, e.g. toluene, styrene **Chlorinated solvents:** trichloroethylene, tetrachloroethylene, 1,1,1 trichloroethylene,	**Inorganic gases and chlorinated solvents:** carboxyhaemoglobin (for methylene chloride and carbon monoxide), trichloroethanol (for trichloroethylene)

Interpretation of data

Units and creatinine correction

- *Blood samples:* in micrograms (µg) or milligrams per litre (mg/L).
- Urine levels: in milligrams per gram (mg/g) of creatinine, or millimoles per millimole (mmol/mmol) of creatinine. Urine concentration can vary widely because of variation in fluid intake and sweat. Concentration/dilution effects are corrected by adjusting for specific gravity or creatinine correction. Creatinine correction is not advised if the creatinine <3 or >30mmol/L.

Biological exposure limits

BM data are usually compared with biological exposure standards set by national authorities. Examples include the following:

- The TLV® list of the ACGIH® contains Biological Exposure Indices (BEIs®).[1] The BEI® are advisory reference values and represent the concentration of a substance that is likely to be found in the sample of a worker who was exposed through inhalation to the TLV®.
- The Deutsche Forschungsgemeinschaft (DFG, the German Research Foundation) publishes an annual list of biological tolerance values (BAT). A BAT is defined as a maximum permissible quantity of a substance which does not generally impair the health of a worker. Thus the BAT value is primarily health based.
- In the UK there is a statutory requirement for monitoring lead under the CLAW Regulations. Under CLAW, action and suspension levels are assigned for lead workers. However, for other substances hazardous to health the HSE has adopted non-statutory biological monitoring guidance values (BMGVs).

Biological monitoring guidance values

- BMGVs are non-statutory. Where the BMGVs are exceeded, this indicates that work practices and controls need to be investigated. It does not imply that health effects will occur or that the WEL is exceeded. Table 31.2 gives a list of chemicals and their assigned BMGV values. For each substance, a free leaflet is available from the HSE describing the analytical method, sampling strategy, quality assurance schemes, and interpretation of results
- BMGVs for different substances may be based on different information types which may include one of the following:
  - relationship between biological concentrations and health effects
  - relationship between biological concentrations and exposure at the level of the workplace exposure limit (WEL) *or*
  - data collected from representative samples of workplaces that are using principles of good occupational hygiene practice to minimize exposure.

---

1 ACGIH (2011). *Threshold Limit Values for Chemical Substances and Physical agents & Biological Exposure Indices.* ACGIH, Cincinnati.

Table 31.2 BMGV values

Substance	BMGV	Sampling time
Butan-2-one	70µmol butan-2-one/Lin urine	Post-shift
2-Butoxyethanol	240mmol butoxyacetic acid/mol creatinine in urine	Post-shift
Carbon monoxide	30ppm carbon monoxide in end-tidal breath	Post-shift
Chromium VI	10µmol chromium/mol creatinine in urine	Post-shift
Cyclohexanone	2mmol cyclohexanol/mol creatinine in urine	Post-shift
Dichloromethane	30ppm carbon monoxide in end-tidal breath	Post-shift
N, N-dimetylacetamide	100mmol N-methylacetamide/mol creatinine in urine	Post-shift
Glycerol trinitrate	15µmol total nitroglycols/mol creatinine in urine	At the end of the period of exposure
Lindane	35nmol/L (10µg/L) of lindane in whole blood (equivalent to 70nmol/L of lindane in plasma)	Random
MbOCA	15µmol total MbOCA/mol creatinine in urine	Post-shift
Mercury	20µmol/mol creatinine in urine	Random
4-Methylpentan-2-one	20µmol 4-methyl pentan-2-one/L in urine	Post-shift
4,4 -Methylene dianiline (MDA)	50µmol total MDA/mol creatinine in urine	Post-shift for inhalation and pre-shift next day for dermal exposure
Polyaromatic hydrocarbons (PAHs)	4µmol 1-hydroxypyrene/mol creatinine in urine	Post-shift
Xylene, o-, m-, p-, or mixed isomers	650mmol methyl hippuric acid/mol creatinine in urine	Post-shift

Interfering factors

The following factors can affect BM results:
- Diet (fish increases arsenic/mercury level)
- Sex (females have higher erythrocyte protoporphyrin levels than males)
- Age (cadmium levels increase with age amongst smokers)
- Alcohol intake affects the metabolism of organic solvents, e.g. styrene
- Ethnic groups: evidence for difference in metabolism of solvents
- A metabolite of interest may be produced by more than one substance.

Further information

HSE (2007). *Workplace exposure limits 2005* (amendments 2007), EH40/2005. HSE Books, Sudbury.

Practical and ethical considerations

Practicalities

Several practical considerations must be taken in to account before start-
ing a BM programme:
- *The reason for collecting samples:* compliance, risk assessment, health
  surveillance, epidemiological studies
- Appointment of a competent person to oversee the development and
  implementation of the programme
- Criteria for selecting individuals for monitoring
- Provision of information for subjects, and obtaining individual consent.
- Development of a suitable biological monitoring strategy:
  - timing of sample collection in relation to the beginning and end of
    shift or working week (see Table 31.3)
  - number of samples to be taken
  - type of biological sample to be collected
  - substance or metabolite to be measured
  - *amount of sample required*
- *Selection of suitable laboratory:* experience of specific analysis, quality
  assurance schemes, validated analysis method
- Any special precautions for the collection, storage, stability, packaging,
  and dispatch of samples to a laboratory
- How the data will be interpreted, including non-occupational
  exposure.
- Feedback of grouped anonymized results to the workforce
- Storage of data, and who has access to the data
- Use of the data and likely benefits to the employees.

Ethical considerations and access to data

- Since BM involves taking samples from individuals it is essential that the
  rights of individuals are safeguarded
- The need for the monitoring, collection of samples, associated risks,
  and the use of data should be discussed and agreed with all concerned,
  employees, employers and workers representatives
- Workers must be made aware of what will be analysed in the sample
  taken and what action may follows based on the results
- Results must be treated as confidential and disclosed only to those
  health professionals the worker has agreed should have the results
- The individual tested is entitled to his/her results together with an
  explanation of them
- Group data can be provided to management and unions ensuring that
  any specific identifiers are removed
- Under the UK COSHH Regulations, the results should be kept for at
  least 40 years from the date of last entry
- When companies cease operation they are advised to offer the data
  (both biological and personal inhalation) to the HSE.

Table 31.3 Half-life of chemicals and optimum sampling time: general relationship as a guide for monitoring

Half-life (h)	Optimum sampling time
<2	End of exposure
~2–10	End of exposure at the end of week shift or beginning of the next shift
~10–100	End of exposure at the end of the working week
>100	Random (sampling time not critical)

Further information

HSE (1997). *Biological monitoring in the workplace*, HSG 167. HSE Books, Sudbury.

Prevention and control of exposure

Exposure prevention and control

Prevention and control

As far as exposure to hazardous substances is concerned, there is a legal duty under the COSHH Regulations to prevent or, where this is not reasonably practicable, to control exposure adequately.

- Where it is not reasonably practicable to prevent exposure, the employer must apply protection measures appropriate to the activity including, in order of priority:
  - design and use of appropriate work processes, systems of work, engineering controls, and the provision of suitable work equipment and materials
  - the control of exposure at source including use of ventilation systems and appropriate organizational measures to minimize the risks
  - where adequate control of exposure cannot be achieved then suitable PPE should be used in addition to measures listed here.
- The measures used to control exposure should include:
  - arrangements for safe handling, storage, transport and disposal (waste materials) of substances hazardous to health
  - suitable maintenance procedures
  - reducing the number of employees exposed, the level and duration of exposure, and the quantity of material used
  - general ventilation
  - appropriate hygiene measures including adequate washing facilities.

Exposure to carcinogens

Where exposure to carcinogens cannot be prevented, the following control measures are required in addition to those described here.

- Total enclosure of process and handling systems
- Prohibition of eating, drinking, and smoking
- Cleaning floors, walls, and other surfaces at regular intervals
- Designating those areas and equipment which may be contaminated
- Storing, handling, and disposing of carcinogens safely, including use of closed and clearly labelled containers.

Personal protective equipment

- PPE provided by the employer should be suitable for the purpose and comply with the Personal Protective Equipment Regulations 2002
- PPE including protective clothing should be properly stored in a well-defined area, checked at suitable intervals, and, if defective, repaired or replaced.

Use of controls

- Every employer who provides control measures is required to take reasonable steps to ensure that they are properly used
- Employees must make full and proper use of any control measures provided and report defects to their employer.

Maintenance, examination, and testing of controls

- Employers are required to maintain plant, equipment, engineering controls, and PPE in an efficient state, in efficient working order, and in clean condition
- All control measures including systems of work and supervision should be reviewed
- All LEV should be examined and tested every 14mths unless another interval is specified, e.g. in Schedule 4 of the COSHH Regulations
- Where RPE (other than disposable RPE) is used to control exposure the employer should ensure that it is examined and, where appropriate, tested at suitable intervals.

Principles of good practice

In the UK a set of principles of good control practice are used as a basis for judging whether control is adequate for hazardous substances. These include:

- Design and operate processes and activities to minimize emission and the spread of agents
- Take in to account all relevant routes of exposure when developing control measures
- Control exposure by means that are proportional to health risk
- Choose the most effective and reliable control options that minimize the emission and spread of health hazards
- Where adequate control cannot be achieved by other means, provide suitable PPE, in combination with other control measures
- Check and review regularly all aspects of control measures for their continuing effectiveness
- Inform and train employees about the hazards and risks from the agents with which they work and the use of control measures developed to minimize risks
- Ensure that the introduction of any control measures does not increase the overall risk to health and safety.

Control hierarchy: source, transmission, and the individual

When controlling exposure to pollutants, the objective is to ensure that safe levels are achieved. The following three components should be considered in turn: (1) control at source; (2) prevent or control transmission of the pollutant to the individual; (3) protect the worker.

(1) Control at source

- Eliminate the hazard by:
  - changing the process or method of work so that the hazard is not created
  - substitute hazardous with non-hazardous substances
- Modify the process to reduce the frequency, intensity or duration of emission
- Substitute substance with one of lower toxicity or different form of the same substance
- Enclose the process/sources of emission
- Provide extraction ventilation
- Improve process/equipment maintenance
- Limit areas of contamination, e.g. spills, leaks.

Hierarchy of control: examples for noise and vibration
- Use alternative tools (altered frequency and amplitude)
- Introduce or increase damping; isolate machine from floor (noise)
- Avoid/cushion impact.

(2) Prevent/control transmission

- Shielding between the worker and source
- Increase distance
- Housekeeping
- Sufficient dilution ventilation.

Hierarchy of control: examples for noise and vibration
- Reflective and absorbent barriers
- Active noise control.

(3) Individual

- Automatic or remote control
- Enclose the worker
- Safer work practice and systems of work
- Education, training, supervision

- Provide PPE
- Reduce exposure time
- Reduce number of workers exposed
- Health surveillance.

Software/organizational solutions

Options for controlling exposure to hazards in the workplace can be categorized broadly as software (management solutions) and hardware (engineering) methods. Selection and use of PPE is discussed on 📖 pp. 652–66.

Hierarchy of software/organizational solutions

Elimination

Complete elimination of processes or substances is usually difficult. Elimination is usually limited to unnecessary operations or poor work practices. In some cases high-risk activities are subcontracted to another operator.

Substitution

- *By a less toxic substance:* e.g. in painting using water-based solvents or organic solvents of lower vapour pressure
- *By the same substance:* but in a form that reduces exposure, e.g. use material in pellet form rather than as a powder.

Designing or redesigning the process

Reductions in exposure may be achieved by adjustments to the way the job is performed or modifying the layout of the process and the operator's work procedures. For example, Fig. 32.1 shows alternative methods for drum filling.

Suppression of the substance

Suppression can be achieved in a number of ways. For example, water is used as dust suppressant. Evaporation of vapour from volatile solvents in tanks can be suppressed by using a refrigerated strip just above the surface, creating a cool layer of concentrated vapour and reducing further evaporation. In electroplating the surfaces of tanks can be covered by floating plastic spheres, which reduce the surface area available for evaporation, or by adding low-density liquid surfactants.

Other software methods

- Good work practice and systems (including good housekeeping)
- Appropriate supervision
- Job rotation
- *Information, instruction, and training:* the worker must be made aware of the following:
  - hazards to which they are exposed, and the risks to health
  - factors (process, equipment, method of work, environment) which may affect their exposure
  - any relevant occupational exposure limits
  - significant findings of risk assessments
  - appropriate precautions and actions to be taken in order to safeguard health
  - the correct use of control measures provided and how to recognize and report defects, e.g. PPE, engineering controls
  - the signs and symptoms associated with the hazards and reporting requirements.

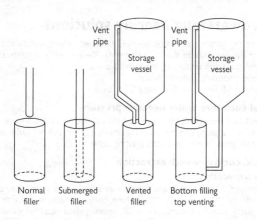

Fig. 32.1 Alternative methods of drum filling. (Reproduced from Sadhra SS, Rampal KG (1999). *Occupational health-risk assessment and management.*) With persmission from Wiley-Blackwell, Oxford.

Hardware/engineering solutions

Engineering controls are often not well designed or well maintained and rely on the operator to use them correctly. The hierarchy of control is:
• Total enclosure under negative pressure
• Partial enclosure with extraction
• General dilution ventilation (see 📖 p. 642).

Total enclosure under negative pressure

To reduce exposure to very toxic substances the contaminants are handled in an enclosure under negative pressure, e.g. hot cells for radio-active materials, glove boxes, and bead blasting cabinets.

Partial enclosure with extraction

Extraction booths

The source of emission is enclosed on all sides, except where access is needed (Fig. 32.2(a)). Examples include chemical fume cupboards and paint spray booths. Air velocity at the opening (face velocity) should be sufficient to prevent escape of substance in to the environment. Typical face velocities for booths are in the range 0.5–2.5m/s.

Canopies

Canopies (Fig. 32.2(b)) are designed to draw upwards, and thus are best designed to capture pollutants from hot processes, but are unsuitable if the worker needs to lean over the process.

Hoods

Hoods are placed at the side or behind the source in relation to the worker (Fig. 32.2(c)). Typical capture velocities for pollutants range from 0.25 to 10m/s.
• For hoods, the velocity decays rapidly with distance from the hood, e.g. for a circular hood the velocity is only approximately 10% of the face velocity one diameter away. For this reason, the process should be conducted close to the hood, i.e. within the capture distance
• Once captured, pollutants need to be kept airborne in the ducting, which is achieved by minimum transport velocities. Transport velocities range from 7 to 10m/s for fumes to >20m/s for heavy and moist dust, e.g. paint-spraying particles
• Hoods with width to length ratios <0.2 are called slots. Slots are commonly used on degreasing tanks, cleaning baths, and electroplating tanks to remove vapours and mists released from the tank surfaces.

High velocity, low volume (HVLV)

[1]HVLV extraction is used to draw particles directly from the point of release by a nozzle handling high air velocities. The chosen velocity must be higher than the tip speed of the tool, e.g. cutting, grinding, sanding.

---

[1]**Definitions** of velocities (face, capture, transport) are given on page 676

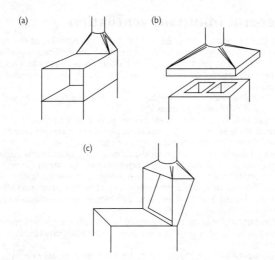

Fig. 32.2
Extraction ventilation devices: (a) extraction booths. (b) Canopy hoods.
(c) Open-face hood.

General (dilution) ventilation

General (or dilution) ventilation reduces the concentration of the contaminant by mixing the contaminated air with clean, uncontaminated air. Air is supplied to and from an area or building via air exhaust fans placed in the walls or roof of a room or building. The air supply may also be filtered and heated.

General ventilation requirements are covered in the Workplace (Health, Safety and Welfare) Regulations 1992:

* Fresh air is required to provide oxygen, remove carbon dioxide, remove excess heat or, if conditioned, provide heat, remove odours, and dilute contaminants arising from workplace activities
* Air introduced into workplaces should be free of contaminants such as engine exhaust emissions or discharges from nearby extract outlets
* Air may be re-circulated to conserve energy costs. Re-circulated air, including air conditioning systems, should be filtered to remove impurities and have fresh air added to it before being reintroduced to the workplace
* Mechanical ventilation systems should be regularly cleaned and tested to ensure that they are kept clean from anything that may contaminate the air
* Insufficient air changes may lead to tiredness, lethargy, dry or itchy skin, and eye irritation
* CIBSE produces recommended fresh air supply rates per person (CIBSE Guide A: Environmental Design). The fresh air supply rate should not normally fall below 5–8L/s/occupant
* HSE has published detailed guidance on measures to avoid Legionnaires' disease caused by *Legionella pneumophila* which grows in water-cooling towers.[1]

Use of general ventilation to control exposure to hazardous substances

General ventilation is used to complement LEV systems in industrial environments. Occasionally, when the installation of LEV is impractical, e.g. in confined space, exposure reduction may be achieved by dilution ventilation. The aim is to dilute a pollutant to a safe level before it reaches the breathing zone of the worker.

When used to control chemical pollutants, dilution ventilation is limited to situations where the pollutants:
* Are produced (released) at a low concentration and uniform rate
* Are of relatively low toxicity
* Not drawn or blown towards the worker(s).

When designing dilution ventilation systems consideration needs to be given to the location of air inlet, position of source of the pollutant and the position of the worker. Dilution ventilation is more effective if the exhaust fan is located close to exposed worker and the air supply (makeup air) is located behind the worker so that contaminated air is drawn away from the worker's breathing zone (Fig 32.3).

1 HSC (2000). *Legionnaires' Disease. The control of legionella Bacteria in Water Systems. Approved Code of Practice and Guidance.* HSE Books, Sudbury. ISBN 0717617726.

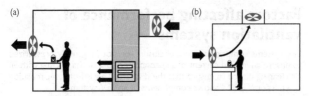

Fig. 32.3 Example of good (a) and poor dilution (b) ventilation design.

Factors affecting performance of ventilation systems

LEV systems comprise a hood, enclosure, or slot (negatively pressurized to ensure an inward current of air) connected to a fan via ducting with an air-cleaning device to ensure that the discharged air is fit for recirculation or emission. Fig.32.4 shows components of an LEV system.

Factors leading to poor performance

LEV performance depends on its design, the integrity of its components and its maintenance and use. Inadequate performance results from:
- Insufficient enclosure
- Low capture velocity
- Extracted air volume is lower than the volume of pollutant released
- Filters and air cleaners blocked
- Restricted, blocked, or damaged ducting
- Ducting too resistant
- Fan of the wrong type or size
- *Fan entry conditions unsatisfactory:* bend or damper close to fan inlet affecting velocity profile
- *Fans badly installed:* the wrong way round or rotating in the wrong direction
- Fan blades dirty or corroded, or motor seized
- *Air discharge to atmosphere affected by wind:* best to discharge vertically. Weather shields must not restrict the airflow from the discharge point
- No provision to allow make-up air to replace that extracted
- Multi-branched system not balanced
- Poor maintenance and care
- New workstation added without adjusting fan performance.

LEV system components
- *Inlets:* such as booths, hood, slot, canopy, or enclosure
- *Ducting:* which may contain bends, junctions, dampers; it may be circular or rectangular in cross section and rigid or flexible
- *Fans:* usually centrifugal type
- *Air cleaners:* such as bag filter, wet scrubber, cyclone, or solvent recovery device
- *Discharge:* to atmosphere via a stack, diffuser, grille, or just open duct.

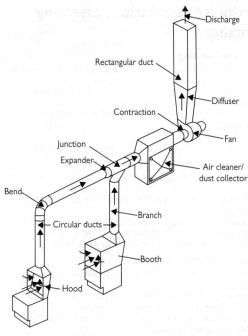

Fig. 32.4 Components of LEV system. © HSE (1998). *Maintenance, examination and testing of local exhaust ventilation*, HSG54, figure 1, p. 2. HSE Books, Sudbury.

Local exhaust ventilation: assessing performance

Examination and testing
According to HSG258 (2011) examination and testing of LEV involves three stages:
- A through visual examination to verify the LEV is in efficient working order, in good repair, and in a clean condition
- Measurement and examination of the technical performance of the system against its specification, i.e. comparison with original commissioning report

Assessment to check the control of worker exposure is adequate.

Visual and structural examination
- External examination of all parts of the systems for damage, wear and tear
- Check filter cleaning devices (e.g. mechanical shake down system) are working correctly
- Check pressure (built in) gauges, e.g. located before and after filter
- Check that the monitors and alert/alarms are working correctly
- Check for deposits of settled dust in and around the LEV hood.

Assessment of the technical performance
- Static pressure measurements taken behind each hood, and across the filter and the fan
- Check velocities (capture, face and transport) of air at various points in the systems (as specified in the system commissioning manual)
- Calculate the airflow rates (q) at the face of the hood or booth and in the duct including at the filter and fan:

$$Q = v \times a,$$

where v is the velocity (m/s), a is the cross-section area of hood or duct (m^2)

- Check speed of fan and motor
- Check the replacement or make-up air supply
- Test the air cleaner performance and any air re-circulating systems.-

Compare the result of testing with the design specification for the system.

The assessment of control effectiveness
- Ensure operator's working zone is within capture zone of the LEV (Fig. 32.5)
- Dust lamp tests to check escape of fine dust or mists
- Smoke tube or leak tests
- Observe the operator and work practice
- Conduct air sampling to determine whether control is achieved.

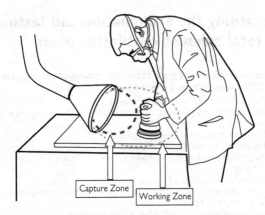

Fig. 32.5 Capture and working zone. Note: The *capture zone* is the space in front of the hood where the air velocity is sufficient to capture the contaminant. The *working zone* is defined as the space where the activity generates the contaminant. For effective control, the working zone must be lie within the capture zone of the hood.

Definitions

- *Capture velocity*: the air velocity required at the source of emission sufficient to cause the pollutant to move towards the mouth of the extractor and thus be successfully captured
- *Face velocity*: the air velocity at the opening of a hood or enclosure
- *Transport velocity*: minimum velocity required in the system, including ductwork and extract devices, to keep collected particles airborne and to prevent them from being deposited in the system
- *Static pressure*: the pressure exerted by a fluid in motion at right angles to the direction of flow
- *Velocity pressure*: the pressure equivalent of the kinetic energy of a fluid in motion. It is calculated from the expression $P_v = 0.5pv^2$ where p is the density of air (kg/m^3) and v is the velocity of air (m/s).
- *Total pressure*: the sum of the static and velocity pressures at a point in an air stream. It can be +ve or −ve relative to atmospheric pressure.

Further information and guidance

HSE (2011). *Controlling airborne contaminants at work—a guide to local exhaust ventilation (LEV)*, HSG258. HSE, Sudbury. Available at: ℘ http://www.hse.gov.uk/pubns/priced/hsg258.pdf

HSE (2008). *Clearing the air—a simple guide to buying and using local exhaust ventilation (LEV)*, INDG408. HSE, Sudbury. Available at: ℘ http://www.hse.gov.uk/pubns/indg408.pdf

Recording the examination and testing of local exhaust ventilation plant

A suitable record of each thorough examination and test of LEV should contain the following details

- The name and address of the employer
- The identification (and location) of the LEV, and the process and substances concerned
- The dates of the examination and test
- The process conditions at the time of test, e.g. normal
- Diagram of the LEV system showing position of hood, filter, fan and test points
- Information about the LEV plant which shows:
  - its intended operation performance for controlling adequately
  - exposure to hazardous substances
  - whether the LEV is still achieving the same performance
  - if not, the adjustment or repairs needed to achieve that performance
- Methods used to make the judgment of performance
- Results of any air sampling relevant to LEV performance
- Name, job title, and employer of the person carrying out the examination and test
- Observation on the way the operator used the LEV
- Signature of person carrying out the test.

- The employer should have a LEV 'user manual' and a system 'logbook'
- These documents should be supplied as part of the design, installation, and commissioning process
- The maximum time between tests for most LEV systems is 14mths (see 🕮 p. 532, Control of Substances Hazardous to Health Regulations Regulations 2002)
- The employer should keep the examination and test report for at least 5yrs.

Personal protective equipment: legal requirements and use

Definition
PPE is defined as all equipment (including clothing) that is intended to be worn or held by a person at work, and which protects him/her against one or more risks to his health or safety.

Legal requirements
See PPE at Work Regulations 1992 (as amended) *Personal protective equipment: legal requirements and use, PPE at Work Regulations 1992.* The law governing the use of PPE in other specific regulations is contained in:
- PPE at Work Regulations 1992 COSHH 2002 (as amended)
- Control of Asbestos at Work Regulations 2002 (as amended)
- Control of Lead at Work Regulations 2002
- Ionizing Radiation at Work Regulations 1999
- Confined Spaces Regulations 1997
- Control of Noise at Work Regulations 2005
- Construction (Head Protection) Regulations 1989.

△ PPE is considered as the last resort to protect against risks to health and safety. Thus there is a need to demonstrate first that the risk cannot be controlled adequately by other means.

Use of PPE
- Effective protection is only achieved by suitable PPE, correctly fitted and maintained, and properly used
- PPE is used widely, but should be considered as the last resort as:
  - it only reduces exposure for the individual wearer, whereas control at source protects all those in the area
  - the actual level of protection is difficult to assess
  - it may interfere with work tasks/practice
  - it may be uncomfortable and restrict the wearer, limiting movement, and visibility.
- PPE should be selected and used after justification for its use has been made in the risk assessment. For example RPE can be used in the following situations:
  - where inhalation exposure remains despite use of other controls, i.e. used minimize residual risk
  - where there is short-term or infrequent exposure and use of other controls is not practical
  - as an interim measure, e.g. when putting in place other controls
  - for emergency response, e.g. safe exit or emergency rescue
  - for emergency work/when there is temporary failure of controls.

Setting up a effective PPE programme
Having assessed the risk and implemented all reasonable control measures, the following steps should be considered when setting up a PPE programme.

- Identify individuals/tasks/environment where PPE is needed
- Select appropriate PPE to control residual exposure
- Involve worker in the PPE selection process
- Match PPE to each individual wearer
- Carry out fit tests for respiratory protective equipment (RPE)
- Ensure the use of PPE does not create additional risks
- Ensure that the PPE is compatible with other PPE
- Minimize PPE use time by defining when it should be used, e.g. particular tasks
- Train the wearer in the correct use of their PPE and supervise use
- Inspect PPE to ensure it is correctly maintained
- Provide suitable storage facilities to prevent contamination
- *Record:* PPE issue, maintenance, inspection, and RPE fit-testing data
- Inform individuals of the need for PPE, consequences of PPE failure and the importance of reporting PPE defects.

Selecting respiratory equipment

The decision to use RPE should be justified in a risk assessment. When selecting RPE consideration must be given to:

- *Individual factors*: health status, e.g. cardiorespiratory problems
- *Contaminant*: form of substance, single substance/mixture, nature of release (energy), concentration and variation, toxicity, OEL
- *Task*: duration, other PPE used, mobility, manual dexterity, visibility, communication, work rate (metabolic rate)
- *Environment*: indoor/outdoor, temperature, humidity
- *Legal requirements*: CE marking, employer and employee duties
- *Costs*: equipment, training, testing, repair/replacing storage, and record keeping.

RPE protection factors

The effectiveness of RPE is indicated by the assigned protection factor (APF). The APF is the level of respiratory protection that the respirator (or class of respirators) is expected to provide to employees when it is used correctly.

> *Example:* A respirator with an APF of 10 should reduce the workers exposure by a factor of 10, i.e. to one-tenth of exposure level in the breathing zone (outside the mask). Therefore the maximum use concentration (MUC) an employee can be expected to be protected when wearing this respirator is 10 times the WEL.

⚠ Whenever the exposure approaches the MUC, then the next higher class of respirator should be selected.

APF values assigned to different types of RPE are given in HSG 53 (HSE, 2005). Examples of RPE are shown on 📖 p. 655, Protective equipment.

Required protection factor

> *Example:* A worker is exposed to dust assigned a WEL 8h TWA = 5mg/m³. The daily TWA exposure is measured to be 20mg/m³. In order to reduce the personal exposure to the WEL, the required protection (PF) is: PF= 20/5 =4.

RPE selector guide

HSG 33 (HSE, 2005) describes a generic guide on the selection of RPE which comprises 5 steps:

- *Step 1:* details about the company and the work environment

- *Step 2:* information on control measures currently in use (other than RPE), reasons for wanting to use RPE, whether work is to be carried out in a confined space, and risk of oxygen deficiency
- *Step3:* determination of the health hazard group (HHG) for the substance and the level of protection needed. The HHG is based on risk phrases assigned to the substance. The required PF is determined from the combination of HHG and the amount of substance used and its dustiness/volatility
- *Step 4:* consideration of tasks and individual factors that may affect the selection of the RPE, e.g. work rate, mobility, medical conditions
- *Step 5:* consider need to test the selected RPE for a good fit over the mouth and nose (fit test).

RPE fit testing

A major cause of leaks for RPE equipment is poor fit. Fit testing will ensure that the RPE selected is suitable to the individual wearer.
- Tight-fitting RPE must be fit tested as part of the initial selection stage
- The fit-test report should include the following:
  - name of the person fit tested
  - make, model, type, and size of face-piece tested
  - exercises performed during the test
  - the test method (qualitative or quantitative)
  - measured fit factor if applicable
  - date of test
  - details of person carrying out the test
- Fit testing should be conducted by a competent person. Competence can be demonstrated through achieving accreditation under the 'Fit2Fit RPE Fit Test Providers Accreditation Scheme' developed by the British Safety Industry Federation (BSIF). For further details on the scheme, see ℘ http://www.fit2fit.org.

Further information

HSE (2005). *Respiratory protective equipment at work. a practical guide,* HSG 53. HSE Books, Sudbury. Available at: ℘ http://books.hse.gov.uk/hse/public/saleproduct.jsf?catalogueCode= 9780717629046

BSI (2005) *Respiratory protective devices—recommendations for the selection, use, care and mainte-nance,* guidance document BSEN529. BSI, London.

Types of respiratory protective equipment

- RPE can be divided in to two main types:
  - *respirator (filtering device)*—i.e. filter used to remove contaminants; do not use for protection in situations with reduced oxygen levels
  - *breathing apparatus (BA)*—requiring a supply of breathing quality air from an independent source, e.g. air compressor, air cylinder
- Both types are available with different face pieces. Masks (Fig. 32.6) rely on a good seal with the wearer's face. Hoods, helmets, and visors (loose-fitting face pieces) rely on clean air being provided to the wearer to prevent leak-in of contaminants (Fig. 32.7).

Filter for respirators

There are three main types of filter: particle filter, gas/vapour filter, and combined filter. Examples of different types of RPE available are shown in Tables 32.1 and 32.2.

- Particle filters are marked with a 'P' sign and filtration efficiency number 1 (low), 2, or 3 (high). If the filter is re-usable with fan-assisted respirators they will also have a sign 'TH' or 'TM'
- Gas/vapour filters are categorized by the substance type they can be used against. The filter is marked with a letter indicating type, a number to indicate capacity (1 = low, 2 = medium, 3 = high) and a colour code. See Table 32.2.

Combined filters are marked for both particles and gas/vapour, e.g. A1P3—organic vapour with capacity class 1 and high efficiency particle filter.

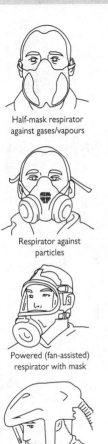

Half-mask respirator
against gases/vapours

Respirator against
particles

Powered (fan-assisted)
respirator with mask

Powered (fan-assisted)
respirator with hood

Fig. 32.6 Types of respirator.

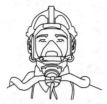

Fresh air hose BA

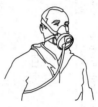

Contant flow air line BA
with mask

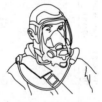

Demand valve BA

Fig. 32.7 Types of breathing apparatus.

Table 32.1 Protection values for different types of RPE

| | Respirators | | | | | | Breathing apparatus | | | |
PF required	Half-mask, particle filters	Half-mask, gas filters	Full face mask, particle filters	Full face mask, gas filters	Powered (fan-assisted) masks	Powered (fan-assisted) hoods	Fresh air hose	Constant flow airline BA	Demand valve BA
4	FFP1, FMP1, P1		P1						
10	FFP2, FMP2, P2	FF gas, FM gas, Gas	P2		TM1	TH1	LDH1		
20	FFP3, FMP3, P3			Gas	TM2	TH2		LDH2, LDM1, LDM2, Half-mask	
40			P3		TM3	TH3	Full face mask, Hood	LDH3, LDM3, Full mask	
200								Suit	
2000									Airline, self-contained

From HSE (2005). *Respiratory protective equipment at work*, HSG 53. HSE Books, Sudbury, p. 30. © Crown copyright, material is reproduced with the permission of HMSO and Queen's Printer for Scotland.

Table 32.2 Gas/vapours filters

Filter type	For use against	Colour code	Other information
A	Organic gases and vapours, boiling point >65°C	Brown	EN 14387
B	Inorganic gases and vapours	Grey	EN 14387. Do not use against carbon monoxide
E	SO_2 and other acid gases	Yellow	EN 14387
K	Ammonia and its organic derivatives	Green	EN 14387
Hg	Mercury	Red and white	EN 14387, includes P3 particle filter. Max. use time 50h
NO	Oxides of nitrogen	Blue and white	EN 14387, includes P3 particle filter. Single use only
AX	Organic gases and vapours, boiling point <65°C	Brown	EN 14387. Single use only
SX	Substance as specified by the manufacturer	Violet	EN 14387

From HSE (2005). *Respiratory protective equipment at work*, HSE 53. HSE Books, Sudbury, p. 28. © Crown copyright, material is reproduced with the permission of the Controller of HMSO and Queen's Printer for Scotland.

Further information
HSE (2005). *Respiratory protective equipment at work: a practical guide*, HSG53. HSE Books, Sudbury.

Hearing protectors

Requirements, types, use, and maintenance

- Guidance on hearing protection can be found in the CNAWR 2005 (📖 p. 548, Control of Noise at Work Regulations 2005). More detailed information can be found in BS EN 458:2004 Hearing protectors, Recommendations for selection, use, care and maintenance
- Under CNAWR the use of personal hearing protectors (HP) is compulsory for employees whose exposure to noise is likely to reach either of the upper exposure action values, i.e. 85dB(A) and 137dB(B) and for any employees working within areas assigned as hearing protection zones
- HP should be used where additional protection is needed above what can be achieved using other methods of noise control (e.g. engineering) and as a short term measure
- Avoid HPs that over protect the worker, i.e. reducing the level at the ear below 70dB
- HPs must be CE marked showing that it meets the European Standard BS EN 352
- HPs include earmuffs and earplugs; the latter can be custom moulded.
- Most HPs provide greater protection at higher frequencies than at lower frequencies.

Earmuffs

Easy to fit, re-usable, clearly visible, and hence easy to monitor. They may be uncomfortable in warm conditions. Long hair, beards, jewellery, or glasses may reduce protection. More expensive than ear plugs.
- *Seals:* check seals for cleanliness, hardening, and damage
- *Cup:* check for cracks, holes, damage
- *Headbands:* avoid over-bending and twisting, check tension
- Store in a clean environment.

Earplugs

More suitable when used with other PPE, e.g. safety glasses. Workers who suffer from recurrent otitis externa may be unable to tolerate earplugs. Custom-made plugs are more comfortable and are easier to fit for some wearers. However, need to conduct fit tests before putting into use.
- *Reusable plugs:* clean regularly, ensure not damaged or degraded
- *Issue to individual:* not to be shared
- Require careful insertion to ensure effective protection
- Provide greater protection at higher than low frequency
- Risk of infection (dirty hands)
- *Disposable plugs:* use only once.

Special protector types

- *Level-dependent (or amplitude-sensitive) protectors:* designed to protect against noise, but allow communication during quieter periods.
- *Flat or tailored frequency protectors:* these provide similar protection across all frequencies which can assist communication. Useful where

it is important to be able to hear high-frequency sound at the correct level relative to lower-frequency sounds, e.g. musicians.

- *Active noise reduction (ANR) protectors:* incorporate an electronic sound-cancelling system enabling additional noise attenuation. Effective at low frequencies (50–500Hz).
- *Protectors with communication facilities:* these use a wire or aerial to rely signals, alarms, and messages to the wearer. The signal level should not be too loud and the microphone should be switched off when not in use.

Selecting hearing protectors

When selecting HPs the following should be considered:

- Noise level (personal) and exposure variation
- Pattern of exposure
- Noise reduction (attenuation) provided by the protector
- Work environment (temperature, humidity, dust, dirt)
- Compatibility with other PPE worn
- Comfort and wearer preference
- *Hearing needs:* communication, hearing warning sounds, conducting tasks
- *Costs:* equipment, maintenance, training
- *Health problems:* ear infections, discharge, etc.
- Legal requirements.

Further information

BS EN 458:2004 Hearing Protectors. Recommendations for Selection, Use, Care and Maintenance. Guidance Documents.

Predicting noise reduction

The noise level at the ear (L'_A) when hearing protection is worn can be estimated using three different methods (octave band method, high, medium, and low frequencies (HML) method, and single rating number (SNR) method). L'_A is estimated by subtracting the estimated noise reduction (using manufacturer's performance data) from measured noise data.

Manufacturers' hearing protection data

The supplier must provide the following information for the HP. An example of supplier data is shown in Table 32.3:
• Mean and standard deviation attenuation values at each octave band centre frequency (63Hz–8KHz)
• Assumed protection values (APrV) at each frequency, i.e. mean protection minus one SD
• H, M, L and SNR values.

Noise level data required for estimating protection

The following types of noise data should be measured depending on the method chosen (one of three) to calculate the attenuation afforded by the ear protector.
• *Octave band analysis:* requires measurement of noise level at each octave centre frequency for the range 63Hz–8kHz
• HML require measurement of the A-weighted (LA) and C-weighted (LC) sound pressure levels
• *SNR:* requires single measurement of LC only.

Predicting attenuation using the HSE electronic spreadsheet

The measured noise levels and manufacturer's data can be entered into an electronic spreadsheet to calculate the attenuation afforded by the chosen ear protector. The spreadsheet is available on the HSE website (🖰 http://www.hse.gov.uk/noise). Of the three methods, the octave band analysis method provides the best estimate for L'_A.

Hearing protectors usually give lower protection than predicted by manufactures data due to, e.g. poor fitting. The difference between manufacturers' data and 'real-world data' is accounted for in the HSE calculator by 'derating' the protection by 4dB.

Protector use time If HP is removed in a noisy area, even for short period, amount of protec tion provided will be reduced (Fig. 32.8).

Information for employees

Employees should be provided with information on HPs including:
• Why and where HPs need to be worn?
• How replacements can be obtained?
• How to wear HPs with other personal protection?
• How to check, store, and report damage to HPs?

Table 32.3 Example of noise attenuation data supplied by manufacturers

	Octave band centre frequency (Hz)							
	63	125	250	500	1000	2000	4000	8000
Mean attenuation	17.3	21	24.5	27.3	27.9	33.8	36.1	40.8
Standard deviation (dB)	5.4	5.3	6.7	6.6	4.8	3.7	5.2	6.5
Assumed Protection Value (APV)	11.9	15.7	17.8	20.7	23.1	30.1	30.9	34.3
Single number values	H	29	M	23	L	20	SNR	27

APV, mean attenuation minus 1 SD.

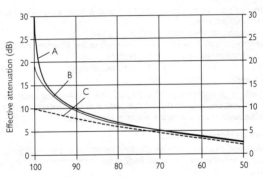

Fig. 32.8 Effectiveness of hearing protectors in relation to time worn. Protectors providing (A) 30dB attenuation, (B) 20dB attenuation, and (C) 10dB attenuation. From HSE (2005). *The Control of Noise at Work Regulations 2005*. HSE Books, Sudbury. Material reproduced with permission from the Controller of HMSO,

Gloves

Glove selection and use

Gloves differ in design, material, thickness, and size. The following factors should be considered when selecting gloves to avoid contact with harmful substances:

- The substance types handled (Tables 32.4 and 32.5) and their dermal effects (local and systemic)
- Type and duration of dermal contact
- *The user:* size (use sizing charts) and comfort.
- *The tasks:* e.g. manual dexterity requirements, need for sterile gloves
- Work environment (temperature and humidity).

Check that correct gloves have been selected using supplier's performance data, and that the glove user is not allergic to the glove material, e.g. powdered latex gloves. The HSE glove selection memory aid (from HSG262) is available on web page ℘ http://www.hse.gov.uk/skin/resources/glove-selection.pdf

Glove failure

Protective gloves can fail to protect the wearer from exposure to chemicals in different ways.

- *Permeation:* chemical migrates through glove
- *Penetration:* bulk flow of chemical through seams, pinholes, closures, porous materials, or other imperfections
- *Degradation:* change in physical properties of glove material as a result of exposure to a chemical agent.

▶ The *breakthrough time* is defined as the time between the initial application of a test chemical to the outside surface of the protective glove and its subsequent presence on the inside of the material.

Glove performance data

Glove suppliers usually provide chemical resistance charts, with glove performance for different chemicals. Performance is rated using the following data:

- *Breakthrough time:* ranges from 1–10 to >480min.
- *Permeation rate:* fast, medium, or slow
- *Degradation:* scale 0–6.

Applications

- Protection from cuts and abrasion, handling sharps
- Keeping hands warm in cold weather when using machines that cause HAVS
- Handling chemicals, radio-active materials, hot or cold materials
- Danger of electrical hazards
- Work involving naked flame, welding.

Gloves should be checked regularly and replaced if they are worn or have deteriorated. Workers should receive training in the correct way to care for, put on, wear, and take off gloves. Need to also ensure that there are adequate facilities for storage, cleaning, replacement, and disposal of gloves.

Table 32.4 Glove selection

Protection against	Glove type (examples)
Penetration and abrasion	Leather, Kevlar
Thermal	Terrycloth (protect against heat and cold) Neoprene (handling oils at low temperature)
Fire	Chromated leather gloves
Chemical protection	Neoprene, natural rubber, nitrile, butyl, PVA, PVC, Vitron

Table 32.5 Glove materials for chemical protection

Glove type	Protection against	Limitations
Nitrile (synthetic rubber)	Oil-based chemicals, lubricants, aliphatic solvents and aqueous chemicals	Prone to swelling with some solvents
PVC	Aqueous chemicals, e.g. acids and alkalis	Protection for some solvents limited because of plasticizers
Neoprene	Petrol, oil, lubricants	
PVA	Most organic solvents	Soluble in water
Butyl	Strong acids	Poor resistance to oils and lubricants
Viton	Chlorinated solvents and aromatic hydrocarbons	Poor resistance to ketones
Latex	Aqueous chemicals	Powdered gloves may cause allergic reactions and sensitization

Further information

HSE (2009). *Managing skin exposure risk at work*, HSG262. HSE Books, Sudbury. Available at: ℅ http://www.hse.gov.uk/pubns/priced/hsg262.pdf

Protective clothing

Protective clothing includes separates (jacket, trousers), aprons, overalls, coveralls, and body suits.

Applications
- *Chemical work protecting against accidental spillages:* use aprons
- *Contact with sprays or jets of chemicals:* use coveralls
- *Wet working:* using water sprays for cleaning, use rubbers, plastic, water-repellent coatings, waterproofs, breathable fabrics
- *Radiant heat from welding, foundries:* flame-retardant, insulating, and heat-resistant fabric
- *Electrical and electrostatic hazards:* materials which resist build-up of static electricity

Precautions
- When selecting protective clothing consider the chemical resistance and protection, protection against mixtures, and breakthrough times recommended by the manufacturer
- Store used/contaminated clothing separate from clean clothing
- Inspect for wear and tear/loose seams and damage
- Do not wear loose protective clothing close to moving machines
- Clean clothing following the manufacturer's instructions.

⚠ If protective gloves or clothes are worn incorrectly this may increase the risk to the individual.
- Contaminant may get inside the protective device (glove) and be occluded, resulting in higher exposure
- Prolonged use may cause moisture (sweat) on skin which can act as an irritant
- Reduces heat loss, which may increase likelihood of heat stress
- Latex gloves may cause an allergic reaction in susceptible individuals (📖 p. 202, Latex allergy)
- Gloves worn near moving equipment and machinery parts may be caught in the equipment, drawing the worker's hand into the moving machinery.

Further information
HSE (1992). *Personal protective equipment at work regulations 1992* (as amended). HSE Books, Sudbury.

HSE (1992). *A short guide to personal protective equipment at work regulations 1992*. HSE, Sudbury. Available at: 🔗 http://www.hse.gov.uk/pubns/indg174.pdf

Eye and face protection

Types of eye and face protection

Eye protection can be divided into three basic types:
- *Safety spectacles:* separate lenses in metal or plastic frame with side shields
- *Goggles:* flexible plastic frame with one or two lenses and flexible headband. With the rim in contact with the face, goggles provide eye protection from all sides
- *Face shields or visors:* one large lens with a frame and adjustable head harness or mounted on helmet. Can be worn with prescription lenses. Protects the face, but eyes are not fully enclosed.

Applications

Eye protection is required for the following hazards:
- Splashes of chemicals, e.g. acids or body fluids
- Chipping and debris from use of power-driven tools on metals, woods, etc.
- Molten metal, radiant heat sparks, or hot liquid splashes from furnaces
- Intense light (lasers) and other optical radiation likely to cause risks to the eye, e.g. UV light from welding.

Selecting eye and face protection

Table 32.6 shows examples of eye protection for different hazard types.

Table 32.6 Eye protection and hazards

Hazard	Eye protection equipment	Examples
Impact	Spectacles with toughened lenses/side screens	Flying swarf Chiselling
Dust	Goggles Air-fed positive pressure hood with visor	Grinding Shot-blasting
Molten metal	Goggles Face shield or visor	Casting and pouring
Radiation (non-ionizing)	Goggles, tinted Face shield or visor with correct protective shade Sunglasses	Welding and lasers (UV radiation) Casting and pouring molten metal/glass (IR radiation) Outdoor work (UV radiation)
Chemical or biological	Goggles Face shield or visor	Exposure to gases, vapours, liquids, dusts, biological agents

Precautions

- Issue eye protection on a personal basis and ensure that it fits properly
- Stored in a protective case
- When cleaning, follow manufacturer's instructions
- Do not use when the visibility (scratched and worn lenses) is reduced or the headband is damaged or worn
- *Lens may mist:* use anti-mist sprays or ventilation eye protection.

Standards for selection, use and maintenance

BS 7028: 1999 *Eye Protection for Industrial and Other Uses. Guidance on Selection, Use and Maintenance.*

Further information and guidance

HSE (2009). *European standards and markings for eye and face protection,* OM 2009/3. Available at: ℘ http://www.hse.gov.uk/foi/internalops/fod/om/2009/03app3.pdf

British Standards on eye protection. Available at: ℘ http://www.bsigroup.co.uk/DualSearch/?q=eye+protection

Section 7

Toxicology

Principles of toxicology

Toxicology and dose–response

Toxicology is the study of the adverse effects of chemicals in humans and other living organisms. It plays a fundamental role in chemical risk assessment.

Dose–response relationship

The dose–response relationship refers to the correlative relationship between exposure to a chemical (dose) and the effect that occurs (response).

Classification of dose–response

Two types of dose–response relationship exist.

Graded dose–response

This relates to the occurrence of effects in an *individual*, with the response varying in severity according to dose.

Quantal dose–response

This relates to the distribution of a specific response within a *population*. For many chemicals, the quantal dose–response relationship is characterized by a normal frequency distribution, represented in a frequency histogram by a bell-shaped curve. This distribution reflects differences in susceptibility to chemicals within a population (biological variation), indicating the presence of *sensitive* individuals and *resistant* individuals.

Dose–response parameters

Several parameters can be derived from the dose–response relationship.
- *NOAEL*: the dose at which no observable adverse effects occur
- *Lowest observable adverse effect level (LOAEL)*: the lowest dose at which adverse effects are observed
- *Threshold*: the dose below which the probability of an individual responding is zero
- *LD50*: median lethal dose, a single dose of substance that can be expected to cause death in 50% of experimentally exposed animals. This value is determined in acute systemic toxicity tests and is used to indicate the relative acute toxicity of a substance.

Patterns of dose–response

- With essential elements and vitamins, the shape of the graded dose–response relationship in an individual is U-shaped, representing adverse effects which occur at low doses (deficiency) and at high doses (toxicity) (Fig. 33.1)
- With genotoxic carcinogens, the response (development of cancer) is considered not to have a threshold (i.e. there is no dose that is associated with zero risk) (Fig. 33.2).

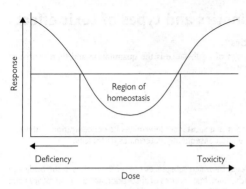

Fig. 33.1 Dose–response relationship for an essential substance.

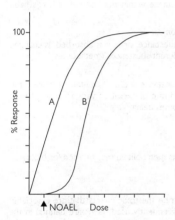

Fig. 33.2 Comparison of dose–response for two compounds (A) with no threshold and (B) with threshold.

Toxicokinetics and types of toxic effect

Toxicokinetics

The toxicokinetics of a substance is the quantitation and time course of four components:

- Absorption
- Distribution
- Metabolism
- Excretion.

The toxicokinetics of a substance determines its concentration at the target organ/tissue and consequently determines its toxicity.

Absorption

This is the process by which substances cross membranes in the body and enter the bloodstream. Main routes of absorption are the respiratory tract (inhalation), the skin (dermal), and the GI tract (oral).

Distribution

This is the translocation of substance within the body after it has been absorbed into the blood.

Metabolism (or biotransformation)

This is the process by which a substance, once it is absorbed, is changed into one or more chemically different substances (metabolites).

Excretion

This is the process by which a substance and/or its metabolites are eliminated from the body. Route and rate of excretion vary according to the substance, the most common routes being:

- Urine
- Faeces
- Exhaled breath.

Excretion of the substance (or its metabolites) may be used for biological monitoring purposes.

Types of toxic effect

Several terms are used to describe the toxic effects that are associated with exposure to a substance. Frequently used terms are defined in the following section.

- *Acute effects*: resulting from short periods of exposure to a relatively high concentration/dose of chemical, e.g. irritation of eyes, skin, and respiratory tract (toluene, arsenic), and central nervous system depression (*n*-hexane)
- *Chronic effects*: caused by repeated or prolonged exposure to a relatively low concentration/dose of chemical, e.g. central nervous toxicity (toluene), cancer of respiratory tract, skin, and liver (arsenic), and peripheral neuropathy (*n*-hexane)
- *Local effects*: occur at the site of first contact with a substance

- *Systemic effects*: occur only after the substance has been absorbed into the body
- *Immediate effects*: these develop soon after exposure takes place. In contrast, *delayed effects* only become apparent some time after exposure has taken place; perhaps months or years later
- *Reversible effects*: subside once exposure ceases
- *Irreversible effects* remain following cessation of exposure; in some cases, irreversible effects may become progressive.

Specific toxic effects

Carcinogenesis

Carcinogenesis is a multistage process in which exposure to a substance leads to genetic damage within the cell, resulting in uncontrolled proliferation of cells and ultimately the occurrence of a tumour. Carcinogenic substances are generally divided into:

- *Genotoxic mechanism:* those which cause cancer by direct damage to the genetic material
- *Non-genotoxic mechanism:* those which cause cancer by indirect damage to the genetic material.

Mutagenesis

This is a permanent change in the genetic material of a cell (DNA), involving a single gene, a block of genes, or an entire chromosome, which is passed on to the next generation of cells. A mutation in germ cells (reproductive cells such as sperm and ova and their precursors) can result in genetic damage that is passed on to offspring (heritable genetic defects). A mutation in somatic cells (non-reproductive cells) may lead to the development of cancer.

Respiratory sensitization

A state of specific airway hyper-responsiveness that is induced in some individuals by certain substances (respiratory sensitizers or asthmagens). Immunological or irritant mechanisms may be involved.

Skin sensitization

An immunologically mediated skin reaction which occurs in some individuals as a result of skin contact with certain substances.

Assessment of toxicity and evaluation of toxicological data

Assessment of toxicity

EU legislation requires that chemicals placed on the market must undergo a risk assessment to determine the risks to humans and the environment. An important part of the risk assessment process involves determining the intrinsic harmful properties of the substance (hazard identification) using toxicological data.

Toxicological testing

Toxicological data may come from animal, human, or *in vitro* studies, or be based on structure–activity relationships (SARs). Toxicological data for new substances and, when necessary, for existing substances are obtained using standardized test methods which are contained in Annex V of Directive 67/548/EEC. The standardized toxicity tests are conducted in laboratory animals or using *in vitro* systems.

- *Existing substances:* any substance listed in the European Inventory of Existing Commercial Chemical Substances (EINECS). All substances which were commercially available in EU between January 1971 and September 1981 appear in EINECS, comprising 100,204 substances. An EINECS number is assigned to each substance.
- *New substances:* any substance that became commercially available in the EU after September 1981. These substances appear in the European List of Notified Chemical Substances (ELINCS), which is periodically updated. Each substance is assigned an ELINCS number.

Toxicological data for the following endpoints are examined:
- Acute systemic toxicity
- Skin irritation
- Eye irritation
- Skin sensitization
- Repeated dose toxicity
- Mutagenicity
- Carcinogenicity
- Reproductive toxicity.

REACH legislation

This legislation (see 🕮 p. 554) emphasizes that unnecessary testing on animals should be avoided. To this end REACH promotes:
- The use of alternative methods for assessing hazards of substances
- The sharing of toxicological data between registrants.

Evaluation of toxicological data

Toxicological data for many substances involve uncertainties that need to be characterized for risk assessment:
- For most substances, toxicological data are based on animal studies, often using levels of exposure that are higher than would be applicable to humans

- The human population is more diverse than would be expected in a group of laboratory animals, and this variability needs to be taken into consideration
- Toxicological data may incorporate several experimental inadequacies (e.g. inappropriate exposure route, short duration of exposure, or deviations from standardized test methods).

Uncertainty or assessment factors

When evaluating toxicological data, these uncertainties are addressed by the use of uncertainty or assessment factors. The intention is that incorporating uncertainty factors will provide some reassurance of protection against the harmful effects of chemicals when limited information is available.

Classification and labelling

Classification and labelling involves:
- Evaluation of the hazards of a substance (or preparation) in accordance with EU legislation
- Communicating the hazard via the label.

Legislation

In the UK, the regulations relating to classification and labelling are called the Chemical (Hazards Information and Packaging for Supply) Regulations 2009, commonly known as CHIP4. These regulations implement the EU Dangerous Substances Directive and the Dangerous Preparations Directive.

The regulations are in the process of being replaced by EU Regulations Classification, Labelling and Packaging of Substances and Mixtures (CLP Regulation), introduced in 2009 and to be fully implemented in June 2015 (see p. 41, Chemical hazards).

The aim of these regulations is to ensure that people who are supplied with any chemical receive information on its hazards and advice on how to protect themselves, others, and the environment. Classification entails evaluating toxicological data for a substance and comparing these against specified classification criteria.

Occupational exposure limits

OEL is a generic term for occupational air standards, used for personal monitoring, as a means of assessing whether or not workers are exposed to unacceptable levels of a substance.

Purpose

The main purposes of OELs are:
- To demonstrate compliance
- To identify individuals at risk
- To select control measures in order to minimize health risks
- To enable enforcement.

Factors considered in setting standards include:
- Where the substance is used
- Identification of critical health effects
- Number of people exposed to the substance
- Typical exposure levels
- Control technology available
- Cost of implementing control systems
- Potential health benefits from exposure reduction.

Workplace exposure limits

- WELs are occupational exposure limits set for substances hazardous to health under the COSHH Regulations. HSE produces an annual list of WELs in the document EH40
- A WEL is the maximum concentration of an airborne substance, averaged over a reference period, to which employees may be exposed by inhalation
- Two limit periods, referred to as the time-weighted average concentration (TWA), are used to express the WELs, i.e. the long term (8h) and the short term (15min)
- Where a substance is not assigned a WEL, this does not indicate that it is safe. Exposure to such substances should be reduced to a level as low as reasonably practicable, taking account of the toxicity of the substance
- In the EH40, chemicals can be assigned the notations 'Sk' and 'Sen':
  - *Sen*—substance capable of causing occupational asthma, including substances assigned a risk phrase R42 (may cause sensitization by inhalation) or R42/43 (may cause sensitization by inhalation and skin contact)
  - *Sk*—substance can be absorbed through skin, i.e. those substances for which there are concerns that dermal absorption will lead to systemic toxicity.

Deriving the WEL value: information and stages

- Assessment of the toxicology, i.e. potential of the substance to produce adverse health effects
- Identification of NOAEL/LOAEL from the dose–response relationship
- Application of uncertainty factors (safety factors)

- Estimate the highest exposure at which no adverse effects would be expected to occur in workers following exposure over a lifetime
- The Advisory Committee on Toxic Substances determines whether the derived exposure level is currently practicable; then WEL is proposed at this level.

Criteria for setting WELs from EH40

- The WEL value is set at a level at which no adverse effects on human health would be expected to occur based on the known/predicted effects of the substance. However, if such a level cannot be identified with reasonable confidence, or if this level is not reasonably achievable
- The WEL value would be based on a level corresponding to what is considered to be good control, taking into account the severity of the likely health hazards and the costs and efficacy of control solutions.

Compliance with WELs

Substances assigned a WEL fall in to two groups:
- Substances defined as carcinogens or mutagens, or that cause occupational cancer
- All other hazardous substances assigned a WEL.

For carcinogens and mutagens, employers must ensure that the exposure is reduced as far below the WEL as is reasonably practicable. For other substances, the employer needs to ensure that the WEL is not exceeded.

Units

- Concentration of airborne particles (dusts, fumes) is expressed in milligrams per cubic metre (mg/m^3)
- In EH40, limits for dusts are usually expressed as the inhalable or respirable fraction
- Limits for fibres are expressed as fibres per millilitre of air (fibres/mL)
- Volatile organic substances are expressed in both parts per million by volume (ppm) and milligrams per cubic metre (mg/m^3).

Airborne concentration can be converted from ppm to mg/m^3 (or vice versa) using the following equation:

$$WEL\ (mg/m^3) = WEL\ (ppm) \times MW/24.05526$$

Where MW is the molecular weight of the substance and 24.05526 is the molar volume of an ideal gas at 20°C and 1atm pressure (101325 Pa, 760mmHg).

Epidemiology in occupational health

Epidemiology

Measures of disease occurrence

Epidemiology is concerned with the distribution and determinants of illness and disease in human populations. Various measures are used to quantify the rates at which disorders occur in defined groups of people. These measures may relate to a population in its entirety (crude rates), or they may be specific to defined subgroups (e.g. sex- and age-specific rates).

Case definition

Defining a case of disease may be relatively straightforward. For example, it is usually not too difficult to decide whether or not someone has recently incurred a hip fracture. For some disorders, the distinction between normality and abnormality may be less clear–cut (e.g. hypertension, diabetes). In these circumstances, case definitions should be explicit, even if somewhat arbitrary. Otherwise, measured rates of disease cannot be meaningfully interpreted.

Incidence

The incidence of a disease is the rate at which new cases occur in a population over time. It is the measure of most relevance to studies of disease causation.

Mortality

Mortality (death) rates refer to the incidence of death from a disease. For diseases in which a large proportion of cases are rapidly fatal (e.g. mesothelioma), mortality serves as a good proxy for incidence.

Prevalence

The prevalence of a disease is the proportion of a population who are cases at a defined point in time (point prevalence) or during a defined period (period prevalence). For example, the point prevalence of rheumatoid arthritis in a population at the time of a survey might be 1%, and the one-month prevalence of low back pain 20%. The prevalence of a disease depends upon its incidence and also on the time for which people remain cases before recovery or death. Prevalence rates may be relevant to the planning of health services. In addition, they are sometimes used as a proxy for incidence in studies of disease causation. However, findings must be interpreted with caution, since associations with prevalent disease could reflect effects on recovery or fatality as well as on incidence.

Proportional rates

Calculation of incidence, mortality, and prevalence rates requires that the population under study be enumerated. Sometimes this is not possible, but the occurrence of a disease can be related to an indirect index of population size. For example, the proportions of deaths attributed to brain cancer might be compared between two populations. Here the total number of deaths in each population serves as an indirect index of its size. Care is needed, however, in the interpretation of proportional rates. A high proportion of deaths from brain cancer could indicate high mortality from the disease, but it could also reflect an unusually low overall death rate in the population under study.

Standardized rates

Rates of most diseases vary importantly with sex and age, but comparing multiple sex- and age-specific rates between two populations may be unduly cumbersome. Standardization is a method of summarizing disease occurrence in a population that takes account of its sex and age distribution, and thereby allows more meaningful comparison with other populations. It can be applied to incidence, mortality, prevalence or proportional rates. Two methods of standardization are widely used.

Direct standardization

Directly standardized rates are simply a weighted average of sex- and age-specific rates. The weighting factors being defined by the sex and age distribution of a standard population (e.g. the national population).

Indirect standardization

Indirect standardization compares the number of cases of disease in a study population with the number that would have been expected had the study population experienced the same sex- and age-specific rates as a specified standard population (e.g. the national population). The comparison is summarized by the ratio of observed to expected cases (sometimes expressed as a percentage). A standardized mortality ratio (SMR) is an example of such a ratio.

Measures of association

Much of epidemiology is concerned with comparing the occurrence of disease between groups of people according to their exposure to 'risk factors'. A risk factor is a characteristic that is associated with an increase or reduction in the risk (rate) of a disease. The association may be directly causal (e.g. asbestos causes lung cancer) or indirect because the risk factor is a marker for a cause (e.g. yellow stained fingers are a risk factor for lung cancer because they are a marker for smoking).

Various measures are used to summarize the association between risk factors and disease. They are defined here in the context of a risk factor that is classed either as present or absent. However, the definitions can readily be extended to associations with different levels of a risk factor.

Attributable (excess) risk

Attributable risk is the difference in risk between people with and without exposure to a risk factor. It is the measure of association that is most relevant to decisions in risk management for individuals. For example, in deciding whether the risk of cancer from a specified occupational exposure to ionizing radiation is acceptable, we need to know the absolute increase in cancer incidence that is caused by the exposure.

Relative risk

Relative risk is the ratio of risks in people exposed and unexposed to a risk factor. It is a commonly reported measure of association from epidemiological studies, and is related to attributable risk by the formula:

$$AR = (RR - 1) \times Rate_{unexp}$$

where AR is the attributable risk, RR the relative risk and $Rate_{unexp}$ the rate of disease in people who are unexposed to the risk factor.

Odds ratio

An odds ratio is defined as the odds of disease in a person exposed to a risk factor divided by the odds in someone who is unexposed. In most situations odds ratios approximate closely to the corresponding relative risks. However, for very common disorders (e.g. low back pain), odds ratios deviate further from the null value of one. In other words, for positive associations they are larger than the corresponding relative risk, and for negative associations they are smaller.

Population attributable risk

Population attributable risk is defined as the rate of disease in a population minus the rate that would apply if everyone in that population were unexposed to the risk factor. It depends on the attributable risk in individuals and also the prevalence of exposure in the population. It is relevant to risk management for populations, giving an indication of the burden of disease that might be prevented by eliminating exposure to a causal factor.

Attributable proportion (aetiological fraction)

Attributable proportion is the proportion of all cases of disease in a population that would be prevented if the risk of disease in exposed persons were reduced to that of the unexposed. Again, its use is in risk management for populations. The attributable fractions for different causes of a disease may sum to more than 100%. This is because where an individual is exposed to more than one cause, removing any one of the exposures might be sufficient to prevent him getting the disease.

Statistical inference

Populations and samples

Most epidemiological studies use observations in a sample of people to draw conclusions, but a wider population from which the sample derived. For example, the odds ratio for welders in a case-control study of pneumonia might be taken as an estimate of the odds ratio in welders more generally. A sample statistic (the odds ratio in the sample of people who participated in the case-control study) is used to estimate a population parameter (the odds ratio in the population of welders more generally).

One of the limitations on this extrapolation is that samples may be unrepresentative of their parent populations simply by chance, especially if the sample is small in size. Statistical inference is the process by which uncertainties from chance variation between samples are taken into account when drawing conclusions about populations. Two methods are commonly used—hypothesis testing and estimation with confidence intervals.

Hypothesis testing

Hypothesis testing starts with an assumption ('null hypothesis') about the population for which conclusions are to be drawn. A calculation is then made of the probability that the findings in a sample of the size studied would deviate from those expected under the null hypothesis as much as was observed. If this probability ('p-value') is sufficiently low (i.e. the observed findings are sufficiently unlikely under the null hypothesis), the findings are deemed to be 'statistically significant', and the null hypothesis may be rejected.

When reporting hypothesis tests, it is more informative to report the level of their statistical significance (i.e. the magnitude of the p-value) than simply that the p-value is below some specified threshold for significance (e.g. $p < 0.05$).

Statistical tests

Statistical tests such as the chi squared (χ^2) and t-tests, are a mathematical means of calculating p-values. The appropriate test varies according to the study design and the nature of the data collected.

One- and two-tailed tests of significance

A two-tailed p-value is the probability of deviation from the null hypothesis in either direction to the extent that was observed in the study sample. For example, if the null hypothesis were of no association between exposure and disease, a two-tailed p-value would be the probability of finding an association, positive or negative, at least as strong as that observed, simply by chance. A one-tailed p-value relates to deviations from the null hypothesis in only one direction. Unless otherwise stated, quoted p-values are normally two-tailed.

Confidence intervals

A confidence interval is a range within which a population parameter might normally be expected to lie, assuming that the findings from a study sample are unbiased. Usually 95% confidence intervals are quoted. The mathematical derivation of a 95% confidence interval is specified in such a way that, on average, (and in the absence of bias) 95% of intervals so calculated will include the true value for the population parameter.

Confidence intervals are more informative than p-values, and are generally the preferred method of statistical inference in occupational health studies.

Interpretation of associations

Epidemiological studies addressing the relationship between an exposure and disease may differ markedly in their findings. There are several possible reasons for this, all of which should be considered when interpreting observed associations.

Nature and extent of exposure

If an agent or circumstance causes disease, risk may vary according to the nature, intensity, and duration of exposure.

Case mix

The strength of an association may vary according to the mix of disease within a specified case definition. For example, the risk of leukaemia from occupational exposure to ionizing radiation will be higher if the case group comprises predominantly acute myeloblastic leukaemia than if it is made up largely of chronic lymphatic leukaemia.

Bias

Bias is a systematic tendency to underestimate or overestimate a parameter of interest because of a deficiency in the design or execution of a study. There are many potential sources of bias, but broadly they arise because the study sample is systematically unrepresentative of the population about which conclusions are to be drawn (e.g. because of inappropriate selection criteria or incomplete participation of selected subjects), or from inaccurate information about participants.

Because of the practical and ethical constraints on research in humans, bias is inevitable in epidemiological studies. The aim should be to minimize its occurrence and then allow for its potential impact when interpreting results.

Chance

Even if there is no systematic bias in the selection of a study sample, it may be unrepresentative simply by chance. Gauging the potential impact of chance variation between samples entails techniques of statistical inference (confidence intervals or hypothesis testing). In addition consideration should be given to what is known from other studies (including relevant non-epidemiological research). If an association is biologically implausible or incompatible with a large body of prior research, it may be reasonable to attribute it to chance even if it is highly significant statistically.

Confounding

Confounding occurs when a risk factor under study is statistically associated with another exposure or characteristic ('confounding factor') that independently determines the risk of disease. It can lead to spurious associations in the absence of direct causation, or cause true causal associations to be under- or over-estimated. For example, lorry drivers might have an unusually high incidence of lung cancer, not because lorry driving causes the disease, but because they tend to smoke more than the average. Here, smoking would be the confounding factor.

Effect modification

Effect modification occurs when the relative risk associated with a risk factor varies according to the presence or level of another characteristic or exposure (an effect modifier). For example, the relative risk of skin cancer from occupational exposure to sunlight might vary according to skin colour.

Routine health statistics

Purpose

Routinely collected health statistics are used for several purposes in occupational health:

- Monitoring the impact of known occupational hazards and the effectiveness of control measures
- As an alert to previously unrecognized hazards
- As a background against which to assess the occurrence of disease in occupational groups (e.g. in cohort studies or in the investigation of occupational clusters of disease).

Reporting schemes and registers of occupational disease

Reporting schemes are used to collect and register information about cases of definite or probable work-related illness. Applicable to health outcomes that can be linked to occupation with reasonable confidence in the individual case. Attribution to work may be made in two ways:

- *On the timing and other clinical features of the illness:* e.g. acute injuries and poisoning may be linked to work through their temporal relation to an exposure incident, and occupational asthma may be diagnosed through the demonstration of sensitization to an agent encountered only at work
- From knowledge that the individual has been exposed to an agent or circumstance that carries a high relative risk of the health outcome.

Sources in the UK

Various sources of routine health statistics may be useful to occupational health professionals practising in the UK:

- *Reporting schemes for occupational injuries and diseases:* these include data reported to the Health and Safety Executive under RIDDOR; and various voluntary reporting schemes co-ordinated by the Centre for Occupational and Environmental Health at the University of Manchester, as part of The Health and Occupation Reporting Network
- Periodic surveys of health and work conducted by the Health and Safety Executive, including the Labour Force Survey and Workplace Health and Safety Survey (WHASS)
- Statistics of social security compensation for occupational injuries and prescribed industrial diseases
- Statistics of mortality and cancer incidence by occupation—these are published periodically by the Office for National Statistics (ONS) and in the past were produced by its predecessor, the Office of Population Censuses and Surveys (OPCS)
- *General statistics of mortality and cancer incidence:* again published by ONS, these may provide useful background data against which to evaluate patterns of disease observed in occupational populations
- *Hospital Episode Statistics:* published by ONS, these relate to hospital admissions by cause and procedure. They do not include information on occupation, but include useful data on, for example, admissions for accidental pesticide poisoning.

⚠ All of the statistical sources listed have their individual strengths and limitations which must be taken into account when they are used.

Voluntary reporting schemes within The Health and Occupation Reporting Network (THOR)

- Occupational Physicians Reporting Activity (OPRA)
- SWORD
- EPI-DERM Occupational Skin Surveillance
- Musculoskeletal Occupational Surveillance Scheme (MOSS)
- Surveillance of Occupational Stress and Mental Illness (SOSMI)
- Surveillance of Infectious Diseases at Work (SIDAW)
- Occupational Surveillance Scheme for Audiological Physicians (OSSA)
- Occupational Surveillance of Otorhinolaryngological Disease (THOR-ENT).

Further information

University of Manchester. Available at: ℘ http://www.medicine.manchester.ac.uk/oeh/research/thor/schemes/

UK National Statistics (2012). Available at: ℘ http://www.statistics.gov.uk

DWP. *Statistics*. Available at: ℘ http://statistics.dwp.gov.uk/asd/index.php?page=iidb

HSE *Workplace health and safety survey (WHASS) programme*. Available at: ℘ http://www.hse.gov.uk/statistics/publications/whass.htm

HSE *Self-reported work-related illness (SWI) and workplace injuries (LFS)*. Available at: ℘ http://www.hse.gov.uk/statistics/publications/swi.htm

Planning epidemiological research

Unlike many other types of occupational health research, epidemiological investigations often do not require expensive equipment or facilities. However, even the simplest studies must be carefully planned and rigorously conducted.

The starting point for any investigation is one or more study question(s). These should be both worthwhile and answerable. In other words, depending on what is found, the information generated by the study should have the potential to affect how things are done in the future.

Protocols

A protocol is essential for any epidemiological study. It is used in seeking ethical approval, permissions, and funding; as a guide to data collection and analysis; and as a reference when preparing reports of the study findings. The original study protocol, together with a note of any deviations that occurred as the study progressed, should be retained so that they are available if required for the purposes of audit and governance.

If the investigator is inexperienced in epidemiological research, or lacks relevant expertise (particularly in statistics), help should be sought in preparing protocols. The main elements of a protocol are:

- *Background:* this sets up the study question(s), summarizing relevant information from earlier research, the current gaps in knowledge, and why it is important to address these gaps. It may also describe new technical advances that allow the gaps in knowledge to be addressed in a way that was not previously possible
- *Study question(s):* these should be explicitly stated
- *Methods:* this section should describe how the study questions will be addressed. It should include details of which subjects will be eligible for study, and how they will be recruited; what data will be collected about participants, and how these data will be analyzed to answer the study question(s). It may also be relevant to include information about the validity of methods for data collection
- Plans for publication
- *Statistical power:* this gives an indication of confidence that the study sample will not be unrepresentative simply by chance
- *Ethical considerations:* are there ethical issues associated with the research, and if so, how will they be addressed?
- Permissions and agreements (if relevant)
- Funding (if relevant).

Ethical review

Most epidemiological studies require formal review by a properly constituted research ethics committee (where there is doubt advice can be sought from the chair of the committee to which the study would be referred). The relevant committee will depend on who is conducting the study and from where subjects will be recruited:

- *NHS-based research:* via the National Research Ethics Service (NRES)[1]
- *Non-NHS research:* HSE have an ethics committee that, although primarily concerned with HSE research, will consider extramural research in the OH field according to set criteria.[2]

Ethics committees normally specify the format in which they wish to receive applications.

Other approvals

Research that will take place within the NHS requires permission from the NHS organization(s) that will be involved. The National Institute for Health Research provides a coordinated system to assist researchers in obtaining the necessary approvals.[3]

Questionnaires

Questionnaires are often used to collect epidemiological data. They may be self-administered or administered at interview. Questions may be open-ended (i.e. with free text answers) or closed–ended (with a finite set of options from which the answer is chosen). Important considerations in the design of questions are their validity (will they provide accurately the information that is sought?), understandability, and the ease with which the answers can be analyzed. Use of previously developed questions (e.g. from widely used questionnaires) is often an advantage. Questionnaires should collect the information that is likely to be needed to address the study question(s), but unnecessary detail should be avoided.

1 ℘ http://www.nres.npsa.nhs.uk/

2 HSE Research Ethics Committee. Available at: ℘ http://www.hse.gov.uk/research/ethics/index. htm

3 NICE (2012). *Gaining NHS Permission for clinical research.* Available at: ℘ http://www.crncc.nihr. ac.uk/about_us/processes/csp

Investigation of disease clusters

A cluster of disease is an unusually high number of cases in a defined population over a time period during which fewer than one or two cases would be expected.

Disease clusters are not infrequent in occupational populations. Occasionally they result from exposure to a hazardous agent or activity in the workplace, but much more often they simply represent a chance coincidence. Nevertheless, they can be a major cause of anxiety for both employees and managers, and require proper assessment.

The assessment of occupational clusters entails a staged approach, the extent of investigation depending on the level of scientific suspicion that an occupational exposure is responsible and also the level of concern in the workforce and management.

Characterization of index cases

A first step is to characterize the index cases that have given rise to concern. The aim should be to establish:
• The precise diagnosis of each case
• The occupational exposures that the cases share in common.

If the cases, in fact, suffer from different diseases that are unlikely to have the same causes, or they do not share any potentially hazardous occupational exposures, then the level of scientific suspicion is low, and more detailed investigation may not be necessary.

Further investigation

If further investigation is required, the next steps are to:
• Search readily accessible sources of information (e.g. company pension files and occupational health records) for any additional cases with the same diagnosis/diagnoses and exposure(s) as the index cases
• Estimate the expected frequency of the relevant diagnosis/diagnoses in all employees with the same exposure(s) as the index cases. This gives an indication of how unusual the cluster is
• Review published scientific literature regarding known and suspected causes of the disease(s) suffered by the index cases. Look for indications that a shared occupational exposure might have a causal role
• Establish how frequently the shared exposures of the index cases occur elsewhere, and what is known about their potential adverse effects.
  • If the same exposures commonly occur in other occupations or circumstances, then any increased risk of disease might be expected to apply also in these other situations.
  • If the shared exposures have known toxic effects that are consistent with an increased risk of the disease(s) in the index cases, then the level of scientific suspicion is increased. (For example, a cluster of cancer would be more suspicious if there were shared exposure to a known mutagen).

Formal epidemiological studies

If additional investigation is required beyond what has already been described, then often it will take the form of a formal epidemiological study. Such a study may be conducted in the workforce that experienced the cluster, with the aim of providing more precise estimates of risk in relation to specific exposures. However, it must be remembered that clusters only come to attention because they are unusual, and therefore a study in a workforce with a disease cluster can be expected to show elevated risks for the disease concerned. For this reason, a stronger design is to conduct a study in a separate population with similar exposures to the index cases. If a study of this sort provides independent evidence of excess disease, the case for an underlying occupational hazard becomes more compelling.

Cross-sectional surveys

In a cross-sectional survey information is collected at a single point in time (or over a short period) about the prevalence of health outcomes and/or their determinants in a defined population.

In occupational health, information from cross-sectional surveys may be used for several purposes:

- *Planning and prioritizing interventions:* e.g. the prevalence of stress-related illness might be assessed in a workforce to decide whether changes were needed in working methods or styles of management
- *Monitoring the impact of measures to control hazardous exposures:* e.g. the prevalence of sensorineural deafness might be assessed to check the effectiveness of controls on noise exposure, or personal exposures to an airborne pollutant might be measured to check that local exhaust ventilation was working as intended
- *Investigating associations between exposures and disease:* e.g. whether the prevalence of dermatitis is unusually high in workers handling a new material.

Cross-sectional studies of disease causation

Cross-sectional surveys are attractive as a means of investigating causes of disease in that they can often be conducted relatively quickly and cheaply. However, special care is needed in their interpretation.

- Risks may be underestimated because of biases in the selection of subjects for study. This is a particular concern when the disease of interest is sufficiently disabling that it causes people to leave the job in which it arose, or where its symptoms are exacerbated by continuing exposure to the causal agent, again leading people to move from the job that caused it. For example, the risk of asthma from an occupational allergen might be missed if sensitized individuals rapidly moved to other work and therefore were not included in a cross-sectional sample of exposed workers
- The cross-sectional design may make it difficult to distinguish cause from effect. For example, a high prevalence of pathological drinking in publicans might occur because heavy consumers of alcohol preferentially seek employment in bars, or because work as a publican makes people more prone to drink heavily, or both.

For these reasons, cross-sectional studies of disease causation work best for less serious diseases that are unlikely to cause a change of job, and are unlikely to impact on the exposures under investigation.

Cohort studies

In a cohort (longitudinal) study, people with known exposure to a risk factor (e.g. a hazardous occupational exposure) are followed up over time, and their subsequent health or mortality is compared with that of controls that were unexposed or exposed at a lower level. Cohort studies can be used to estimate both attributable and relative risks. The method has been widely used to investigate known and suspected causes of occupational cancer, but can be applied to many other types of health outcome.

Assessment of exposure

Exposures must be assessed not only to the risk factor(s) of prime interest, but also to potential confounding factors. Depending on the study question and the practicality of data collection, the exposure ascertained may be at a single point in time (most often the time of entry to follow-up), over a period up to a specified point in time, or right through to the time of exit from follow-up (this requires repeated assessment of exposures throughout the follow-up period). Many different methods of exposure assessment may be employed, including the use of questionnaires, employment records, occupational hygiene measurements, and bio-monitoring data. Often a job-exposure matrix is applied to translate job titles into agent-specific exposures.

Assessment of health outcome

The methods by which health outcomes are ascertained will depend on the study question, and on practical and ethical limitations. They may be assessed continuously throughout follow-up or at one or more time points during the follow-up period. Methods include the use of death certificates, cancer registrations, and follow-up questionnaires, physical examinations, and clinical investigations. To prevent bias, methods for ascertaining health outcome should not vary in relation to the risk factors under study.

Retrospective cohort studies

Particularly in the study of occupational carcinogens, (where prolonged follow-up is usually required to obtain statistically meaningful results), cohort studies are often conducted retrospectively. This requires that cohort members can be identified retrospectively and their exposures assessed in a way that it is not biased in relation to subsequent health outcome. It is also necessary that the relevant health outcomes can be reliably assessed in retrospect.

Comparisons with the general population

Occupational cohort studies of mortality and cancer incidence commonly use disease rates in the general population (national or regional) as a comparison. This has the advantage of giving statistically robust control data at relatively low cost, and is valid provided it can reasonably be assumed that the exposures of interest are negligible in the general population when compared with those in the study cohort.

Healthy worker effect

In cohort studies that compare mortality in an occupational group with that in the general population, bias may arise from a 'healthy worker effect.' This occurs because employed people tend on average to be healthier than the population at large. In particular, people with chronic disabling disease are liable to be selectively excluded from employment. Thus, when followed up over time, employed populations tend to have lower than average death rates from causes, such as chronic respiratory disease, for which death is often preceded by a prolonged period of disability.

Statistical analysis

Various statistical methods are applied in the analysis of cohort studies, depending in part on the exact study design and the type of health outcome. One technique that is widely used when comparing mortality or cancer incidence in an occupational cohort with that in the general population is the 'person-years method'. This entails first summing the number of years for which cohort members were under follow-up in different combinations of age and calendar period. The age- and calendar period-specific disease rates in the general population are then applied to these person-years of follow-up to obtain an 'expected number' of cases for each combination of age and calendar period. Next, the expected numbers are summed across all combinations of age and calendar period. Finally, the observed number of cases is divided by the total expected number to give a SMR or standardized incidence ratio (SIR).

Case-control studies

In a case-control (case-referent) study people with a disease of interest (cases) are identified, and their past exposure to known or suspected causes is compared with that of controls (referents) that do not have the disease, associations generally being summarized by odds ratios. Sometimes case-control studies are 'nested' within a larger cohort investigation, but even where they are not; they can be viewed as an efficient method of sampling from a theoretical cohort investigation. Essentially, exposure information is collected about all of the cases of disease in the study population and time period, but about only a representative sample of those who are not cases.

Recruitment of cases

The source of cases and method of ascertainment should be explicitly defined. Ideally, cases should have incident (newly presenting or newly diagnosed) disease. Prevalent or fatal cases may be used as an alternative, but associations may then reflect influences on recovery or fatality as well as on incidence. Often an attempt is made to recruit all cases in a defined study population and time period, but this is not essential, and the source population for the case group may only be notional (e.g. the catchment population of a hospital).

Selection of controls

Controls should be representative (in terms of their exposures to risk factors and potential confounders) of the non-cases in the population (defined or notional) that gave rise to the cases. A second objective is that they should provide information on exposures of similar quality to that for cases (the ideal of perfect accuracy is rarely achievable). Often it is impossible to achieve both of those aims simultaneously, and compromise is necessary. Two sources of controls, commonly employed are patients with other diseases and people selected at random (or effectively at random) from the study population.

Matching

The control of confounding in case-control studies is through appropriate statistical analysis, but this is sometimes made more efficient by matching controls to cases (either individually or in groups) according to the presence or levels of potential confounding factors such as sex and age. Where matching is used, the exposures of controls should represent those of all non-cases in the source population with the relevant matching criteria.

Ratio of controls to cases

Where exposure information can be obtained as easily from cases as controls and there is no practical limit to the available pool of cases, statistical efficiency will be maximized by recruiting equal numbers of cases and controls. Where cases are in limited supply or control data can be ascertained more easily than data from cases, the statistical power of a study may usefully be enhanced by taking a higher ratio of controls to cases. However, the return from this diminishes as the ratio increases, and control—case ratios greater than four are rarely worthwhile.

Exposure ascertainment

Exposures must be assessed both to risk factors of interest, and also to potential confounding factors. Various sources of information are used, including questionnaires, historical records, and biomarkers (provided these reflect exposures before disease onset and are not modified by the occurrence of disease). If exposures are ascertained by questionnaire and the recall of cases is more complete than that of controls, bias may result with spurious inflation of risk estimates.

Experimental studies

An experimental study assesses the effect of a planned intervention on outcomes of interest. Outcomes that may be relevant in occupational health research include:

- Disease incidence, prevalence or mortality
- Incidence of other adverse events (e.g. dangerous occurrences or near-miss accidents)
- Biomarkers of sub-clinical health effects (e.g. acetyl cholinesterase activity)
- Biomarkers of exposure to hazardous agents
- Measures of attitude or behaviour.

Occasionally, an intervention may involve deliberately exposing subjects to a hazardous agent at low levels, looking for evidence of minor subclinical effects. Mostly, however, it is ethical to study the impact only of potentially beneficial interventions (e.g. aimed at controlling a hazardous exposure or practice). Comparisons may be between a new intervention and standard practice, or between two or more different interventions.

Study designs

Various study designs may be employed, depending on the nature of the intervention(s) and outcome(s) of interest.

Simple 'before and after comparisons'

Outcome measures are assessed in the same subjects or groups before and after an intervention, looking for changes that might be attributable to the intervention. The weakness of this design is that results may be confounded by other determinants of outcome that change over time in parallel with the intervention.

Non-randomized, controlled comparisons

Subjects or groups receiving an intervention are compared with controls that receive a different intervention or are managed according to standard practice. At baseline (i.e. prior to the intervention), controls should be as similar as possible to the subjects receiving the intervention in characteristics that are known or likely to predict the outcomes under study. This may be easier to achieve if the outcome is the change in a parameter following the intervention rather than its absolute value.

Randomized controlled interventions

People or groups with similar baseline characteristics are randomly assigned to receive the intervention or to serve as controls, and their subsequent outcomes are compared. If there is marked heterogeneity of subjects or groups at baseline, they should be stratified before randomization according to likely predictors of outcome, and then randomized within strata. The advantage of randomized controlled interventions is that when randomization is applied to large numbers of individuals or groups; it tends to eliminate confounding effects even for unrecognized confounders. However, when only a few individuals or groups are available for study, the benefits of randomization are minimal, and it is usually better to use a non-randomized companion.

Blinding

Sometimes it is possible to 'blind' subjects, those implementing an intervention, and/or those assessing outcome measures as to whether an individual or group received a particular intervention. This can have two advantages:

- Prevention of confounding that might occur if knowledge of the intervention led to other parallel changes (either deliberate or subconscious)
- Reduction of potential bias in the assessment of outcomes (e.g. from placebo effects).

Blinding is particularly important where the assessment of outcomes depends on subjective judgment by the participant or an investigator.

Section 9

Environmental medicine

Environmental protection

Environmental medicine

General principles

- Environmental exposures, while sharing many attributes with occupational exposures, are often more subtle. They are generally of much lesser degree (e.g. pesticide exposure in farming communities, outdoor air pollution) and the effects are not so easily attributable to the exposure
- Where an environmental exposure is recognized to affect health, the aim of the physician or regulator is to protect the individual by removing or reducing exposure, e.g. reducing ambient air pollution by improvements in engine and fuel technology
- This *exposure, effect, control paradigm* (Fig. 35.1):
  - provides a framework for understanding how a specific exposure might lead to an individual health effect
  - identifies where control measures might be instituted, e.g. by reducing personal exposure or reducing emissions by legislation.

Exposures

- *Routes of exposure:*
  - inhalation
  - through the skin
  - ingestion
  - other exposures (noise, vibration, UV light)
- *Quantification of exposures:*
  - questionnaire or structured interview, but relies on memory, often of distant events
  - direct measurement, e.g. air quality
  - biomarkers, e.g. blood lead (Pb) levels
- Modelling, by using existing information to develop predictions of exposure where direct measurement cannot be made.

Exposure and outcome

- Once an estimate of exposure has been made, this needs to be matched against a specified outcome. During this process all recognized confounders must be identified and measured (where possible), so that interpretation is valid
- *Vulnerable groups* within any population are the young (including the unborn child), the elderly, and the infirm. These groups may show adverse effects of environmental exposures at lower exposures than healthy adults of working age.

Control

- Control measures depend on route(s) of exposure and may be multiple (e.g. pesticides). An understanding of the proportion of the total dose from each route is essential when considering control
- The *precautionary approach* is usually used, where, without waiting for cast-iron proof that exposure A via route B causes disease C, action is taken to reduce overall exposure.

Practicalities of assessing environmental exposures and health impacts

The effect of an environmental exposure may come to notice through the following:

- *Increased exposure*: recognition that a population is exposed to a specific substance or pollutant mix, e.g. particulate air pollution in cities
- *Disease clustering*: recognition of a cluster of a specific disease in time and/or place (e.g. outbreaks of infectious disease)
- *By analogy:* with exposure to other proven exposure/outcome situations elsewhere, e.g. current concerns around exposure to nanomaterials bearing in mind the proven adverse effects of asbestos and the considerable delays in accepting the true health impact of that material.

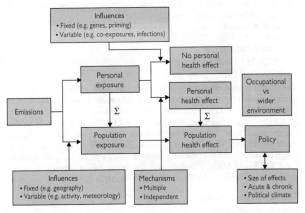

Fig. 35.1 Health effects of an environmental hazard.

Health Protection Agency

Structure of the Health Protection Agency

The HPA was set up in 2003, as a Special Health Authority. However, it became an independent public body in 2005, when it was combined with the then NRPB. It is made up of five main elements:

- HPA headquarters
- Centre for Infections
- Centre for Emergency Preparedness and Response
- Centre for Radiation, Chemical and Environmental Hazards
- National Institute for Biological Standards and Controls.

Role of the Health Protection Agency

The Health Protection Agency's role is to protect the public health. It covers chemical, biological, radiological or nuclear threats. The role of the Health Protection Agency (% http://www.hpa.org.uk/AboutTheHPA/) is divided into the following areas:

- Chemical hazards
- Biological hazards
- Radiation hazards
- Emergency response
- Infectious diseases.

The Health Protection Agency is the UK's lead body on health protection, but it also has responsibility to provide local health protection services in England. This local health protection role is fulfilled by Health Protection Scotland (HPS) in Scotland, the National Public Health Service in Wales and by the Department of Health, Social Services and Public Safety in Northern Ireland. The HPA has to work closely with other relevant agencies in order to fulfill their work, notably the Department for Environment, Food and Rural Affairs (DEFRA) and the Environment Agency. Its work will be subsumed into the Department of Health in 2011–12.

Remit of the centres

- *Centre for infections:*
  - communicable disease surveillance
  - advising government on infectious diseases
  - microbiological reference laboratory
  - outbreak investigation for major epidemics or unusual infections
- *Centre for Emergency Preparedness and Response:*
  - monitoring and assessment of new, emerging or re-emerging infectious illnesses
  - developing and maintaining Britain's capacity to deal with emergencies such as disease outbreaks or chemical releases including acts of terrorism. This includes training emergency services, and running exercises to test responses
  - Providing advice on the management of chemical, biological, radiological or nuclear incidents (CBRN)
- *Centre for Radiation, Chemical and Environmental Hazards:*
  - Radiation Protection Division

- Chemical Hazards and Poisons Division—offering advice on chemical incidents including fires, chemical leaks and pollution (the Air Quality and Noise section is part of HPA); the National Poisons Information Service (NPIS) provides advice to NHS staff on the management of individual patients.
- *National Institute for Biological Standards and Controls:* the National Institute for Biological Standards and Controls (NIBSC) mission is to assure the quality of biological medicines.

Relevant legislation

The Health Protection Agency Act 2004.

Outdoor air pollution

- Air pollution is a mix of different particles, gases, and chemicals, the proportions of which vary by source and by site
- The major contributors are anthropogenic, although there can be major contributions from natural sources under some circumstances
- Control of air quality is exercised at national government level, but can only deal with locally produced anthropogenic emissions as natural sources are uncontrollable as, to a certain extent, is transport of air pollution from one country to another
- Continued exposure to polluted air confers a greater risk to health than episodes, although the Great London Smog of December 1952, which killed at least 4000 individuals, was critical as it led to the introduction of the Clean Air Act 1956.

Content and sources

Particles

Sources
- Vehicle emissions
- Industry
- Power generation
- *Natural:* sea salt, disturbed dust, volcanoes

Measures
- Mass (expressed as μg/m^3 of air)
  - gravimetrically
  - *PM*10—particulate matter <10μm in diameter
  - *PM*2.5—particulate matter <2.5μm in diameter
  - *reflectance*—i.e. by measurement of blackness of a filter (Black Smoke)
  - *light scattering*—expressed as PM_{10}, $PM_{2.5}$
  - *numbers*—expressed as particle numbers per cubic centimetre of air.
- These measures are usually expressed as 24-h or annual means.

Gases

- *Sulphur dioxide:* largely from industry or power generation
- *Nitrogen dioxide:* 2° pollutant from vehicles
- *Ozone:* 2° pollutant from action of UV light on oxides of nitrogen and hydrocarbons
- *Carbon monoxide:* from vehicles.

Gases are expressed as ppb or μg/m3 and for the timescale relevant to their air quality standard.

Other substances

- Carcinogens:
  - benzene
  - 1,3-butadiene
  - PAHs
- Lead.

Health effects

Diffuse pollution
- ↑ Particles are associated with ↑ mortality and ↑ hospital admissions for cardiopulmonary disease on a day-to-day basis
- Similar effects are seen with ozone and sulphur dioxide, but of lesser degree
- Effects on asthma are limited to hospital admissions and, inconsistently, to symptoms and lung function
- Effects of long-term exposure on disease prevalence and severity may be more marked
- Association with incidence of lung cancer but not other cancers shown in the USA.

Point source pollution
- Emissions from point sources can cause clusters of disease (e.g. soyabean dust emissions from the docks in Barcelona in the 1980s led to outbreaks of acute asthma)
- The worst recorded peacetime incident occurred in Bhopal, India, in 1984 when an incident at the Union Carbide (India) Ltd plant led to the release of a cloud of methyl isocyanate gas causing over 3800 deaths
- More usually, concerns arise about the potential for an identified source to be a cause of disease clusters. See Chapter 34 in Investigation of disease clusters
- Many disease clusters are chance events unrelated to point sources of pollution, but understandably generate considerable public concern.

Control

- Air quality standards are based on health effects worldwide even though air pollution also impacts on crop yields and the integrity of buildings
- Responsibility for air quality falls to local councils in the UK.

Relevant guidance and legislation

- Clean Air Act 1993 (c. 11). Stationery Office, London
- Air Quality Limit Values Regulations 2001. Stationery Office, London. Similar regulations apply across the UK
- The UK's archive of air pollution measurements. Available at: ℜ http://www.airquality.co.uk/archive/index.php
- The UK's air quality strategy can be viewed at: ℜ http://www.defra.gov.uk/environment/quality/air/air-quality/approach/

Indoor air pollution

- In the developed world 90% of time is spent indoors
- In parts of the developing world much greater time is spent outdoors
- Indoor air quality is not subject to legislation except in the workplace, where occupational exposure standards apply in some settings.

Indoor pollutants

- Environmental tobacco smoke (ETS)
- Allergens, including moulds
- Indoor penetration of pollutants from outside (notably particles)
- Cooking fume
- Settled dust
- Micro-organisms
- Endotoxins
- Nitrogen dioxide (NO_2) from gas cookers and fires
- Carbon monoxide (CO) faulty gas appliances
- Ozone
- Kerosene products
- Biomass fuel combustion, e.g. plant material or agricultural waste
- VOCs, e.g. formaldehyde
- Radon.

Health effects

- *ETS exposure:*
  - respiratory symptoms in children
  - lung cancer
- *Biomass fuel:*
  - lung cancer
  - chronic bronchitis/chronic obstructive pulmonary disease (COPD)
- *Cooking fume:*
  - lung cancer
  - possibly exacerbation of asthma
- *Radon:* lung cancer
- *Sick building syndrome occurs in artificially ventilated buildings:* the exact cause is unknown but it appears to relate to air exchange rates and temperature. It presents with a range of symptoms (see 📖 p. 334, Sick building syndrome):
  - headaches
  - tiredness
  - poor concentration
  - sore throats
  - nasal symptoms
  - tight chest
  - inability to wear contact lenses/dry eyes.

Control
- There are no indoor air quality standards. Such controls would raise issues of individual civil rights
- By law anyone installing or servicing gas appliances must be Gas Safe registered
- Landlords are required to have gas appliances serviced annually, keep records for two years and give new or existing tenants a copy of the current safety certificate.

Relevant legislation and guidance
Gas Safety (Installation and Use) Regulations 1998. Stationery Office, London.

Water pollution

Safe drinking water[1] is essential for life. Microbiological contamination is well recognized, but contamination by metals, etc., also occurs. Pollution follows spills, industrial discharges, mining (especially abandoned mines), agricultural run-off and leachate from landfill. Naturally occurring metals may affect water quality. Pollutants may be point sources such as industrial discharges or diffuse pollutants including agricultural run-off of animal wastes. Contamination of estuarine and inland seas may lead to severe impacts e.g. the Aral Sea disaster. Water is divided into surface waters (streams, rivers, lakes) and ground water (~98% of available fresh water). These are closely linked and exchange occurs between them.

Arsenic

Groundwater contamination is often from natural sources with ↑ arsenic in parts of Bangladesh, Chile, India, etc. Chronic ingestion causes;
- thickening of the skin (hyperkeratosis) and ↑ pigmentation
- bladder cancer
- pancreatic cancer
- skin cancer
- peripheral neuropathy
- diabetes
- 'Blackfoot disease'; peripheral vascular disease (Taiwan).

Arsenic remediation
- Test water for arsenic and mark supplies with ↑ arsenic
- Educate people as to risks of drinking high arsenic water
- Source low arsenic water:
  - rain water harvesting
  - deep boreholes to aquifers with low arsenic,
  - sand filtration.

Fluoride
- High fluoride levels occur in areas near mountain ranges worldwide
- Fluoride in drinking water at ~1ppm prevents dental caries
- Exposure to fluoride >2ppm as a child < 8-yr-old → dental fluorosis
- Children > 8yrs cannot develop dental fluorosis
- Mild dental fluorosis → white spots on teeth (hypomineralized enamel)
- Severe dental fluorosis is rare → heavily mottled and stained teeth
- Chronic ingestion of water with >10ppm fluoride → osteofluorosis.
- Endemic osteofluorosis: back pain, calcified ligaments, bone thickening
Severe cases of osteofluorosis resemble ankylosing spondylitis.

Fluoride remediation
- Fluoride removal from water is expensive
- Use low fluoride water supplies where possible
- Defluoridation may be carried out using contact precipitation.

---

1 WHO (2011). *Guidelines for drinking-water quality*, 4th edn. WHO, Geneva.

Lead (Pb)

- Water may be contaminated by inorganic lead in houses with lead pipes (pre-1970's UK housing) or copper pipes joined with lead-solder
- Soft water areas → ↑ lead levels as acidic water ↑ plumbo-solvency
- ~40% of UK houses still have lead water pipes[2]
- 10–20% of human Pb. exposure is from water.

Lead remediation

- Water suppliers ↓ plumbo-solvency by adding lime to low pH supplies (to ↑ pH) and/or orthophosphate (a corrosion inhibitor), if water at the consumer's kitchen tap is likely to have lead >10μg/L
- Remove all lead pipes and tanks from potable water supplies
- Run kitchen tap for 1min if it hasn't been used for >6h
- Never use water from hot water taps for drinking or cooking
- Do not use water from bathroom taps for drinking.

Organic chemicals

Pesticides

- Spills or run-off from agriculture → ground water contamination
- Main threat is to aquatic life, rather than human health.

Solvents

Contamination of ground water by organic solvents may occur where chemicals spill or underground fuel storage tanks leak.

Polychlorinated biphenyls

PCBs are persistent organic pollutants (POPs) that may contaminate water supplies e.g. PCBs from abandoned electrical equipment.

Other contaminants

Nitrates

- Occur in ground water due to fertilizers and animal wastes
- Nitrates → nitrites → methaemoglobinaemia ('blue baby syndrome') in bottle-fed infants <3 months age (see 📖 p. 328, Methaemoglobinaemia)
- Nitrate remediation; reverse osmosis, distillation or anion exchange.

By-products of water treatment

- Water is often treated with chemicals such as chlorine or chloramines
- Trihalomethane is generated by organic material reacting with chlorine. Whether exposure causes birth defects or bladder cancer is disputed.

Endocrine disruptors

- Phthalates, human sex hormones and pharmaceutical agents in water have been linked with abnormal sexual developmental in some species
- Whether exposure leads to adverse effects in humans is unclear.

---

2 Chartered Institute of Water and Environmental Management. *Position on Lead in Drinking Water*, August 2005.

Soil pollution

Introduction

- Soil pollution may occur due to industrial, military, or agricultural releases of pollutants
- Municipal waste disposal is a significant source of soil pollution in many countries
- The source may be:
  - a point source or
  - diffuse, e.g. run-off from roads contaminated with lead, oils
- Contamination may arise locally, but deposition of pollutants from distant sources may also occur, e.g. acid rain
- Industrial activities in an area may leave a legacy of soil pollution for future generations:
  - mining, e.g. mine tailings
  - metal refining
  - leather tanning (chrome)
  - demolition (asbestos)
  - town gas production
- Poor or non-existent records of waste disposal further complicate remediation in such cases.

Soil contaminants

- *Heavy metals:*
  - arsenic
  - chromium
  - cadmium
  - lead
  - mercury
  - nickel
- Cyanide
- *Persistent organic pollutants:*
  - pesticides
  organic solvents—chlorinated hydrocarbons, benzene
  - PCBs
  - PAHs
  - dioxins
- Asbestos.

Examples of soil pollution

Love canal

- One of the best known examples of soil pollution occurred in Love Canal (now called Black Creek Village) in upstate New York
- Approximately 21,000 tons of chemicals, including 200 tons of trichlorophenol, were buried in a disused canal near a residential area over many years
- Chemicals leached into the basements of some of the homes

- Epidemiological studies of residents showed ↑ miscarriages
- Hundreds of families had to be evacuated
- One consequence of the Love Canal episode was the creation of 'Superfund' sites by the US Congress in 1980 set up to deal with contaminated land sites.

Waste incinerators

- Waste incinerators may be a point source of soil pollution downwind
- Incinerators, if poorly run, may discharge heavy metals and dioxins into the atmosphere which contaminate the soil by deposition.

Disposal of sludge and sediments

- Disposal of sewage sludge which may contain heavy metals, e.g. lead, on soil by direct application or soil injection → contamination
- Use of growth promoters containing copper in pig farming can lead to significant copper contamination of soils when slurry is applied to land
- Similar concerns regarding heavy metal contamination arise in the disposal of silt and sediment dredged from harbours or river estuaries.

Food contamination

Food may be contaminated at any stage during production, processing, or distribution. The potential for contamination of food by bacteria, viruses, fungi, parasites, or toxins is well recognized and will not be considered further. Less commonly, chemical or metal contaminants lead to food poisoning outbreaks. Thus, food acts as one pathway for pollutants in the environment to act on human health. Animals may be affected by pollutants (e.g. lead-poisoned wildfowl), become ill and so easier to catch, and pose a hazard to human health if eaten.

Groups at ↑ risk

- Producers and their families who largely consume their own produce
- Children and unborn children are at ↑ risk if exposed to neurodevelopmental toxins, e.g. methyl mercury.

How pollutants enter the food chain

- Pollutants enter the food chain through contamination of air, soil, or water:
  - discharges from factories
  - mines (e.g. heavy metals)
  - agriculture (e.g. pesticides)
  - waste dumps
- Food may be contaminated during:
  - production
  - processing
  - distribution
  - storage
  - preparation/cooking
- Sale of food not intended for human consumption
- Intentional adulteration of foodstuffs.

Agents implicated

- *Cadmium*-contaminated mine discharges entered the Jinzu River basin in Japan. Use of this water for irrigation of rice paddies led to cadmium entering the food chain. Consumption of cadmium-contaminated rice has led to *itai-itai* ('ouch ouch') disease, principally among post-menopausal women. Sufferers developed osteoporosis and proximal renal tubular dysfunction
- Fish may absorb *methyl mercury*. Fishermen and their families who consume these catches are at special risk
  - in the Great Lakes area of North America mercury contamination has lead to health advice being issued on fish consumption
  - in the 1950s, fishermen's families around Minamata Bay, Japan, ate fish contaminated with methyl mercury → neurological illness. For several years an electronics factory had discharged mercury in the bay, so contaminating marine life
  - lead—rarely, lead poisoning may arise from food contamination (e.g. spices, flour). Flour can be contaminated when a damaged millstone is repaired with lead. Illegal alcohol (moonshine) may be

lead contaminated; life-threatening poisoning can occur in heavy drinkers

- Consumption of *adulterated oil* sold as olive oil in 1981 led to Spanish toxic oil syndrome: severe myalgia, eosinophilia, and pulmonary infiltration. Research points to the toxin being fatty acid esters of 3-(N-phenylamino)-1,2-propanediol (PAP). Approximately 20,000 people were affected and 300 died. Others were left with chronic paraesthesia and musculoskeletal and skin complaints
- 'Rice oil disease', termed yusho in Japan and yucheng in Korea, due to PCBs accidentally contaminating rice oil occurred in Japan in 1968 (1800 cases) and Korea in 1978 (~2000 cases). Unborn children exposed to PCBs and their breakdown products, polychlorinated dibenzofurans (PCDFs), showed developmental delay, behavioural problems, and ↓ growth. Chloracne and liver disease occurred.

Pesticides entering the food chain

Organomercurials

Following a series of bad harvests in the late 1960s and early 1970s, Iraq imported wheat treated with mercurial fungicides. The wheat arrived too late for planting that year and so the people consumed seed never intended for human consumption. More than 10,000 people died and ~100,000 people suffered long-term health effects.

Adulteration of foods

Unscrupulous producers, wholesalers, and shopkeepers may adulterate foodstuffs to maximize profits; this kind of fraud flourishes where food testing and enforcement are weak. Activities such as adding illegal dye-stuffs to spices occasionally come to light. Food adulteration is principally an economic issue, but depending on the adulterant used such food may affect human or animal health.

Safety science

Safety science

Health and safety management framework

Employers are required to show evidence of operating an effective health and safety management system (see 🕮 p. 520, Management of Health and Safety at Work Regulations 1999).

A framework for managing health and safety is provided by the HSE in the document *Successful Health and Safety Management*. The five key elements of successful health and safety management are shown in Fig. 36.1, which also illustrates the relationship between them. Further details about some of the key steps are covered Chapter 9, Policies, and on 🕮 pp. 352–55, Quality and audit in OH, and 🕮 p. 737, Measuring performance.

Key elements of successful health and safety management

- Effective health and safety policies set a clear direction for the organization to follow
- Effective management structure and arrangements should be in place to deliver the policy
- Need for a planned and systematic approach to implementing the health and safety policy
- Need to measure performance against agreed standards to show when and where improvements are needed
- Through audits and reviews learn from relevant experiences and apply lessons.

Further information

HSE (1997). *Successful health and safety management*, HSG65. HSE Books, Sudbury. Available at: ℘ http://www.hse.gov.uk/pubns/priced/hsg65.pdf

HSE (2011). *Managing health and safety- Five steps to success.* Available at: ℘ http://www.hse.gov.uk/pubns/indg275.pdf

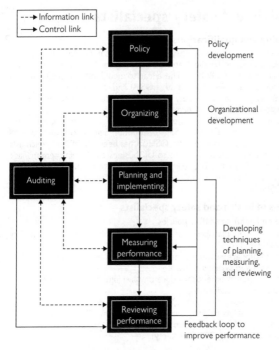

Fig. 36.1 Key elements of successful health and safety management. Reproduced from HSE (1997). *Successful health and safety management*, HSG65, p. 4. HSE Books, Sudbury). © Crown copyright material is reproduced with the permission of the Controller of HMSO and Queen's Printer for Scotland.

Health and safety specialists

Training and qualifications

There are several routes of entry into health and safety. Most common are courses, accredited by the National Examination Board in Occupational Safety and Health (NEBOSH). These lead to membership of the Institution of Occupational Safety and Health (IOSH) and, after further experience, to chartered health and safety practitioner status. Occupational health professionals can also gain membership of IOSH.

Recently, the UK Government accepted the recommendations outlined in the report 'Common Sense, Common Safety' to professionalize health and safety consultants. An OSHCR has been established which lists consultants who can offer advice to UK businesses to help them manage health and safety risks. The register is only open to health and safety consultants who have met certain standards within their professional bodies, e.g. IOSH, BOHS.

Duties of health and safety specialists

Advice on health and safety policies

Health and safety managers, advisers, and safety officers help to formulate policies related to:
- Organizational assessment and management of health and safety risks
- Safe plant and systems of work
- Safe work environment to reduce physical injuries and ill health
- Emergency procedures
- Accident investigation and reporting procedures
- Monitoring safety performance
- Health and safety training programmes

Fire safety (see 📖 p. 738, Fire safety).

Other duties

- Advising management on the design and safe use of plant and equipment
- Periodic inspections to identify unsafe plant, unsafe working conditions, and unsafe practices
- Communicating with safety reps or representatives of employee safety (📖 p. 516) through the Health and Safety Committee
- Facilitating or undertaking risk assessments (including fire risks)
- Advising on compliance with current and new legislation
- Promoting and delivering safety education programmes through toolbox talks, etc.
- Providing information on accident prevention techniques
- Recording accident statistics
- Accident investigation
- Advising about the need to report incidents to HSE in compliance with RIDDOR (see 📖 Appendix 4)

- Assessment of the work environment and work equipment
- Audit of safety systems against international systems (BS 8800/OSHAS 18001)
- Presenting information on safety performance to management
- Liaison with occupational health departments, government inspectors, local authorities, (including fire services), and environmental protection agencies.

Further information

OSHCR. Available at: ℘ http://www.oshcr.org/

Common Sense, Common Safety. ℘ http://www.number10.gov.uk/wpcontent/uploads/402906_ CommonSense_acc.pdf

Accident investigation and management

Definitions

Accidents

Accidents are defined as any unplanned events that give rise to ill health or injury, damage to property, plant, or products, production losses, or increased liabilities (HSE, 1997). Types of accidents include:

- Near miss
- Minor injury
- Major injury
- Property damage.

Incidents

Incidents are all undesired circumstances and near misses, which could cause (potential) accidents.

Purpose of accident investigation

Accidents need to be investigated for the following reasons:

- To collect data required for accident reporting/notification
- To collate information required to defend an insurance claim
- To establish causes
- To identify and take appropriate actions to prevent reoccurrence.

Causes of accidents

Most accidents involve multiple, interrelated causal factors and occur as a result of deficiencies, errors, omissions, or unexpected changes.

- *Personal factors:*
  - knowledge and skill deficiencies
  - physical and mental incapacities
- *Unsafe act:*
  - operating at unsafe speed
  - operating without knowledge or authority
  - using equipment unsafely
  - taking unsafe position
  - failure to use protection
  - failure to warn or signal
  - failure to make secure
- *Unsafe condition:*
  - inadequate guards
  - inadequate warning systems
  - poor housekeeping
  - unsafe equipment
  - excessive exposure to hazards.

Consequences of accidents

- Fatalities
- Ill health and injuries
- Loss of production
- Damage to plant and machinery, raw materials, and products
- Breach of legislation and prosecution

- Civil claims
- *Environmental impact:* spillages, discharge
- Damaged reputation
- Lowered employee morale.

Outcome of accident investigation

Accident prevention programmes should be designed with the aim of reducing danger in the workplace (safe workplace) and increasing workers' perception of risks (safe person).

Management actions as a result of accident investigation include the following:

- Identification of specific training needs
- Need for detailed job safety analysis to identify the hazards and precautions
- Improving systems of work (safe design, safe work procedures, permit to work, safety rules, and review of risk assessments)
- Improve the level of supervision
- Identify areas/tasks where PPE is required
- Preparation of safety guidance notes for particular activities
- Setting up committees and feedback to all concerned
- Improvement in the working environment, e.g. lighting levels, ventilation
- Improvement in information and its provision
- Review health and safety responsibilities.

Cost and reporting of accidents

All organizations should determine the costs of accidents. This process helps to identify causes and consequences, as well as providing useful information on strategies and drivers for future accident prevention.

All accidents have both direct and indirect costs, and incur insured and uninsured costs.

- *Insured costs include:*
  - claims on employers and public liability insurance
  - damage to building, equipment, or premises
- *Uninsured costs include:*
  - lost time
  - extra wages for overtime
  - sick pay
  - production delays
  - fines
  - legal costs, and excess on any claims
  - investigation time.

The total cost of an accident can be determined by considering both direct and indirect costs.

Direct costs

- Increase in liability premiums
- Claims for injury, or for defective or unsafe products
- Fines and damages awarded in criminal courts for breaches of law
- Court and legal costs.

Indirect costs

- *Treatment:*
  - first aid
  - transport
  - hospital attendance
- *Lost time:*
  - injured person
  - management
- *Production:*
  - loss of production
  - damage to plant
  - training
  - supervision
- *Investigation (time and manpower):*
  - management
  - safety advisors
  - safety representatives
  - liaison with external agencies
- *Others:*
  - administration
  - costs incurred by witnesses attending court.

Legal requirements to notify accidents and incidents

- *Reporting accidents, injuries, and dangerous occurrences:*
    - notifiable and reportable major accidents are listed in schedule 1 of RIDDOR
    - dangerous occurrence is a major incidence which has the potential for loss of life and significant damage; these are listed in schedule 2 of RIDDOR
- *Fatal and major injury accidents:* as well as dangerous occurrences must be:
    - reported to the enforcing authority by the quickest practicable means, i.e. telephone, *and* reported in writing within 10 days to the enforcing authority on Form 2508.

Reports to authorities

- *Over 7 day injuries to person at work:* a written report must be sent to the enforcing authority within 15 days of the accident on Form 2508
- Following receipt of a written report from a doctor, occupational diseases (schedule 2 of RIDDOR) are reported using Form 2508A. See 🕮 Appendix 4: List of Reporting of Injuries, Diseases, and Dangerous Occurrence Regulations for a list of RIDDOR reportable diseases
- Gas incidents are reported on Form 2508G.

Documentation

Copies of all forms sent to the authorities must be kept.

Further information

See RIDDOR, 🕮 Appendix 4: List of Reporting of Injuries, Diseases, and Dangerous Occurrence Regulations

HSE Costing accidents and ill health. Available at: ℘ http://www.hse.gov.uk/economics/costing.htm

HSE (2008). The cost to employers in Britain of workplace injuries and work related ill health 2005/06. Available at: ℘ http://www.hse.gov.uk/economics/research/injuryill0506.pdf

Costs to Britain of workplace injuries and work-related ill health: 2009/10 update. . Available at: ℘ http://www.hse.gov.uk/statistics/pdf/cost-to-britain.pdf

Accident data

Accident rates enable analysis of trends, facilitating comparison between one organization and another, or between different parts of the same organization.

Examples of accident rate measures

- Incidence rate = (total number of accidents/number of persons employed) × 1000
- Frequency rate = (total number of accidents/total number of man-hours worked) × 100,000
- Severity rate = (total number of days lost/total number of man hours worked) × 1000
- Duration rate = No. of man-hours worked/total number of accidents

Standardization of accident data

When comparing accident rates it is important to ensure that the following elements are standardized:
- Definitions of what has to be reported
- Reporting procedures
- Methods of calculation.

In addition to the industry data, certain industry associations provide their members with accident statistics, which may be used for 'benchmarking', i.e. comparing performance data with competitors.

National accident statistics

The HSE produces the *Safety Statistics Bulletin* which contains summary data on fatal injuries to workers, subdivided into employees and self-employed. Non-fatal injuries to workers are subdivided into:
- Over 3-day injuries to workers
- Injuries to the member of the public
- Dangerous occurrences
- Gas safety.

Further information

HSE (2011). *Health and Safety Statistics.* Available at: ℘ http://www.hse.gov.uk/statistics/

Measuring performance in health and safety management

Performance needs to be measured to assess how well risks are controlled. Monitoring also reinforces management commitment to health and safety. Two types of monitoring systems are used:

- Active systems, which monitor the design, development, implementation, and operation of management systems and compliance with standards, i.e. monitoring achievement of specific plans and providing feedback on performance before accidents or ill health occur
- Reactive systems involve monitoring incidents, accidents, cases of ill health, damage to property, and other evidence of deficient health and safety performance, i.e. monitoring is triggered after an event.

Active (proactive) monitoring data

- Staff perception of management commitment to health and safety
- Periodic review of documents, e.g. risk assessments, maintenance programmes
- Exposure and health surveillance data to assess adequacy of controls
- Extent of compliance with standards
- Observation of work and behaviour
- *Training in health and safety:* numbers trained and its effectiveness
- Knowledge among staff of risks and controls
- Time taken to implement actions
- Actual use of personal protective equipment
- Frequency of inspections, safety tours, audits
- Competence of staff with responsibilities for health and safety
- Number of staff suggestions for health and safety improvements
- Staff attitudes to risk and use of controls.

Reactive monitoring data

- Regulatory agency enforcement action
- Sickness absence data
- Reported accidents and injuries (lost time, property damage)
- Damage to property.

Outcome of performance assessment

For the risks that are identified during active and reactive monitoring, actions should include the following:

- Identify reasons for under-performance
- Identify underlying failure in health and safety management systems
- Prevent recurrence
- Satisfy legal requirements, e.g. reporting under RIDDOR.

Further information

HSE website. Available at: ℘ http://www.hse.gov.uk. Information about health and safety management, including risk assessment tools for slips, trips, and falls, industry-specific advice on machine safety, and other aspects.

Fire safety

- Fire is a constant threat to all premises. In the UK in 2008 there were ~1800 fires in industrial premises
- For a fire to start there must be adequate fuel, a source of oxygen, and an ignition source
- Fires may start accidentally, but the threat of arson should also be considered and appropriate measures taken to reduce this risk
- Good housekeeping, effective maintenance (especially of electrical equipment), rigorous health and safety procedures, and effective fire detection, warning, and firefighting systems all reduce fire risks.

Fire regulations

- Current regulations governing fire prevention in England and Wales came into force from October 2006—the Regulatory Reform (Fire Safety) Order 2005. Similar legislation applies in Scotland—the Fire (Scotland) Act 2005
- Fire authorities no longer issue fire certificates
- *The regulations cover non-domestic premises:*
  - offices and shops
  - factories and warehouses
  - residential care
  - sleeping accommodation
  - education
  - places of assembly
  - theatres/cinemas
  - outdoor events
  - health care
  - transport facilities
- Enforcement of the Fire Safety Regulations is the responsibility of the local fire and rescue service, except for Crown property where HM Fire Safety inspectors take this role.

Other relevant regulations

Where a workplace contains dangerous substances which can create an explosive atmosphere, e.g. petrol, gas, solvents, paints, flour or wood dusts then DSEAR 2002 and the Equipment and Protective Systems intended for use in Potentially Explosive Atmospheres Regulations 1996 will likely also apply.

Main requirements

The main requirement is to carry out a fire risk assessment. The Department for Communities and Local Government guidance on fire safety identifies five steps for fire risk assessment.

Identify hazards

- The person in control of premises must undertake a fire risk assessment
- *This assessment should identify sources of:*
  - fuel
  - ignition
  - oxygen.

Identify people at risk

- Employers need to consider all persons who may be affected in the event of a fire on their premises, including staff, visitors, and the public
- Particular consideration needs to be given to making adequate provision for those at special risk:
  - disabled people
  - elderly people
  - children or parents with babies
  - lone workers.

Evaluate, reduce, and remove risks

The employer must provide adequate fire prevention measures and maintain them.

Record, plan, inform, instruct, and train

- The main findings of the risk assessment, including those regarding people at special risk, must be recorded in writing
- Employers must prepare an emergency fire plan
- Staff must be provided with sufficient information, instruction, and training on fire prevention and the actions necessary in the event of a fire. This may include measures such as training in the use of fire extinguishers, fire safety briefings, and regular fire drills to rehearse fire evacuation procedures.

Review

Any significant changes, e.g. to premises or work practices, requires review of the fire plan.

Legislation and guidance

- National Archives. Available at: ℘ http://webarchive.nationalarchives. gov.uk/+/http://www.communities.gov.uk/pub/394/Fireguidesseries_ id1500394.pdf
- Scottish Government. Available at: ℘ http://www.infoscotland.com/ firelaw

Electrical safety

Epidemiology

According to HSE figures approximately 25 people die from electric shock or electrical burns at work each year.

General principles

- Electrical equipment should be suitable for the environment in which it is used
- In environments that are damp or wet, electrical equipment should be suitably insulated to prevent electrocution
- Where electrical equipment is to be used in areas where there is a potential for explosion, suitable equipment should be employed
- Only competent persons should be allowed to work on electrical equipment or installations
- The normal policy should be that work is only undertaken on equipment or installations known to be dead and electrically isolated
- Live system/equipment working should be the exception rather than the rule. It should only be carried out where it is unreasonable for work to be done on dead systems/equipment and where a suitable risk assessment has been carried out by a competent person
- Any equipment provided, e.g. voltage meters, should be suitable for use and adequately maintained
- Before commencing work on electrically isolated equipment it should be confirmed, through the use of a suitable test procedure by a competent person, that the equipment is dead
- Wherever possible, equipment should be disconnected (and protected against accidental reconnection) from electrical power before any work is attempted
- Any equipment to be worked on should be isolated and secured by 'locking out' using an inter-lock. In addition, a notice should be posted at the point of disconnection so that all personnel are aware that electrical work is being undertaken on the dead system
- As a final precaution, any high-voltage equipment should be earthed so that, in the event of equipment failure, the operator will be protected
- Where work has to be carried on any high-voltage electrical equipment/installations a permit to work system will be required.

Legislation and guidance

HSE (2004). *Electricity at work: safe working practices*, HSG 85. HSE Books, Sudbury. Available at: http://www.hse.gov.uk/electricity/precautions.htm

Road safety

Epidemiology

The independent Work-Related Road Safety Task Group estimated that;
- One-third of all road accidents involve someone at work
- ~1000 people die in work-related road crashes in the UK each year
- 250 people are seriously injured each week in work-related road crashes.

General principles

- All road users must comply with road traffic legislation
- The Health and Safety at Work, etc. Act 1974 places duties on employers to manage occupational risks to prevent harm to workers and the public and this includes road safety. The organization's health and safety policy should address road safety—a specific road safety policy may be required
- Commuting to and from a worker's home is not covered by the Health and Safety at Work, etc., Act 1974
- Employers should undertake a risk assessment of their work-related road safety, consult with employees and their representatives and act on their findings
- Interventions should initially focus on high risk drivers based on:
  - annual business mileage
  - accident records
  - young drivers
- Employers should consider induction training on road safety for new employees

The need for road travel should be reviewed and either safer transport methods such as rail be substituted or teleconferences be used instead.

Vehicles

- Vehicles should be fit for purpose
- Well maintained
- Safety and ergonomic features should be considered when purchasing new vehicles
- Tachographs, where fitted, should be regularly inspected to confirm drivers are complying with legislation, e.g. speed limits
- Privately owned vehicles must be insured for business use and if over 3yrs old, have a valid MOT.

Drivers

- Drivers should be competent
- Medically fit to drive that category of vehicle
- Licenses should be inspected at employment and regularly reviewed thereafter
- *Drivers should be:*
  - trained in the safe operation of their vehicle, e.g. pre-journey checks of warning lights, tyre pressures
  - trained in adjusting seating and head restraints

- trained in securing loads and ensuring their correct distribution in the vehicle
- aware of their vehicle height, width and weight (laden and unladen)
- trained to respond to a vehicle breakdown safely.

Journeys

- The journey plan should take an appropriate route (e.g. large vehicles should avoid low bridges, narrow roads)
- Where possible avoid rush hours
- Should take account of prevailing weather and road conditions
- Work patterns and delivery timetables should be realistic to avoid placing inappropriate demands on drivers, which might lead them to speed
- Driving rosters should take account of total hours worked and not just hours at the wheel to reduce driver fatigue
- Long journeys should be broken by an overnight stop.

Legislation and guidance

- HSE *Driving at work: managing work-related road safety*, HSE INDG 382. Available at: ᐩ http://www.hse.gov.uk/pubns/indg382.pdf
- HSE Report of the Work-related Road Safety Task Group. Available at: ᐩ http://www.hse.gov.uk/roadsafety/report.htm

Clinical tasks and procedures

Recording an occupational health consultation

Every new consultation should start with an explanation to the patient/employee of the role of occupational health and the rules of communication (see 📖 p. 360, Ethical principles in clinical occupational health practice, 📖 p. 362, Confidentiality, consent, and communication, 📖 p. 444, General principles of fitness for work assessments).

Checklist for clinical consultations

Handwritten notes

- Notes should be written clearly (preferably in black ink) or dictated and typed
- *Every* sheet should be labelled with the patient/client's name, and at least one other identifier (e.g. DOB or address) or preferably a unique serial number
- *Essential details of referral:*
  - by whom? (self, manager, other)
  - reason (short-term absence, long-term absence, performance issues, other)
  - job title, employer, duration of employment
  - membership of pension scheme if applicable
- Clinical history with a focus on current symptoms and function: ask about day-to-day activities in sufficient detail to judge whether the Equality Act applies.

  ⚠ Ask routinely about alcohol and recreational drug intake. Alcohol is often used as a maladaptive coping strategy by those with anxiety or depression.
- Previous medical history and sickness absence history
- Details of the current job including information about tasks, or preferably a job description: remember to consider psychosocial (demand, control, support, job satisfaction) as well as physical aspects of the job
- *Occupational history including duration of previous similar jobs or exposures:* episodes of job change or loss because of health problems; any applications for compensation or Industrial Injuries Benefit. Be alert for relevant co-exposures
- *Clinical examination:* relevant physical examination, and mental state examination where appropriate
- *Summary and conclusions:* it is useful to include a brief formulation or justification of conclusions, especially where there is likely to be dispute
- *Output:*
  - list in hand written record all outputs from the consultation including telephone calls, other conversations, written reports, or letters

- always record a brief summary of the content of verbal outputs
- See 🕮 p. 406, Long-term sickness absence, 🕮 p. 444, General principles of fitness for work assessments, for the content of outputs to the referring manager
- Print your name and job title
- Sign and date every record
- Record that the employee has been informed about their rights of access to the report from the consultation, whether they wish to have a copy of the report, and (if so) if they wish to see the report before it is released.

File copies of the following documents

- *Informed consent for referral:* this is sometimes included on a referral *pro forma.* Where consent has not been gained prior to referral, it is good practice to obtain it at the beginning of the consultation. This is particularly important if the OH physician is concerned that the employee is unhappy or poorly informed about the referral. An example of an information sheet for referred clients is given in 🕮 p. 839, Appendix 2: Consent for an occupational health assessment
- Written referral from employer
- *Supporting material where appropriate:* e.g. job description, musculoskeletal or mental health symptoms questionnaires if used in the clinical assessment, relevant test results (e.g. lung function)
- Reply to manager
- Letters to GP or specialist consultant where applicable
- Written consent for reports (see 🕮 p. 580, Access to Medical Reports Act 1988).

Workplace visits

- Workplace visits should be carried out where indicated by the initial clinical assessment. Functional assessment in the workplace can be very useful in offering practical advice about adjustments to work
- File handwritten notes of the visit (including interview with manager or co-workers) and typed report
- File any supporting material, e.g. COSHH or other risk assessments, occupational hygiene data.

Assessing mental health: tools

Things to ask yourself before using assessment tools

- Why am I using a tool?
- Am I clear about the distinction between a screening tool and a diagnostic tool?
- Do I refer a patient just because of their score?
- What will I do if my clinical impression differs from the score on the tool?

Advantages of using assessment tools

- *As an aide memoire:* ensure all important questions asked
- To provide an 'objective' measure of severity
- To generate a score to assist communication with other health professionals
- To measure response over time, e.g. following treatment
- Can be completed by the patient at home or in waiting room

Disadvantages of using assessment tools

- *Crude measures:* patients can score highly without being especially 'ill'
- *Falsely reassuring:* distinction between screening and diagnosis
- Don't take into account your own clinical impression of the patient
- Have the potential to lead to unnecessary referrals
- Only examine symptoms in one (occasionally two) domains, e.g. most depression tools ignore anxiety and vice versa
- Tools assess symptoms rather than function
- Many tools are under copyright

Checks and calibration

Depression and anxiety assessment tools have not been validated in the occupational health setting. *Ad hoc* use is to be discouraged. Many psychiatrists do not use rating scales at all. There is a recognition, for example in medico-legal circles, that a number of factors, including occasionally frank exaggeration, can contribute to the score on a questionnaire.

The choice of rating scale needs consideration; the choice will vary depending on why a scale is thought necessary. The use of assessment tools may be best considered as part of a wider strategy for identifying and managing depression in the workplace. Training might be needed. Policies for how to respond to high scores or unexpected scores should be established before they occur.

Examples of assessment questionnaires

- *Patient Health Questionnaire (PHQ9):* commonly used in 1° care in the UK so may assist communication with GP. Is free and accessible online. Limited range of questions and possibility of over-scoring—false positive. No anxiety questions
- *Beck Depression Inventory (BDI-II):* lengthier more detailed questionnaire, but takes longer to complete. Includes questions about somatic symptoms. No anxiety questions. Copyright
- *Hospital Anxiety and Depression Scale (HADS):* specifically designed for use in hospital settings where patients have several possible causes for somatic symptoms such as fatigue—*is this your patient population?* Includes anxiety symptoms which can be scored separately. Utility of cut-offs (8 and 10) not clear. Copyright.

Further information

Mitchell AJ, Coyne JC (eds) (2010). *Screening for depression in clinical practice: an evidence-based guide.* Oxford University Press, New York.

Psychological therapies

Overview

Psychological interventions are best viewed in the same way as pharmacological or physical interventions. There are many to choose from:
- An evidence-based approach, where available, is recommended
- Benefits and adverse effects need to be carefully weighed
- Specific interventions are effective for specific disorders
- Cost is likely to be part of any treatment decision.

▶ One difference to consider is that the effectiveness of many psychological therapies depends in part on the relationship between the patient and the therapist.

Counselling

Pros
- Readily available
- Can be relatively inexpensive
- High reported levels of patient satisfaction

Cons

Little good evidence to suggest effective in treatment of psychiatric disorder (compared to lower levels of distress or upset).

Further information

BACP. Available at: ℜ www.bacp.co.uk

Henderson M, Hotopf M, Wessely S (2003). Workplace counselling *Occup Environment Med*, **60**, 899–90.

McLeod J (2010). The effectiveness of workplace counselling: a systematic review. *Counsel Psychother Res*, **10**, 238–48.

Cognitive behavioural therapy

Pros
- Excellent evidence base
- Effective for a wide range of common mental disorders including depression, phobias, post-traumatic stress disorder
- Also effective for chronic fatigue syndrome and irritable bowel syndrome
- Provides patients with 'tools' they can use should difficulties recur
- Can be delivered effectively online (e.g. beating the blues).

Cons
- Is hard work! Patients need to do homework and keep detailed diaries
- Trained therapists in short supply
- Can be expensive
- Patients require a minimum of 6–8 sessions; some need many more.

Further information

Royal College of Physicians (2012). *Cognitive behavioural therapy*. Available at: ℜ http://www.rcpsych.ac.uk/mentalhealthinfoforall/treatments/cbt.aspx

Beating the Blues (2006–2012). *Beat depression and anxiety*. Available at: ℜ http://www.beatingtheblues.co.uk

Gilbert P (2009). *Overcoming depression: a guide to recovery with a complete self-help programme.* Constable & Robinson, London.
LTTFF. *Living life to the full.* Available at: ⊗ http://www.llttf.com

Psychodynamic psychotherapy

Pros

- Can help with complex and longstanding difficulties
- Allows patients time to think *why* things might have happened as well as how they might make changes.

Cons

- *Is a major commitment:* sessions are at least weekly and continue for many months or longer
- Model not necessarily easily understood
- Many different forms (e.g. Freudian, Jungian, Lacanian, etc.) and not always clear which is indicated
- Can be expensive
- Relatively little evidence of benefit for diagnosable psychiatric disorders.

Further information

Royal College of Physicians. Psychotherapies. Available at: ⊗ http://www.rcpsych.ac.uk/mental-healthinfo/treatments/psychotherapies.aspx
Tavistock and Portman. Available at: ⊗ www.tavistockandportman.nhs.uk

Improving access to psychological therapies

- NHS programme to improve the delivery of treatment for common mental disorders according to NICE guidelines
- Since 2011 its remit has broadened to include support to patients of all ages, and patients with long-term physical conditions
- Widely though not yet universally available in England
- CBT and other talking therapies available in a range of different intensities
- Keeping patients in, or returning patients to, work is a priority and trial of employment advisors working alongside Improving access to psychological therapies (IAPT) therapists underway.

Further information

Improving access to Psychological Therapies (2012). *Relieving distress, transforming lives.* Available at: ⊗ www.iapt.nhs.uk

Chronic pain

Persistent pain in the absence of signs of tissue injury is now recognized as reflecting a dysfunctional sensory system. Changes occur at receptor level in both the peripheral and central nervous system. Although there is no specific predisposing personality type, pain is associated with catastrophizing (excess worry about a situation).

Classification of pain
- Somatic
- Visceral
- Neuropathic (nerve injury)
- Idiopathic.

Epidemiology of chronic pain
- In the UK, 7.8 million people have chronic pain; 50% have depression
- 50% of loss of quality of life is attributable to pain
- Low back pain is the commonest pain-related cause of work loss
- Of the top ten health problems impacting productivity, three specifically relate to pain (back/neck pain, other chronic pain, and arthritic pain).

Risk factors for disability and sickness absence
- High pain intensity
- High perceived disability
- Beliefs and fears about the harmful effect of work
- High physical job demands
- Inability to modify work
- High job stress
- Poor workplace social support or dysfunction
- Poor job satisfaction.

New Zealand Yellow Flags system Predicts absence risk:
- Have you had time off work in the past with pain?
- What do you understand is the cause of your pain?
- What are you expecting will help you?
- How is your employer responding to your pain? Your co-workers? Your family?
- What are you doing to cope?
- Do you think that you will return to work? When?

⚠ If the worker expects the pain to be a sign of harm or they are reliant on passive behaviours to manage pain, then they are at risk of long term absence from work.

The Keele STarT Back Tool identifies those at risk of chronic disability.

Pain management
Based on three key principles—reassurance it is safe to move, rehabilitation to support movement and relief of pain. General approach includes:

- Referral to local exercise initiatives and simple analgesia
- Paracetamol for mild to moderate pain
- Anti-inflammatories for inflammatory pain (⚠ but side effects)
- Amitriptyline, and other tricyclics or anticonvulsants (gabapentin or pregabalin) as first line medication for neuropathic pain
- Referral to specialist pathways and services for those who fail to improve or have complex pain issues
- CBT approach if significant psychosocial factors are present
- Unless specific serious medical pathology is suspected (red flags), diagnostic tests such as x-ray or MRI scans are not appropriate
- Facilitate modifications to work, including limits to the duration of concentrating on a task or a reduction in physical demands
- The Pain Toolkit describes 12 steps to managing pain.

▶ The prognosis for return to work falls dramatically after 12 weeks, so the focus should be on early, rapidly phased, goal-based, rehabilitation.

The pain toolkit
- *0–2 weeks:* provide support and reassurance to stay active
- *2–6 weeks:* develop a specific plan which identifies obstacles and provides a structure to return to work, including modifications
- *6–12 weeks shift up a gear:* provide vocational rehabilitation and cease ineffective healthcare interventions
- *12+ weeks:* establish communication between all players, avoid unnecessary medical interventions and ensure social solutions in place.

Difficult cases

These should be managed by a multidisciplinary pain service.
- *Pain medications:*
  - Opioids ⚠ There is little evidence for the efficacy of strong opioids in many pain conditions. Long acting preparations are recommended and avoidance of variable effect medications, such as pethidine
- Radiofrequency denervation can be cost effective in highly selected cases
- Management of depression including CBT and other cognitive approaches, including meditation techniques
- If struggling at work, explore reduction in hours, retraining/ redeployment or (as a last resort) ill health retirement.

Further guidance

NICE. *Management of long-term sickness and incapacity for work*, PH19. Available at: ℘ http://www.nice.org.uk/PH19

NICE. *Low back pain: early management of persistent non-specific low back pain*, CG88. Available at: ℘ http://publications.nice.org.uk/low-back-pain-cg88

Keele University. *Keele STarT Back Tool*. Available at: ℘ http://www.keele.ac.uk/sbst/

Night worker health assessment

Under the European Working Time Directive employers must offer a health assessment to night workers (📖 p. 574, Working Time Regulations 1998).

Process

A night worker's assessment is a two-stage process, consisting of:
- A screening questionnaire (see Fig. 37.1)
- A medical examination for those in whom the screening questionnaire identifies a medical problem that might be caused or made worse by night work, and which needs further detailed assessment.

Role of occupational health

This will depend upon the arrangements for access to OH services:
- Where there is an in-house OH department, both screening questionnaires and subsequent examinations will usually be carried out by the OH team
- However, in organizations which have contracted or ad hoc access to OH advice, the screening questionnaire is often administered by the HR department or a manager. This is permissible under the Working Time Regulations, provided that the advice of an appropriate health professional is sought when designing the questionnaire
- Medical examinations (where appropriate) must be carried out by a suitably medically qualified person.

Communication of results

- The rules that apply to all OH reports are relevant for communicating the outcome of night worker health assessments. Medical or confidential information should not normally be disclosed (and if so, only with the individual's consent). Conclusions should be confined to practical advice about fitness for night work and any adjustments required, including transfer to day work
- Where there is no OH department (and the screening questionnaires are handled by HR officers or others), the screening questionnaire should be designed to protect confidentiality. One method is to ask workers to tick a single box (following a checklist of health problems that are relevant for night work) to declare the *existence* of a health problem, but not to disclose its *nature*. This approach is supported by the Department of Trade and Industry.

PERSONAL DETAILS

Surname: --

Forename(s):   -------- -----------------------

Date of birth: --

Gender: delete: M/F
Job title: -------------------------------

Manager: --

Contact address (internal or home address):

------------------------------ -------------------------------
----

HEALTH DECLARATION

Please tick this box if you have any of the following health disorders:

[   ]

- Diabetes
- Heart or circulatory disorders
- Depression/anxiety
- Stomach or intestinal disorders
- Chronic chest conditions
- Any condition that causes difficulty with sleeping
- Any medical condition for which you are taking medicines
  according to a strict timetable

NEXT STEPS

If you have declared a health problem, you may be referred to a
doctor or nurse for further assessment. This will be done in
confidence, and no medical details will be passed to your employer
without your consent. The medical adviser will make a simple
declaration of your fitness for night work, and the need for any
adjustment to working hours on health grounds.

SIGNATURE :------------------------------------ DATE :--------------------

Fig 37.1 Example of night worker health assessment questionnaire.

Methods for alcohol and drug screening

Managers are responsible for the health, safety, and welfare of those working under their supervision. This responsibility includes ensuring employee fitness for work.

Managers must be alert to intoxication from alcohol or drug misuse. This can be established by simple observations and assessment of cognition, speech, posture, and movements without recourse to screening tests.

Screening tests

▶ Testing for drugs and alcohol should not be undertaken lightly, and must be part of a substance abuse policy (see 📖 p. 378, Substance abuse policies).

- There are many different forms of screening tests for alcohol and drugs of misuse that may be conducted (see Table 37.1);
  - directly at the 'point of contact'
  - indirectly using specialist laboratory services
- Alcohol may be measured by breath, saliva or urine testing
- Drug testing may use blood, saliva, hair or urine with differing considerations as shown in Table 37.1.

⚠ All test subjects must be invited to pre-declare any prescribed or over-the-counter medicines and any special foods or supplements that they have taken, to enable accurate test interpretation.

Table 37.1 Summary of screening methods

	Breath	Saliva	Urine	Blood	Hair
Advantages					
Easy to collect	+	+	+		+
Observable test	+	+		+	+
Minimal training	+	+	+		
Equipment readily available	+	+	+	+	+
Low cost	+	+	+		
Long-term detection					+
Disadvantages					
Difficult to collect				+	
Potential for deliberate interference by subject			+		
Limited application (substances that can be tested)	+	+			+

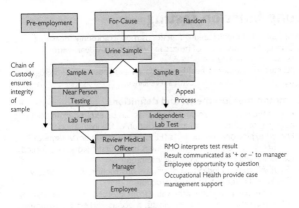

Fig. 37.2 Alcohol and drug screening process.

Chain of custody

- This is the process for managing the collection, handling, storage, and testing of biological samples to prevent any possible contamination or interference (see Fig. 37.2)
- Normally, the sample is divided at collection into samples A and B and sealed, with a tamper evident seal, in the presence of the test subject. In the event of a positive sample A test result, the test subject has the opportunity to arrange an independent test of sample B.

Who should be tested?

- The selection of test subjects must be clearly defined in the policy and selection procedures should avoid any possible discrimination
- *Possible options may include:*
  - announced or unannounced testing of all employees
  - only those in defined safety critical roles
  - those involved in accidents ('for cause').

Positive test results

- Alcohol testing often uses the Road Traffic Act standards to define fitness for work
- Drug testing reports only the presence of an illicit drug as a marker for drug-taking behaviour
- The Review Medical Officer (RMO) will interpret and report test results, but managers are responsible for deciding possible employment implications.

Further information

Faculty of Occupational Medicine (2006). *Guidance on Alcohol and Drug Misuse in the Workplace.* FOM, London.

Lung function testing

In occupational medicine lung function is most commonly measured:
- During the assessment of fitness for work in individuals with respiratory disorders
- As part of respiratory health surveillance and subsequent investigation (📖 p. 428, Respiratory health surveillance).

Common measurements and definitions
- FVC is the maximum volume of gas that can be expired from the lungs during a forced expiration from a position of full inspiration
- Forced expiratory volume in 1s (FEV_1) is the maximum volume of gas that can be expired from the lungs in the first second of a forced expiration from a position of full inspiration
- FEV_1/FVC gives an indication of airways obstruction. A ratio below 70–75% indicates significant obstruction
- PEF is the maximum flow achievable from a forced expiration starting at full inspiration with an open glottis. It occurs early in the expiratory manoeuvre when the lungs are expanded and the airway diameter is large
- Simple self-paced tests of walking distance (e.g. the 6-min walk test) can be used in the objective assessment of functional disability. However, such tests depend on motivation. In the shuttle walk test the subject increases his/her walking speed each minute. This test is more reproducible than simple paced walk tests. The gold standard test uses a bicycle ergometer to measure VO_2 max and other physiological parameters. However, this requires standardized testing in a laboratory and is not usually practicable for routine clinical OH work.

Nomograms
FEV_1, FVC, and PEF vary with height, age, and sex, and with ambient temperature and pressure. Conversely, FEV_1/FVC is useful because it is self-normalizing (unaffected by height, age, and sex). Individual recordings of lung volumes should be compared with nomograms (reference graphs of the normal readings in healthy adults for a given age, height, and sex). This can be done manually using standard graphs (given in Appendix 6: Lung volumes). However, most modern automated spirometers provide a print-out that includes a comparison with normal 'expected' values.

Quality control in lung function testing
It is important that measurements are reproducible. This is particularly important for health surveillance, where serial measurements are used to identify temporal changes in function. Therefore, lung function testing should be governed by a written protocol. The British Thoracic Society recommends the following.
- *Standard training and procedures for staff who carry out testing:*
  - record patient's height, weight, age
  - record medication including timing of latest dose of bronchodilators

- record temperature and barometric pressure for BTPS standard[1] corrections
- patient should be seated for 5–10min prior to testing, and sit upright in a chair for the test
- standard set of instructions for the patient, including standardized encouragement for maximum inspiration and to maintain effort throughout expiration
- Spirometers and peak flow meters must be maintained according to the manufacturer's instructions
- Spirometers must be calibrated regularly according to the manufacturer's instructions[2]
- Quality check on the flow volume print-out and guidelines for rejection, and repeat if unsatisfactory
- Record the greatest FEV_1, FVC, and PEF from at least three technically acceptable manoeuvres. The variability between readings should be ≤5%.

Rejection criteria for lung function measurements

- Leak at the mouthpiece
- Poorly co-ordinated start to the manoeuvre
- Cough during the manoeuvre
- Early termination of the expiration
- Submaximal effort

Further information and guidance

British Thoracic Society and the Association of Respiratory Technicians and Physiologists (1994). *Guidelines for the measurement of respiratory function*, Recommendations of the British Thoracic Society and the Association of Respiratory Technicians and Physiologists. *Resp Med*, **38**, 165–94.

American Thoracic Society (2002). Guidelines for the six-minute walk test. *Am. J Resp Crit Care Med*, **166**, 111–17. Available at: http://ajrccm.atsjournals.org/cgi/content/full/166/1/111

---

1 Body temperature and pressure standard.

2 Since 2004, new peak flow meters have a corrected scale (EU scale). Old mini-Wright peak flow readings must be converted using a standard scale.

Serial peak flow testing

Method of choice for suspected cases of occupational asthma.

Protocol

Initial training

It is important that readings are as reproducible as possible. Therefore, the patient should first be instructed in basic PEF technique. This should be taught by an OH professional, or a technician who has been trained in standard procedures. The patient should be observed, and corrected on poor technique. Readings taken at the same time should be within 5% before the technique is deemed satisfactory.

Recording regime

- The best of three PEF readings should be recorded every 2h during waking time. Measurements should be continued at home and at work
- Reading should continue for a period of at least 4wks: including at least a 1-wk period away from work
- A standardized sheet should be used by the patient to record the timing of:
  - symptoms
  - medication, in particular bronchodilators
  - significant exposures, e.g. work activity (noting that co-exposure to more than one allergen can occur), leisure time exposure to smoky rooms, cold air, exercise
- Patients should be instructed not to enter missing or very late readings, but to leave blanks in the event that readings are inconvenient or inadvertently forgotten.

Tampering Although rare in practice, it is theoretically possible for patients to tamper with or fabricate serial peak flow readings. Moreover, non-compliance is not uncommon. It is more difficult to tamper and to disguise non-compliance if digital data-logging peak flow meters are used.

Recording and interpreting results

- Serial PEF charts are usually plotted graphically to show the minimum, maximum, and mean peak flow readings each day. Treatments and exposures, and presence at work or home can be noted on the graph (see Fig. 37.3)
- Research evidence suggests that the consistency of diagnostic interpretation of serial PEF records by physicians using basic visual examination of graphical plots is poor; so physicians have tried to standardize interpretation using criterion-based computer software. Various computer programmes are used by specialist centres. Some are freely available for use by OH practitioners, including the OASYS software. OASYS uses a scoring system to assess serial PEF records, and preset cut-off scores to determine occupational asthma cases (94% specificity and 75% sensitivity).

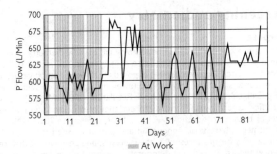

Fig. 37.3 Example of a serial peak flow record from a trout processing worker showing occupational asthma. (Reproduced by kind permission of Dr Keith Palmer.)

- The diagnostic features of occupational asthma on a serial PEF record are:
  - variable airflow obstruction, with >20% variation in PEF values
  - consistent falls in peak flow on work days compared with non-work days.

Further information and guidance

OASYS. Oasys and occupational asthma. Available at: ℘ http://www.occupationalasthma.com/default.aspx

Screening audiometry

Purpose

Hearing conservation programmes employ industrial audiometry to confirm the effectiveness of existing noise control measures. Health surveillance is required for all employees exposed at the upper action value and those workers at ↑ risk between the lower and upper action values (see 📖 p. 548, Control of Noise at Work Regulations 2005). Most OH services offer screening, rather than diagnostic audiometry. The latter involves tests of both air conduction (AC) and bone conduction (BC), whereas the former only tests air conduction and cannot be used for diagnosis. By measuring hearing thresholds (the faintest sound perceived at that frequency) the aim is to detect deterioration before the individual is aware of any deficit.

▶ The test–retest reliability of industrial audiometry is limited. There are many causes of hearing loss other than noise-induced hearing loss (NIHL) (see 📖 p. 302, Noise-induced hearing loss). Do not assume that hearing loss in a noise-exposed worker is necessarily NIHL (see 📖 p. 430, Classification of hearing loss, and 📖 p. 432, Patterns of hearing loss).

How to perform screening audiometry

Tools required

- *Pure tone audiometer:* a number of audiometers are available for industrial audiometry including the Bekesy self-recording audiometer and computer-based automatic systems. Frequencies tested are 500Hz and 1, 2, 3, 4, 6, and 8kHz, and intensity of tone ranges from 0 to 120dB HL
- Matched earphones with insulating ear muffs.

▶ Ideally audiometry tests are carried out in a soundproof booth or room to ↓ ambient noise. Background noise should not exceed that stated in EN 26189.

Screening questionnaire

- The employee should complete a short questionnaire to record:
  - occupational and hobby noise exposure (e.g. music, shooting, motor sport) and use of hearing protection
  - risk factors for hearing loss (use of ototoxic drugs, head injury, meningitis, ear disease, ear surgery, family history of deafness)
  - symptoms, such as dizziness, tinnitus, ear discharge, or communication difficulties due to hearing impairment.

Clinical examination

- The external ears should be examined for evidence of previous surgery, followed by otoscopy looking for impacted cerumen and to inspect the tympanic membrane
- Record evidence of otitis externa, tympanic perforations, etc.
- Tuning fork testing (Rinne and Weber tests) may assist in the interpretation of any hearing loss identified on a pure-tone screening audiogram (See 📖 p. 302, Noise-induced hearing loss).

Exposure enquiry

▶ Employees should not be noise exposed in the 16h prior to test to reduce the risk of temporary threshold shift (TTS). Alternatively, wear PPE if noise exposed prior to testing.

• Record noise exposure in the 16h before testing
• Where there is doubt as to the presence of TTS, repeat audiometry at a later date when not noise exposed.

Procedure

Detailed information on audiometry methods is available in EN 26189.

• Explain the procedure to the employee and give clear instructions: 'We are going to test your hearing. You will hear a series of tones of varying loudness and pitch. Each time you hear a tone, please press the button once and once only. Please listen carefully'
• The tester should check to confirm that the employee has understood
• The employee should don the earphones and the tester should check that the earphones are well fitted
• Once test commences, observe the employee's performance to confirm that he/she is correctly responding to the screening audiometry
• Problems may arise where people are not motivated (poor attention) or have not grasped what is required of them
• If audiogram is at odds with speech communication, repeat the test
• Once the test is complete it should be reviewed with the employee.

Checks and calibrations

• Test ambient noise level with a noise meter to confirm that background noise is within recommended limits
• A three-stage approach to calibration is advised:
  • *Stage A*—daily inspection (e.g. loose/damaged headphone wires); self-test audiogram identifies gross changes in performance.
  • *Stage B*—3-monthly on-site objective test of calibration
  • *Stage C*—annual workshop calibration check/recalibration if required. If daily/quarterly checks raise doubts, recalibration is indicated.

Retention of audiometry records

Records of health surveillance should be retained for as long as the employee remains in employment. As claims for NIHL may arise many years after employment ends, it is prudent to retain records for longer.

Relevant standards and guidance

• *EN 26189*: 1991 Specification for pure tone air conduction threshold audiometry for hearing conservation purposes
• *BS EN 60645–1*: 2001 Audiometers. Pure-tone audiometers
• HSE (2005). *Controlling noise at work. The Control of Noise at Work Regulations 2005*, L108. HSE Books, Sudbury.
• The British Society of Audiology. Available at: ℜ http://www.thebsa. org.uk/

Colour vision testing

Pre-employment or pre-placement testing for colour vision deficits may be required in safety critical jobs (aviation, fire-fighting, railways) or in jobs requiring good colour matching (printing, textiles). One example of a safety critical job is seafaring, where deck crew must distinguish other ships' red and green navigation lights at night to avoid collisions.

Congenital red–green colour vision deficits occur in 8% of men and 0.4% of women, reflecting the X-linked inheritance of this condition. Although such people are often termed 'colour blind' this is a misnomer as most show altered colour recognition.

Procedure

The accuracy of colour vision testing is influenced by the test employed, the individual's visual acuity, and the adequacy of lighting. There are many colour vision tests, but few are widely used in occupational health practice.

▶ What matters is whether an employee's colour perception is adequate, in terms of safety and performance, for the proposed role. In recent years some industry bodies have reviewed colour vision demands in their industry and revised guidance on colour vision standards and testing for specific occupations; notably the UK's Maritime and Coastguard Agency for seafarers, the Civil Aviation Authority for flight crew and the Fire Services for firefighters. These revised standards should avoid unnecessarily excluding some individuals with colour vision deficits who are, in fact, fit for that work.

Ishihara test

- Ishihara plates were designed as a screening test for congenital red–green colour vision deficits. This test is the one most commonly employed in the occupational setting
- A number of different versions of this test exist, including the full 38 plate, an abbreviated 24 plate, and a concise 14 plate edition
- The 38 plate edition consists of an introductory plate, transformation plates (2–9), vanishing plates (10–17), hidden digit plates (18–21) and classification plates (22–25). The numbers on transformation plates are read as different numbers by those with colour vision deficits when compared with those with normal colour vision. Vanishing plate numbers are invisible to those with red–green deficits. Classification plates are used to classify those screening positive on plates 2–17. Birch recommends that the hidden digit plates are unhelpful and should be omitted
- The 24 plate edition has an introductory plate, transformation plates (2–8), and vanishing plates (9–13)
- The Ishihara test should be viewed at arm's length. Although the recommended lighting is a MacBeth easel lamp, this is now difficult to obtain. Daylight is a reasonable substitute
- Many with normal colour vision will misinterpret some plates, and these misinterpretations should be distinguished from true errors

- The individual should be asked to read and identify the number on each plate
- Undue delay (>4s) in identifying a number suggests a mild deficit. Three or more errors on plates 2–17 of the 38 plate edition or two errors on plates 2–13 of the abbreviated 24 plate test indicate red–green colour deficit.

City University test

- The City University test (3rd edn) is a two-part test. Part 1 is a sensitive screening test of four pages, with four lines of coloured dots arranged in columns of three. The individual is asked to identify differences in colour (where they exist) in each column. It may be used to identify tritan deficits based on specific errors made on the lower half of pages 2, 3, and 4
- Part 2 is a series of six plates, each of which has a central coloured dot and four coloured dots arranged around the central dot. The individual has to identify which of the four surrounding dots is the closest colour match to the central dot
- Part 2 will classify subjects as protan, deutan, tritan, or normal colour perception
- Those with mild deficits score normally or make few errors in Part 2.

Lantern tests

The Maritime and Coastguard Agency vision standards indicate that those deck officers and ratings failing the Ishihara test may undergo a lantern test. This must be done at one of the three MCA marine offices, using a Holmes Wright B lantern.

Relevant standards and guidance

HSE (1987). *Colour vision examination: a guide for occupational health providers*, MS7. HSE Books, Sudbury. Available at: ℘ http://www.hse.gov.uk/pubns/ms7.pdf

Further information

Birch J (2001). *Diagnosis of defective colour vision*, 2nd edn. Butterworth Heinemann, Oxford.

Clinical assessment of hand–arm vibration syndrome

Clinical grading

The vascular and neurological components of HAVS are graded according to 2 scales developed by a workshop in Stockholm (see Tables 37.2 and 37.3).

These scales are used internationally and by the HSE and UK Faculty of Occupational Medicine to frame advice on avoidance and career counselling. (Some assessors now combine these clinical features with the output from objective tests—see *HAVS clinical assessment and diagnosis*).

Table 37.2 Stockholm workshop scale for classifying VWF

Stage*	Grade	Description
0		No attacks
1	Mild	Occasional attacks affecting only the tips of one or more fingers
2	Moderate	Occasional attacks affecting distal and middle (rarely also proximal) phalanges of 1/more fingers
3	Severe	Frequent attacks affecting all phalanges of most fingers
4	Very severe	As in stage 3, with trophic skin changes in the finger tips

Table 37.3 Stockholm workshop scale for classifying sensorineural HAVS

Stage*	Symptoms
0SN	Exposed to vibration but no symptoms
1SN	Intermittent numbness, with or without tingling
2SN	Intermittent or persistent numbness, reduced sensory perception
3SN	Intermittent or persistent numbness, reduced tactile discrimination and/or manipulative dexterity

*The sensorineural stage is established separately for each hand.

Additionally, the vascular effects are sometimes allotted a score, based on the phalanges in which blanching symptoms are reported (see Fig. 37.4).

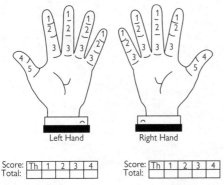

Fig. 37.4 Griffin blanching score.

Non-clinical tasks and procedures

Document a workplace inspection

Part A. Background information
- Name of factory
- Department(s) inspected
- Purpose of inspection
- Name and qualifications of inspector
- Date of inspection.

Part B. Inspection checklist
1. Plant, process, materials
- Site plan
- Processes and tasks conducted (routine and non-routine)
- Hazard types identified (including methodology). (*Hazard types:* physical, chemical, biological, psychosocial, ergonomic/mechanical)
- Materials handled (raw materials, products, by-products, waste products)
- Control measures available and their use, e.g. personal protective equipment, engineering controls, and administrative controls.

2. Personnel
- *Workforce:* number, job titles, gender
- Working hours, shift patterns
- Sickness absence, risk assessment, RIDDOR reports, health surveillance data.

3. Services and records
- Welfare facilities (canteen, changing rooms, showers, etc.)
- Occupational health staff and clinical facilities
- Occupational health services provided
- *Record:* types, safe keeping, and access.

Part C. Findings
- Activities conducted on site
- *Hazards:* type, location, number exposed and timing of exposure
- Significant hazards identified
- Ranking/prioritization of risks
- Agreed list of actions, responsibilities, and timescale.

Signature
Review data

Write an occupational hygiene report

Title page

Introduction

Information on processes assessed

Assessment methodology

Discussion

Assess an occupational hygiene report

OH professionals must be able to assess the quality and relevance of occupational hygiene reports, interpret them, and advise the employer on further action. This checklist summarizes the items that should be included in a good-quality (and fairly detailed) hygiene report.

Title page
- Name and address of client
- *Consultant:*
  - name (printed legibly)
  - qualifications
  - signature
- Date of issue
- Report reference number.

Introduction
- Background to the investigation
- Who requested the survey
- Purpose of survey
- Information provided by client
- Date on which the work was conducted
- Description of plant, layout, and main processes.
Shift patterns.

Information on processes assessed
- Types of processes and/or tasks assessed
- Equipment/tools/chemical substances used by workforce
- Patterns of work
- Control measure available and whether they are used
- Relevant health and safety legislation
- Occupational exposure limits
- Summary of potential health effects, e.g. acute and chronic.

Assessment methodology
- Techniques used to evaluate exposure; both sampling and analysis, and reference to standard validated methods, e.g. MDHS published by the HSE
- Limitations of the technique methods used (if appropriate)
- Sampling strategy, including selection of individuals for sampling and sampling periods
- Techniques used for evaluating control measures
- Instrument type used and their calibration.

Discussion
- Interpretation of results with reference to objectives and relevant legislation and exposure standards
- Explanation for the following:
  - variations in measured exposure levels
  - exposure patterns/trends
  - outliers

- Sources of error in data collection and uncertainties in estimating exposure levels.

Recommendations
- Key points for action, including reasons and implications of taking no action
- Prioritization of action including resources, expertise, and timescale
- Address any specific concerns expressed by the client and mentioned in the Introduction.

⚠ Remember that if you are not an occupational hygienist, you should only interpret hygiene data to the extent of your competence. Most OH professionals have general training in the principles of occupational hygiene. However, always ask for clarification or explanation of results from the occupational hygienist who produced the report if the conclusions are not clear and/or well justified.

Carry out an ergonomics assessment

A comprehensive ergonomics assessment covers the range of ergonomics hazards, including physical (posture, loading, repetition), psychosocial, and organizational factors.

Monitoring and analysis techniques

There are numerous methods for assessing ergonomics risks (Table 38.1). The simplest combinations for most basic assessments are a self-administered questionnaire to a population of exposed workers (or a sample thereof) plus direct observation of work tasks. Further information about specific aspects of risk assessment is given on 📖 p. 120, Lifting and handling; 📖 p. 124, Posture; 📖 p. 128, Repetitive work; 📖 p. 780, Carry out a display screen equipment assessment; 📖 p. 134, Organizational psychosocial factors; 📖 p. 308, Stress 1: recognition and assessment; 📖 p. 311, Stress 2: interventions/risk controls.

Ergonomics assessment tools

A number of generic ergonomics assessment tools are available for use in workplace and task assessment. As with most practical methods of risk assessment, there is a compromise between scientific validity and usability. The tools listed here have been developed by ergonomics experts and are widely used.

HSE tools

- Manual Handling Assessment Chart (MAC). Available at: ℘ http://www.hse.gov.uk/msd/mac/index.htm
- Are you making the best use of lifting and handling aids? Available at: ℘ http://www.hse.gov.uk/pubns/indg398.pdf
- *Pushing and pulling of loads*: assessment and example checklists. Available at: ℘ http://www.hse.gov.uk/msd/pushpull/ppchecklists.pdf; and ℘ http://www.hse.gov.uk/msd/pushpull/ppexample.pdf
- Tools linked to HSG (60) Upper limb disorders in the workplace. Available at: ℘ http://www.hse.gov.uk/msd/pdfs/riskfilter.pdf; and ℘ http://www.hse.gov.uk/msd/pdfs/worksheets.pdf

Other ergonomics assessment tools

- The Assessment of repetitive tasks (ART) tool. Available at: ℘ http://www.hse.gov.uk/msd/uld/art/index.htm
- The Rapid Upper Limb Assessment (RULA) tool:
  - *original reference*—McAtamney L, Corlett EN (1993). RULA: a survey method for the investigation of work-related upper limb disorders, *Appl Ergon*, **24**, 91–9.
  - *download form*—℘ http://ergo.human.cornell.edu/ahRULA.html

Table 38.1 Monitoring and analysis techniques

Method	Advantages	Disadvantages
Self-administered questionnaire or checklist about specific exposures or risk factors	Quick to complete and inexpensive	Subjective Confined to the items in the questionnaire; therefore ↓ scope for recognizing new or unexpected risks
Interviewer administered questionnaire or checklist	Opportunity for standardized explanation from interviewer	Subjective
Direct observation in the workplace, recording the exposures in real time. Computer technology can be used to facilitate recording	Objective	Intrusive Difficult to check that all risks have been captured, as there is no permanent record of the actual activity
Video recording in the workplace, with later indirect observation and recording of exposures	Objective Repeatable measurements from a permanent record of the actual activity	Intrusive Ethical issues around recording if sensitive subjects are inadvertently included on the video, e.g. when videoing a health care worker lifting and handling patients
Observing experimental reconstructions of tasks under laboratory conditions	Objective Allows closer measurements that might be too intrusive to be used in an actual workplace (e.g. attachment of a spinal motion monitor, or use of an inclinometer)	Always a 'proxy' for workplace exposures, so may not recreate the task or working environment accurately

Carry out a noise assessment

The noise assessment can be divided into three stages.

Background information

- Define purpose of the survey, e.g. collection of noise exposure data for compliance with the Control of Noise at Work Regulations 2005
- Gather background information:
  - plan of work/layout to be assessed
  - tasks performed and patterns of work
  - time spent on specific tasks and variability in exposure time
  - previous records of noise surveys/assessments
  - control measures available, e.g. ear muffs, noise refuge and control rooms, acoustic screens
  - any recent relevant health concerns/reported symptoms.

Preliminary site visit and static noise measurements

- Systematically identify all noise sources
- *Collect exposure information:* who is exposed, when, for how long, and how often
- Identify control measures used and their effectiveness
- Take measurements with a hand-held sound-level meter at workers' position(s) relative to a noise source
- Plot noise levels on a site map (noise mapping) showing position of machines and workers. This helps to understand the distribution of noise levels for the area being assessed
- Estimate the LAeq for the job/task levels from information on tasks performed by workers and exposure time
- The LAeq for each job/task is then combined with its duration during the working day to determine the $L_{EP,d}$. The calculation can be performed using the electronic spreadsheet available on the HSE website ℘ www.hse.gov.uk/noise

Detailed noise survey: personal dosemetry

- In certain situations the $L_{EP,d}$ and peak sound pressure level are best determined by personal dosemetry:
  - fluctuating noise exposure levels
  - high exposure variability
  - sources of impulse noise
- Where $L_{EP, d}$ is likely to exceed the noise exposure limits, carry out octave band analysis (noise frequency pattern) for tasks performed by the workers. These data will assist with the selection and design of control measures
- Identify steps needed to reduce noise exposure as far as reasonably practicable by examining in turn the noise source, the transmission of noise from the source, and the individual exposed
- Keep records of assessment (see Table 38.2) and review.

Table 38.2 Noise monitoring survey data form

a. Premises—name, address

b. Survey—conducted by, date of survey

c. Survey equipment—type, model, calibration, sound level meter settings e.g. weighting, response time

d. Workplace—layout, processes, noise sources

e. Individuals exposed—number, shift pattern, tasks conducted

f. Ear defenders—type available, actual use time, protection afforded by ear defender

Estimate of personal exposure levels

Tasks and location	Individual (name)	Noise level L_{Aeq}	Exposure duration	$L_{EP,d}$ dB(A)	Peak pressure (L_{Cpeak})
Octave band analysis—dB levels at different frequencies					
Frequency	63Hz	125Hz	500Hz	1KHz 2KHz	4KHz 8KHz
dB level					

▶dB values, e.g. for a noise source (machine) need to measure using an octave band analyser as part of the survey, and record on the form for each frequency.

Carry out a display screen equipment assessment

All organizations are likely to possess at least some equipment that falls under the terms of the Health and Safety (DSE) Regulations 1992 as amended (see 📖 p. 528, Health and Safety (DSE) Regulations 1992). These regulations require that every employer shall perform an assessment of workstations to assess and reduce risk for DSE users.

Procedure

- The assessor should be trained regarding the requirements of the DSE regulations and how to undertake a DSE assessment
- Use a checklist or on-line questionnaire to gather operator feedback
- Record the key findings for retention until the next DSE assessment.

▶ A home worker's workstation should be assessed even if the employer did not provide the workstation.

Elements to be considered in a DSE assessment

Equipment

- Workstation should be of sufficient size to permit adjustment of the equipment and should be non-reflective
- Chair should be height adjustable with an adjustable backrest that offers good lumbar support
- A footrest should be provided if the user so desires
- Display screen/monitor should give a clear image with adjustable contrast and brightness
- Keyboard should be adjustable, with sufficient space in front of the keyboard to support wrists/arms
- Keys should be legible and the keyboard layout should facilitate use
- Document holder should be provided where required
- Keyboard and mouse should be regularly cleaned as a build-up of dirt ↑ risk of work-related upper limb disorder
- Non-keyboard input devices (mouse/tracker ball, etc.) should be suitable for the task and the user.

Environment

- Adequate space
- Keep workstation tidy and free from clutter
- Adequate room/task lighting
- No direct glare or reflections on screen
- Adjustable window blinds
- Comfortable humidity levels
- Low noise levels from equipment
- Avoid trailing cables.

Equipment/user interface

- Software should be fit for purpose
- 'Help' functions should be provided
- User must be adequately trained in:
  - use of equipment/software
  - setting up the workstation correctly

- Poor user posture ↑ risk of musculoskeletal disorders (MSDs) (see 📖 p. 256, Work-related upper limb disorders 1; 📖 p. 258, Work-related upper limb disorders 2);
  - avoid slouching
  - avoid work at an angle
  - avoid very small fonts; use 'zoom' function
  - minimize keystrokes by use of 'macro' functions
  - regular breaks from keyboarding ↓ fatigue
  - keyboarding skills course ↓ risk of MSDs.

Frequency of review

The DSE assessment should be reviewed where:
- The workstation is moved
- The hardware or software is upgraded
- There is a substantial change to task demands
- The environment around the workstation is changed, e.g. new lighting
- There is a change to the user's capacity/abilities due to injury or ill health.

Relevant legislation and guidance

HSE (2003). *Work with Display Screen Equipment: Health and Safety (Display Screen Equipment) Regulations 1992 as amended by the Health and Safety (Miscellaneous Amendments) Regulations 2002. Guidance on Regulations.* L26, HSE Books, Sudbury.

Assess and interpret a research paper

In order to make the best use of research evidence, and avoid being misled by poor science, it is advisable to appraise published original research papers critically.

The majority of research papers in occupational medicine are observational studies.[1] A checklist for identifying common problems with cohort and case-control studies, divided by each main section of a paper, is given here. The list is intended for readers of single scientific papers following publication, rather than as a guide for peer reviewers at the stage when a manuscript can be revised, or for those who are compiling evidence tables for guideline development.

Introduction
- Is the existing state of knowledge adequately described?
- Is the study well justified?
- Is it relevant for your own practice?

Methods
Study sample
- Are the target population and the sample well defined?
- Is the sample sufficiently large?
  - ideally, a power calculation should be shown
  - wide confidence intervals are an important clue to inadequate sample size
- Are there any obvious sources of bias in the selection of subjects (e.g. volunteers, patients seen for medico-legal purposes)?

Selection of controls
Are the comparison groups appropriate?
- Controls in case-control studies should be selected from the same population as the cases (e.g. clinic attenders from the same hospital catchment area)
- Care should be taken that unexposed groups in cohort studies are not inadvertently exposed, e.g. through proximity to exposed workers.

Tools
Are the methods of case ascertainment standardized?
- Case definitions should be stated clearly. It is useful if definitions are used widely, as the results are more easily compared with previous literature
- Methods should be valid and repeatable. It is not always possible to validate subjective outcomes, e.g. pain or mental ill health, as there is no gold standard. However, questionnaires and other tools should at least have acceptable repeatability
- *Confounding:* have possible confounding factors been considered, and attempts made to measure them for inclusion (adjustment) in later analysis?

1 Randomized controlled trials (RCTs) are rare in occupational medicine research and are not covered here. Methods for assessing RCTs are available. Improving the quality of reporting of RCTs: The CONSORT statement. Available at: ◌ http://www.biomedcentral.com/1471–2288/1/2/

Exposure assessment

Consider the quality and accuracy of exposure assessment.

- Using job title as a proxy for exposure is common, but rather inaccurate
- Retrospective exposure assessment from hygiene records varies in quality
- Recalled exposure can be subject to bias if the subject has the disease of interest.

Statistical methods

Statistical techniques must be stated clearly (but not necessarily described in detail). Check that they are appropriate for the format of data presented.

Results

Response rates

Rates >55% are desirable. Lower response rates are acceptable, but the impact of response bias on the results should be discussed.

Presentation of results

- Look for an indication of the magnitude of effect or risk (odds ratio, relative risk, prevalence rate ratio). Consider whether an increased risk is likely to be important clinically
- Look for an estimate of statistical uncertainty (the likelihood that the results could have occurred by chance). Traditionally, *P*-values have been used to express statistical significance, but they do not give a feel for the size of an effect. Confidence intervals around a risk estimate give more information about the scale of a finding.

Discussion and conclusions

- Were limitations acknowledged and discussed? These must be borne in mind when making the link to practice
- Are the conclusions drawn appropriate?
- Are the results related to other evidence from the existing literature?
- If a study has added new knowledge, is this generalizable to your local population?
- Do the results suggest that a change in practice is indicated?

Writing a press release

Purpose

Press releases are issued to draw the attention of journalists to new information which may be of interest to their readership/audience. They may be directed at specialist publications (e.g. trade magazines) as well as the more general media (newspapers, radio, and television). They help to maximize publicity, and also give the instigator some control over its timing.

Sources of assistance

Occupational health professionals normally issue press releases with assistance from experts in media relations, who can advise on their format, and optimize their circulation to journalists. Depending on the circumstances, assistance may come from:

- *The editorial staff of a scientific journal:* many journals these days like to publicize their content beyond specialist readers, and have well-developed systems for promoting publicity
- *Academic institutions:* most major academic institutions have a press office
- *Conference organizers:* it is common practice to highlight selected presentations at medical and scientific conferences, which may be of wider interest
- *Media relations departments of employing companies:* many larger companies have such departments

Government press offices: relevant to occupational health professionals working for government departments, agencies, and advisory committees.

Advance preparation

In planning a press release, several questions should be considered.

- What is the main message?
- Who is the message for? This will influence both the content, and also the way in which the press release is circulated
- What will be the best timing? There may be little choice about this (e.g. because there is a need to coincide with publication of a paper or a presentation at a meeting). However, where there is flexibility, factors to consider include the timing of other events that are likely to compete for media attention (e.g. a royal wedding) and the availability of an appropriate person to answer any follow-up questions from journalists (which usually come over several days).

Format

In compiling a press release, it is important to bear in mind the way in which journalists work. Some may wish to interview the originators to get additional information, but others will prepare their piece simply from the content of the press release, perhaps supplemented by readily available information from the internet. Requirements include:

- An attention-grabbing headline
- A clear statement of the main message in understandable language

- A short amplification of the main message. It is often helpful to include attributable quotes that can be incorporated into articles
- Useful background information (e.g. brief details of the committee that has issued a report or the conference where paper will be presented)
- Useful references for further information (particularly to websites)
- Contact details for someone who can give further information.

Press conferences

Where it is anticipated that new information will be of special interest to the general media, it may help to accompany a press release with a press conference. Such conferences are best organized by media professionals. The important thing for participating health professionals is to ensure that they are well prepared to answer questions.

Conducting a media interview

Circumstances

The press may question occupational health professionals because they are named as a contact in a press release, or are participants at a press conference. In addition, a journalist pursuing a story may approach them without advance warning. Contacts may take various forms:

- Requests for non-attributable background information
- Interviews to be used in the preparation of written articles
- Live or recorded interviews on radio or television.

Preparation

As for a professional examination, when dealing with the media, it is important to be adequately prepared. In particular, it is essential to have a good understanding of the relevant facts. If you get things wrong, you lose credibility. Where media contact is expected (e.g. following a press release or because a newsworthy event has occurred), it is helpful to anticipate the questions that might be asked. And when an approach is received from a journalist, it is useful to establish at the outset the intended readership/audience, and the planned scope and format of the communication.

Talking to journalists from the written media

- Assume that anything you say is 'on record' and attributable, unless otherwise agreed (most journalists can be trusted to respect such agreements)
- If you do not know the answer to a question, an offer to find out may be appreciated (but be sensitive to the journalist's deadline)
- If you are unable to answer a question (e.g. because of confidentiality), try to explain why rather than simply decline to comment
- Most journalists are happy to let you check quotes that they wish to attribute to you (often they are paraphrases of what was actually said)
- Where deadlines allow, some journalists are happy to receive feedback on the draft text of their article (but remember that final responsibility for the content is theirs)
- Check that your name and affiliation are correctly noted
- Remember that once you are quoted in one article, follow-up enquiries may come from other journalists.

Broadcast interviews

- Pre-recorded interviews have the advantage that if you lose your thread you can start again. However, be mindful that your contribution may be edited and interspersed with other material. Consider whether you trust the producer to do this sympathetically
- Establish in advance the planned format of the programme, including its length, who will be the other participants, and in what capacity you are contributing (representing a group or giving your personal view)
- Think through your main message in advance, and try to ensure that you get it across as early as possible in the interview
- Use language appropriate to the audience and do not talk too fast
- Practical examples may help to illustrate theoretical points

- Avoid appearing defensive
- Avoid saying things that you might regret, even after completion of the interview (if in doubt, assume that the tape is still running)
- Ensure that your name and affiliation have been correctly noted
- Dress appropriately for television appearances, (wear plain, muted, colours)
- Maintain eye contact with the interviewer and avoid fidgeting.

Training

Various courses are available for health professionals on interactions with the media. They provide a good opportunity to develop and practise techniques, and are strongly recommended for those who expect frequent or difficult media contacts.

Emergencies in occupational health

Acute poisoning

General principles and contact details for specialist advice

All substances are poisons: there is none which is not a poison. The right dose differentiates a poison and a remedy.

Paracelsus (1493–1541)

Role of occupational health

- Be aware of the general principles of first aid. OH should lead in this
- In the workplace, adequate numbers of staff should be trained first aiders. This depends on the hazards identified on site (see 📖 p. 536, First Aid at Work Regulations 1981)
- It may be sensible to have staff trained in immediate life support (ILS)
- Know your workplace/work area
- Identify possible sources of chemical exposures/poisoning
- Identify remedial actions needed
- Liaise with nearest acute admitting hospitals for specific hazards, e.g. cyanide, hydrofluoric acid
- Formulate and document immediate first aid/treatment protocols with respect to ambulance call-out times and transfer times to acute hospitals.

Contact details for specialist advice

- Telephone advice from NPIS if needed:
  - *UK NPIS*—0870 600 6266
  - *Ireland NPIC*—(01) 809 2566

Register with TOXBASE® (the primary clinical toxicology database of the NPIS. Available at: 🖰 http://www.toxbase.org/)

Immediate management of poisoning in the workplace

- *Assess the situation:* risk assessment
- Is it safe to approach the casualties?
- ⚠ Remove the casualties from further exposure *if it is safe* to do so
- Contact the emergency services
- *Assess the route of exposure:*
  - inhalation
  - skin contamination/burns
  - eye contamination/burns
  - ingestion (unlikely in the occupational setting)
  - injection
- Assess the need for PPE
- Start decontamination if necessary
- Start first aid
- With known or suspected case of exposure/poisoning instigate *ABCs*:
  - airway
  - breathing
  - cardiac support.

Management of chemical exposures to the eye

⚠ Chemicals splashed or sprayed into the eyes are an emergency.

Features
- Pain, blepharospasm, lacrimation, conjunctivitis, palpebral oedema, and photophobia
- Acidic and alkaline solutions may cause corneal burns
- Alkaline solutions may penetrate all layers of the eye and cause:
  - iritis
  - anterior and posterior synechia
  - corneal opacification
  - cataracts
  - glaucoma
  - retinal atrophy.

⚠ Alkali burns to the eyes are an ophthalmic emergency.

Management of chemical exposures to the eye
- Remove contact lenses if necessary and immediately irrigate the affected eye thoroughly with water or 0.9% saline for at least 10–15min. Continue until the conjunctival sac pH is normal (7.5–8.0). Use pH-sensitive paper, retest after 20min, and re-irrigate if necessary
- Any particles lodged in the conjunctival recesses should be removed
- Repeated instillation of local anaesthetics (e.g. amethocaine) may reduce discomfort and help more thorough decontamination
- Corneal damage may be detected by instillation of fluorescein
- Mydriatic and cycloplegic agents (e.g. cyclopentolate, tropicamide) may reduce discomfort. Do not use in patients with glaucoma
- Patients with corneal damage, exposed to strong acids or alkalis and those whose symptoms do not resolve rapidly should be referred for ophthalmological assessment.

Carbon monoxide poisoning

Properties
- Colourless odourless gas
- Unlikely to be encountered in the occupational setting in isolation
- Product of incomplete combustion including diesel oils, petroleum products and domestic gas.
▶ Leaks of <u>domestic gas</u> do *not* involve CO.

Mechanism of toxicity
- CO combines with haemoglobin to ↓ oxygen-carrying capacity of the blood
- This causes the oxyhaemoglobin dissociation curve (see Fig. 24.1) to shift to the left, impairing tissue oxygen delivery
- CO may also inhibit cytochrome oxidase
- The short-term exposure limit is 200ppm (232mg/m³)
- The long-term exposure limit is 30ppm (35mg/m³).

Poisoning features
Immediate features
- Headache
- Nausea
- Irritability
- Weakness
- Tachypnoea.

Intermediate features
- Dizziness
- Ataxia
- Agitation
- Impairment of consciousness
- Respiratory failure.

▶ Cerebral oedema and metabolic acidosis may develop in serious cases. Less common features include skin blisters, rhabdomyolysis, acute renal failure, pulmonary oedema, myocardial infarction, retinal haemorrhages, cortical blindness, choreoathetosis, and mutism.

Late features
- The majority recover uneventfully.
- Rarely, neuropsychiatric features after periods of several weeks free of symptoms. More common in those >40 years age and includes memory impairment, disorientation, apathy, mutism, irritability, inability to concentrate, personality change, parkinsonism, and parietal lobe lesions. Urinary and/or faecal incontinence and gait disturbance are common. Fortunately, the great majority will recover completely or to a considerable extent within a year.

Indication of severity
- Severity increases with one or more of the following
- Any new objective acute neurological signs, e.g. ↑ tone, upgoing plantar reflexes

- Coma
- Need for ventilation
- ECG indication of infarction or ischaemia
- Clinically significant acidosis
- Initial carboxyhaemoglobin > 30%

▶ The link between carboxyhaemoglobin level and clinical outcome is weak.

Management of carbon monoxide poisoning

- Remove from exposure
- Maintain a clear airway and adequate ventilation
- Give oxygen in as high a concentration as possible
- Transfer to hospital if severely compromised
- Correct metabolic acidosis by increasing oxygen delivery to the tissues
- Give mannitol 1g/kg (as 20%) IV over 20min if cerebral oedema suspected
- Monitor the heart rhythm
- Measure the carboxyhaemoglobin concentration as an emergency. A carboxyhaemoglobin percentage of 30% indicates severe exposure. However, concentrations less than this do not exclude significant poisoning, and the relationship between carboxyhaemoglobin and severity of poisoning and/or clinical outcome is poor
- In patients who have been unconscious look for extrapyramidal features and retinal haemorrhages to assess the severity of CNS toxicity
- The role of hyperbaric oxygen therapy is controversial.

Further information

Heath Protection Agency (2009). *Diagnosing poisoning: carbon monoxide (CO)* (amended October 2010). Available at: ℛ http://www.hpa.org.uk/webc/HPAwebFile/HPAweb_C/1236845874045

Department of Health (2010). Carbon monoxide poisoning: needless deaths, unnecessary injury, Letter from the Chief Medical Officer/Chief Nursing Officer. Available at: ℛ http://www.dh.gov.uk/en/Publicationsandstatistics/Lettersandcirculars/Professionalletters/Chiefmedicalofficerletters/DH_121502

Cyanide 1: poisoning

Properties
- Naturally occurring toxin in a variety of forms
- Important examples are hydrogen cyanide (HCN) gas, salts, e.g. potassium and sodium cyanide (KCN, NaCN), and nitriles (R–CN), which are used widely as solvents and in the manufacture of plastics.

Sources of exposure
- *Industrial:* metal treatment and ore processing, printing, electroplating, photoengraving, electronics, production of acrylics, plastics, and nylon, petrochemical industry
- Fumigants and rodenticides
- Acrylic nail remover and metal polishes
- Fires: combustion of polyurethane, rubber, nylon, etc.
- Tobacco smoke
- Drugs, e.g. sodium nitroprusside
- *Natural sources:* cassava, some grasses, flax, lima beans, linseed.

Toxicity
- Highly toxic by inhalation, ingestion, or dermal or eye exposure
- Soluble cyanide salts (e.g. Na, K, Ca, NH_3) are more toxic than lower-solubility salts (mercury, gold, copper, and silver cyanide).

Onset of toxicity
- Toxicity can occur within a few seconds of HCN gas inhalation, with death occurring within minutes
- Ingestion of soluble cyanide salts can cause toxicity within minutes, but continued absorption can cause toxicity for several hours
- Toxicity from skin exposure requires a large surface area to be affected. Onset of toxicity may be delayed for several hours.

Estimated lethal doses
- Hydrocyanic acid, 50mg
- NaCN/KCN ingestion, 150–300mg (~3mg/kg)
- Median lethal dose for skin contamination, 100mg/kg.

UK short-term occupational exposure limits (15min)
HCN, 10 ppm (11mg/m³)

Cyanogen chloride 0.3 ppm (0.77mg/m³)

UK long-term occupational exposure limits (8-h TWA)
Cyanogen, 10ppm (22mg/m³)

Other cyanides, except HCN and cyanogen chloride 5mg/m³.

Clinical findings
- Rapid respiration
- Hypotension
- Convulsions
- Coma.

⚠ It can be difficult to diagnose cyanide poisoning.

Acute poisoning

Cyanide, cyanogen chloride, acetonitrile, and other cyanide releasing substances.

Ingestion or inhalation of large amounts

Cyanide concentration > 3mg/L (>114µmol/L)

- Immediate unconsciousness
- Convulsions
- Death within 1–15min.

Ingestion, inhalation, or skin absorption of moderate amounts

Cyanide concentration 1–3mg/L (38–114µmol/L)

- Dizziness
- Rapid respiration
- Vomiting
- Flushing
- Headache
- Drowsiness
- Hypotension
- Rapid pulse
- Unconsciousness
- Death in convulsions within 4h except sodium nitroprusside where death may be delayed for 12h.

Ingestion, inhalation, or skin absorption of small amounts

Cyanide concentration < 1mg/L (<38µmol/L)

- Nausea
- Dizziness
- Drowsiness
- Hyperventilation
- Anxiety.

Acute poisoning: acrylonitrile

Inhalation

- Nausea and vomiting
- Diarrhoea
- Weakness
- Headache
- Jaundice.

Note that skin contact can cause epidermal necrosis.

Cyanide 2: treatment

⚠ Rescuers should not put themselves at risk. Moisture on some cyanide salts can liberate HCN.

Immediate first aid

- Maintain clear airway and adequate ventilation
- Give 100% oxygen to all patients
- Monitor pulse, blood pressure, respiratory rate, oxygen saturation, and cardiac rhythm
- Transfer all definite cases to hospital as rapidly as possible
- Consider starting treatment on site if transfer to hospital is likely to be prolonged, and depending on severity of exposure.

Diagnosis

In the absence of a blood cyanide concentration the following features suggest cyanide poisoning:
- Lactate >7 mmol/L
- Elevated anion gap acidosis
- Reduced arteriovenous oxygen gradient.

Mild poisoning

- Observe asymptomatic and mildly symptomatic patients for at least 6 hours after ingestion of cyanide salt and at least 12h after ingestion of acetonitrile
- Give 50mL of 25% sodium thiosulphate (12.5g) IV over 10min.

Moderate and severe poisoning

- Patients with moderate or severe poisoning should be managed in a critical care environment
- Treatment with antidote therapy is necessary in all cases
- It is important that the admitting hospital is informed if any antidote therapy has been given in the pre-hospital setting since repeat doses of some antidotes can cause unwanted side effects
- ⚠ If treatment is started on site the doctor should accompany the casualties to the admitting hospital
- Give 20mL of 1.5% dicobalt edetate solution (300mg) IV over 1min followed immediately by 50mL of 50% dextrose. If there is only a partial response to dicobalt edetate 300mg or the patient relapses after recovery, a further dose of dicobalt edetate 300mg should be given. If a second dose of dicobalt edetate is administered, there is a danger of inducing cobalt toxicity, if the diagnosis is *not* cyanide poisoning
- In addition, the administration of 50mL of 25% sodium thiosulphate (12.5g) IV over 10min may be beneficial
- *Or*, if dicobalt edetate is not available, give 10mL of 3% sodium nitrite solution (300mg) IV over 5–20min *and* 50mL of 25% sodium thiosulphate (12.5g) IV over 10min

- A further dose of sodium thiosulphate 12.5g IV over 10min may be needed. A second dose of sodium nitrite should *not* be given because of the risk of excessive methaemoglobinaemia
- Response to treatment in the pre-hospital setting can be assessed by improved haemodynamic status
- Single brief convulsions do not require treatment. If frequent or prolonged, control with IV diazepam (10–20mg) or lorazepam (4mg)
- Correct hypotension by raising the legs of the patient and/or expanding the intravascular volume.

Hydrogen sulphide poisoning

Properties
- Colourless gas with characteristic 'rotten egg' smell
- CAS Number 7783–06–4
- UN 1053.

Synonyms
- Sulphuretted hydrogen
- Sulphur hydride
- Hydrosulphuric acid.

Toxicity
- Irritant gas with systemic asphyxiant effects
- Reversibly inhibits cytochrome oxidase, which impairs cell respiration
- Rapidly absorbed by inhalation
- Little absorption occurs through the skin
- Irritating to the eyes
- Occupational short-term exposure limit is 10ppm ($14mg/m^3$)
- Long-term exposure limit is 5ppm ($7mg/m^3$).

0.02–0.025ppm	Odour threshold
10ppm	Unpleasant smell, sore eyes
100ppm	Loss of smell after 3–15min, eyes, and throat sting
250ppm	Prolonged exposure—pulmonary oedema
1000ppm	Rapid collapse, respiratory paralysis, coma, and death within minutes

Features
Prolonged exposure causes:

• Respiratory tract irritation	• Bronchitis
• Rhinitis	• Dyspnoea
• Pharyngitis	• Pulmonary oedema

Systemic effects

• Vomiting	• Drowsiness
• Diarrhoea	• Tremor
• Headache	• Muscular weakness
• Nystagmus	• Seizures
• Dizziness	• Tachycardia
• Agitation	• Hypotension

Inhalation of high concentrations

Leads rapidly to:

• Collapse	• Coma
• Respiratory paralysis	• Cardiac arrhythmias
• Cyanosis	• Death within minutes
• Convulsions	

Eye effects

May be delayed and include:

• Irritation	• Photophobia
• Inflammation	• Conjunctivitis
• Lacrimation	• Keratitis
• Conjunctival hyperaemia	• Blepharospasm

Recovery is usually complete, but there may be permanent damage.

Skin effects
- Skin discoloration
- Pain, itching, erythema
- Local frostbite.

Management of H_2S poisoning
- Remove from exposure (rescuers must wear PPE)
- Oxygen in as high a concentration as possible, if necessary via an endotracheal tube
- Skin decontamination is usually not necessary because it is a gas. Removing patient's clothing and washing the skin with water and a mild detergent may reduce the risk of odour-related complaints in rescuers, but this is *not* a priority if dealing with a critically ill patient
- Maintain a clear airway and adequate ventilation
- Monitor pulse, blood pressure, and oxygen saturation
- If the patient has clinical features of bronchospasm treat conventionally with nebulized bronchodilators and steroids
- Transfer to hospital
- Correct hypotension with IV fluids
- Convulsions are unlikely to require treatment by the time the patient reaches medical care but IV diazepam 10–20mg could be given if necessary.

Organophosphate poisoning

See also 📖 p. 298.

Immediate management and decontamination

- ⚠ Avoid contaminating yourself: organophosphates are rapidly absorbed through skin
- Wear appropriate protective clothing
- Supportive measures are vitally important.

▶ Most products are dissolved in hydrocarbon solvents. Aspiration of these products will cause severe aspiration pneumonia with high mortality, and for this reason gastric aspiration should be avoided.

Management of organophosphate poisoning

- Prevent further absorption according to route of exposure:
- remove to fresh air
- remove soiled clothing and wash contaminated skin with washing-up liquid in water (see 📖 p. 803)
- Consider hospital transfer early
- Protect the airway
- Gain IV access
- Monitor BP and pulse
- In symptomatic patients establish intravenous access
- Collect blood samples in an EDTA tube for measurement of erythrocyte and plasma cholinesterase activities to confirm the diagnosis
- If bronchorrhoea develops, administer atropine 0.6–2mg IV every 10–15min until secretions are minimal and the patient is atropinized (dry skin and sinus tachycardia). In severe cases very large doses of atropine may be required if hospital admission is likely to be delayed
- Moderately or severely poisoned patients should be given pralidoxime mesilate 2g IV over 4min to reactivate phosphorylated enzyme
- IV diazepam 5–10mg is useful in controlling apprehension, agitation, fasciculation, and convulsions. The dose may be repeated as required.

Skin decontamination: pesticides

- ⚠ Safety first
- Avoid contaminating yourself
- Wear protective clothing
- Do *NOT* allow smoking nearby. There may be a risk of fire if a solvent is involved
- Carry out decontamination in a well-ventilated area, preferably with its own ventilation system
- The patient should remove soiled clothing and wash him/herself if possible
- Put soiled clothing in a sealed container to prevent escape of volatile substances
- Wash hair and all contaminated skin with liberal amounts of water (preferably warm) and soap
- Pay special attention to skin folds, fingernails, and ears.

Note: The intensity of the odour is not necessarily an indication of the toxicity of the pesticide. It may be due to the solvent or have been added as a deterrent against ingestion.

Mercury poisoning

Properties

Mercury occurs in three forms:
- *Elemental mercury:* highly mobile silvery liquid, volatile even at room temperatures. Rapidly absorbed by lungs. Usually only toxic by inhalation
- *Inorganic mercurial salts or minerals:* e.g. mercuric chloride, mercuric iodide, mercuric oxide, mercuric sulphide, mercurous chloride
- *Organic mercury:* e.g. ethylmercury, methylmercury, merthiolate.

Toxicity

Can occur from ingestion, injection, inhalation, or dermal absorption.

Acute inhalation of mercury vapour

- Cough
- Breathlessness
- Chest tightness
- Pulmonary irritation
- Pneumonitis, pulmonary oedema, necrotizing bronchiolitis, and ARDS
- 'Influenza-like' symptoms with muscle pains, fever, and tachycardia
- GI upset may occur within a few hours.

Elemental mercury

- *Inhalation of elemental mercury globules may cause:*
  - pneumonitis
  - haemoptysis
  - respiratory distress
- Systemic mercury toxicity is unlikely to occur following ingestion.

Management of elemental mercury poisoning

- Remove from source of exposure
- Give supplemental oxygen
- Transfer to hospital if appropriate.

Inorganic mercurial salts or minerals

Toxicity

- Inorganic salts are highly *corrosive*
- Fatalities have occurred after ingestion of 0.5g of mercuric chloride.

Features

- GI mucosa and kidney are the main target sites
- Burning of the mouth and throat
- Abdominal pain
- Nausea
- Vomiting followed by haematemesis
- Bloody diarrhoea
- Colitis
- Intestinal mucosal necrosis.

Management of inorganic mercury poisoning

- Remove from source of exposure
- Give supplemental oxygen
- Give pain relief if necessary
- Transfer to hospital as soon as possible

Organomercury compounds

Toxicity

Systemic mercury poisoning results typically from acute inhalational exposure or chronic/repeated ingestion of contaminated foods.

Features

- Ingestion causes:
  - retching, coughing and choking
  - ingestion of aryl mercury salts causes nausea, vomiting and abdominal pain
  - systemic mercury poisoning may ensue
- *Inhalation may cause:*
  - mucous membrane irritation
  - repeated or substantial exposures can result in systemic toxicity.

Skin exposure

Mucous membrane irritant at high concentrations.

Management of organomercury poisoning

Ingestion

- Supportive measures provide the mainstay of therapy
- Save blood and urine for mercury concentration determination in symptomatic patients
- Specialist referral is indicated in patients with systemic features of mercury poisoning. Chelation therapy with DMPS may be required in these cases.

Inhalation

- Remove from exposure
- Oxygen/bronchodilators may be required
- Symptomatic and supportive measures dictated by patient's condition.

Skin exposure

Decontamination priority: use standard decontamination procedures.

Phenol poisoning

Properties
Phenols are industrial chemicals, used in disinfectants, which have a characteristic sweet odour:
- CAS 108–95–2
- UN 2821 phenol (solutions)
- UN 2312 phenol (molten)
- UN 1671 phenol (solid).

Synonyms

Carbolic acid	Phenolum
Hydroxybenzene	Phenyl hydrate
Phenic acid	Tar oils
Phenylic acid	Tar acids

Toxicity
- Corrosive to body tissues
- Rapidly absorbed following skin contact, leading to systemic toxicity
- Inhalation is not the normal route of exposure
- Ingestion is *very toxic*.

Occupational exposure limits
Long-term exposure limit: 2ppm.

Phenols and cresols: features and management
- Exposure by any route can cause irritation, burns, and systemic effects.
- *Ingestion:*
  - causes irritation of mucous membranes and the GI tract.
  - significant ingestion causes white/brown skin and mucosal burns which may be painless
  - laryngeal oedema can occur, and oesophageal stricture may be a late complication
- *Skin contact:* even dilute solutions (1%) can cause irritation, dermatitis, and burns to the skin following prolonged contact. Often presents as relatively painless white or brown necrotic lesions. The brown discoloration may remain after healing
- *Eye contact:* causes irritation, conjunctival and corneal oedema, and blindness.

Systemic features
- Nausea
- Vomiting
- Diarrhoea
- Hypotension
- Tachycardia

- Cardiac arrhythmias
- Metabolic acidosis
- Pallor
- Sweating
- Shock.

▶ CNS stimulation is followed by drowsiness, respiratory depression, cyanosis, convulsions, coma, bronchospasm, rapid-onset pulmonary oedema, and death.

Management of acute poisoning with phenols

- Remove patient from exposure
- Ensure a clear airway and adequate ventilation
- Give oxygen if clinically indicated
- Monitor pulse, BP, and cardiac rhythm
- Transfer to hospital
- Single brief convulsions do not require treatment. If frequent or prolonged control with IV diazepam 10–20mg or lorazepam 4mg.

Phenol: skin contamination

Wash all contaminated areas of the skin with copious quantities of water.

Phenol splashed or sprayed into the eyes

See p. 792, General principles of acute poisoning and contact details for specialist advice for eye decontamination procedures.

Methaemoglobinaemia (acute treatment)

Characterized by increased quantities of haemoglobin in which the iron of haem is oxidized to the ferric (Fe^{3+}) form, i.e. leads to oxidation of haemoglobin. Methaemoglobin causes a variable degree of cyanosis. See 📖 p. 328, Methaemoglobinaemia for clinical features and causal exposures.

Exposure to a large amount of these agents can lead to the development of 50–60% methaemoglobin. The symptoms of acute anaemia develop because methaemoglobin lacks the capacity to transport oxygen.

Treatment of acute methaemoglobinaemia

Acute toxic methaemoglobinaemia presents a serious medical emergency:
- Remove from the toxic agent
- Arrange for immediate admission to hospital
- Assessment with ABCs
- Methylene blue (methylthioninium chloride) should be administered in a dose of 1–2mg/kg IV over 5min. Repeated doses may be needed
- Methylene blue (methylthioninium chloride) should not be used if the methaemoglobinaemia is due to chlorate poisoning as it may convert the chlorate to hypochlorite which is an even more toxic compound
- In cases of acute methaemoglobinaemia with intravascular haemolysis, haemodialysis with exchange transfusion is the treatment of choice.

Hydrofluoric acid exposure

Properties
A colourless fuming liquid used in metal extracting, refining, polishing, and glass etching. An industrial chemical but also present in some household rust removers. A solution of hydrogen fluoride in water.

Synonyms
Hydrogen fluoride.

Toxicity
See Table 39.1:
- *Corrosive (acid):* readily penetrates intact skin, nails, and deep tissue layers
- Skin exposure or ingestion of any quantity can be dangerous and can result in severe hypocalcaemia
- Ingestion or skin contact alone or with inhalation has led to death
- There may be sudden deterioration and fatal arrhythmias can occur within 90min.

Concentration	Time to symptom onset
Anhydrous or > 50%	Immediate
20–50%	Up to 8h
< 20%	Up to 24h

⚠ Solutions with concentrations as low as 2% may cause burns if they remain in contact with the skin for long enough.

Further information
True B-L, Dreisbach RH (eds) (2002). *Dreisbach's handbook of poisoning prevention, diagnosis and treatment*, 13th edn. Parthenon Publishing, Lancaster.

Warrell DA, Cox TM, Firth JD, Benz EJ (2005). *Oxford textbook of medicine*, 4th edn. Oxford University Press, Oxford.

Table 39.1 Toxicity of hydrofluoric acid

Mode of entry	Signs/symptoms	Management (all transfer to hospital)	Possible systemic effects to be aware of
Ingestion	Burning of mouth, throat Retrosternal/abdominal pain Laryngeal burns Hypersalivation Vomiting 9 haematemesis Hypotension Oesophageal/gastric perforation	Urgent assessment of airway, intubation/tracheostomy may be needed Transfer to hospital Treat hypocalcaemia Calcium gluconate 10–30mL of 10% sol IV Treat hypovolaemia Opiates may be needed	Hypocalcaemia Hypomagnesaemia Hyperkalaemia Metabolic acidosis Myoclonus Tetany Convulsions CNS depression
Inhalation	Irritation upper airway Cough Chest tightness Headache Ataxia Confusion Dyspnoea 9 stridor Haemorrhagic pulmonary oedema—late sign	As above	Cardiac arrthythmias: Prolonged QT VT/VF

Table 39.1 (Cont'd)

Mode of entry	Signs/symptoms	Management (all transfer to hospital)	Possible systemic effects to be aware of
Skin contact	Severe and deep burns Pain disproportionate Blue-grey discoloration in severe cases Time for burn to develop: Anhydrous or >50% immediate 20–50% up to 8h <20% up to 24h	Remove clothing Irrigate with water for 15–30min Opiates may be needed Apply calcium gluconate gel in surgical glove for hand burns	See ingestion
Eye contact	Conjunctivitis Chemosis Corneal epithelium coagulation ± necrosis	Remove contact lenses Irrigate with water or 0.9% saline for at least 30min Calcium gluconate solution should not be used Local anaesthetics (e.g. amethocaine) may help decontamination Mydriatic and cycloplegic agents (e.g. tropicamide), may help (avoid in glaucoma)	See ingestion

Non-chemical emergencies

Management of anaphylaxis

General considerations

In OH practice, anaphylaxis can occur in association with the administration of immunizations. All OH departments that administer vaccines must have adequate facilities for resuscitation. Resuscitation equipment should be latex free, particularly in the health care industry where the incidence of type 1 hypersensitivity to latex among employees is significant. OH staffs who administer vaccines should be retrained in resuscitation protocols annually.

Prevention of anaphylaxis

- Seek history of known allergy to vaccine components prior to immunization
- Vigilance in individuals who have a strong history of atopy, although immunization is not contraindicated.

Diagnosis of anaphylaxis

Rapid onset (variable, but usually within minutes of immunization) of:
- Generalized itching, urticaria
- Peri-orbital oedema
- Peri-oral oedema, oedema of the tongue and pharynx (with stridor)
- Wheezing and dyspnoea
- Collapse with hypotension, tachycardia.

Treatment of anaphylaxis

- Mild (itching, but no features of angio-oedema or shock). Oral anti-histamines
- Moderate to severe:
  - maintain airway and circulation if cardiovascular collapse (30 chest compressions to two ventilations if cardiorespiratory arrest)
  - 100% oxygen, via mask, insert airway if unconscious
  - adrenaline 0.5–1mL of 1:1000 (0.5–1mg) IM; can be repeated at 5min intervals according to pulse and blood pressure
  - establish venous access and start IV colloids
  - give hydrocortisone 200mg by IM or slow IV injection (can be repeated) and chlorpheniramine 10mg IM or slow IV injection
- Moderate to severe cases will require admission because of risk of prolonged reactions and recurrence. Individuals who experience mild reactions can be discharged with oral antihistamines.

Reporting adverse reactions

- Report to Committee on Safety of Medicines (CSM) using yellow card scheme. ℘ http://medicines.mhra.gov.uk/
- Record in OH notes and counsel individual about avoidance
- Report to GP with the individual's consent.

Further information

Resuscitation Council (UK). Available at: ℘ http://www.resus.org.uk/

Department of Health (2006). *Immunization against infectious disease* (The Green Book). DH, London. Available at: ℘ http://www.dh.gov.uk/prod_consum_dh/groups/dh_digitalassets/@ dh/@en/documents/digitalasset/dh_128623.pdf

Management of needlestick and contamination incidents 1

Hazards associated with needlestick injury

- *Main hazards:* HBV, HCV, HIV (📖 p. 152, Hepatitis B; 📖 p. 154, Hepatitis C; 📖 p. 156, Human immunodeficiency virus)
- Any blood-borne infection (e.g. malaria) can be transmitted by needlestick injury (NSI)
- For prevention of NSIs see 📖 p. 104, Human tissue and body fluids.

Classification of contamination incidents

- *Percutaneous:* when a contaminated sharp breaches intact skin
- *Mucocutaneous:* when blood or body fluids splash onto mucous membranes or non-intact skin
- ▶ Intact normal skin is an effective barrier against BBV.

Immediate first aid

- Wash wound with soap and water; encourage bleeding gently
- Irrigate exposed mucous membranes copiously with water.

Risk assessment (see Tables 40.1–40.3)

Table 40.1 Risk estimates derived from historical data on occupational transmissions

Specific BBV	Risk of transmission after percutaneous exposure to infected source material
HBV	Up to 30% for HBeAg positive source
HCV	1.9%
HIV	0.3%

Source testing

Source patients should generally be tested for HBV, HCV, and HIV:

- *Pre-test discussion and informed consent:* are essential, and may be carried out by any appropriately trained and competent health care worker
- *The unconscious source patient:* should not normally be tested until consent has been obtained. If necessary, PEP should be commenced until the patient awakes. If a source patient has died, consent should normally be obtained from a relative.

Table 40.2 Risk estimates can be refined according to two aspects of the NSI

	Higher risk	Lower risk
Injury details	Hollow needle	Solid needle
	Exposure to blood	Exposure to other fluids*
	Puncture to ungloved hands	Puncture through gloves
	Deep wound	Superficial wound
	Sharp visibly blood-stained	Sharp not visibly blood-stained
	Needle had been directly in the source's blood vessel	Mucocutaneous exposure
Source infectivity	HBeAg positive	HBeAg negative, anti-HBe positive
	High HIV viral load/ low CD4 count (terminal AIDS)	Low/undetectable HIV viral load/ high CD4 count

*There is no evidence of transmission from non-blood-stained urine, saliva, faeces, or tears.

Table 40.3 Follow-up of NSI recipients

NSI (high risk or known +ve source)	Baseline	6wks	12wks	24wks
HbsAg		HbsAg	HBsAg	HBsAg
HCV		HCV RNA	HCV RNA	Anti-HCV
		LFTs	Anti-HCV	
HIV			Anti-HIV	*
All	Store serum (for 2yrs)			

Follow-up highlighted in bold is quoted in published guidance from the Health Protection Agency or Expert Advisory Group on AIDS.

*Co-infection (HIV + HCV) in the source patient has been associated with late seroconversions in the recipient HCW, so 24-wk follow-up should be considered in these cases.

Post-exposure prophylaxis

- *HBV, HIV:* see 📖 p. 820, Management of needlestick injury 2: hepatitis B virus post-exposure prophylaxis, 📖 p. 822, Management of needlestick injury 3: human immunodeficiency virus post-exposure prophylaxis.
- *HCV:* at present there is no effective PEP against HCV, but follow-up aims to identify seroconversion early so that intervention with interferon can be offered.

Counselling and psychological support

Despite the generally low risk of infection, NSIs are extremely anxiety-inducing. Careful risk communication, counselling, and support are vital.

Restrictions from work

Recipients of high risk NSIs should not be restricted from work (or EPPs) during follow-up, but advised to practice safe sex and avoid blood donation. Fitness for EPPs (if seroconversion occurs) is covered in Chapter 24.

Reporting procedures

Exposure incidents from sources that are positive for BBV are reportable
* To HSE under RIDDOR 1995
* To the HPA Centre for Infections (or to Health Protection Scotland)
* In England, as a serious untoward incident to the Strategic Health Authority.

Further information and guidance

HPA (2012). *Bloodborne viruses (BBVs) and occupational exposure.* Available at: ℛ http://www.hpa.org.uk/infections/topics_az/bbv/guidelines.htm

GMC (2012). Guidance on issues regarding consent. GMC, London. Available at: ℛ http://www.gmc-uk.org/guidance/ethical_guidance.asp

Management of needlestick and contamination incidents 2: hepatitis B post-exposure prophylaxis

Indications

Significant occupational exposure to HBV positive source material.

Regime

- Treatment depends on whether the recipient has been immunized against HBV and (if so) whether they have achieved adequate immunity. See Table 40.4.
- Hepatitis B specific immunoglobulin (HBIG) is usually provided by the local HPA laboratory. If you provide cover for managing NSIs, ensure that clear arrangements are in place to access HBIG promptly if indicated.

Further information and guidance

Department of Health (2006). Hepatitis B. In: *Immunization against infectious disease: The Green Book*. DH, London. Available at: ℘ http://www.dh.gov.uk/prod_consum_dh/groups/dh_digitalassets/@ dh/@en/documents/digitalasset/dh_108820.pdf

HPA. *Immunoglobulin handbook*. Available at: ℘ http://www.hpa.org.uk/webc/HPAwebFile/ HPAweb_C/1194947401259

Table 40.4 Summary of post-exposure treatment for hepatitis B

HBV status of person exposed	Significant exposure			Non-significant exposure	
	HBsAg positive source	Unknown source	HBsAg negative source	Continued risk	No further risk
≤1 dose HB vaccine pre-exposure	Accelerated course of HB vaccine* HBIG × 1	Accelerated course of HB vaccine*	Initiate course of HB vaccine	Initiate course of HB vaccine	No HBV prophylaxis Reassure
≥2 doses HB vaccine pre-exposure (anti-HBs not known)	One dose of HB vaccine followed by second dose 1mth later	One dose of HB vaccine	Finish course of HB vaccine	Finish course of HB vaccine	No HBV prophylaxis Reassure
Known responder to HBV vaccine (anti-HBs >10mIU/mL)	Consider booster dose of HB vaccine	Consider booster dose of HB vaccine	Consider booster dose of HB vaccine	Consider booster of HB vaccine	No HBV prophylaxis Reassure
Known non-responder to HB vaccine (anti-HBs <10mIU/mL 2–4mths post-vaccination)	HBIG × 1 Consider booster dose of HB vaccine. A second dose of HBIG should be given at 1mth	HBIG × 1 Consider booster dose of HB vaccine. A second dose of HBIG should be given at 1mth	No HBIG Consider booster dose of HB vaccine	No HBIG Consider booster dose of HB vaccine	No prophylaxis Reassure

* An accelerated course of vaccine consists of doses spaced at 0, 1, and 2mths. A booster dose may be given at 12mths to those at continuing risk of exposure to HBV. Reproduced from Public Health Lab Service, Hepatitis Subcommittee, Communicable Disease Report. 1992: 2, R97–R101. Permission granted. (Further details and explanation of terms used are contained in this article.)

Management of needlestick and contamination incidents 3: human immunodeficiency virus post-exposure prophylaxis

Indications

Significant occupational exposure to source material that is known to be infected with HIV, or high risk of infection and HIV test is not obtainable.

Drug regime

A combination of at least three oral anti-retroviral agents for 4wks, including both nucleoside analogue reverse transcriptase inhibitors (NRTIs) and protease inhibitors (PIs).

The Expert Advisory Group on AIDS (EAGA) recommends the following standard regime

Truvada one tablet (245mg tenofovir and 200mg emtricitabine (FTC)) once daily (od)
plus
Kaletra two film-coated tablets (200mg lopinavir/50mg ritonavir) bd.

Other combinations of NRTIs and PIs are used in particular circumstances:
• Where there is a suspicion of antiretroviral drug resistance in the source patient
• If the recipient is pregnant or has a medical condition
• Where there is difficulty in sourcing starter packs containing Truvada, Combivir plus Kaletra may be used. However, Truvada packs are now available from a number of sources.

If the source patient has been treated with anti-retrovirals, OH professionals are strongly recommended to seek advice from an expert genitourinary physician with experience in treating HIV disease.

Timing of PEP

The EAGA recommends that PEP is given as soon as possible after exposure and certainly within 48–72h of exposure, and continued for at least 28 days. It is not generally recommended to commence PEP beyond 72h post-exposure, but this is a matter for the judgement of local experienced clinicians.

Side effects of PEP

- Serious side effects are rare, but one death has been reported with a previous PEP regime for an occupational exposure
- Unpleasant minor side effects (GI upset, headache) common; treatment with adjuvant anti-emetics and anti-diarrhoeals often required
- The newer PEP regime generally better tolerated than previous combination therapy, but there is still a high incidence of failure to adhere.

Efficacy of PEP

- Advice on HIV PEP is based on indirect evidence of efficacy in the prevention of vertical transmission of HIV, and on surveillance data following occupational exposures
- PEP with Zidovudine has been shown (in a case control study) to reduce the risk of occupational transmission by 80%
- There have been documented cases of occupational transmission of HIV despite appropriate PEP.

Further information and guidance

Chief Medical Officers' Expert Advisory Group on AIDS (2008). HIV post-exposure prophylaxis: Guidance from the UK Chief Medical Officers' Expert Advisory Group on AIDS. Available at: ℜ http://www.dh.gov.uk/en/Publicationsandstatistics/Publications/PublicationsPolicyAndGuidance/ DH_088185

Psychiatric emergencies

General points

- Psychiatric emergencies are relatively common among people who have an established diagnosis of serious mental disorder, but unusual in the general working population
- A situation can be considered as an emergency when there is a serious and current risk to the safety of the person and/or others. This danger may be:
  - a consequence of deliberate planning
  - or the risk can be unintentional.

Immediate assessment of emergencies

- Ensure the safety of the person
- Try to speak with the person, recognizing that it is usually impractical to carry out a detailed psychiatric assessment in these circumstances
- Ensure the safety of others (including yourself) while doing so

⚠ When there is an immediate and serious risk of harm, there should be no delay in calling the police

- If possible, try to establish some dialogue with the person. However, avoid confrontation and disagreement. This may calm the situation, enable further evaluation of the problem, and perhaps give an initial indication whether there is an underlying psychiatric disorder
- A more detailed assessment of the person's mental state can be arranged thereafter in a more secure and specialist setting
- When talking with the person, it may be useful to ask about:
  - what they are planning to do?
  - why they wish to harm themselves or others?
  - what, if anything, has happened very recently to them to prompt the crisis?
  - whether they have had previous mental health problems?
- ⚠ Take any account of suicidal thoughts seriously. Particular concern is raised when a person makes clear statements of intent to kill themselves, particularly:
  - if they have made firm plans of how to kill themselves
  - if they have current significant symptoms of depression and/or if they have experienced recent serious loss-
- Colleagues and management may have some knowledge, ask about:
  - recent stress (whether or not work-related)
  - and any history of previous mental disorder.

▶ A person whose behaviour is considered dangerous as a result of a current mental disorder does not need to be detained using the Mental Health Act in order for them to be restrained in an emergency. This can be carried out under common law. Subsequent specialist assessment and treatment may require the person to be legally detained in hospital.

Lower risk situations

Some situations that cause alarm may not be regarded as medical emergencies that require immediate and assertive intervention. However, they may make it impossible for the person to continue working, and they would benefit from early medical assessment. Such situations may include:

- Acts of self-harm without suicidal intent
- Symptoms of mild or moderate mood disorder
- Overwhelming symptoms of anxiety.

It will be useful to ensure the person agrees to be seen urgently by their GP, out-of-hours medical services or at the A&E department, and if necessary to make arrangements for them to be transported there.

Particular psychiatric disorders

- Behaviour that is dangerous to self or others does not in itself indicate that a person is mentally ill. In many situations, such behaviour arises at times of crisis, and the person may well have behaved similarly in the past when faced with overwhelming difficulties
- Current intoxication with alcohol and/or drugs may increase impulsivity and disinhibition
- In a minority of situations, current symptoms of an untreated serious mental disorder present a serious risk
  - people who have delirium may be disorientated, aroused, hallucinated, and irrational
  - those who have acute schizophrenia may be violent as a result of command hallucinations, or because of their persecutory beliefs
  - symptoms of acute mania may include irrational thinking and extreme excitement and irritability
  - symptoms of severe depression may result in acts of serious self-harm
- It is very unlikely that a confident diagnosis can be made in the setting of an acute emergency. This will usually be possible only after further assessment and observation, physical examination and appropriate investigations, interviews with others who know the person, and knowledge of any previous psychiatric and medical history.

Chapter 41

Terrorism

Terrorism (deliberate use of chemical or biological weapons, or radiation and nuclear weapons)

Small groups of terrorists have the ability to cause massive damage and extensive human suffering with little or no warning. Emergency services must be able to respond rapidly and appropriately to such scenarios.

- Rescue and treatment of victims, and control and containment of fire or other hazards are complicated. Sites may be contaminated with nuclear, chemical, biological, or radiological substances
- The impact of weapons may stretch much further than the scene of disaster. Exposed personnel can spread contamination into other areas as they depart from the scene
- As well as the physical injuries, there is major public fear over any use of such weapons, with the risk of significant psychological casualties. Public reassurance and health risk communication forms an essential part of the management of any incident
- Thorough contingency planning is necessary by all organizations likely to be involved.

Routes of exposure

- Radiation and chemical agents can enter the body by:
  - inhalation
  - absorption through skin or eyes
  - injection by flying glass or shrapnel
  - ingestion
- Biological agents are usually transmitted through inhalation.

Other factors

As well as the direct and indirect health effects from the terrorist agent, the effect of risk controls on responding forces must be considered. Protective equipment limits movement and carries risks of hyperthermia in its own right.

Specific terrorist weapons

Each main class of weapon is covered as a separate topic (see 📖 p. 829, Chemical weapons; 📖 p. 830, Biological weapons; 📖 p. 832, Radiation and nuclear weapons).

Further information and guidance

Guidance is available from the Health Protection Agency. Available at: 🔗 http://www.hpa.org.uk/Topics/EmergencyResponse/CBRNAndDeliberateRelease/

Chemical weapons

Terrorists have used chemical weapons in the past, and it is likely to happen again. There is the potential for large numbers of casualties. Numerous chemical agents exist, each with different symptoms and effects. Although some may require extensive laboratory facilities to manufacture, others can be fabricated relatively simply. Much of the efficacy of such a weapon depends on its ability to disperse the material.

Types of chemical weapons

- *Blood agent/cyanides:* attack the capacity of the blood to hold and deliver oxygen, causing the victim to suffocate. Cyanide gases and compounds are most common
- *Nerve agents:* affect the individual's nervous system. Most belong to the family of organophosphates, and have similarities to some pesticides
- *Blister agents:* also known as vesicants, they attack exposed skin, resulting in blisters and skin burns e.g. mustard gas and lewisite
- *Choking agents:* attack lungs, causing pulmonary oedema, e.g. chlorine and phosgene
- *Incapacitating agents:* usually irritate skin, mucous membranes, eyes, nose, lips and mouth; causing vomiting or intolerable pain. Whilst this may lead to serious medical situations, it is not designed to kill or cause permanent harm. Used alone, the intention is to temporarily incapacitate and force people to leave an area. However, these agents can be used in combination with other chemical weapons to force removal of protective equipment. Examples include pepper spray, Tear/CS gas and other riot control agents.

Risks to emergency personnel

Chemical contamination can offer a major and immediate hazard to responders who must be correctly trained and equipped. All agents have the potential for 2° contamination of ambulances, fire, and medical equipment, thereby affecting anyone who comes in contact with them. Therefore, proper decontamination is necessary before casualties leave the area.

Management of casualties

- *Decontamination:* must take place rapidly often within minutes of exposure
- Stabilization
- Assess cause
- Give antidotes/treat symptoms
- Seek specialist advice.

Biological weapons

Bioterrorism presents serious challenges. Biological weapons can be easy to develop and have utility across the spectrum of conflicts and targets.
- Their release may be:
  - *overt*—announced openly by the perpetrators
  - *covert*—i.e. unannounced without a warning or indication of the organism
- Many organisms could be used deliberately and distributed through food, water, or air
- Depending on the organism, deliberate use may be indistinguishable from natural outbreaks, either through the use of naturally occurring pathogens or because symptoms are identical. Therefore, early recognition of outbreaks can only be achieved if clinicians are aware of the possibility and take appropriate measures before a definite diagnosis is reached
- Agent used and mechanism of delivery will depend on whether terrorists are sponsored by a government. A state sponsored group with access to biotechnology and laboratory infrastructure is much more likely to have the ability to cause casualties on a large scale. However, an unsupported single operative involved in deliberate contamination of food may still have devastating impact, albeit on a smaller scale
- These weapons may be much more effective when used against civilian populations. The latter comprise more vulnerable groups at the extremes of age, the immune compromised and the un-vaccinated, rather than fast moving, relatively healthy military organizations. There is a real risk that public panic will lead to swamping of medical care.

Types of biological weapons

Pathogens
- Disease-causing organisms that can reproduce and keep spreading long after the attack
- Potential for many thousands of casualties, but likely to be much less because of difficulty in efficiently spreading material to reach large populations
- Plague, smallpox, anthrax, and haemorrhagic fever are known to be possible biological weapons.

Toxins
- Poisonous substances produced by living things
- Many are lethal in small quantities and can kill very large numbers of people
- More like a chemical attack than a biological one
- Include ricin, botulism toxin, and aflotoxin
- Again the main problem for the terrorist is one of dispersion.

Recognition of a bioterrorism incident

Any case of smallpox, plague, pulmonary anthrax, glanders, Venezuelan equine encephalitis, or viral haemorrhagic fever in the UK should be assumed to be the effect of a deliberate release unless proven otherwise.

Bioterrorist attack

The following findings indicate the possibility of a bioterrorist attack:
- Unusual illness
- Unusual numbers of patients with same symptoms
- Illness unusual for time of year
- Illness unusual for patient age group
- Illness in an unusual patient
- Illness acquired in an unusual place
- Unusual clinical signs or disease progression.

Prophylaxis and treatment

- Prophylactic vaccination is possible for certain agents. Once the threat is known, vaccination may be used to contain spread of a weapon used strategically. However, it will always involve risk–benefit assessments, and post-exposure measurements may be more relevant
- The delay in detection means those handling initial casualties will be unaware of hazard, and may be unprotected.

Management of biological exposures

- *Dependent on the pathogen:* identification of the agent is critical, and will facilitate measures to protect responders (such as vaccination)
- A suspected casualty should be isolated, and medical staff should wear full protective clothing
- Treatment of the condition depends on the specific agent and symptoms
- Specialist help should be sought. In the UK this is available from the Health Protection Agency
- Monitoring of others exposed and if appropriate post exposure prophylaxis/will be necessary.

Radiation and nuclear weapons

Although terrorist access to functional nuclear weapons cannot be ruled out, it is thought to be very unlikely. More probable scenarios include the use of conventional explosives to attack nuclear facilities, or to spread radioactive materials directly over a large area, and the targeted use of small quantities of radioactive material (e.g. Litvinenko polonium poisoning 2006). In most such cases, it is the fear of the unknown effects of these weapons (rather than any short-term health risks) that is likely to be the major problem.

Radiation sources

- Radiation can present an external or internal hazard
- The terrorist scenario can involve alpha, beta or a gamma radiation (but not neutrons which would only be released from operating nuclear reactors of nuclear weapon yields)
- External hazards, which are predominantly gamma and penetrating, are removed when the source is taken away
- However, contamination by radioactive dust will persist and can damage the skin (beta and gamma only) and internal 'target' organs from inhalation, ingestion, or skin penetration. In these circumstances (unless internal contamination is very major), the main effects are likely to be long term, predominantly involving excess risk of malignancy.

Monitoring

- The presence of radiation in the environment is readily measurable. Many medical physics, nuclear medicine departments and front line services are able to measure beta and gamma radiation, although alpha measurement requires more specialized equipment
- Quantification of an individual's personal exposure is much more difficult.

Risk controls

- It is important that first responders use respiratory protection to avoid breathing in the radioactive dust, and full clothing to prevent contamination of skin
- In the case of an incident involving radioactive iodine, there may be benefit in early use of potassium iodide (KI) as a blocking agent for both responders and casualties.

Management of casualties with radiation exposure

- Provide respiratory protection
- Remove from hazard area
- Decontaminate externally by showering
- Control movement to avoid spread of contamination

▶ However, management of conventional injuries must take priority over radioactive contamination, as the latter will not present an immediate threat to life for either casualty or medical personnel.

- Those who have been exposed to an external radiation hazard present no risk to responding forces once removed from radiation.

In UK radiation casualties should be moved to an appropriate hospital designated by the Strategic Health Authority. Advice can be sought from the ambulance service.

Further information and guidance

Health Protection Agency. Available at: ℜ http:www.hpa.org.uk,

US Radiation Emergency Assistance Centre/Training Centre. Available at: ℜ http://www.orau.gov/reacts

Appendices

Hazard statements for 'health effects' used under classification, labelling, and packaging of substances and mixtures regulations

H300: Fatal if swallowed
H301: Toxic if swallowed
H302: Harmful if swallowed
H303: May be harmful if swallowed
H304: May be fatal if swallowed and enters airways
H305: May be harmful if swallowed and enters airways
H310: Fatal in contact with skin
H311: Toxic in contact with skin
H312: Harmful in contact with skin
H313: May be harmful in contact with skin
H314: Causes severe skin burns and eye damage
H315: Causes skin irritation
H316: Causes mild skin irritation
H317: May cause an allergic skin reaction
H318: Causes serious eye damage
H319: Causes serious eye irritation
H320: Causes eye irritation
H330: Fatal if inhaled
H331: Toxic if inhaled
H332: Harmful if inhaled
H333: May be harmful if inhaled
H334: May cause allergy or asthma symptoms or breathing difficulties if inhaled
H335: May cause respiratory irritation
H336: May cause drowsiness or dizziness
H340: May cause genetic defects
H341: Suspected of causing genetic defects
H350: May cause cancer
H351: Suspected of causing cancer
H360: May damage fertility or the unborn child
H361: Suspected of damaging fertility or the unborn child
H362: May cause harm to breast-fed children

H370: Causes damage to organs
H371: May cause damage to organs
H372: Causes damage to organs through prolonged or repeated exposure
H373: May cause damage to organs through prolonged or repeated exposure

Consent for occupational health assessment

Essential information about your assessment

What is the purpose of an OH assessment?

The purpose is to assess health problems that may be caused (or made worse) by work, or are having an effect on your ability to work. We aim to give fair and impartial advice to *both you and your manager* about:

- Your fitness for your job
- Any risks to your health that arise from your duties or your workplace.

Unlike a normal doctor (or nurse)–patient encounter, an OH assessment does NOT aim to diagnose or treat disease. However, in some circumstances we may just help to ensure that you are receiving the right medical tests or treatment.

When is an OH assessment needed?

Depending on your circumstances, it might be needed:

- When starting a new job
- When returning to work after a period of time off work due to illness
- If you have problems carrying out your job or are not performing as well as would be expected
- If you have a high level of absence from work due to sickness
- If there is a concern that you might have a health problem that is caused or made worse by work.

Who will carry out the assessment?

Your appointment will be with an OH doctor or nurse. The OH doctors and nurses who carry out assessments have skills in assessing the relationship between health and work.

What will happen at my appointment?

The doctor or nurse will ask you questions about your health and your job, and may carry out a medical examination.

- They will sometimes arrange to visit your workplace and see your activities for themselves
- They may ask for your written permission to obtain further medical information from a GP or other doctor who has been treating you. If they ask to do this, the doctor or nurse will explain the reason for requesting a report, and what will happen to the information that your doctor provides.

What will happen after my assessment?

At the end of the consultation we will usually send a report to the person who referred you (usually your manager or a personnel officer).

If you referred yourself, we may or may not want to send a report to your manager, but this would depend on your own situation and wishes.

What information will be sent to my manager?

The sort of information that will be included in the manager's report depends on the reason for your referral, but would usually include practical advice about fitness for work, e.g.

- Whether you are fit for work
- If not fit now, an estimate of how long it might be before you are fit
- Whether adjustments or changes need to be made to your job in order to help you to return to work, or to protect your health. These changes may be short term (for rehabilitation) or longer term
- The likelihood of further health problems leading to absence from work in the future
- The report does not usually contain confidential personal or medical information. Rarely, it might be useful to include some medical details, but this is exceptional and is only done with your consent.

Will I know what is being said about me in a report?

Yes, you have open access to all information that will pass from OH as a result of your assessment. At the end of your appointment, the doctor or nurse will tell you what they are going to say in the report and to whom it will be sent. You will have an opportunity to discuss the report with the doctor or nurse. You can also have a copy of the report if you wish. You can choose to have a copy either before it is released or at the same time.

Can I refuse to see the doctor or nurse, or refuse to have a report released to my manager?

Yes, you are quite free to decline the assessment. You can also refuse to have a report released at the end of the consultation. However, it is often not in your best interest to do so, as your employer will not be able to take your health problem into account properly. If you are worried about the OH consultation or report, please discuss with someone in the OH team. They will help you to understand the likely consequences of consenting or refusing in your own particular case.

Finally

It is important to remember that the OH Professionals do not take sides with either an employee or their manager—but aim to give careful advice to both.

Please do not hesitate to ask for more information or explanation if you need it.

Please sign below to indicate that you have read this information sheet and consent to your occupational health assessment.

Name (in capitals): _____

Signature _____

Date: _____

List of prescribed diseases

List of diseases that are covered and the kinds of jobs that are included. This is not a complete list of jobs, and you should not be put off claiming just because your job is not listed. If in doubt, claim.

Disease no.	Name of disease or injury	Type of job
	Conditions due to physical agents (physical cause)	**Any job involving**
A1	Leukaemia (other than chronic lymphatic leukaemia) or cancer of the bone, female breast, testis or thyroid	Exposure to electromagnetic radiations (other than radiant heat) or to ionizing particles where the dose is sufficient to double the risk of the occurrence of the condition, e.g. people working in the nuclear industry and hospital X-ray departments
A2	Cataract	Frequent or prolonged exposure to radiation from red-hot or white-hot material, e.g. glass and metal workers, stokers
A3	Dysbarism, including decompression sickness, barotrauma and osteonecrosis. For example, the bends	Subjection to compressed or rarefied air or other respirable gases or gaseous mixtures, e.g. underwater or tunnel workers
A4	Task-specific focal dystonia of the hand or forearm. For example, writer's cramp	Prolonged periods of handwriting, typing or other repetitive movements of the fingers, hand or arm
A5	Subcutaneous cellulitis of the hand	Manual labour causing severe or prolonged friction or pressure on the hand, e.g. miners and road workers using picks and shovels
A6	Bursitis or subcutaneous cellulitis arising at or about the knee due to severe or prolonged external friction or pressure at or about the knee, e.g. housemaid's knee	Manual labour causing severe or prolonged external friction or pressure at or about the knee, e.g. workers who kneel a lot
A7	Bursitis or subcutaneous cellulitis arising at or about the elbow due to severe or prolonged external friction or pressure at or about the elbow	Manual labour causing severe or prolonged external friction or pressure at or about the elbow. For example, jobs involving continuous rubbing or pressure on the elbow

A8	Traumatic inflammation of the tendons of the hand or forearm, or of the associated tendon sheaths. Tenosynovitis	Manual labour, or frequent or repeated movements of the hand or wrist, e.g. routine assembly workers
A10	Occupational deafness. Sensorineural hearing loss amounting to at least 50dB in each ear, being the average of hearing losses at 1, 2 and 3kHz frequencies, and being due in the case of at least one ear to occupational noise	The use of, or work wholly or mainly in the immediate vicinity of the use of, a:
		(a) Band saw, circular saw or cutting disc to cut metal in the metal founding or forging industries, circular saw to cut products in the manufacture of steel, powered (other than hand powered) grinding tool on metal (other than sheet metal or plate metal), pneumatic percussive tool on metal, pressurized air arc tool to gouge metal, burner or torch to cut or dress steel-based products, skid transfer bank, knock out and shake out grid in a foundry, machine (other than a power press machine) to forge metal including a machine used to drop stamp metal by means of closed or open dies or drop hammers, machine to cut or shape or clean metal nails, or plasma spray gun to spray molten metal
		(b) Pneumatic percussive tool to drill rock in a quarry, on stone in a quarry works, underground, for mining coal, for sinking a shaft, or for tunnelling in civil engineering works
		(c) Vibrating metal moulding box in the concrete products industry, or circular saw to cut concrete masonry blocks
		(d) Machine in the manufacture of textiles for weaving man-made or natural fibres (including mineral fibres), high speed false twisting of fibres, or the mechanical cleaning of bobbins

(Cont'd)

Disease no.	Name of disease or injury	Type of job
	Conditions due to physical agents (physical cause)	Any job involving
A10 (Cont'd)		(e) Multi-cutter moulding machine on wood, planing machine on wood, automatic or semiautomatic lathe on wood, multiple cross-cut machine on wood, automatic shaping machine on wood, double-end tenoning machine on wood, vertical spindle moulding machine (including a high speed routing machine) on wood, edge banding machine on wood, bandsawing machine (with a blade width of not less than 75mm) on wood, circular sawing machine on wood including one operated by moving the blade towards the material being cut, or chain saw on wood
		(f) Jet of water (or mixture of water and abrasive material) at a pressure above 680 bar, or jet channelling process to burn stone in a quarry
		(g) Machine in a ship's engine room, or gas turbine for performance testing on a test bed, installation testing of a replacement engine in an aircraft, or acceptance testing of an Armed Service fixed wing combat aircraft;
		(h) Machine in the manufacture of glass containers or hollow ware for automatic moulding, automatic blow moulding, or automatic glass pressing and forming
		(i) Spinning machine using compressed air to produce glass wool or mineral wool
		(j) Continuous glass toughening furnace
		(k) Firearm by a police firearms training officer; or
		(l) Shot-blaster to carry abrasives in air for cleaning

A11	(a) Intense blanching of the skin, with a sharp demarcation line between affected and non-affected skin, where the blanching is cold-induced, episodic, occurs throughout the year and affects the skin of the distal with the middle and proximal phalanges, or distal with the middle phalanx (or in the case of a thumb the distal with the proximal phalanx), of:	(a) The use of hand-held chain saws on wood; or
		(b) The use of hand-held rotary tools in grinding or in the sanding or polishing of metal, or the holding of material being ground, or metal being sanded or polished, by rotary tools; or
	(i) in the case of a person with 5 fingers (including thumb) on one hand, any 3 of those fingers, or	
	(ii) in the case of a person with only 4 such fingers, any 2 of those fingers, or	
	(iii) In the case of a person with less than 4 such fingers, any one of them or, as the case may be, the one remaining finger	(c) The use of hand-held percussive metalworking tools, or the holding of metal being worked upon by percussive tools, in riveting, caulking, chipping, hammering, fettling or swaging; or
	Where none of the person's fingers was subject to any degree of cold-induced, episodic blanching of the skin prior to the person's employment in an occupation described in the third column in relation to this paragraph, or	

(Cont'd)

Disease no.	Name of disease or injury	Type of job
	Conditions due to physical agents (physical cause)	Any job involving
A11 (Cont'd)	(b) significant, demonstrable reduction in both sensory perception and manipulative dexterity with continuous tingling or continuous numbness all present at the same time in the distal phalanx of any finger (including thumb) where none of the person's fingers was subject to any degree of reduction in sensory perception, manipulative dexterity, numbness or tingling prior to the person's employment in an occupation described in the second column in relation to this paragraph where the symptoms in paragraph (a) or paragraph (b) were caused by vibration	(d) The use of hand-held powered percussive drills or hand-held powered percussive hammers in mining, quarrying, demolition, or on roads or footpaths, including road construction; or (e) The holding of material being worked upon by pounding machines in shoe manufacture
A12	Carpal tunnel syndrome	(a) The use, at the time the symptoms first develop, of hand-held powered tools whose internal parts vibrate so as to transmit that vibration to the hand, but excluding those tools which are solely powered by hand; or (b) Repeated palmar flexion and dorsiflexion of the wrist for at least 20h/week for a period or periods amounting in aggregate to at least 12mths in the 24mths prior to the onset of symptoms. We use 'repeated' to mean once or more often in every 30s
A13	Osteoarthritis of the hip	Work in agriculture as a farmer or farm worker for a period of, or periods which amount in aggregate to, 10yrs or more

A14	Osteoarthritis of the knee	Work underground in a coal mine for a period of, or periods which amount in aggregate to, at least 10yrs in any one or more of the following occupations:
		(a) before 1 January 1986 as a coal miner; or
		(b) on or after 1 January 1986 as a:
		(i) face worker working on a non-mechanized coal face
		(ii) development worker
		(iii) face salvage worker
		(iv) conveyor belt cleaner; or
		(v) conveyor belt attendant
		A 'non-mechanized coal face' means a coal face without either powered roof supports or a power loader machine which simultaneously cuts and loads the coal or without both
		Work wholly or mainly fitting or laying carpets or floors, (other than concrete floors) for a period of, or periods which amount in aggregate to, 20yrs or more

(Cont'd)

Disease no.	Name of disease or injury	Type of job
	Conditions due to biological agents (caused by animal, plant or other living organism)	**Any job involving**
B1	Anthrax	(a) Contact with anthrax spores, including contact with animals infected by anthrax; or
		(b) Handling, loading, unloading or transport of animals of a type susceptible to infection with anthrax or of the products or residues of such animals
B2	Glanders	Contact with equine animals or their carcasses, e.g. farm and slaughterhouse workers, and grooms handling horses
B3	Infection by leptospira. For example, swamp fever, swineherd's disease, and Weil's disease	(a) Work in places which are, or are liable to be, infested by rats, field mice or voles, or other small mammals; or
		(b) Work at dog kennels or the care or handling of dogs; or
		(c) Contact with bovine animals or their meat products or pigs or their meat products. For example, farm, veterinary, sewerage and slaughterhouse workers
B4	Ankylostomiasis	Contact with a source of ankylostomiasis
B5	Tuberculosis. TB infection	Contact with a source of tuberculous infection. For example, doctors, nurses, ambulance crews, pathology technicians and social workers
B6	Extrinsic allergic alveolitis (including farmer's lung)	Exposure to moulds or fungal spores or heterologous proteins by reason of employment in:
		(a) Agriculture, horticulture, forestry, cultivation of edible fungi or malt-working; or

		(b) Loading or unloading or handling in storage mouldy vegetable matter or edible fungi; or
		(c) Caring for or handling birds; or
		(d) Handling bagasse
		(e) Work involving exposure to metalworking fluids mists
B7	Infection by organisms of the genus brucella, Brucellosis	Contact with:
		(a) Animals infected by brucella, or their carcasses or parts thereof, or their untreated products; or
		(b) Laboratory specimens or vaccines of, or containing, brucella. For example, farm, veterinary, slaughterhouse, animal laboratory workers
B8A	Infection by hepatitis A virus	Contact with raw sewage
B8B	Infection by hepatitis B or C virus	Contact with:
		(a) Human blood or human blood products; or
		(b) Any other source of hepatitis B or C virus
B9	Infection by *Streptococcus suis*. A very rare form of meningitis from exposure to infected pigs or pork products	Contact with pigs infected by *Streptococcus suis*, or with the carcasses, products or residues of pigs so infected, e.g. pork butchers, pig breeders, slaughterhouse workers
B10(a)	Avian chlamydiosis	Contact with birds infected with *Chlamydia psittaci*, or with the remains or untreated products of such birds, e.g. duck farm workers, feather processing workers, abattoir workers, poultry meat inspectors, pet shop owners and assistants

(Cont'd)

Disease no.	Name of disease or injury	Type of job
	Conditions due to biological agents (caused by animal, plant or other living organism)	**Any job involving**
B10(b)	Ovine chlamydiosis	Contact with sheep infected with *Chlamydia psittaci*, or with the remains or untreated products of such sheep, e.g. sheep farm workers, veterinary surgeons
B11	Q fever	Contact with animals, their remains or their untreated products, e.g. farm workers involved in the rearing of sheep, abattoir workers, veterinary surgeons
B12	Orf	Contact with sheep or goats, or with the carcasses of sheep or goats, e.g. farm workers, abattoir workers, meat inspectors
B13	Hydatidosis	Contact with dogs, e.g. shepherds, veterinarians and people who care for dogs
B14	Lyme disease	Exposure to deer or other mammals of a type liable to harbour ticks harbouring *Borrelia* bacteria
B15	Anaphylaxis	Employment as a healthcare worker having contact with products made with natural rubber latex

Disease no.	Name of disease or injury	Type of job
	Conditions due to chemical agents (chemical cause)	**Any job involving**
C1(a)	Anaemia with a haemoglobin concentration of 9g/dL or less, and a blood film showing punctate basophilia	The use or handling of, and exposure to the fumes, dust or vapour of, lead or a compound of lead, or a substance containing lead
C1(b)	Peripheral neuropathy	For example, plumbers, painters, enamellers, pottery glazing workers
C1(c)	CNS toxicity	

C2	CNS toxicity characterized by parkinsonism	The use or handling of, or exposure to the fumes, dust or vapour of, manganese or a compound of manganese, or a substance containing manganese, e.g. dry battery, pottery glazing and soap workers
C3(a)	Phossy Jaw	Work involving the use or handling of, or exposure to, white phosphorous
C3(b)	Peripheral polyneuropathy or peripheral polyneuropathy with pyramidal involvement of the CNS, caused by organic compounds of phosphorous which inhibit the enzyme neuropathy target esterase	Work involving the use or handling of, or exposure to, organic compounds of phosphorous
C4	Primary carcinoma of the bronchus or lung	Exposure to the fumes, dust or vapour of arsenic, a compound of arsenic or a substance containing arsenic
C5(a)	CNS toxicity characterized by tremor and neuropsychiatric disease	Exposure to mercury or inorganic compounds of mercury for a period of, or periods which amount in aggregate to, 10yrs or more
C5(b)	Central nervous system toxicity characterized by combined cerebellar and cortical degeneration	Exposure to methyl mercury
C6	Peripheral neuropathy	The use or handling of, or exposure to the fumes or vapour of, carbon disulphide (also called carbon disulfide)
C7	Acute non-lymphatic leukaemia	Exposure to benzene
C12(a)	Peripheral neuropathy	Exposure to methyl bromide (also called bromomethane)
C12(b)	CNS toxicity	
C13	Cirrhosis of the liver	Exposure to chlorinated naphthalenes
C16(a)	Neurotoxicity	Exposure to the dust of gonioma kamassi
C16(b)	Cardiotoxicity	

(Cont'd)

Disease no.	Name of disease or injury	Type of job
	Conditions due to chemical agents (chemical cause)	Any job involving
C17	Chronic beryllium disease	Inhalation of beryllium or a beryllium compound
C18	Emphysema	Inhalation of cadmium fumes for a period of, or periods which amount in aggregate to, 20yrs or more
C19(a)	Peripheral neuropathy	Exposure to acrylamide
C19(b)	CNS toxicity	
C20	Dystrophy of the cornea (including ulceration of the corneal surface) of the eye. Wasting and ulceration of corneal surface of the eye	Exposure to quinone or hydroquinone
C21	Primary carcinoma of the skin	Exposure to arsenic or arsenic compounds, tar, pitch, bitumen, mineral oil (including paraffin), or soot
C22(a)	Primary carcinoma of the mucous membrane of the nose or paranasal sinuses	Work before 1950 in the refining of nickel involving exposure to oxides, sulphides or water-soluble compounds of nickel
C22(b)	Primary carcinoma of the bronchus or lung	

C23	Primary neoplasm of the epithelial lining of the urinary tract	(a) The manufacture of 1-naphthylamine, 2-naphthylamine, benzidine, auramine, magenta or 4-aminobiphenyl (also called biphenyl-4-ylamine)
		(b) Work in the process of manufacturing methylene-bis-orthochloroaniline (also called MbOCA) for a period of, or periods which amount in aggregate to, 12mths or more
		(c) Exposure to 2-naphthylamine, benzidine, 4-aminobiphenyl (also called biphenyl-4-ylamine) or salts of those compounds otherwise than in the manufacture of those compounds
		(d) Exposure to orthotoluidine, 4-chloro-2-methylaniline or salts of those compounds; or
		(e) Exposure for a period of, or periods which amount in aggregate to, 5yrs or more, to coal tar pitch volatiles produced in aluminium smelting involving the Soderberg process (that is to say, the method of producing aluminium by electrolysis in which the anode consists of a paste of petroleum coke and mineral oil which is baked *in situ*)
C24	(a) Angiosarcoma of the liver; or	Exposure to vinyl chloride monomer in the manufacture of PVC
	(b) Osteolysis of the terminal phalanges of the fingers; or	
	(c) Sclerodermatous thickening of the skin of the hands; or	
	(d) Liver fibrosis due to exposure to vinyl chloride monomer	
C24A	Raynaud's phenomenon due to exposure to vinyl chloride monomer	Exposure to vinyl chloride monomer in the manufacture of PVC before 1 January 1984

(Cont'd)

Disease no.	Name of disease or injury	Type of job
	Conditions due to chemical agents (chemical cause)	**Any job involving**
C25	Vitiligo	The use or handling of, or exposure to, paratertiarybutylphenol (also called 4-tertbutylphenol), paratertiarybutylcatechol (also called 4-tertbutyl(catechol), para-amylphenol (also called p-pentyl phenol isomers), hydroquinone, monobenzyl ether of hydroquinone (also called 4-benzyloxyphenol) or mono-butyl ether of hydroquinone (also called 4-butoxyphenol)
C26(a)	Liver toxicity	The use or handling of, or exposure to, carbon tetrachloride (also called tetrachloromethane)
C26(b)	Kidney toxicity	
C27	Liver toxicity	The use or handling of, or exposure to, trichloromethane (also called chloroform)
C29	Peripheral neuropathy	The use or handling of, or exposure to, n-hexane or n-butyl methyl ketone
C30(a)	Dermatitis	The use or handling of, or exposure to, chromic acid, chromates or dichromates
C30(b)	Ulceration of the mucous membrane or the epidermis	
C31	Bronchiolitis obliterans	The use or handling of, or exposure to, diacetyl (also called butanedione or 2,3-butanedione) in the manufacture of: (a) diacetyl; or (b) food flavouring containing diacetyl; or (c) food to which flavouring containing diacetyl is added
C32	Carcinoma of the nasal cavity or associated air sinuses	(a) the manufacture of inorganic chromates; or (b) work in hexavalent chrome plating

Disease no.	Name of disease or injury	Type of job
	Miscellaneous conditions not included elsewhere in the list	Any job involving
D1	Pneumoconiosis. Includes silicosis and asbestosis	(1) (a) The mining, quarrying or working of silica rock or the working of dried quartzose sand or any dry deposit or dry residue of silica or any dry admixture containing such materials (including any occupation in which any of the aforesaid operations are carried out incidentally to the mining or quarrying of other minerals or to the manufacture of articles containing crushed or ground silica rock)
		(b) The handling of any of the materials specified in the foregoing subparagraph in or incidental to any of the operations mentioned therein, or substantial exposure to the dust arising from such operations
		(2) The breaking, crushing or grinding of flint or the working or handling of broken, crushed or ground flint or materials containing such flint, or substantial exposure to the dust arising from any such operations
		(3) Sand blasting by means of compressed air with the use of quartzose sand or crushed silica rock or flint, or substantial exposure to the dust arising from sand and blasting.
		(4) Work in a foundry or the performance of, or substantial exposure to the dust arising from, any of the following operations:
		(a) the freeing of steel castings from adherent siliceous substance

(Cont'd)

Disease no.	Name of disease or injury	Type of job
	Miscellaneous conditions not included elsewhere in the list	Any job involving
D1 (Cont'd)		(b) the freeing of metal castings from adherent siliceous substance:
		(i) by blasting with an abrasive propelled by compressed air, by steam or by a wheel, or
		(ii) by the use of power-driven tools
		(5) The manufacture of china or earthenware (including sanitary earthenware, electrical earthenware and earthenware tiles), and any occupation involving substantial exposure to the dust arising therefrom
		(6) The grinding of mineral graphite, or substantial exposure to the dust arising from such grinding
		(7) The dressing of granite or any igneous rock by masons or the crushing of such materials, or substantial exposure to the dust arising from such operations
		(8) The use, or preparation for use, of a grindstone, or substantial exposure to the dust arising therefrom
		(9) (a) The working or handling of asbestos or any admixture of asbestos
		(b) the manufacture or repair of asbestos textiles or other articles containing or composed of asbestos
		(c) the cleaning of any machinery or plant used in any foregoing operations and of any chambers, fixtures and appliances for the collection of asbestos dust

(d) substantial exposure to the dust arising from any of the foregoing operations

(10)(a) Work underground in any mine in which one of the objects of the mining operations is the getting of any mineral;

(b) the working or handling above ground at any coal or tin mine of any minerals extracted therefrom, or any operation incidental thereto;

(c) the trimming of coal in any ship, barge, or lighter, or in any dock or harbour or at any wharf or quay;

(d) the sawing, splitting or dressing of slate, or any operation incidental thereto

(11) The manufacture of carbon electrodes by an industrial undertaking for use in the electrolytic extraction of aluminium from aluminium oxide, and any occupation involving substantial exposure to the dust arising therefrom

(12) Boiler scaling or substantial exposure to the dust arising therefrom

(13) Exposure to dust if the person employed in it has never at any time worked in any of the other occupations listed

| D2 | Byssinosis. A respiratory condition | Work in any room where any process up to and including the weaving process is performed in a factory in which the spinning or manipulation of raw or waste cotton or of flax, or the weaving of cotton or flax, is carried on, e.g. cotton or flax workers |

(Cont'd)

Disease no.	Name of disease or injury	Type of job
	Miscellaneous conditions not included elsewhere in the list	Any job involving
D3	Diffuse mesothelioma (primary neoplasm of the mesothelium of the pleura or of the pericardium or of the peritoneum). A cancer starting in the covering of the lungs or the lining of the abdomen	Exposure to asbestos, asbestos dust or any admixture of asbestos at a level above that commonly found in the environment at large
D4	Allergic rhinitis which is due to exposure to any of the following agents: (a) isocyanates (b) platinum salts (c) fumes of dusts arising from the manufacture, transport or use of hardening agents (including epoxy resin curing agents) based on phthalic anhydride, tetrachlorophthalic anhydride, trimellitic anhydride or triethylenetetramine (d) fumes arising from the use of rosin as a soldering flux (e) proteolytic enzymes (f) animals including insects and other anthropods used for the purposes of research or education or in laboratories	Exposure to any of the agents set out in column 2 of this paragraph. Wide range of occupations for example, metal plating industry, food processing, laboratory workers, grain processing, drug manufacture, washing powder manufacture, hair dressing, electronics industry, welders, dye tea and coffee processing

(g) dusts arising from the sowing, cultivation, harvesting, drying, handling, milling, transport or storage of barley, oats, rye, wheat or maize, or the handling, milling, transport or storage of meal or flour made therefrom

(h) antibiotics

(i) cimetidine

(j) wood dust

(k) ispaghula

(l) castor bean dust

(m) ipecacuanha

(n) azodicarbonamide

(o) animals including insects and other arthropods or their larval forms used for the purposes of pest control or fruit cultivation, or the larval forms of animals used for the purposes of research, education or in laboratories

(p) glutaraldehyde

(q) persulphate salts or henna

(r) crustaceans or fish or products arising from these in the food processing industry

(Cont'd)

Disease no.	Name of disease or injury Miscellaneous conditions not included elsewhere in the list	Type of job Any job involving
D4 (Cont'd)	(s) reactive dyes	
	(t) soya bean	
	(u) tea dust	
	(v) green coffee bean dust	
	(w) fumes from stainless steel welding. For example, hay fever symptoms.	
	(x) products made with natural rubber latex	
D5	Non-infective dermatitis of external origin (excluding dermatitis due to ionizing particles or electromagnetic radiations other than radiant heat). For example, skin rash, dermatitis	Exposure to dust, liquid or vapour or any other external agent except chromic acid, chromates or bi-chromates, capable of irritating the skin (including friction or heat but excluding ionizing particles or electromagnetic radiations other than radiant heat), e.g. any job involving exposure to a substance which can irritate the skin except for jobs involving exposure to chromium compounds (see C30) and radiation
D6	Carcinoma of the nasal cavity or associated air sinuses (nasal carcinoma). Cancer of the nose	(a) Attendance for work in or about a building where wooden goods are manufactured or repaired; or (b) Attendance for work in a building used for the manufacture of footwear or components of footwear made wholly or partly of leather or fibreboard; or (c) Attendance for work at a place used wholly or mainly for the repair of footwear made wholly or partly of leather or fibreboard

D7	Asthma which is due to exposure to any of the following agents:	Exposure to any of the agents set out in column 2 of this section
	(a) isocyanates	
	(b) platinum salts	
	(c) fumes or dusts arising from the manufacture, transport or use of hardening agents (including epoxy resin curing agents) based on phthalic anhydride, tetrachlorophthalic anhydride, trimellitic anhydride or triethylenetetramine	
	(d) fumes arising from the use of rosin as a soldering flux	
	(e) proteolytic enzymes	
	(f) animals including insects and other arthropods used for the purposes of research or education or in laboratories	
	(g) dusts arising from the sowing, cultivation, harvesting, drying, handling, milling, transport or storage of barley, oats, rye, wheat or maize, or the handling, milling, transport or storage of meal or flour made therefrom	
	(h) antibiotics	
	(i) cimetidine	
	(j) wood dust	
	(k) ispaghula	

(Cont'd)

Disease no.	Name of disease or injury	Type of job
	Miscellaneous conditions not included elsewhere in the list	Any job involving
D7 (Cont'd)	(l) castor bean dust	
	(m) ipecacuanha	
	(n) azodicarbonamide	
	(o) animals including insects and other arthropods or their larval forms, used for the purposes of pest control or fruit cultivation, or the larval forms of animals used for the purposes of research, education or in laboratories	
	(p) glutaraldehyde	
	(q) persulphate salts or henna	
	(r) crustaceans or fish or products arising from these in the food processing industry	
	(s) reactive dyes	
	(t) soya bean	
	(u) tea dust	
	(v) green coffee bean dust	
	(w) fumes from stainless steel welding	

(wa) products made with natural rubber latex	
(x) any other sensitizing agent (occupational asthma)	
D8	Primary carcinoma of the lung where there is accompanying evidence of asbestosis	(a) The working or handling of asbestos or any admixture of asbestos; or
		(b) The manufacture or repair of asbestos textiles or other articles containing or composed of asbestos; or
		(c) The cleaning of any machinery or plant used in any of the foregoing operations and of any chambers, fixtures and appliances for the collection of asbestos dust; or
		(d) substantial exposure to the dust arising from any of the foregoing operations
D8A	Primary carcinoma of the lung	Exposure to asbestos, in the course of:
		(a) The manufacture of asbestos textiles; or
		(b) Spraying asbestos; or
		(c) Asbestos insulation work; or
		(d) Applying or removing materials containing asbestos in the course of ship building
		where all or any of the exposure occurs before 1 January 1975, for a period of, or periods which amount in aggregate to, 5yrs or more, or otherwise, for a period of, or periods which amount in aggregate to, 10yrs or more
D9	Unilateral or bilateral diffuse pleural thickening with obliteration of the costophrenic angle	As D8 above

(Cont'd)

Disease no.	Name of disease or injury	Type of job
	Miscellaneous conditions not included elsewhere in the list	Any job involving
D10	Primary carcinoma of the lung	(a) Work underground in a tin mine; or
		(b) Exposure to bis (chloromethyl) ether produced during the manufacture of chloromethyl methyl ether; or
		(c) Exposure to zinc chromate, calcium chromate or strontium chromate in their pure forms; or
		(d) employment wholly or mainly as a coke oven worker:
		(i) for a period of, or periods which amount in aggregate to, 15yrs or more; or
		(ii) in top oven work, for a period of, or periods which amount in aggregate to, 5yrs or more; or
		(iii) in a combination of top oven work and other coke oven work for a total aggregate period of 15yrs or more, where one year working in top oven work is treated as equivalent to 3yrs in other coke oven work.

D11	Primary carcinoma of the lung where there is accompanying silicosis.	Exposure to silica dust in the course of:
		(a) the manufacture of glass or pottery
		(b) tunnelling in, or quarrying sandstone or granite
		(c) mining metal ores
		(d) slate quarrying or the manufacturing of artefacts from slate.
		(e) mining clay
		(f) using siliceous materials as abrasives
		(g) cutting stone
		(h) stonemasonry
		(i) work in a foundry
D12	Chronic bronchitis or emphysema; or both where, with maximum effort, where there is evidence of a forced expiratory volume in one second which is: (i) at least 1L below the appropriate mean value predicted, obtained from the following prediction formulae which give the mean values predicted in litres: For a man, where the measurement is made without back-extrapolation, $(3.62 \times height (m)) - (0.031 \times age (yrs)) - 1.41$; or, where the measurement is made with back-extrapolation, $(3.71 \times height (m)) - (0.032 \times age (yrs)) - 1.44$	Exposure to coal dust (whether before or after 5 July 1948) by reason of working: (a) Underground in a coal mine for a period or periods amounting in aggregate to at least 20yrs (b) On the surface of a coal mine as a screen worker for a period or periods amounting in aggregate to at least 40yrs before 1 January 1983; or (c) Both underground in a coal mine, and on the surface as a screen worker before 1 January 1983, where 2yrs working as a surface screen worker is equivalent to 1yr working underground, amounting in aggregate to at least the equivalent of 20yrs underground

(Cont'd)

Disease no.	Name of disease or injury	Type of job
	Miscellaneous conditions not included elsewhere in the list	Any job involving
D12 (Cont'd)	For a woman, where the measurement is made without back-extrapolation, (3.29 × height (m)) – (0.029 × age (yrs)) – 1.42; or, where the measurement is made with back-extrapolation (3.37 × height (m)) – (0.030 × age (yrs)) –1.46	
or	(ii) Less than 1L	
D13	Primary carcinoma of the nasopharynx	Exposure to wood dust in the course of the processing of wood or the manufacture or repair of wood products, for a period or periods which amount in aggregate to at least 10yrs

Reproduced with kind permission from the Department of Work and Pensions. Found online at ℅ http://www.dwp.gov.uk

List of RIDDOR reportable diseases

Occupational diseases

Conditions due to physical agents and physical demands of work

- Inflammation, ulceration, or malignant disease of the skin due to ionizing radiation
- Malignant disease of the bones due to ionizing radiation
- Blood dyscrasia due to ionizing radiation. *Activity:* work with ionizing radiation
- Cataract due to electromagentic radiation. *Activity:* work involving exposure to electromagnetic radiation (including radiant heat)
- Decompression illness
- Barotrauma resulting in lung or other organ damage
- Dysbaric osteonecrosis. *Activity:* work involving breathing gases at increased pressure (including diving)
- Cramp of the hand or forearm due to repetitive movements. *Activity:* work involving prolonged periods of handwriting, typing or other repetitive movements of the fingers, hand, or arm
- Subcutaneous cellulitis of the hand (beat hand). *Activity:* physically demanding work causing severe or prolonged friction or pressure on the hand
- Bursitis or subcutaneous cellulitis arising at or about the knee due to severe or prolonged external friction or pressure at or about the knee (beat knee). *Activity:* physically demanding work causing severe or prolonged friction or pressure at or about the knee
- Bursitis or subcutaneous cellulitis arising at or about the elbow due to severe or prolonged external friction or pressure at or about the elbow (beat elbow). *Activity:* physically demanding work causing severe or prolonged friction or pressure at or about the elbow
- Traumatic inflammation of the tendons of the hand or forearm or of the associated tendon sheaths. *Activity:* physically demanding work, frequent or repeated movements, constrained postures or extremes of extension or flexion of the hand or wrist
- Carpal tunnel syndrome. *Activity*: work involving the use of hand-held vibrating tools
- Hand–arm vibration syndrome. *Activity:* work involving:
  - the use of chain saws, brush cutters, or hand-held or hand-fed circular saws in forestry or woodworking
  - the use of hand-held rotary tools in grinding material or in sanding or polishing metal
  - the holding of material being ground or metal being sanded or polished by rotary tools

- the use of hand-held percussive metal working tools or the holding of metal being worked upon by percussive tools in connection with riveting, caulking, chipping, hammering, fettling, or swaging
- the use of hand-held powered percussive drills or hand-held powered percussive hammers in mining, quarrying, or demolition, or on roads or footpaths (including road construction) or
- the holding of material being worked upon by pounding machines in shoe manufacture.

Infections due to biological agents

- *Anthrax:* activity
  - work involving handling infected animals, their products, or packaging containing infected material or
  - work on infected sites
- *Brucellosis:* activity—work involving contact with
  - animals or their carcasses (including any parts thereof) infected by Brucella or the untreated products of same or
  - laboratory specimens or vaccines of or containing Brucella
- Chlamydiosis:
  - Avian chlamydiosis—activity: work involving contact with birds infected with *Chlamydia psittaci*, or the remains or untreated products of such birds
  - Ovine chlamydiosis—activity: work involving contact with sheep infected with *chlamydia psittaci* or the remains or untreated products of such sheep
- *Hepatitis:* activity—work involving contact with
  - human blood or human blood products or
  - any source of viral hepatitis
- *Legionellosis:* activity—work on or near cooling systems which are located in the workplace and use water; or work on hot water service systems located in the workplace which are likely to be a source of contamination
- *Leptospirosis:* activity—
  - work in places which are or are liable to be infested by rats, field mice, voles, or other small mammals
  - work at dog kennels or involving the care or handling of dogs; or
  - work involving contact with bovine animals or their meat products or pigs or their meat product- s
- *Lyme disease:* activity—work involving exposure to ticks (including in particular work by forestry workers, rangers, dairy farmers, gamekeepers, and other persons engaged in countryside management)
- *Q fever:* activity—work involving contact with animals, their remains, or their untreated products
- *Rabies:* activity—work involving handling or contact with infected animals
- *Streptococcus suis:* activity—work involving contact with pigs infected with Streptococcus suis, or with the carcasses, products, or residues of pigs so affected
- *Tetanus:* activity—work involving contact with soil likely to be contaminated by animals

- *Tuberculosis:* activity—work with persons, animals, human or animal remains, or any other material which might be a source of infection
- Any infection reliably attributable to the performance of the work specified in the entry opposite hereto. *Activity:* work with micro-organisms; work with live or dead human beings in the course of providing any treatment or service or in conducting any investigation involving exposure to blood or body fluids; work with animals or any potentially infected material derived from any of these activities.

Conditions due to substances

- Poisoning by any of the following:
  - acrylamide monomer
  - arsenic or one of its compounds
  - benzene or a homologue of benzene
  - beryllium or one of its compounds
  - cadmium or one of its compounds
  - carbon disulphide
  - diethylene dioxide (dioxan)
  - ethylene oxide
  - lead or one of its compounds
  - manganese or one of its compounds
  - mercury or one of its compounds
  - methyl bromide
  - nitrochlorobenzene, or a nitro-, amino-, or chloro-derivative of benzene or of a homologue of benzene
  - oxides of nitrogen
  - phosphorus or one of its compounds

Activity: any activity

- *Cancer of a bronchus or lung. Activity:*
  - work in or about a building where nickel is produced by decomposition of a gaseous nickel compound or where any industrial process which is ancillary or incidental to that process is carried on; or
  - work involving exposure to bis (chloromethyl) ether or any electrolytic chromium processes (excluding passivation) which involve hexavalent chromium compounds, chromate production, or zinc chromate pigment manufacture
- Primary carcinoma of the lung where there is accompanying evidence of silicosis. *Activity:* any occupation in—
  - glass manufacture
  - sandstone tunnelling or quarrying
  - the pottery industry
  - metal ore mining
  - slate quarrying or slate production
  - clay mining
  - the use of siliceous materials as abrasives
  - foundry work
  - granite tunnelling or quarrying; or
  - stone cutting or masonry

- *Cancer of the urinary tract. Activity:* work involving exposure to any of the following substances—
  - beta-naphthylamine or methylene-bis-orthochloroaniline
  - diphenyl substituted by at least one nitro or primary amino group or by at least one nitro and primary amino group (including benzidine)
  - any of the substances mentioned in the subparagraph above if further ring substituted by halogeno, methyl, or methoxy groups, but not by other groups or
  - the salts of any of the substances mentioned in the subparagraphs above; or
  - the manufacture of auramine or magenta
- *Bladder cancer*: activity—work involving exposure to aluminium smelting using the Soderberg process
- *Angiosarcoma of the liver:* activity;
  - work in or about machinery or apparatus used for the polymerization of vinyl chloride monomer, a process which, for the purposes of this subparagraph, comprises all operations up to and including the drying of the slurry produced by the polymerization and the packaging of the dried product or
  - work in a building or structure in which any part of the process referred to in the foregoing subparagraph takes place
- *Peripheral neuropathy*: activity—work involving the use of handling of or exposure to the fumes of or vapour containing n-hexane or methyl-n-butyl ketone
- Chrome ulceration of:
  - the nose or throat or
  - the skin of the hands or forearm

Activity: work involving exposure to chromic acid or to any other chromium compound.

- *Folliculitis:* activity—work involving exposure to mineral oil, tar, pitch, or arsenic
- *Acne:* activity—work involving exposure to mineral oil, tar, pitch, or arsenic
- *Skin cancer*: activity—work involving exposure to mineral oil, tar, pitch, or arsenic
- *Pneumoconiosis (excluding asbestosis)*: activity—
  - the mining, quarrying or working of silica rock or the working of dried quartzose sand, any dry deposit or residue of silica, or any dry admixture containing such materials (including any activity in which any of the aforesaid operations are carried out incidentally to the mining or quarrying of other minerals or to the manufacture of articles containing crushed or ground silica rock) or
  - the handling of any of the materials specified in the foregoing sub-paragraph in or incidentally to any of the operations mentioned therein or substantial exposure to the dust arising from such operations
  - The breaking, crushing, or grinding of flint, the working or handling of broken, crushed, or ground flint or materials containing such

flint, or substantial exposure to the dust arising from any of such operations
- Sand blasting by means of compressed air with the use of quartzose sand or crushed silica rock or flint or substantial exposure to the dust arising from such sand blasting
- Work in a foundry or the performance of, or substantial exposure to, the dust arising from any of the following operations:
  — the freeing of steel castings from adherent siliceous substance or
  — the freeing of metal castings from adherent siliceous substance:
  — by blasting with an abrasive propelled by compressed air, steam, or a wheel or
  — by the use of power-driven tools
- The manufacture of china or earthenware (including sanitary earthenware, electrical earthenware, and earthenware tiles) and any activity involving substantial exposure to the dust arising therefrom
- The grinding of mineral graphite or substantial exposure to the dust arising from such grinding
- The dressing of granite or any igneous rock by masons, the crushing of such materials, or substantial exposure to the dust arising from such operations
- The use or preparation for use of an abrasive wheel or substantial exposure to the dust arising therefrom
- Work underground in any mine in which one of the objects of the mining operations is the getting of any material
- the working or handling above ground at any coal or tin mine of any materials extracted therefrom or any operation incidental thereto
- the trimming of coal in any ship, barge, lighter, dock, or harbour, or at any wharf or quay or
- the sawing, splitting, or dressing of slate or any operation incidental thereto
- The manufacture of work incidental to the manufacture of carbon electrodes by an industrial undertaking for use in the electrolytic extraction of aluminium from aluminium oxide and any activity involving substantial exposure to the dust therefrom
- Boiler scaling or substantial exposure to the dust arising therefrom
- *Byssinosis*: *activity*— the spinning or manipulation of raw or waste cotton or flax or the weaving of cotton or flax, carried out in each case in a room in a factory, together with any other work carried out in such a room
- Mesothelioma
- Lung cancer
- *Asbestosis*: activity—
  - the working or handling of asbestos or any admixture of asbestos
  - the manufacture or repair of asbestos textiles or other articles containing or composed of asbestos
  - the cleaning of any machinery or plant used in any of the foregoing operations and of any chambers, fixtures, and appliances for the collection of asbestos dust; or
  - substantial exposure to the dust arising from any of the foregoing operations

- *Cancer of the nasal cavity or associated air sinuses*: activity—
  - work in or about a building where wooden furniture is manufactured or
  - work in a building used for the manufacture of footwear or components of footwear made wholly or partly of leather or fibre board; or
  - work at a place used wholly or mainly for the repair of footwear made wholly or partly of leather or fibre board or
  - work in or about a factory building where nickel is produced by decomposition of a gaseous nickel compound or in any process which is ancillary or incidental thereto
- *Occupational dermatitis*: activity—work involving exposure to any of the following agents:
  - epoxy resin systems
  - formaldehyde and its resins
  - metalworking fluids
  - chromate (hexavalent and derived from trivalent chromium)
  - cement, plaster, or concrete
  - acrylates and methacrylates
  - colophony (rosin) and its modified products
  - glutaraldehyde
  - mercaptobenzothiazole, thiurams, substituted para-phenylene-diamines and related rubber processing chemicals
  - biocides, antibacterials, preservatives, or disinfectants
  - organic solvents
  - antibiotics and other pharmaceuticals and therapeutic agents
  - strong acids, strong alkalis, strong solutions (e.g. brine), and oxidizing agents including domestic bleach or reducing agents
  - hairdressing products including in particular dyes, shampoos, bleaches, and permanent waving solutions
  - soaps and detergents
  - plants and plant-derived material including in particular the daffodil, tulip, and chrysanthemum families, the parsley family (carrots, parsnips, parsley, and celery), garlic and onion, hardwoods and the pine family
  - fish, shell-fish, or meat
  - sugar or flour or
  - any other known irritant or sensitizing agent including in particular any chemical bearing the warning 'may cause sensitization by skin contact' or 'irritating to the skin'
- *Extrinsic alveolitis (including farmer's lung)*: activity—exposure to moulds, fungal spores, or heterologous proteins during work in:
  - agriculture, horticulture, forestry, cultivation of edible fungi, or malt-working
  - loading, unloading, or handling mouldy vegetable matter or edible fungi whilst the same is being stored
  - caring for or handling birds or
  - handling bagasse

- *Occupational asthma*: activity—work involving exposure to any of the following agents:
  - isocyanates
  - platinum salts
  - fumes or dust arising from the manufacture, transport, or use of hardening agents (including epoxy resin curing agents) based on phthalic anhydride, tetrachlorophthalic anhydride, trimellitic anhydride or triethylene-tetramine
  - fumes arising from the use of rosin as a soldering flux
  - proteolytic enzymes
  - animals including insects and other arthropods used for the purposes of research or education or in laboratories
  - dusts arising from the sowing, cultivation, harvesting, drying, handling, milling, transport, or storage of barley, oats, rye, wheat, or maize or the handling, milling, transport or storage of meal or flour made therefrom
  - antibiotics
  - cimetidine
  - wood dust
  - ispaghula
  - castor bean dust
  - ipecacuanha
  - azodicarbonamide
  - animals including insects and other arthropods (whether in their larval forms or not) used for the purposes of pest control or fruit cultivation or the larval forms of animals used for the purposes of research or education or in laboratories
  - glutaraldehyde
  - persulphate salts or henna
  - crustaceans or fish or products arising from these in the food processing industry
  - reactive dyes
  - soya bean
  - tea dust
  - green coffee bean dust
  - fumes from stainless steel welding
  - any other sensitizing agent, including in particular any chemical bearing the warning 'may cause sensitization by inhalation'.

Appendix 4 is reproduced with permission from HSE.

Informatics in occupational health

The use of information technology in occupational medicine is continually increasing. A great deal of practical information is available on the worldwide web. Wherever possible, useful websites and web references for guidance documents have been quoted within specific topics throughout this handbook. Listed here are websites that are useful for OH practice.

UK professional bodies in OH
- Faculty of Occupational Medicine (FOM).
  Available at: ℘ www.fom.ac.uk
- Society of Occupational Medicine (SOM).
  Available at: ℘ http://www.som.org.uk/
- British Occupational Hygiene Society (BOHS).
  Available at: ℘ http://www.bohs.org
- Institution of Occupational Safety and Health (IOSH).
  Available at: ℘ http://www.iosh.co.uk

Specialist /industry-specific practitioner groups
Some require a membership subscription, but selected material is free.
- Association of NHS Occupational Physicians (ANHOPS).
  Available at: ℘ http://www.anhops.com/
- Association of Local Authority Medical Advisers (ALAMA).
  Available at: ℘ http://www.alama.org.uk/
- Commercial Occupational Health Providers Association (COHPA).
  Available at: ℘ http://www.cohpa.co.uk/

Discussion forum
Occenvmed. Available at: ℘ http://www.occmed.free-online.co.uk/page5.html

Academic departments of occupational medicine
- The Institute of Occupational and Environmental Medicine, University of Birmingham.
  Available at: ℘ http://www.birmingham.ac.uk/schools/haps/departments/ioem/index.aspx
- Centre for Occupational and Environmental Health, University of Manchester.
  Available at: ℘ http://www.medicine.manchester.ac.uk/oeh/
- Medical Research Council Epidemiology Resource Centre, University of Southampton.
  Available at: ℘ http://www.mrc.soton.ac.uk/index.asp?page=33

- Department of Occupational and Environmental Medicine, National Heart and Lung Institute.
  Available at: ℘ http://www.lungsatwork.org.uk/clinical.php
- Other university departments of occupational and environmental medicine can be located through the respective university websites.

Occupational and environmental medicine journals

- *Occupational and Environmental Medicine*.
  Available at: ℘ http://oem.bmjjournals.com/
- *Occupational Medicine*.
  Available at: ℘ http://occmed.oxfordjournals.org/
- *Scandinavian Journal of Work, Environment and Health*.
  Available at: ℘ http://www.sjweh.fi/
- *Journal of Occupational and Environmental Medicine*.
  Available at: ℘ http://www.joem.org/pt/re/joem/home
- *Annals of Occupational Hygiene*.
  Available at: ℘ http://annhyg.oxfordjournals.org/

Links to other occupational health disciplines

- British Thoracic Society.
  Available at: ℘ http://www.brit-thoracic.org.uk/
- Ergonomics Society.
  Available at: ℘ http://www.ergonomics.org.uk/

Other useful UK websites

- Health, Environment and Work (HEW).
  Available at: ℘ http://www.agius.com/hew/index.htm
- UK Health and Safety Executive (HSE).
  Available at: ℘ http://www.hse.gov.uk
- HSE statistics.
  Available at: ℘ http://www.hse.gov.uk/statistics/
- UK Health Protection Agency.
  Available at: ℘ http://www.hpa.org.uk
- Clinical evidence.
  Available at: ℘ http://www.clinicalevidence.com/ceweb/conditions/index.jsp
- National Institute for Health and Clinical Excellence (NICE).
  Available at: ℘ http://www.nice.org.uk/
- NHS Plus.
  Available at: ℘ http://www.nhsplus.nhs.uk/
UK Department for Work and Pensions.
  Available at: ℘ http://www.dwp.gov.uk/

International websites

- European Agency for Safety and Health at Work.
  Available at: ℘ http://europe.osha.eu.int/OSHA
- National Institute for Occupational Health and Safety (USA).
  Available at: ℘ http://www.cdc.gov/niosh/homepage.html
- World Health Organization (WHO).
  Available at: ℘ http://www.who.int/en/
- International Research on Cancer (IARC).
  Available at: ℘ http://www.iarc.fr/

Lung volumes

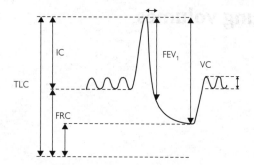

Fig. A6.1 Subdivisions of lung volume illustrated by spirometric recording of volume against time during tidal breathing for three breaths, followed by maximal inspiration and then maximal forced expiration, before returning to tidal breathing in a normal subject. RV, residual volume; FRC, functional residual capacity; IC, inspiratory capacity; TLC, total lung capacity; FEV1, forced expiratory volume in 1 s; VC, vital capacity; VT, tidal volume. Note that TLC = FRC + IC = VC + RV. Reproduced with permission from the Warrell DA, et al (2003). *Oxford Textbook of Medicine*, 4 edn, vol. 2. By permission of Oxford University Press.

Height and weight converter and body mass index (BMI) calculator

BMI calculator

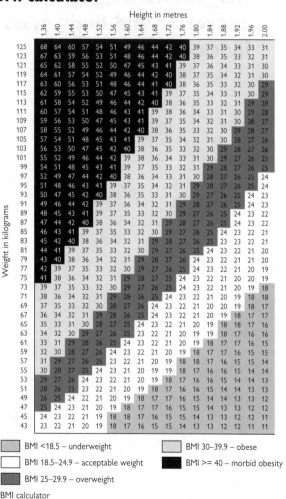

Fig A7.1 BMI calculator.

Height converter

Table A7.1 Height converter

Height (ft and in)	Height (m)
5'0"	1.52
5'1"	1.55
5'2"	1.58
5'3"	1.60
5'4"	1.63
5'5"	1.65
5'6"	1.68
5'7"	1.70
5'8"	1.73
5'9"	1.75
5'10"	1.78
5'11"	1.80
6'0"	1.83
6'1"	1.85
6'2"	1.88
6'3"	1.90
6'4"	1.93
6'5"	1.96
6'6"	1.98

Weight conversion chart

Table A7.2 Weight conversion chart

kg	lbs	St/	pounds	kg	lbs	St/	pounds	kg	lbs	St/	pounds
38.1	84	6	0	54.0	119	8	7	69.9	154	11	0
38.6	85	6	1	54.4	120	8	8	70.3	155	11	1
39.0	86	6	2	54.9	121	8	9	70.8	156	11	2
39.5	87	6	3	55.3	122	8	10	71.2	157	11	3
39.9	88	6	4	55.8	123	8	11	71.7	158	11	4
40.4	89	6	5	56.2	124	8	12	72.1	159	11	5
40.8	90	6	6	56.7	125	8	13	72.6	160	11	6
41.3	91	6	7	57.2	126	9	0	73.0	161	11	7
41.7	92	6	8	57.6	127	9	1	73.5	162	11	8
42.2	93	6	9	58.1	128	9	2	73.9	163	11	9
42.6	94	6	10	58.5	129	9	3	74.4	164	11	10
43.1	95	6	11	59.0	130	9	4	74.8	165	11	11
43.5	96	6	12	59.4	131	9	5	75.3	166	11	12
44.0	97	6	13	59.9	132	9	6	75.7	167	11	13
44.5	98	7	0	60.3	133	9	7	76.2	168	12	0
44.9	99	7	1	60.8	134	9	8	76.7	169	12	1
45.4	100	7	2	61.2	135	9	9	77.1	170	12	2
45.8	101	7	3	61.7	136	9	10	77.6	171	12	3
46.3	102	7	4	62.1	137	9	11	78.0	172	12	4
46.7	103	7	5	62.6	138	9	12	78.5	173	12	5
47.2	104	7	6	63.0	139	9	13	78.9	174	12	6
47.6	105	7	7	63.5	140	10	0	79.4	175	12	7
48.1	106	7	8	64.0	141	10	1	79.8	176	12	8
48.5	107	7	9	64.4	142	10	2	80.3	177	12	9
49.0	108	7	10	64.9	143	10	3	80.7	178	12	10
49.4	109	7	11	65.3	144	10	4	81.2	179	12	11
49.9	110	7	12	65.8	145	10	5	81.6	180	12	12
50.3	111	7	13	66.2	146	10	6	82.1	181	12	13
50.8	112	8	0	66.7	147	10	7	82.6	182	13	0
51.3	113	8	1	67.1	148	10	8	83.0	183	13	1
51.7	114	8	2	67.6	149	10	9	83.5	184	13	2
52.2	115	8	3	68.0	150	10	10	83.9	185	13	3
52.6	116	8	4	68.5	151	10	11	84.4	186	13	4
53.1	117	8	5	68.9	152	10	12	84.8	187	13	5
53.5	118	8	6	69.4	153	10	13	85.3	188	13	6

Table A7.2 (Cont'd)

kg	lbs	St/	pounds	kg	lbs	St/	pounds	kg	lbs	St/	pounds
85.7	189	13	7	99.8	220	15	10	113.9	251	17	13
86.2	190	13	8	100.2	221	15	11	114.3	252	18	0
86.6	191	13	9	100.7	222	15	12	114.8	253	18	1
87.1	192	13	10	101.2	223	15	13	115.2	254	18	2
87.5	193	13	11	101.6	224	16	0	115.7	255	18	3
88.0	194	13	12	102.1	225	16	1	116.1	256	18	4
88.4	195	13	13	102.5	226	16	2	116.6	257	18	5
88.9	196	14	0	103.0	227	16	3	117.0	258	18	6
89.4	197	14	1	103.4	228	16	4	117.5	259	18	7
89.8	198	14	2	103.9	229	16	5	117.9	260	18	8
90.3	199	14	3	104.3	230	16	6	118.4	261	18	9
90.7	200	14	4	104.8	231	16	7	118.8	262	18	10
91.2	201	14	5	105.2	232	16	8	119.3	263	18	11
91.6	202	14	6	105.7	233	16	9	119.7	264	18	12
92.1	203	14	7	106.1	234	16	10	120.2	265	18	13
92.5	204	14	8	106.6	235	16	11	120.7	266	19	0
93.0	205	14	9	107.0	236	16	12	121.1	267	19	1
93.4	206	14	10	107.5	237	16	13	121.6	268	19	2
93.9	207	14	11	108.0	238	17	0	122.0	269	19	3
94.3	208	14	12	108.4	239	17	1	122.5	270	19	4
94.8	209	14	13	108.9	240	17	2	122.9	271	19	5
95.3	210	15	0	109.3	241	17	3	123.4	272	19	6
95.7	211	15	1	109.8	242	17	4	123.8	273	19	7
96.2	212	15	2	110.2	243	17	5	124.3	274	19	8
96.6	213	15	3	110.7	244	17	6	124.7	275	19	9
97.1	214	15	4	111.1	245	17	7	125.2	276	19	10
97.5	215	15	5	111.6	246	17	8	125.6	277	19	11
98.0	216	15	6	112.0	247	17	9	126.1	278	19	12
98.4	217	15	7	112.5	248	17	10	126.6	279	19	13
98.9	218	15	8	112.9	249	17	11	127.0	280	20	0
99.3	219	15	9	113.4	250	17	12	127.5	281	20	1

Agents classified by the IARC monographs, volumes 1–106

CAS No.	Agent	Group	Volume	Year
000075–07–0	Acetaldehyde associated with consumption of alcoholic beverages	1	100E	2012
	Acid mists, strong inorganic	1	54, 100F	2012
001402–68–2	Aflatoxins	1	56, 82, 100F	2012
	Alcoholic beverages	1	44, 96, 100E	2012
	Aluminium production	1	34, Sup 7, 100F	2012
000092–67–1 4	Aminobiphenyl	1	1, Sup 7, 99, 100F	2012
	Areca nut	1	85, 100E	2012
000313–67–7	Aristolochic acid (NB: Overall evaluation upgraded to Group 1 based on mechanistic and other relevant data)	1	82, 100A	2012
000313–67–7	Aristolochic acid, plants containing	1	82, 100A	2012
007440–38–2	Arsenic and inorganic arsenic compounds	1	23, Sup 7, 100C	2012
001332–21–4 013768–00–8 012172–73–5 017068–78–9 012001–29–5 012001–28–4 014567–73–8	Asbestos (all forms, including actinolite, amosite, anthophyllite, chrysotile, crocidolite, tremolite) (NB: Mineral substances (e.g. talc or vermiculite) that contain asbestos should also be regarded as carcinogenic to humans.)	1	14, Sup 7, 100C	2012
	Auramine production	1	Sup 7, 99, 100F	2012
000446–86–6	Azathioprine	1	26, Sup 7, 100A	2012
000071–43–2	Benzene	1	29, Sup 7. 100F	2012
000092–87–5	Benzidine	1	29, Sup 7, 99, 100F	2012
	Benzidine, dyes metabolized to (NB: Overall evaluation upgraded to Group 1 based on mechanistic and other relevant data)	1	99, 100F	2012

CAS No.	Agent	Group	Volume	Year
000050–32–8	Benzo[a]pyrene (NB: Overall evaluation upgraded to Group 1 based on mechanistic and other relevant data)	1	92, 100F	2012
007440–41–7	Beryllium and beryllium compounds	1	58, 100C	2012
	Betel quid with tobacco	1	85, 100E	2012
	Betel quid without tobacco	1	85, 100E	2012
000542–88–1 000107–30–2	Bis(chloromethyl)ether; chloromethyl methyl ether (technical-grade)	1	4, Sup 7, 100F	2012
000055–98–1	Busulfan	1	4, Sup 7, 100A	2012
000106–99–0 1,3	Butadiene	1	97, 100F	2012
007440–43–9	Cadmium and cadmium compounds	1	58, 100C	2012
000305–03–3	Chlorambucil	1	26, Sup 7, 100A	2012
000494–03–1	Chlornaphazine	1	4, Sup 7, 100A	2012
018540–29–9	Chromium (VI) compounds	1	49, 100C	2012
	Clonorchis sinensis (infection with)	1	61, 100B	2012
	Coal, indoor emissions from household combustion of	1	95, 100E	2012
	Coal gasification	1	92, 100F	2012
008007–45–2	Coal-tar distillation	1	92, 100F	2012
065996–93–2	Coal-tar pitch	1	35, Sup 7, 100F	2012
	Coke production	1	92, 100F	2012
000050–18–0 006055–19–2	Cyclophosphamide	1	26, Sup 7, 100A	2012
059865–13–3 079217–60–0	Cyclosporine	1	50, 100A	2012
000056–53–1	Diethylstilbestrol	1	21, Sup 7, 100A	2012
	Engine exhaust, diesel	1	46, 105	in prep
	Epstein-Barr virus	1	70, 100B	2012
066733–21–9	Erionite	1	42, Sup 7, 100C	2012

CAS No.	Agent	Group	Volume	Year
	Estrogen therapy, postmenopausal	1	72, 100A	2012
	Estrogen-progestogen menopausal therapy (combined)	1	72, 91, 100A	2012
	Estrogen-progestogen oral contraceptives (combined) (NB: There is also convincing evidence in humans that these agents confer a protective effect against cancer in the endometrium and ovary)	1	72, 91, 100A	2012
000064–17–5	Ethanol in alcoholic beverages	1	96, 100E	2012
000075–21–8	Ethylene oxide (NB: Overall evaluation upgraded to Group 1 based on mechanistic and other relevant data)	1	97, 100F	2012
033419–42–0	Etoposide (NB: Overall evaluation upgraded to Group 1 based on mechanistic and other relevant data)	1	76, 100A	2012
033419–42–0 015663–27–1 011056–06–7	Etoposide in combination with cisplatin and bleomycin	1	76, 100A	2012
	Fission products, including strontium-90	1	100D	2012
000050–00–0	Formaldehyde	1	88, 100F	2012
	Haematite mining (underground)	1	1, Sup 7, 100D	2012
	Helicobacter pylori (infection with)	1	61, 100B	2012
	Hepatitis B virus (chronic infection with)	1	59, 100B	2012
	Hepatitis C virus (chronic infection with)	1	59, 100B	2012
	Human immunodeficiency virus type 1 (infection with)	1	67, 100B	2012
	Human papillomavirus types 16, 18, 31, 33, 35, 39, 45, 51, 52, 56, 58, 59 (NB: The HPV types that have been classified as *carcinogenic to humans can differ by an order of magnitude* in risk for cervical cancer)	1	64, 90, 100B	2012

CAS No.	Agent	Group	Volume	Year
	Human T-cell lymphotropic virus type I	1	67, 100B	2012
	Ionizing radiation (all types)	1	100D	2012
	Iron and steel founding (occupational exposure during)	1	34, Sup 7, 100F	2012
	Isopropyl alcohol manufacture using strong acids	1	Sup 7, 100F	2012
	Kaposi sarcoma herpesvirus	1	70, 100B	2012
	Leather dust	1	100C	2012
	Magenta production	1	57, 99, 100F	2012
000148–82–3	Melphalan	1	9, Sup 7, 100A	2012
000298–81–7	Methoxsalen (8-methoxypsoralen) plus ultraviolet A radiation	1	24, Sup 7, 100A	2012
000101–14–4 4,4'	Methylenebis (2-chloroaniline) (MOCA) (NB: Overall evaluation upgraded to Group 1 based on mechanistic and other relevant data)	1	57, 99, 100F	2012
	Mineral oils, untreated or mildly treated	1	33, Sup 7, 100F	2012
	MOPP and other combined chemotherapy including alkylating agents	1	Sup 7, 100A	2012
000091–59–8 2	Naphthylamine	1	4, Sup 7, 99, 100F	2012
	Neutron radiation (NB: Overall evaluation upgraded to Group 1 with supporting evidence from other relevant data)	1	75, 100D	2012
	Nickel compounds	1	49, 100C	2012
016543–55–8	N'-Nitrosonornicotine (NNN) and 4-(N-	1	89, 100E	2012
064091–91–4	Nitrosomethylamino)-1-(3-pyridyl)-1-butanone (NNK) (NB: Overall evaluation upgraded to Group 1 based on mechanistic and other relevant data)			
	Opisthorchis viverrini (infection with)	1	61, 100B	2012
	Painter (occupational exposure as a)	1	47, 98, 100F	2012

CAS No.	Agent	Group	Volume	Year
057465–28–8 3,4,5,3',4'	Pentachlorobiphenyl (PCB-126) (NB: Overall evaluation upgraded to Group 1 based on mechanistic and other relevant data)	1	100F	2012
057117–31–4 2,3,4,7,8	Pentachlorodibenzofuran (NB: Overall evaluation upgraded to Group 1 based on mechanistic and other relevant data)	1	100F	2012
000062–44–2	Phenacetin (NB: Overall evaluation upgraded to Group 1 with supporting evidence from other relevant data)	1	24, Sup 7, 100A	2012
	Phenacetin, analgesic mixtures containing	1	Sup 7, 100A	2012
014596–37–3	Phosphorus-32, as phosphate	1	78, 100D	2012
007440–07–5	Plutonium	1	78, 100D	2012
	Radioiodines, including iodine-131	1	78, 100D	2012
	Radionuclides, alpha-particle-emitting, internally deposited (NB: Specific radionuclides for which there is sufficient evidence in humans are also listed individually as Group 1 agents)	1	78, 100D	2012
	Radionuclides, beta-particle-emitting, internally deposited (NB: Specific radionuclides for which there is sufficient evidence in humans are also listed individually as Group 1 agents)	1	78, 100D	2012
013233–32–4	Radium-224 and its decay products	1	78, 100D	2012
013982–63–3	Radium-226 and its decay products	1	78, 100D	2012
015262–20–1	Radium-228 and its decay products	1	78, 100D	2012
010043–92–2	Radon-222 and its decay products	1	43, 78, 100D	2012
	Rubber manufacturing industry	1	28, Sup 7, 100F	2012
	Salted fish, Chinese-style	1	56, 100E	2012

CAS No.	Agent	Group	Volume	Year
	Schistosoma haematobium (infection with)	1	61, 100B	2012
013909–09–6	Semustine [1-(2-Chloroethyl)-3-(4-methylcyclohexyl)-1-nitrosourea, Methyl-CCNU]	1	Sup 7, 100A	2012
068308–34–9	Shale oils	1	35, Sup 7, 100F	2012
014808–60–7	Silica dust, crystalline, in the form of quartz or cristobalite	1	68, 100C	2012
	Solar radiation	1	55, 100D	2012
	Soot (as found in occupational exposure of chimney sweeps)	1	35, Sup 7, 100F	2012
000505–60–2	Sulfur mustard	1	9, Sup 7, 100F	2012
010540–29–1	Tamoxifen (NB: There is also conclusive evidence that tamoxifen reduces the risk of contralateral breast cancer in breast cancer patients)	1	66, 100A	2012
001746–01–6 2,3,7,8	Tetrachlorodibenzo-para-dioxin	1	69, 100F	2012
000052–24–4	Thiotepa	1	50, 100A	2012
007440–29–1	Thorium-232 and its decay products	1	78, 100D	2012
	Tobacco, smokeless	1	89, 100E	2012
	Tobacco smoke, second-hand	1	83, 100E	2012
	Tobacco smoking	1	83, 100E	2012
000095–53–4	ortho-Toluidine	1	77, 99, 100F	2012
000299–75–2	Treosulfan	1	26, Sup 7, 100A	2012
000079–01–6	Trichloroethylene	1	63, 106	in prep
	Ultraviolet radiation (wavelengths 100–400 nm, encompassing UVA, UVB, and UVC)	1	100D	2012
	Ultraviolet-emitting tanning devices	1	100D	2012
000075–01–4	Vinyl chloride	1	97, 100F	2012
	Wood dust	1	62, 100C	2012
	X- and Gamma-Radiation	1	75, 100D	2012

Index

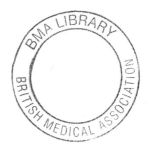

FEV₁/VC Caucasian <u>MALES</u> (courtesy of Vitalograph)

Prediction Nomogram

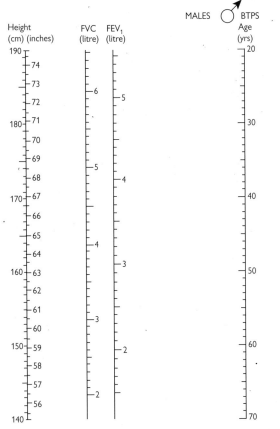

From Oxford Handbook of Respiratory Medicine by Chapman *et al* (2004), with permission from Oxford University Press.